Handbook of Urology
Diagnosis and Therapy

Third Edition

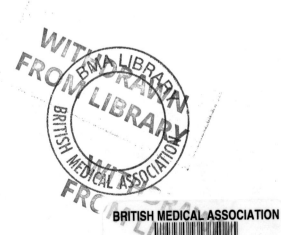

Handbook of Urology
Diagnosis and Therapy

Third Edition

Editors

Mike B. Siroky, M.D.
Professor of Urology, Boston University School of Medicine; Chief of Urology, Veterans Affairs Medical Center, Boston, Massachusetts

Robert D. Oates, M.D.
Professor of Urology, Boston University School of Medicine; Attending Urologist, Boston Medical Center, Boston, Massachusetts

Richard K. Babayan, M.D.
Professor and Chairman of Urology, Boston University School of Medicine; Attending Urologist, Boston Medical Center, Boston, Massachusetts

LIPPINCOTT WILLIAMS & WILKINS
A **Wolters Kluwer** Company

Philadelphia • Baltimore • New York • London
Buenos Aires • Hong Kong • Sydney • Tokyo

Acquisitions Editor: Brian Brown
Developmental Editor: Michelle M. LaPlante
Production Editor: Thomas Boyce
Manufacturing Manager: Colin Warnock
Cover Designer: Christine Jenny
Compositor: Circle Graphics
Printer: R. R. Donnelley–Crawfordsville

© 2004 by LIPPINCOTT WILLIAMS & WILKINS
530 Walnut Street
Philadelphia, PA 19106 USA
LWW.com

Printed in the USA

Library of Congress Cataloging-in-Publication Data

Handbook of urology : diagnosis and therapy / editors, Mike B. Siroky,
    Robert D. Oates, Richard K. Babayan.--3rd ed.
        p. ; cm.
    Rev. ed. of: Manual of urology. 2nd ed. c1999.
    Includes bibliographical references and index.
    ISBN 0-7817-4221-8
    1. Urology--Handbooks, manuals, etc. I. Siroky, Mike B.
(Mike Benjamin), 1946- II. Oates, Robert D. III. Babayan, Richard K.
IV. Manual of urology.
    [DNLM: 1. Urologic Diseases--diagnosis--Handbooks. 2. Urologic
Diseases--therapy--Handbooks. 3. Genital Diseases, Male--diagnosis--
Handbooks. 4. Genital Diseases, Male--therapy--Handbooks.
WJ 39 H2363 2004]
RC872.9.M36 2004
616.6--dc22

                                                                2003065995

Care has been taken to confirm the accuracy of the information presented and to describe generally accepted practices. However, the authors, editors, and publisher are not responsible for errors or omissions or for any consequences from application of the information in this book and make no warranty, expressed or implied, with respect to the currency, completeness, or accuracy of the contents of the publication. Application of this information in a particular situation remains the professional responsibility of the practitioner.

The authors, editors, and publisher have exerted every effort to ensure that drug selection and dosage set forth in this text are in accordance with current recommendations and practice at the time of publication. However, in view of ongoing research, changes in government regulations, and the constant flow of information relating to drug therapy and drug reactions, the reader is urged to check the package insert for each drug for any change in indications and dosage and for added warnings and precautions. This is particularly important when the recommended agent is a new or infrequently employed drug.

Some drugs and medical devices presented in this publication have Food and Drug Administration (FDA) clearance for limited use in restricted research settings. It is the responsibility of the health care provider to ascertain the FDA status of each drug or device planned for use in their clinical practice.

10 9 8 7 6 5 4 3 2 1

To the memory of

Robert J. Krane, M.D.
January 15, 1943–November 17, 2001

Former Chairman of the Department of
Urology at Boston University

A colleague, a friend, and a mentor to us all

Contents

Contributing Authors ix
Preface xi

1. The Abnormal Urinalysis. 1
    Luke M. O'Connell and Mike B. Siroky

2. Imaging of the Genitourinary Tract 16
    Charles Hyde and Rebecca K. Schwartz

3. Radionuclide Imaging. 30
    Rachel A. Powsner and Dean J. Rodman

4. Evaluation of Renal Mass Lesions 51
    Juan P. Litvak and Robert D. Oates

5. Instrumentation of the Lower Urinary Tract. 63
    C. Charles Wen and Richard K. Babayan

6. Upper Tract Instrumentation
    and Visualization 79
    Luke M. O'Connell and Richard K. Babayan

7. Urodynamic Studies 87
    C. Charles Wen and Mike B. Siroky

8. Lower Urinary Tract Symptoms 98
    *Peter A. Zeman, Mike B. Siroky,
    and Richard K. Babayan*

9. Urinary Incontinence 122
    Elise De and Tracey Wilson

10. Male Sexual Dysfunction 143
    *Ronald E. Anglade, Ricardo M. Munnariz,
    and Irwin Goldstein*

11. Genitourinary Trauma and Emergencies. 164
    Meir Daller and Gennaro Carpinito

12. Endoscopic Surgery of the Lower Urinary Tract
    and Laparoscopy 188
    *C. Charles Wen, Juan P. Litvak,
    and Richard K. Babayan*

13. Genitourinary Infection 206
    Joseph Alukal, Julita Mir, and Colm Bergin

14. Urinary Calculi and Endourology 232
    *Ronald E. Anglade, David S. Wang,
    and Richard K. Babayan*

15. Neoplasms of the Genitourinary Tract 249
    Andrew Kramer and Mike B. Siroky

16. Medical Management of
    Genitourinary Malignancy 300
    Ignacio F. San Francisco and Ken Zaner

17. Radiation: External Beam and Brachytherapy 328
    Anthony L. Zietman

18. Neurourology 341
    C. Charles Wen and Mike B. Siroky

19. Pediatric Urology 355
    Elise De and Stuart B. Bauer

20. Male Reproductive Dysfunction 380
    Ronald E. Anglade and Robert D. Oates

21. Priapism 407
    *Meir Daller, Ricardo M. Munnariz,
    and Irwin Goldstein*

22. Sexually Transmitted Diseases 414
    Khalid Badwan and Mike B. Siroky

23. Surgical Disorders of the Adrenal Gland 426
    Meir Daller and Mike B. Siroky

24. Fluid and Electrolyte Disorders 441
    Peter A. Zeman and Mike B. Siroky

25. Renal Failure, Dialysis, and
    Renal Transplantation 457
    *Ricardo M. Munnariz, Andrew Kramer,
    and Gennaro Carpinito*

26. Perioperative Care of the Patient 491
    Rie Aihara

Appendix I. American Urological Association
Symptom Score Index 508

Appendix II. Modified Partin Table for
Predicting Pathological Stage in
Prostate Cancer 510

Subject Index 511

Contributing Authors

Rie Aihara, M.D. *Assistant Professor of Surgery, Boston University School of Medicine, Department of Surgery / Division of Trauma and Critical Care, Boston, Massachusetts*

Joseph Alukal, M.D. *Resident, Department of Urology, Boston University Medical Center, Boston, Massachusetts*

Ronald E. Anglade, M.D. *Chief Resident and Fellow, Department of Urology, Boston University Medical Center, Boston, Massachusetts*

Richard K. Babayan, M.D. *Professor and Chairman of Urology, Boston University School of Medicine; Attending Urologist, Boston Medical Center, Boston, Massachusetts*

Khalid Badwan, M.D. *Resident, Department of Urology, Boston University Medical Center, Boston, Massachusetts*

Stuart B. Bauer, M.D. *Associate Professor of Surgery (Urology), Harvard Medical School, Senior Associate in Surgery, Department of Urology, The Children's Hospital, Boston, Massachusetts*

Colm Bergin, M.D. *Fellow in Infectious Disease, Boston Medical Center, Boston, Massachusetts*

Gennaro Carpinito, M.D. *Associate Professor, Department of Urology, Boston University School of Medicine; Attending Urologist, Boston Medical Center, Boston, Massachusetts*

Meir Daller, M.D. *Chief Resident, Department of Urology, Boston University Medical Center, Boston, Massachusetts*

Elise De, M.D. *Chief Resident, Department of Urology, Boston University Medical Center, Boston, Massachusetts*

Irwin Goldstein, M.D. *Professor of Urology, Boston University School of Medicine; Attending Physician in Urology, Boston Medical Center, Boston, Massachusetts*

Charles Hyde, M.D. *Assistant Professor of Radiology, Boston University School of Medicine; Chief, Ultrasound Section, Veterans Affairs Medical Center, Boston, Massachusetts*

Andrew Kramer, M.D. *Chief Resident, Department of Urology, Boston University Medical Center, Boston, Massachusetts*

Juan P. Litvak, M.D. *Chief Resident, Department of Urology, Boston University Medical Center, Boston, Massachusetts*

Julita Mir, M.D. *Clinical Instructor in Medicine, Boston University School of Medicine, Boston, Massachusetts*

Ricardo M. Munnariz, M.D.   *Assistant Professor of Urology, Boston University School of Medicine, Boston Medical Center, Boston, Massachusetts*

Luke M. O'Connell, M.D.   *Chief Resident, Department of Urology, Boston University Medical Center, Boston, Massachusetts*

Robert D. Oates, M.D.   *Professor of Urology, Boston University School of Medicine; Attending Urologist, Boston Medical Center, Boston, Massachusetts*

Rachel A. Powsner, M.D.   *Associate Professor of Radiology, Boston University School of Medicine; Staff Physician, Department of Radiology, Boston Medical Center, Boston, Massachusetts*

Dean J. Rodman, M.D.   *Senior Attending Physician, Department of Nuclear Medicine, Sibley Memorial Hospital, Washington, D.C.*

Ignacio F. San Francisco, M.D.   *Fellow, Department of Urology, Beth Israel Medical Center, Brookline, Massachusetts*

Rebecca K. Schwartz, M.D.   *Instructor in Radiology, Boston University School of Medicine; Section Head, Computed Tomographic Imaging, Veterans Affairs Medical Center, Boston, Massachusetts*

Mike B. Siroky, M.D.   *Professor of Urology, Boston University School of Medicine, Chief of Urology, Veterans Affairs Medical Center, Boston, Massachusetts*

David S. Wang, M.D.   *Assistant Professor of Urology, Boston University School of Medicine; Attending Physician, Boston Medical Center, Boston, Massachusetts*

C. Charles Wen, M.D.   *Resident, Department of Urology, Boston University Medical Center, Boston, Massachusetts*

Tracey Wilson, M.D.   *Assistant Professor of Urology, Boston University School of Medicine; Attending Physician, Boston Medical Center, Boston, Massachusetts*

Ken Zaner, M.D., Ph.D.   *Boston Medical Center, Hematology/Oncology, Boston, Massachusetts*

Peter A. Zeman, M.D.   *Resident, Department of Urology, Boston University Medical Center, Boston, Massachusetts*

Anthony L. Zietman, M.D.   *Associate Professor of Radiation Oncology, Harvard Medical School; Associate Radiation Oncologist, Massachusetts General Hospital, Boston, Massachusetts*

Preface

The purpose of the third edition of the *Handbook of Urology: Diagnosis and Therapy* remains to serve as a daily companion to the house officer and medical student responsible for the surgical care of the urology patient. The emphasis of the book remains the diagnosis and therapy of urological disorders. Open surgical procedures are not described in great detail but endoscopic, medical and diagnostic procedures are well described. Most chapters were written by current and past residents and trainees associated with the Boston University Training Program in Urology, with input and advice from the faculty.

Although the third edition remains true to its original purpose, it represents a complete revision of the second edition published in 1999. We have added new chapters on upper urinary tract instrumentation and laparoscopy. Advances in understanding priapism have warranted a separate chapter for this entity. A new chapter on perioperative care has been added to reflect the current practice of risk assessment prior to surgery. The chapter on incontinence was completely re-written to reflect current understanding in this area. In the other chapters, emphasis was placed on detailing new diagnostic techniques and describing emerging therapies. For example, the role of thermotherapy in treating prostatic obstruction is given more emphasis, as is the use of laser energy to treat urinary calculi.

The second edition was well received in North America and abroad. We hope that medical students, residents and fellows find the third edition equally useful in the day-to-day care of urologic patients. We are extremely grateful to our contributing authors for their superb effort in completing this work. We also wish to thank everyone associated with Lippincott Williams & Wilkins for their support, in particular Michelle M. LaPlante.

Mike B. Siroky, M.D.
Robert D. Oates, M.D.
Richard K. Babayan, M.D.

The Abnormal Urinalysis

Luke M. O'Connell and Mike B. Siroky

I. Collection of the urine specimen should be carried out in the clinic or hospital rather than at home. Urine that is not freshly voided or has been collected from a urine drainage bag is unreliable for urinalysis.

A. Male adults. The clean-catch midstream method is most reliable in adult males. In uncircumcised patients, the foreskin must be retracted and the meatus cleansed with an antiseptic solution such as povidone–iodine, benzalkonium chloride, or hexachlorophene. The first 30 mL is passed without collection. The sterile specimen container is then placed into the urinary stream, and approximately 50 to 100 mL is collected. The specimen container is capped immediately, and the urinalysis is performed as soon as possible after collection. The portion not used for urinalysis may be used for culture, if indicated.

B. Female adults. The midstream clean-catch technique in female patients requires more effort and attention to detail than in males. In females, collection is usually done by the patient sitting on the toilet. After the labia are separated with one hand, an antiseptic solution is applied to cleanse the perimeatal area. A wiping motion *toward the perineum* is used. After the first 25 mL is passed, the next 50 to 100 mL is collected in a sterile specimen container. If a satisfactory specimen cannot be obtained, catheterization should be used.

C. Children. In very young patients, urine is usually obtained by cleansing the meatus with an antiseptic solution and placing a sterile plastic bag over the penis or vulva. Suprapubic needle aspiration of the bladder may be required to obtain a reliable urine specimen, and this is easily accomplished in young children because the bladder is located in a more intraabdominal position than in adults.

II. Physical characteristics of the urine

A. Color. The normal yellow color of urine is caused by various amounts of urochrome, a product of hemoglobin degradation. The most important color abnormality is red or reddish brown urine, suggesting the presence of erythrocytes, hemoglobin, myoglobin, or pigments derived from medications or other substances (Table 1.1).

B. Turbidity or nontransparency of the urine may be a consequence of phosphaturia, pyuria, chyluria, or bacteriuria. It is important not to confuse turbidity with pyuria.

C. Specific gravity and osmolality are closely related measures of urine concentration. Specific gravity varies from 1.000 to 1.040, whereas osmolality varies from 50 to 1,200 mOsm/L. Presence of radiologic contrast media or heavy proteins may raise the specific gravity but not the osmolality of urine. Dilute urine may be seen in diabetes insipidus, diabetes mellitus, chronic renal failure, and polydipsia. Excessively concentrated urine may occur in dehydration and congestive heart failure.

Table 1.1.   Common causes of discolored urine

Red or red–brown
  Erythrocyturia
  Hemoglobinuria
  Myoglobinuria
  Porphyruria
  Natural food pigments (beets, berries)
  Food coloring (rhodamine B)
  Drugs
    Phenothiazines
    Phenazopyridine
    Laxatives (phenolphthalein, senna)
    Adriamycin
    Rifampin
    Phenytoin

Amber or dark yellow
  Bilirubin
  Foods (carrots, riboflavin, vitamin A)
  Drugs
    Sulfonamides
    Chloroquine
    Phenacetin

Orange
  Phenazopyridine
  Laxatives containing phenolphthalein
  Rifampin
  Sulfasalazine

Blue or green
  Pseudomonas infection
  Drugs
    Amitriptyline
    Indomethacin
    Promethazine
    Triamterene

III.   Chemical characteristics of urine may be tested by means of reagent dipsticks and include pH, urine nitrite, leukocyte esterase, glucose, protein, and blood.

  A.   The **pH** is a measure of renal acidifying ability and of reactions occurring in the urine after it is produced by the kidney. **Alkaline urine** (pH > 6.5) is seen in renal tubular acidosis as well as in specimens obtained within 2 hours of a large meal or left standing at room temperature for several hours. Patients with infections caused by urea-splitting organisms (*Proteus* sp, some *Escherichia coli*) tend to have particularly alkaline urine. Ingestion of bicarbonate as well as some diuretics (acetazolamide) may produce an alkaline urine. **Acid urine** (pH < 6.0) is seen in respiratory acidosis, starvation, loss of alkali due to diarrhea, and ingestion of acidifying agents such as ammonium chloride.

B. Bacteriuria is detected by measuring urine nitrite levels. Many common intestinal bacteria contain nitrate reductase, an enzyme that converts urine nitrate to nitrite when exposed to urine for a minimum of 4 hours. Thus, best results are obtained on first-voided morning urine specimens. The test may produce a false negative if the patient is voiding frequently, if the bacteria do not contain nitrate reductase, or if the urine contains low levels of nitrate or has a high specific gravity. The presence of ascorbic acid in the urine may also produce a false-negative nitrite reaction. False-positive readings for urinary nitrite may occur in the presence of hematuria.

C. Leukocytes may be detected by measuring leukocyte esterase, an enzyme released when white cells lyse. A positive test result indicates the presence of six leukocytes per high-power field or more. False-negative tests can occur in the presence of heavy proteinuria, glycosuria, high specific gravity, blood, tetracycline, cephalexin, gentamicin, phenazopyridine, ascorbic acid, or nitrofurantoin in the urine. Low specific gravity, oxalic acid, or traces of oxidizing agents may cause false positives.

D. Glucose is spilled in the urine when the serum glucose level is 180 mg/dL or higher. Glycosuria may occur during pregnancy even with normal serum glucose levels. False-positive results may occur in the presence of aspirin and cephalosporins. Sensitivity may decrease with urine of high specific gravity (>1,030) and with high ascorbic acid concentrations.

E. Protein excretion is estimated by measuring urinary albumin levels. The dipstick reaction is positive at albumin concentrations of 30 mg/dL or higher. The degree of proteinuria may be overestimated if the urine is extremely concentrated. Normal urine of high specific gravity may cause higher than normal readings, as will alkaline urine (pH ≥ 9) and urine containing chlorhexidine.

F. Blood. The dipstick reagent reacts to hemoglobin (in red cells and free) as well as myoglobin. Thus, the reagent strip reaction is not specific for red cells. In general, more than three to five red cells per high-power field will produce a positive reagent strip reaction. A false-positive test result may be caused by contamination with povidone–iodine. Ascorbic acid in the urine may interfere with the reagent strip reaction and give a false-negative result for hemoglobin. Microscopic examination of the urine can easily differentiate true erythrocyturia from other causes of positive reagent strip reactions (Table 1.2).

IV. Microscopic examination is performed after centrifuging 10 mL of urine at 2,000 rev/min for 5 minutes, discarding the

Table 1.2. Differentiating the causes of red-colored urine

Cause	Dipstick Result	Microscopic Result
Erythrocyturia	Positive	Positive
Myoglobinuria	Positive	Negative
Hemoglobinuria	Positive	Negative
Pigmenturia	Negative	Negative

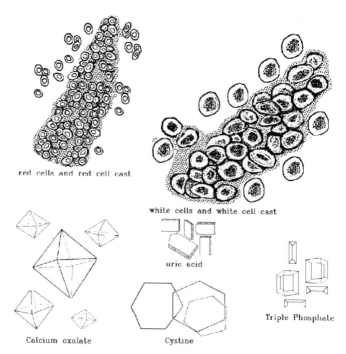

red cells and red cell cast

white cells and white cell cast

uric acid

Triple Phosphate

Calcium oxalate   Cystine

Fig. 1.1.   Most common findings on microscopic examination of the urine.

supernatant, resuspending the sediment, and placing a drop of sediment on a glass slide for microscopy under both low- and high-power lenses (Fig. 1.1).

A.   Red blood cells are easily seen under the high-power (×400) lens of the microscope. Microscopic hematuria is usually quantified as the number of red blood cells per high-power field. The finding of five or more red blood cells per high-power field is abnormal. Red blood cell casts (Fig. 1.1) are cylindrical clumps of red cells in the shape of the renal tubules or collecting ducts and are indicative of a renal source. Dysmorphic red cells are also highly suggestive of a glomerular source of hematuria.

B.   White blood cells in the urine are indicative of inflammation anywhere along the genitourinary tract or even contiguous with genitourinary organs. More than five white blood cells per high-power field should be considered abnormal. White cell casts (Fig. 1.1) indicate a renal source. Leukocytes are often present in the urine without bacteriuria. The persistent presence of "sterile" pyuria suggests the possibility of genitourinary tuberculosis.

C.   Other cells that may be seen include squamous epithelial cells shed from the vagina and renal tubular cells.

D.   Crystals are commonly seen on urine microscopy and are not pathologic as an isolated finding (Fig. 1.1). **Calcium oxalate** crystals look like small pyramids or squares and are seen in patients with calcium oxalate calculi or chronic inflammatory bowel disease. **Uric acid** crystals appear in acidic urine as small rectangular or rhomboid-shaped flat plates. So-called **triple-phosphate** or **struvite** crystals are composed of magnesium–ammonium phosphate and look like domed rectangles or coffin lids. These crystals precipitate only in urine that has a pH above 8. Such high pH levels generally occur only with infection caused by urea-splitting organisms. **Cystine** crystals occur in cystinuria when the urine pH falls below 7. The crystals appear as small plates with five or six sides, similar to a stop sign.

E.   Bacteria and other organisms include gram-negative and gram-positive bacteria, yeast, trichomonads, and *Schistosoma* sp. Spermatozoa are commonly seen in male urine.

F.   Artifacts include starch granules from gloves, hair, and clothing fibers. The finding of food particles or stool indicates the presence of an enteric–urinary fistula.

V.   Hematuria

The finding of hematuria is one of the most common and most important signs of disease in urology. The causes of hematuria range from benign (exercise related) to malignant (bladder carcinoma) (Table 1.3). Because the degree of hematuria bears no relation to the seriousness of the underlying cause, hematuria should always be considered a symptom of serious disease until proved otherwise. Hematuria is usually categorized as **gross** (visible to the unaided eye) or **microscopic** (more than three red cells per high-power microscopic field on two of three properly collected specimens). Hematuria may be further characterized as initial, terminal, or total. Initial hematuria is said to indicate a source distal to the external sphincter, terminal hematuria has a source in the proximal urethra or bladder neck, and total hematuria has a source in the bladder or upper tract. Needless to say, the source of hematuria cannot be determined accurately from the history alone. **False hematuria** is discoloration of the urine from pigments such as food coloring and myoglobin. **Factitious hematuria** is the presence of red blood cells in the urine from a source outside the urinary tract (e.g., malingering). Patients attempting to obtain narcotic drugs often present with a history of renal colic substantiated by factitious hematuria. They may add blood to their urine after voiding and before presenting it for urinalysis.

Some causes of hematuria are summarized in Table 1.3. Because of the large number of diseases that may cause hematuria, it is helpful to categorize them as glomerular, renal, urologic, and hematologic. Approximately 10% to 20% of patients presenting with microscopic hematuria will have no source of bleeding identified (idiopathic hematuria) even after exhaustive evaluation. Among patients with an identifiable cause, about one-third are of renal origin and two-thirds are caused by middle or lower urinary tract lesions. The bladder is the source in 40% of patients with gross hematuria. Overall, about 2.5% of patients with microscopic hematuria will be found to have a urologic malignancy; however, the risk increases rapidly with aging (Fig. 1.2) and in certain

Table 1.3. Some important causes of hematuria

Glomerular
  Acute glomerulonephritis
  Lupus nephritis
  Benign familial hematuria
  Benign essential hematuria (Berger's disease)
  Goodpasture's syndrome
  Exercise hematuria

Renal
  Polycystic kidney disease
  Medullary sponge kidney
  Papillary necrosis
  Renal infarction or embolus
  Lymphoma
  Multiple myeloma
  Amyloidosis
  Inflammation and infection
  Vascular malformations

Urologic
  Neoplasms
  Calculi
  Benign prostatic hypertrophy
  Urethral stricture
  Endometriosis
  Diverticulitis, appendicitis
  Abdominal aortic aneurysm
  Foreign body
  Infection

Hematologic
  Congenital and acquired coagulopathies
  Therapeutic anticoagulation
  Sickle cell disease and trait
  Sickle cell thalassemia
  Sickle cell–hemoglobin C disease

Factitious
  Vaginal bleeding

False hematuria
  Food pigments
  Drug metabolites

groups such as smokers and those who work with certain industrial chemicals (e.g., aniline dyes). Women under the age of 40 and nonsmokers are at lower risk.

The age, sex, and race of the patient are important indicators of the likely cause. In children, one should consider acute glomerulonephritis, urinary infection, and Wilms' kidney tumor. In men older than 60, bladder carcinoma and benign prostatic hyperplasia (BPH) are the most common causes of hematuria. In young female patients, cystitis is the most common cause. Hematuria is the most common presenting complaint of patients with sickle cell trait. This

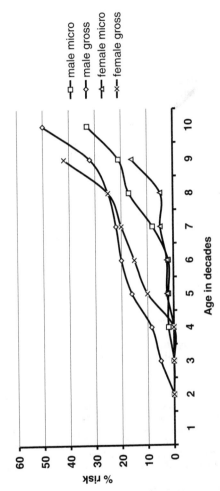

Fig. 1.2. Risk of finding malignancy in patients with hematuria according to patient age. (Adapted from data in Khadra et al. A prospective analysis of 1,930 patients with hematuria to evaluate current diagnostic practice. *J Urol* 2000;163:524.)

hematologic disorder accounts for approximately one-third of instances of hematuria in blacks.

A.   Diagnosis of hematuria. When a patient presents with hematuria or a screening urinalysis shows a positive result for blood, the initial step is to establish the presence of red blood cells in the voided urine. This may not always be straightforward, as red coloration of the urine may be caused by erythrocyturia, hemoglobinuria, myoglobinuria, or pigmenturia (Table 1.1). Test results with the commonly available dipstick reagent strips will be positive in the presence of red cells, hemoglobin, or myoglobin, and thus they are not specific for erythrocyturia (Table 1.2). Only the microscopic examination can document the presence of red cells in the urine.

1.   Urine culture and sensitivity should be ordered to rule out infection.

2.   Screening imaging studies. Computed tomography (CT) scan with intravenous contrast agent has become the radiologic test of choice for the evaluation of both microscopic and gross hematuria. CT has largely replaced the intravenous pyelogram (IVP) for evaluation of the upper urinary tract. CT is readily available and quickly performed. In addition to imaging the genitourinary tract, it can also provide information on other abdominal pathology that may be present. CT has a higher sensitivity for stones (94% to 98%) than does IVP (52% to 59%). In patients with a contrast allergy or renal insufficiency who cannot tolerate contrast media, ultrasound can be used as the screening test. Combined with urinary cytology and retrograde ureterograms, ultrasound allows for evaluation of the entire upper tract in such cases.

3.   Cystourethroscopy *is indicated in all instances of hematuria.* It is helpful in some instances to perform cystoscopy while the patient is bleeding to determine the site of bleeding. Biopsy specimens should be taken from any suspected lesions or areas. Retrograde pyelography, brush biopsy, or ureteroscopy may be performed in conjunction with cystoscopy.

4.   Ureteroscopy should be considered in instances of hematuria that can be localized to the upper urinary tract. A small biopsy forceps or a brush can be used to obtain tissue from any suspected areas.

5.   Urinary cytology can be very helpful in diagnosing urothelial malignancy. Cytologic results may be difficult to read in the presence of large amounts of blood in the urine. Urine cytology specimens from the upper tracts may be obtained by ureteral catheterization and barbotage with saline solution. The sensitivity of urine cytology is lower in low-grade tumors and excellent in high-grade tumors and carcinoma in situ.

6.   Cancer-related proteins specific for genitourinary malignancies have been developed in recent years. NMP-22 (Matritech) detects the nuclear matrix proteins shed during cell turnover in papillary transitional cell carcinoma, including carcinoma in situ. In patients with sterile urine, this test has a sensitivity approaching 86%. However, the specificity falls off dramatically in the presence of inflammation (i.e., stones or infection). The bladder tumor antigen test offers similar results and can be easily performed in the clinic or office in about 5 minutes. These tests may prove to be effective in following patients with known prior bladder tumors, but their usefulness as initial screening tests to replace cystoscopy has not yet been proven.

B.   Hematuria of obscure origin. In approximately 10% to 20% of patients with microscopic hematuria, no cause of hematuria can be identified even after extensive urologic evaluation. The question then becomes how to follow these patients. Never tell patients that there is "nothing wrong" or that their examination findings are "normal," because an abnormality may turn up on future examination. It should be explained that the long-term significance of their persistent hematuria is unknown and that close follow-up is required. If an episode of gross hematuria develops, cystoscopy should be performed urgently in an attempt to visualize the source of bleeding. If the bleeding can be localized to one side, angiography or ureteroscopy should be considered. A careful drug history should be taken, with particular attention to occasional use of aspirin and nonsteroidal analgesics, which can induce coagulopathy. As long as microscopic hematuria persists, the patient must be followed by urinalysis and urinary cytology every 6 months. If cytology becomes abnormal, irritative voiding symptoms develop in the absence of infection, or gross hematuria occurs, then a full evaluation should be repeated, including cystoscopy and imaging.

C.   Renal causes of hematuria are characterized by red cell casts, dysmorphic red cells, and presence of >500 mg of protein in the urine/24 h.

   1.   Nephropathy and nephritis. In children, glomerulonephritis accounts for about one-half of instances of hematuria. Most of the glomerulopathies cause hematuria and usually proteinuria as well. Proteinuria of significant degree (more than 2+) is very suggestive of glomerular disease, as is the presence of casts of red cells.

      a.   Acute poststreptococcal glomerulonephritis occurs when circulating antibody–antigen complexes are trapped in the glomeruli. This type of glomerulonephritis occurs most commonly in children aged 3 to 10 years following streptococcal pharyngitis or impetigo. Approximately 2 weeks after the initial infection, the patient usually presents with fever, headache, and mild hypertension. Urinalysis reveals erythrocyturia, mild proteinuria, and casts. Frequently, serum antistreptolysin-O titers are elevated and total serum complement levels are decreased. More than 95% of instances resolve spontaneously; serious renal insufficiency may develop in 58%.

      b.   Benign essential hematuria (Berger's disease) is a form of acute focal glomerulonephritis seen predominantly in male patients between the ages of 12 and 55 (mean age at presentation 25 years). This disorder, which is associated with the deposition of immunoglobulin (Ig) A and occasionally IgG in the glomerular mesangium, is also called **IgA nephropathy.** Typically, the patient presents within 1 to 3 days after an acute upper respiratory infection or other viral illness with a presenting complaint of gross hematuria

(45%), incidentally discovered microscopic hematuria (30%), or proteinuria (20%). Almost all patients have proteinuria in excess of 0.5 g/day. Patients with Berger's disease tend to suffer recurrent episodes of gross hematuria with repeated viral infections and show persistent microscopic hematuria (often with casts of red cells) between relapses. Unlike the urine specimens of family members of patients with benign familial hematuria, the urine specimens of family members in this case are normal. Although most patients suffer no loss of renal function, in approximately 25%, a slowly progressive renal failure associated with hypertension develops over a period of years. No specific treatment is available for this disorder.

c.   Benign familial hematuria. Between 25% and 50% of children investigated for idiopathic hematuria are found to have family members with microscopic hematuria. The disorder may affect patients of any age (mean age 32 years), has a two-to-one female predominance, and is inherited as an autosomal dominant trait. The only means of making this diagnosis is by obtaining a urinalysis from the siblings and parents of patients found to have idiopathic hematuria. Proteinuria may be found in approximately 50% of patients; however, this condition, unlike Berger's disease, is usually associated with a minimal degree of proteinuria. The condition appears to have no long-term implications of renal disease.

d.   Alport's syndrome, also called progressive familial nephropathy, is characterized by familial renal failure and deafness. The disease predominantly affects younger male patients (mean age 13 years). Hematuria occurs in about one-third of patients, and significant proteinuria is very common.

e.   Goodpasture's syndrome is characterized by hemoptysis, malaise, headache, and hematuria. The urine shows gross or microscopic hematuria, and renal function is abnormal. The disorder is thought to be caused by the deposition of antibodies against glomerular basement membrane in glomeruli and in the lung. Treatment involves high-dose corticosteroids and immunosuppressive agents.

2.   Exercise. Hematuria accompanied by proteinuria and casts of red cells in the urinary sediment may occur after strenuous exercise such as swimming, running, and team sports. All patients should be questioned regarding exercise when the history is taken. Even if exercise is temporally related to the onset of hematuria, exercise hematuria remains a diagnosis of exclusion after a complete workup has been performed.

D.   Sickle cell anemia. This congenital disorder is caused by replacement of hemoglobin A with hemoglobin S, a less soluble molecule that is prone to polymerization (sickling) when exposed to low oxygen tension, low pH, or both. Patients with the homozygous form (hemoglobin SS; **sickle cell disease**), encountered rarely by urologic physicians, have severe anemia; intermittent vascular crises involving the chest, abdomen, and skeleton; and repeated infections (pneumococcal pneumonia, gram-negative osteomyelitis). There is no specific treatment, and these patients usually do not survive past the age of 30. The heterozygous form (hemoglobin SA, S-thalassemia, and SC; **sickle cell trait**) is present in approximately 8% of African Americans and can occur in white persons as well. Except for causing a mild renal tubular concentrating defect, sickle cell trait is generally asymptomatic; however, these patients are prone to episodes of hematuria of renal origin. The bleeding is probably related to the hypoxic, hypertonic, and acidotic conditions that prevail in the renal medulla. With onset of the sickling phenomenon, arteriolar obstruction leads to papillary necrosis and hematuria. For reasons not understood, bleeding occurs four times more often from the left kidney than the right and is slightly more common in female patients. In approximately 50% of instances, the patient will give a past history of episodes of self-limited gross hematuria.

   1.   Diagnosis is easily accomplished by the sickle cell preparation. If the result of this test is negative and sickle cell trait is still suspected, hemoglobin electrophoresis should be ordered; however, the presence of sickle cell trait in a black patient does not establish this as the sole cause of bleeding. In one series, approximately 30% of patients with sickle trait hematuria were found to have infection or malignancy as a cause of bleeding. Thus, one must guard against ascribing all hematuria in black patients to the presence of sickle cell trait and carry out a complete urologic investigation, including appropriate radiologic studies and cystoscopy. At the same time, one must consider the possibility of sickle cell trait in white patients with hematuria of obscure origin.

   2.   Treatment of sickle cell–associated hematuria involves nonspecific measures in many instances because the hematuria often resolves spontaneously. Such measures include bed rest, intravenous fluids, and oral or parenteral alkali therapy. Oxygen by nasal cannula probably has little effect on the oxygen tension in the renal medulla but is widely used nevertheless. For patients who do not respond to these measures, specific modalities aimed at reducing the tonicity, acidity, and low oxygen tension in the renal medulla have been described.

   a.   Infusion of distilled water (500 mL over 15 minutes IV) is a safe procedure that reportedly can quickly terminate an episode of hematuria caused by sickling. For reasons that are not clear, the risk of producing intravascular hemolysis in patients with hemoglobin S is minimal.

   b.   Urinary alkalinization has a sound physiologic basis in this disorder. Two grams of sodium bicarbonate orally four times daily or one ampule per 1,000 mL of intravenous fluid should adequately alkalinize the urine.

   c.   Diuretics act to decrease the hypertonicity of the renal medulla. Both loop diuretics (ethacrynic acid, furosemide) and osmotic diuretics (mannitol, urea) are effective.

   d.   ε-Aminocaproic acid (EACA) is a potent inhibitor of urokinase, an enzyme that causes fibrinolysis in the urinary tract. EACA prevents dissolution of clots in the urinary tract and thus promotes hemostasis. For this reason, it has been used widely in many forms of urologic hemorrhage, including that caused by sickle hemoglobinopathies. The presence of disseminated intravascular coagulation must be ruled out before EACA is used. EACA is equally effective orally or intravenously for bleeding caused by sickle cell trait. An initial dose of 5 g IV is followed by a continuous infusion of 1 g/h. Hematuria usually ceases within 2 to 3 days of initiation of therapy. Maintenance therapy of 4 g PO four times daily should be continued for at least 6 weeks. The major side effect of EACA therapy has been ureteral obstruction from clots.

e.   Local irrigation with hemostatic agents such as oxychlorosene or silver nitrate may be effective in difficult cases. Irrigation through a ureteral catheter with 100 mL of 0.1% oxychlorosene or 1% silver nitrate has been reported to stop bleeding quickly.

E.   Hemorrhagic cystitis associated with cyclophosphamide, ifosfamide, and radiation therapy may sometimes cause life-threatening bladder hemorrhage. **Radiation cystitis** occurs in approximately 10% of patients who have received pelvic radiation, but only a small number experience severe bladder hemorrhage. **Cyclophosphamide (Cytoxan)** and **ifosfamide** are alkylating agents whose toxic metabolite (acrolein) is excreted in the urine. Gross hematuria occurs in about 12% of patients receiving these agents and is dose dependent. In most instances, the bleeding is self-limited (48 hours in duration), and the patients require transfusion of only 2 units. **MESNA** (2-mercaptoethanesulfonic acid) may provide prophylaxis against hemorrhagic cystitis caused by ifosfamide. The dose is 20% of the ifosfamide dose intravenously and is given 4 to 8 hours after each chemotherapy infusion. The **treatment** of hemorrhagic cystitis is as follows:

1.   Cystoscopy under anesthesia (spinal or general) should be performed if bleeding persists. All clots must be evacuated and whatever bleeding can be identified cauterized.

2.   One percent alum in sterile water is often effective. Alum is an aluminum salt that causes precipitation of proteins without systemic effects. Anesthesia is not required to administer intravesical alum, and it may be used at the bedside. The solution is administered continuously through a large-caliber three-way Foley catheter at a rate of 1 L/8 h.

3.   EACA may be effective in controlling bladder hemorrhage. The presence of disseminated intravascular coagulation must be ruled out before EACA is used. The drug is given orally (loading dose of 5 g followed by 1 g/h for 8 hours), intravenously (loading dose of 5 g in 250 mL of diluent over the first hour followed by 1 g/h over 8 hours), or intravesically (5 g in 1 L of saline solution for bladder irrigation infused over 3 to 4 hours).

4.   Silver nitrate induces thrombosis in bleeding vessels in the bladder mucosa but is milder than formalin. Under general or spinal anesthesia, 200 mL of 1% silver nitrate solution is placed in the bladder through a urethral catheter and drained after 15 minutes. The bladder is continuously irrigated with normal saline solution over the next 48 hours.

5.   Formalin is a solution of gaseous formaldehyde in water. Because the maximum solubility of formaldehyde in water is

38%, such a solution is called 100% formalin. A 1% formalin (0.38% formaldehyde) solution is recommended for bladder irrigation; higher concentrations are likely to cause severe bladder necrosis and fibrosis. The following protocol is recommended:

   a. Under anesthesia (general or spinal), **all clots are evacuated** and a **cystogram is obtained** to assess the integrity of the bladder and rule out vesicoureteral reflux. Intravesical formalin is contraindicated in the presence of reflux but may be used if occlusive ureteral catheters are placed.

   b. With the Foley catheter drawn tightly against the bladder neck, 1% formalin is poured into the barrel of a Toomy (catheter tip) syringe held 15 cm above the pubis and allowed to run into the bladder by gravity drainage. After 3 minutes, the bladder is drained completely by gravity. The formalin irrigation may be repeated until a total of 1,000 mL of formalin solution has been used.

   c. After formalin irrigation is completed, the bladder is washed with 1,000 mL of distilled water.

6. **Urinary diversion.** If the measures described are not successful, the patient should be returned to the cystoscopy room under anesthesia (preferably epidural or spinal) for placement of bilateral ureteral catheters or stents to divert the urine. For reasons that are not clear, urinary diversion has been observed to reduce or eliminate urinary bleeding. Cutaneous ureterostomy should be considered if permanent diversion is required.

F. Hematuria associated with anticoagulation. Hematuria occurs in 5% to 10% of patients receiving anticoagulation with heparin or sodium warfarin despite the fact that the coagulation levels are well within therapeutic range in most of these patients. About 25% of such patients have urologic cancer diagnosed on investigation of their hematuria. An additional 50% have benign urologic lesions causing hematuria, such as BPH, urethral stricture, and ureteral calculus. Thus, the onset of hematuria in a patient receiving anticoagulation has the same (if not greater) significance as in another patient and mandates a complete urologic evaluation.

G. Coagulopathies presenting as hematuria. Patients with hematuria of obscure origin should be screened for the presence of a coagulopathy. The prothrombin time, partial thromboplastin time (PTT), thrombin time, platelet count, and bleeding time should be determined. If coagulopathy is suspected, hematologic consultation is indicated. Although any coagulopathy may present as hematuria, the most common problems are the following:

1. **Thrombocytopenia.** In general, bleeding problems are not encountered in patients with platelet counts above 50,000/µL. Decreased production of platelets in bone marrow may be drug induced (antineoplastic agents, thiazide diuretics, estrogens, alcohol) or may be caused by replacement by malignancy (prostate cancer). Increased peripheral destruction of platelets occurs in idiopathic thrombocytopenic purpura and in disseminated intravascular thrombosis. In instances of splenomegaly, platelets may be sequestered in the spleen, causing peripheral thrombocytopenia (hypersplenism).

2.   Hemophilia is caused by congenital deficiency of factor VIII or factor IX. Deficiency of factor VIII is five times more common than deficiency of factor IX. Although hemarthrosis is the most common problem, approximately 30% of patients with hemophilia have hematuria, which can be a severe problem, causing ureteral obstruction by clots. Both conditions are treated by infusion of fresh frozen plasma or cryoprecipitate. Factor VIII and factor IX concentrates are reserved for patients with severe hemophilia.

3.   von Willebrand's disease is a congenital deficiency of factor VIII characterized by prolongation of PTT and bleeding time with a normal platelet count. Spontaneous bleeding is rarer than in hemophilia. Treatment is administration of cryoprecipitate or fresh frozen plasma.

4.   Disseminated intravascular coagulation may result from sepsis, metastatic carcinoma (prostate, breast, gastrointestinal), liver disease, surgery, obstetric complications, massive trauma, or burns. Laboratory diagnosis is based on consumption of coagulation factors and platelets with elevated titers of fibrin degradation products. Treatment is based on correcting the underlying disorder and use of heparin in some instances.

5.   Primary fibrinolysis implies the destruction of fibrin in the absence of underlying coagulation and is extremely rare. It is said to occur in carcinoma of the prostate and during extracorporeal circulation. Treatment involves a combination of EACA and heparin because there is frequently an accompanying thrombotic process. Fresh frozen plasma is used to replace coagulation factors that have been consumed.

SUGGESTED READING

Abarbanel J, Benet AE, Lask D, et al. Sports hematuria. *J Urol* 1990; 143:887–890.

Blumenthal SS, Fritsche C, Lemann J, Jr. Establishing the diagnosis of benign essential hematuria. *JAMA* 1988;259:2263–2266.

Grossfeld GD, Litwin MS, Wolf JS, et al. Evaluation of asymptomatic microscopic hematuria in adults: the American Urological Association Best Practice Policy Panel, part I: definition, detection, prevalence, and etiology. *Urology* 2001;57:599.

Grossfeld GD, Litwin MS, Wolf JS, et al. Evaluation of asymptomatic microscopic hematuria in adults: the American Urological Association Best Practice Policy Panel, part II: patient evaluation, cytology, voided markers, imaging, cystoscopy, nephrology evaluation, and follow-up. *Urology* 2001;57:604.

Khadra MH, Pickard RS, Charlton M, et al. A prospective analysis of 1,930 patients with hematuria to evaluate current diagnostic practice. *J Urol* 2000;163:524.

Kraus SE, Siroky MB, Babayan RK, et al. Hematuria and the use of nonsteroidal anti-inflammatory drugs. *J Urol* 1984;132:288–290.

Lynch TH, Waymont B, Dunn JA, et al. Repeat testing for hematuria and underlying urological pathology. *Br J Urol* 1994;74:730–732.

McInnes BK III. The management of hematuria associated with sickle hemoglobinopathies. *J Urol* 1980;124:171–174.

Mokulis JA, Arndt WF, Downey JR, et al. Should renal ultrasound be performed in the patient with microscopic hematuria and a normal excretory urogram? *J Urol* 1995;154:1300–1301.

Murakami S, Igarashi T, Hara S, et al. Strategies for asymptomatic microscopic hematuria: a prospective study of 1,034 patients. *J Urol* 1990;144:99–101.

Nicolle LE, Orr P, Duckworth H, et al. Gross hematuria in residents of long-term-care facilities. *Am J Med* 1993;94:611–618.

Shaw ST Jr, Poon SY, Wong ET. Routine urinalysis: is the dipstick enough? *JAMA* 1985;253:1596–1600.

Van Savage JG, Fried FA. Anticoagulant-associated hematuria: a prospective study. *J Urol* 1995;153:1594–1596.

Woolhandler S, Pels RJ, Bor DH, et al. Dipstick urinalysis screening of asymptomatic adults for urinary tract disorders: 1. Hematuria and proteinuria. *JAMA* 1989;262:1214–1219.

Imaging of the Genitourinary Tract

Charles Hyde and Rebecca K. Schwartz

An extensive array of modalities and procedures is available for imaging of the genitourinary tract. Selection of the appropriate modality depends on the clinical question at hand in addition to considerations of patient safety, patient comfort, and cost. To make a good choice, one needs a thorough understanding of the utility of the various imaging modalities (Table 2.1). In our discussion, we focus mainly on the technique and indications for urologic imaging. Interpretation of these studies is beyond the scope of this chapter.

I. Plain abdominal radiograph

The frequently used acronym KUB (kidneys, ureters, and bladder) is a misnomer, as the plain abdominal radiograph does not demonstrate the ureters and only rarely demonstrates the bladder. It is only moderately useful to demonstrate the renal contours. These can be assessed on technically optimal films, which hint at abnormalities such as renal masses and abnormalities of renal size or position.

A. Technique. No preparation is needed. A single supine view is usually adequate; "upright" views, useful in evaluating the bowel, are rarely useful in evaluating the genitourinary system.

B. Indications. The greatest utility of the abdominal radiograph in urology is to evaluate for the presence and position of calculi, catheters, and stents and to obtain a preliminary view before performing other examinations. The plain radiograph of the abdomen should, additionally, be routinely used to evaluate abnormalities of the bones, including congenital, posttraumatic, and postoperative changes and the presence of osteoblastic metastases (typical of prostate carcinoma) and osteolytic metastases (the majority of solid tumors). In addition, gas collections, both normal (bowel) and abnormal (renal parenchyma, intrarenal collecting system, bladder, etc.), should be routinely sought.

II. Ultrasound

Ultrasound (US) is very useful in evaluating the urinary tract. Widely available, relatively inexpensive, and entailing no use of radiation, US provides generally excellent visualization of the kidneys, intrarenal collecting systems, and bladder. US is used as an initial screening examination of the urinary tract and has assumed much of the role once played by intravenous urography (IVU) in this regard. One significant drawback of US in comparison with other modalities such as computed tomography (CT), magnetic resonance imaging (MRI), and IVU is that no direct information is obtained about renal function. US can also be of limited use in obese patients or in patients with a very large amount of bowel gas.

US plays a lesser role in ureteral evaluation. Although US can sometimes visualize a dilated proximal or distal ureter, most of the ureter will be obscured by overlying bowel gas, and a nondilated

Table 2.1.   Utility of various imaging modalities

	KUB	IVP	Retrograde Pyelogram	US	I– CT	I+ CT	MRI	NM-MAG3
Renal parenchyma	+	++	0	+++	+++	++++	++++	++
Renal calculi	++	+++	++–++++	+++	++++	++ to +++	0	0
Renal function	0	++	0	0	0	++	++++	++++
Intrarenal collecting system	0	+++	+++–++++	+++	++	+++	+++	++
Ureter	0	++	++++	0 (nondilated) ++ (dilated)	++	+++	+	++
Bladder	+	+++	Usually performed with cystoscopy	++++	+++	++++	+++	++

IVP, intravenous pyelogram; I– CT, non-contrast-enhanced computed tomography; I+ CT, contrast-enhanced CT; NM-MAG3, nuclear renal scan with mercaptoacetyltriglycine; (0), no use; (+), minimally or rarely useful; (++), occasionally useful; (+++), useful; (++++), very useful.

ureter generally cannot be seen at all. The prostate is moderately well seen on transabdominal US and is very well visualized on transrectal US (TRUS). Another US examination frequently of interest to the urologist is scrotal US.

A.   Technique. No special preparation is required. Because the kidneys are retroperitoneal, renal US, unlike general abdominal US, does not require the patient to be fasting. Images are obtained in longitudinal and transverse planes. Whenever possible, the patient is imaged with a urine-distended bladder to improve visualization of the bladder and prostate. The postvoid residuum is calculated after the patient voids. A quick and useful approximation of the bladder volume is the formula (height × width × depth × 0.5); the same formula is used to calculate the prostate weight in grams.

Because US examination is performed in real time, it is particularly useful for imaging children or patients who are uncooperative. With a portable machine, US examinations can be performed at the patient's bedside or in the operating room.

B.   Indications. US is useful for general screening of the urinary tract. It is the examination of choice in defining renal cysts and in differentiating solid masses from cysts. It is particularly useful for detecting renal masses, kidney size and contour, diagnosing and following hydronephrosis, and evaluating the bladder. It is a useful adjunct in demonstrating renal calculi. It is less useful in evaluating lesions of the intrarenal collecting system, perirenal spaces, adrenals, and ureters and in the setting of trauma.

C.   Renal transplant. US of renal transplants is a special case. Because of the superficial location of a transplant and the lack of interposition of bowel gas, visualization of the transplant is usually excellent. Doppler tracings of the iliac artery, main renal artery, and intralobar and arcuate arteries give excellent insight in the evaluation of transplant failure and rejection and are routinely performed (see Chapter 25).

D.   Scrotal US is the single best radiologic method for evaluating the scrotal contents, including the testicles and extratesticular structures, and it is an invaluable part of the evaluation of scrotal pathology. Testicular pathology (including masses and inflammation), extratesticular pathology (including hydroceles), and epididymal pathology (including spermatoceles, epididymal masses, and inflammatory conditions) are all routinely imaged. In terms of technique, no preparation is needed. A high-frequency (5- to 12-MHz) linear transducer is used to image the scrotum directly.

E.   TRUS. Transabdominal US of the prostate is generally limited to quantifying prostate size. A detailed image of the prostate and periprostatic structures is obtained by prostate TRUS, in which a high-frequency transducer is placed in the rectum. The prostatic zones are usually well seen, prostatic pathology is frequently identified, and the prostate size can be accurately measured.

1.   Indications for TRUS include an abnormality on digital rectal examination, elevated prostate-specific antigen, or previously abnormal results of a prostate biopsy. It must be emphasized that TRUS is neither sensitive nor specific; a normal result on TRUS examination does not exclude prostate carcinoma, and an abnormal examination result can be seen despite the absence of significant pathology. One of the major indications for TRUS is to guide a needle biopsy of the prostate. Important but less frequently applied indications for TRUS are examination of the seminal vesicles and ejaculatory ducts in the evaluation of infertility and imaging of the prostate for abscess. TRUS can also be used to diagnose or drain a prostatic abscess.

2. Technique. The patient is given a Fleet enema and is asked to void before the examination. We currently give 400 mg of gatifloxacin PO 1 hour before the biopsy and then repeat the dose 12 and 24 hours after the biopsy. Some literature suggests that a single oral dose 30 to 60 minutes before biopsy gives equally good results in low-risk populations (nondiabetic, no history of urinary tract infections, age under 70). Biopsies are obtained with the patient in the left lateral position, although the lithotomy position can also be used. We obtain six segmental biopsy specimens with an 18-gauge spring-loaded needle. The number of biopsies should be increased to increase the sampling rate in glands larger than 50 g. If a focal abnormality is identified, one to three additional biopsy specimens should be obtained. Some bleeding—usually self-limited—from the rectum or urethra is common following the procedure. Complications (with approximate incidence) include mild hematuria (60%), severe hematuria (<1%), dysuria (5% to 10%), urinary tract infections (1% to 2%), urosepsis (0.1%), rectal bleeding (2%), rectal bleeding requiring treatment (0.1%), hematospermia (10%), vasovagal episode (1%), and prostatic infection (<0.5%). In summary, we have a 1% incidence of bleeding significant enough to require observation and a <0.5% incidence of serious postbiopsy infection.

III.   CT

CT, like US, has revolutionized the radiologic evaluation of the genitourinary tract. CT allows the radiologist to assess directly the morphology and function of the kidneys, the appearance of the surrounding retroperitoneal soft tissues (lymph nodes, adrenals, aorta, inferior vena cava), and the patency of vascular structures (renal veins and arteries). In the pelvis, CT can evaluate the bladder, prostate, and surrounding soft tissues and lymph nodes as well as the ureters. CT is limited for the evaluation of the penis and scrotum, and these structures are generally better assessed by US or MRI.

A. Technique. CT examinations can be performed with or without oral contrast medium and with or without intravenous contrast medium. It is important that the specific indications—the specific question to be answered—be discussed with the radiologist before a CT is performed, as the technique used may vary significantly.

The technique used must also vary with the capabilities of the CT scanner. Until recently, most scanning was performed with conventional axial CT, with stepped table movement between tomographic slices. This imaging process is relatively slow, with a scanning time of approximately 2 seconds and an interscan delay of 2 to 8 seconds. At least 1 minute is required to scan through the kidneys. Problems with this method include motion artifacts, gaps in scanning, and limited ability to evaluate the entire kidney in a uniform phase of enhancement. **Partial volume artifacts,** a particular problem when small peripheral masses are evaluated, occur if the lesion being studied is not in the center of the slice. The CT number calculated for any tissue slice will be an average of the different types of tissue included.

More recently, helical (spiral) scanning has replaced axial scanning as the preferred method for many indications, including the genitourinary tract. In helical scanning, the CT table moves continuously, and images are continuously obtained. Thus, an entire sequence is obtained in a single breath-hold. The pitch is the ratio of table speed to collimation. At a pitch of 1:1, an average kidney can typically be scanned at 5-mm collimation in fewer than 30 seconds. Neither motion artifacts nor gaps are a problem when patients are able to cooperate and hold their breath. "Partial voluming" is minimized with images reconstructed in the center of a lesion.

  1. Intravenous contrast agent is routinely used for most indications. Patients should fast for 4 hours before administration of intravenous contrast to reduce the risk of emesis and aspiration. After adequate intravenous access has been obtained, approximately 100 mL of contrast material is given at the rate of 2.0 to 4.0 mL/s, depending on the specific indication. After contrast material is given, several phases of renal enhancement occur. Knowledge of these different phases allows one to optimize the scanning protocols and interpret the findings intelligently.

  a. The **angiographic phase** occurs 15 to 40 seconds after contrast injection begins. The number, location, and patency of the renal arteries and the location and patency of the renal veins can be assessed.

  b. The **cortical phase** of renal enhancement normally occurs between 25 and 80 seconds after the initial exposure to contrast material. The renal cortex is maximally enhanced, and the corticomedullary differences are greatest. Enhancement of the cortex is often uneven, and both the sensitivity and the specificity for detecting renal lesions are diminished.

  c. The **nephrographic phase** usually begins 90 to 120 seconds after the injection of contrast medium and is characterized by the homogeneous enhancement of the entire renal parenchyma as a consequence of enhancement of the medulla. It is in this phase that detection of renal lesions, particularly smaller lesions, is greatest.

  d. The **excretory** or **urographic phase** begins when contrast material is visualized in the collecting system, including calyces, infundibula, and renal pelvis. This typically begins 3 to 5 minutes after injection and persists for several minutes. A nephrogram can be seen through much of the excretory phase.

B. Protocols. We use the following CT protocols in our institution. Modified protocols may be used in different institutions.

1. Renal/ureteral calculi. Helical CT scanning has replaced IVU as the primary imaging modality for the evaluation of renal colic. Helical scanning is performed with 5-mm collimation, reconstructed at 4-mm intervals, *without* intravenous or oral contrast agent. Oral contrast should not be used, as it may lead to difficulties in defining bowel diverticula and distinguishing the appendix from calculi. Densities that may represent calculi are searched in the kidneys and along the ureters. Repeat scanning with intravenous contrast and delayed images (10 minutes after injection) can be performed if scanning without intravenous contrast fails to demonstrate a calculus or if qualitative information about renal function is desired, particularly in a patient with an identified renal or ureteral stone.

2. Renal masses. CT scanning to search for renal masses or to evaluate suspected renal masses identified by other imaging modalities should be performed initially without intravenous contrast. This is followed by a bolus of 100 to 120 mL of intravenous contrast agent. Scanning of the kidneys should begin approximately 100 seconds after initiating the contrast injection to visualize the kidney in the nephrographic phase. As some tumors are better seen in the urographic phase, scanning should be repeated 5 to 10 minutes after contrast administration. With helical scanners that allow for rapid, repetitive sequential imaging, an additional earlier scan is performed in the angiographic phase to obtain more information about the renal vasculature. With this protocol, invasion of the renal vein and inferior vena cava can be assessed, and the number and location of renal arteries can be shown. Additional imaging of the abdomen and pelvis facilitates staging by determining lymph node spread and the presence of metastatic disease. If a renal mass is identified, a chest CT is also recommended.

3. CT angiography of the kidneys. CT angiography is a new technique developed to image the renal arteries and veins without catheter angiography. Contrast agent is injected through an antecubital vein, as in a routine enhanced CT scan, but at a more rapid rate, typically 3 mL/s or more. Scanning commences within 20 to 25 seconds. Delayed scanning may be performed to obtain anatomic images of the kidneys. Two- and three-dimensional reconstructed images of the renal vasculature demonstrate anomalies such as accessory renal arteries and retroaortic or circumaortic renal veins and pathologic entities such as renal artery stenoses, occlusions, and aneurysms.

4. Renal infection. Generally, pyelonephritis is a clinical diagnosis, and CT is used to define complications or response to treatment in complex cases. Routine scanning of the kidneys without intravenous contrast can demonstrate renal enlargement; diffuse, focal, or multifocal areas of low attenuation (abscess or focal pyelonephritis); and perinephric inflammation or fluid collections. CT following intravenous administration of contrast also depicts all these abnormalities and can be used if questions remain.

5. Bladder and ureters. Scanning of these structures must be performed 5 to 10 minutes after contrast injection and can be supplemented by prone positioning and the Valsalva maneuver. Helical scanning with 5-mm collimation, reconstructed at 4-mm intervals, allows for two-dimensional reconstructions. CT urography has allowed CT to replace IVU, in many cases, for detection and exclusion of upper tract involvement by transitional cell carcinoma (TCCA). Ureteral obstruction and periureteric inflammation and masses can be demonstrated. US is the preferred modality for evaluating the bladder, although CT is preferred for visualizing the perivesical fat and pelvic lymph nodes. Even in patients who cannot receive intravenous contrast medium, there may be intrinsic contrast between the urine-filled ureter or bladder and its wall that will allow assessment of wall thickness and contour as well as hydroureter.

IV.   Excretory urogram, intravenous urogram, and intravenous pyelogram

The above three terms are used interchangeably, although we prefer intravenous urogram (IVU). The first edition of this manual noted that "the IVU is still the initial examination in most instances for the evaluation of the genitourinary tract," but we no longer feel this is correct. Although there remains a role for IVU, the IVU is no longer the cornerstone of urologic imaging. The IVU is able to evaluate, to some degree, all aspects of the urinary tract—kidney parenchyma, renal function, intrarenal collecting system, ureters, and bladder; however, it is not the best means of evaluating any of these (Table 2.1).

A.   Technique. The patient should preferably be fasting to minimize emesis. Some radiologists routinely give a laxative. The patient should not be excessively hydrated. The patient should void immediately before the examination. There are many acceptable protocols for obtaining images in an IVU. In fact, as emphasized for many years, it is important to "tailor" the urogram to attempt to answer the clinical questions raised. Nevertheless, the following is the "standard" set of films obtained at our institution, with the understanding that departures from this protocol are common:

1. Scout abdomen and tomogram
2. Injection of contrast material by bolus intravenous injection
3. Tomograms at consecutive levels through the middle of the kidney at 1, 2, and 3 minutes after injection
4. A 5-minute supine abdominal radiograph
5. Placement of abdominal compression
6. Ten-minute anteroposterior (AP) and bilateral 30-degree posterior oblique coned views of the kidneys
7. Abdominal film after compression device released ("release film")
8. AP and oblique views of the bladder
9. AP postvoid bladder

An initial plain radiograph, called a **scout film,** is used to check for excessive bowel gas and internal or external radiodense objects, including contrast material in the gastrointestinal tract (barium or contrast from recent CT) and to check radiographic technique. A bolus injection gives superior images and is preferred. Drip infusion is used only when a bolus is impossible. Contrast is given according to the guidelines in Table 2.2.

Table 2.2. Guidelines for contrast administration

Newborns	2.0–3.0 mL/kg
Children	1.0–2.0 mL/kg
Adults	1.0 mL/kg (up to 100 mL)

Tomograms, which we routinely perform, increase the radiation exposure but also improve the visualization of the renal parenchyma and collecting system, predominately by "separating" the kidneys from adjacent bowel gas.

Abdominal compression is performed by inflating a rubber balloon over each side of the sacrum or at the pelvic brim, causing partial obstruction of the ureters. When properly performed, it can significantly improve visualization of the intrarenal collecting system and ureters. When improperly performed, it is uncomfortable for the patient and worthless. Contraindications for abdominal compression include recent abdominal surgery, aortic aneurysm, and an acutely obstructed urinary tract. A release abdominal film obtained after the compression device has been removed offers the best opportunity to visualize the ureters by IVU. A prone view can occasionally be helpful, as can a film with the patient upright.

Views of the bladder must be tailored depending on the indication for the IVU and can be partially or completely eliminated if further evaluation of the bladder (e.g., by cystoscopy or US) is planned or has already been performed. A complete evaluation on IVU includes AP and oblique views of the filled bladder and a postvoid image.

B.   Indications. The current indications for IVU are for evaluation of the calyces and ureters, especially in cases of known or suspected urothelial malignancy, for postoperative evaluation of the ureter, and for detailed evaluation of the calyces, ureteropelvic junction, and ureterovesical junction. Although IVU can be used in the evaluation of calculi and hydronephrosis, it is no longer the initial test of choice for either of these indications. Further, it no longer has a primary role in the evaluation of trauma, noncalculous hematuria, suspected renal malignancy, infections, renal failure, polycystic kidney disease, hypertension, and prostate disorders. An absolute contraindication to performing an IVU is the inability of the patient to tolerate contrast material because of renal insufficiency or allergy history.

C.   Iodinated contrast material. The use of iodinated contrast material is so important to the practice of urologic imaging that a more detailed discussion of contrast agents seems appropriate, including pharmacology, complications, and the treatment and prevention of complications (Table 2.3). Most radiographic contrast material can be classified into low-osmolarity contrast material (LOCM) and high-osmolarity contrast material (HOCM). High-quality images can be obtained with both HOCM and LOCM, with small differences in contrast enhancement unlikely to be clinically important. LOCMs have lower rates of all reactions, particularly acute reactions. Adverse

**Table 2.3.   Characteristics of commonly
used radiographic contrast media**

Generic Name	Trade Name	% Weight	Osmolality (mOsm/kg)	Ionic
Meglumine diatrizoate	Cystografin	30	600	Yes
Meglumine iothalamate	Cysto-Conray	43	1,000	Yes
Sodium diatrizoate 50	Hypaque 50	50	1,550	Yes
Meglumine diatrizoate 60	Hypaque 60	60	1,400–1,500	Yes
Reno-M-60	—	—	—	—
Conray 60	—	—	—	—
Iopamidol 128	Isovue 128	26	300	No
Iohexol 180	Omnipaque 180	39	450	No
Iopromide 240	Ultravist 240	50	500	No
Iohexol 300	Omnipaque 30	65	700	No

reactions occurred in 12.7% of patients injected with HOCM and
3.1% of patients injected with LOCM. Severe reactions occurred
in 0.2% of HOCMs and 0.04% of LOCMs. Multiple studies con-
cluded that the risk of an adverse reaction is approximately
four to six times greater with HOCMs. The issue of whether
LOCM should be used for all patients versus selective use in
high-risk populations is largely a function of the differential
cost of LOCM to HOCM, reimbursement rates, and the cost of
treating contrast reactions. Many articles have discussed both
the economic and the safety issues. Despite the literature having failed to consistently prove the cost effectiveness of the universal use of LOCMs, most hospitals have tended to convert to
universal use of LOCMs as the differential cost of contrast
material has fallen.

   1.   Systemic reactions to contrast material. The exact
   pathogenesis of contrast reactions is unknown but include
   effects from osmolality, chemotoxicity, and complement activation. It is a consistent finding that systemic contrast
   reactions are considerably more common following intravenous injections than intraarterial injections. Reactions to
   contrast agents can be classified as idiosyncratic or nonidiosyncratic, based on known or presumed cause. Idiosyncratic
   reactions, also called anaphylactoid reactions, include reactions that resemble allergic reactions and are presumed to
   be immunoglobulin E mediated. They can occur in anyone
   and are not dose dependent. Typical reactions include nasal
   congestion, urticaria, laryngeal edema, and bronchospasm.
   Nonidiosyncratic reactions are believed to result from direct
   chemotoxic effects (nausea, vomiting, cardiac arrhythmias,
   depressed cardiac function) or from hyperosmolality (local

pain, vasomotor instability, vasovagal reaction). Nonidiosyn-cratic reactions can occur in anyone, are more common in sick or debilitated patients, and are relatively dose dependent.

2. Contrast-mediated nephrotoxicity. Contrast-mediated nephrotoxicity is a significant consideration when considering administering intravenous contrast material in patients with diminished renal function. The incidence is small in patients with normal baseline renal function. Elevation of serum creatinine by >50% over baseline is seen in 1.6% of patients, and elevation of serum creatinine by >150% is seen in 0.15% of patients. When seen, nephrotoxic effects usually occur within 24 to 36 hours and peak within 48 to 72 hours, with gradual recovery to baseline renal function within a week. The etiology is multifactorial and not completely understood. Predisposing factors include renal insufficiency, diabetes, dehydration, age over 70 years, multiple myeloma (some disagree), proteinuria, and concomitant administration of aminoglycosides. These effects are additive, and those at greatest risk are diabetics with preexisting renal insufficiency. Although serum creatinine is a somewhat insensitive indicator of renal function, most radiology departments base their contrast protocols on it. In patients with a creatinine level above 1.5 to 1.7 mg/dL, contrast material should be used rarely or not at all. There are few differences in contrast-mediated nephrotoxicity between types of contrast agents; LOCMs may be minimally less nephrotoxic. Prophylaxis is achieved by adequate hydration (intravenous saline at 75 mL/h) before, during, and after exposure to radiocontrast agents. Recent attempts to lessen nephrotoxicity in at-risk populations with prophylactic theophylline (oral or intravenous) or with acetylcysteine (Mucomyst; 600 mg PO bid the day before and the day of contrast material administration) are interesting, but these agents are not routinely used.

3. Local effects. Extravasation is a function of intravenous technique and, as such, can occur with any contrast material. LOCM extravasation may cause fewer complications. The risks are predictable and include large volumes of contrast material, rapid infusions, poorly placed catheters, and patients who are very old or very young, are unconscious, or have "poor veins." Rapid infusions can rupture both veins and catheters, and it is important to be aware that a power injector can easily exceed the pressure limit of a small catheter. Symptoms include burning and pain that are usually felt immediately but may be delayed. Skin blistering, paresthesias, and persistent pain are serious signs. Extravasation can develop into ulceration and tissue necrosis. The acute inflammatory process peaks in 24 to 48 hours, but the time course is highly variable; tissue necrosis has been seen in as little as 6 hours after injection. Extravasation must therefore be taken seriously, and close follow-up is appropriate. There is no treatment protocol that has been demonstrated to be consistently effective. Many apply local cooling or heat, but these are of unclear benefit.

4. Delayed reactions. These occur 1 hour to 7 days after contrast administration. Most reactions are mild, are often difficult to differentiate from the patient's underlying condition, and include rash, nausea, vomiting, headache, and chills. Incidence is difficult to assess owing to differences in definitions, doses, and patient populations but is quoted as 2% to 8%, with the incidence being similar among contrast agents.

5.   Prophylaxis. There was a 31% reduction in the incidence of acute reactions when oral corticosteroids were taken both 2 and 12 hours before intravenous HOCM was administered. No protective effect was identified when steroids were given as a single dose 1 to 2 hours before contrast material, and there is no additional protective effect when steroids are administered for >24 hours. Common pretreatment protocols include 40 mg of prednisone 2 and 12 hours before contrast agent or prednisone 20 mg q6h for four doses before contrast material. Pretreatment with antihistamines probably reduces the chance of urticaria; pretreatment with a histamine-2 (H_2) blocker is logical but unproven. It is difficult to weigh the relatively small risk of low doses of steroids versus the small risk of a contrast reaction. Even though most symptoms reduced are mild to moderate, the balance might favor pretreatment if there are no contraindications to oral corticosteroids. Some examinations can be performed with a lower dose of contrast material. More importantly, when a patient presents with a relative or absolute contraindication to contrast material, one should always explore utilizing other imaging studies, including MRI, US, or CT scans, without intravenous contrast material.

6.   Treatment of contrast material reactions. Contrast reactions agents can be clinically classified by severity (mild, moderate, severe, or fatal). Most adverse reactions develop within 5 minutes, and certainly within 1 hour. Urticaria, facial edema, laryngeal edema, bronchospasm, and seizures are considered severe reactions.

   a.   Mild or moderate reactions. Pruritus or a scant urticaria is usually self-limited. More severe reactions can be treated with 25 to 50 mg of diphenhydramine IV, IM, or PO. As urticaria can be part of a generalized anaphylactoid reaction, close observation is mandatory.

   b.   Severe reactions. If **laryngeal edema** is present, 0.1 to 0.3 mL of 1:1,000 epinephrine should be given subcutaneously every 15 minutes to a total dose of 1 mg, in addition to hydration and oxygen (6 to 10 L/min). Diphenhydramine and H_2 blockers may be considered. If **bronchospasm** is present, a β-adrenergic agonist inhaler may provide symptomatic relief. If persistent, parenteral β-adrenergic agonists or aminophylline, 6.0 mg/kg IV over 10 to 20 minutes, should be considered. **Hypotension** may be seen as an isolated symptom or associated with sneezing, urticaria, watery eyes, or any other symptoms of an anaphylactoid syndrome. Rapid fluid replacement, frequently several liters, is the most important treatment. If life threatening, epinephrine 1:10,000 can be given intravenously, 1.0 mL slowly up to 10 mL. A **vasovagal reaction** may present with hypotension and bradycardia and may be accompanied by diaphoresis, abdominal cramps, and generalized anxiety. Besides rapid fluid resuscitation (aided by Trendelenburg's position), 0.5 to 1.0 mg IV of atropine may be given, up to 2 mg.

   c.   Fatal reactions. Fatal reactions do occur. There are minimal data on the relative mortality because of the very low incidence. The best data indicate the rate of fatal reactions to be 0.00043% for HOCM and 0.00029% for LOCM.

   7.   Drug interactions. Contrast material can potentially interfere with a number of other drugs. Two deserve special attention.

   a.   Metformin. Lactic acidosis, a rare complication but one with 50% mortality, has been reported in patients on metformin (Glucophage) who have received contrast material. The drug should be temporarily withheld at the time of contrast material injection and should be reinstated 48 hours later when the patient's renal function has been documented to have returned to baseline.

   b.   Interleukin-2. Patients treated with interleukin-2 immunotherapy, either concurrently or in the past, may develop delayed reactions after administration of contrast material.

V.   MRI

MRI has many uses in the genitourinary system, particularly in patients who, because of renal insufficiency or allergy history, cannot safely tolerate intravenous contrast administration. The outstanding soft tissue resolution offered by MRI makes it well suited for evaluating renal masses, and its potential for noninvasive vascular imaging has revolutionized the radiologic evaluation of vascular anatomy. Tissue contrast in MRI depends on the relaxation properties of protons in varying magnetic fields, rather than on ionizing radiation, which makes MRI a comparatively risk-free examination. Imaging protocols vary significantly, however, based on the indication for the examination; hence, MRI nearly always has a more restricted field of view and scope than CT for answering general questions about the status of other structures, and it is imperative to define the goal of MRI before the examination begins.

MRI of the kidneys is performed with a variety of pulse sequences, depending on the indication for the examination. In general, T1-weighted images are best for defining anatomy and are often performed in multiple planes, usually axial and coronal. If appropriate for optimal depiction of a mass or other pathology of interest, sagittal or oblique imaging may also be useful. T1-weighted images with a fat saturation pulse will null the signal from fat and help to identify lesions such as angiomyolipomas, which often have a significant macroscopic fat content. Microscopic fat, as seen in adrenal adenomas, can be detected with gradient echo "in-phase" and "out-of-phase" techniques.

T2-weighted images are better for demonstrating pathology and help to differentiate between cysts, which are very bright, and solid masses, which are only somewhat bright. Imaging after administration of gadolinium is crucial to discriminate between solid enhancing lesions and cystic nonenhancing lesions. As in CT scanning, serial MR sequences after gadolinium administration can help define masses seen in different phases of enhancement (cortical, nephrographic, and urographic). Image quality is enhanced in high magnetic field strength systems with improved gradients that allow for rapid imaging during breath-holding. It is often useful to obtain rapid sequential series of images during the angiographic, nephrographic, and urographic phases following gadolinium administration, as well as breath-hold T2-weighted images that minimize respiratory motion artifacts.

MR angiography makes possible a detailed evaluation of the renal vasculature. Flowing blood has different signal characteristics than thrombus or tumor within a vessel. Both "black-blood" (spin echo) and "bright-blood" (gradient echo) techniques have been developed to evaluate vascular patency and morphology. In addition, gadolinium-enhanced scans offer better contrast and spatial resolution of vascular abnormalities, especially when performed as rapid breath-hold sequences.

A.   Indications. Indications for MRI of the genitourinary system include evaluation of renal masses, renal vasculature, prostate cancer, and adrenal masses. Experimental uses include MR urography. **Contraindications** include the presence of ferromagnetic intracranial vascular clips, cardiac pacemakers, and certain prosthetic cardiac valves. Relative contraindications, sometimes amenable to pharmacologic intervention, include severe claustrophobia and the patient's inability to lie still for 30 to 45 minutes of imaging.

B.   MRI of renal masses. Renal masses can be characterized by MRI as solid, hemorrhagic, or cystic. Postgadolinium images, performed in a dynamic fashion, are an essential component of the MRI protocol. Visualization of small masses is enhanced by high-resolution imaging in multiple phases of enhancement. Urographic-phase imaging can help exclude the diagnosis of a calyceal diverticulum, which can on occasion be confused with a renal mass on earlier images. As with CT, anatomic imaging of the remainder of the abdomen can reveal lymph node and adrenal metastases. MRI is readily suited to the determination of vascular (renal vein, inferior vena cava) patency with either gadolinium-enhanced or nonenhanced techniques and of the number and origin of renal arteries, which may be useful in surgical planning.

C.   MR angiography of the renal vasculature. Both the status and number of the renal arteries and the position of the renal veins can readily be assessed with MRI. Many scanners allow for breath-hold, high-resolution, gadolinium-enhanced MR arteriography, which has proved to be nearly as accurate as conventional angiography for the assessment of renal artery number and morphology, without the associated risks of femoral artery puncture and complications of iodinated contrast administration. Renal vein and inferior vena cava patency can generally be assessed without the use of gadolinium, with either black-blood (spin echo) or bright-blood (gradient echo) techniques.

D.   MRI of prostate cancer. With the use of endorectal MR coils, high-resolution imaging of the prostate can be obtained. Foci of suspected neoplasm can be demonstrated, as well as extracapsular spread and involvement of the neurovascular bundle. During the same examination, an additional set of anatomic images of the pelvis can be obtained with the body coil to assess for pelvic adenopathy and metastatic disease to bone.

E. MRI of adrenal masses. Adrenal masses can be readily characterized with MRI. In-phase and out-of-phase imaging can be performed, without gadolinium administration, to assess for the presence of microscopic amounts of fat in an adrenal mass noted on CT or US. The presence of microscopic fat in a lesion strongly favors the diagnosis of adrenal adenoma rather than metastatic disease, and such lesions can potentially be followed with a biopsy being performed. Pheochromocytomas are extremely bright on T2-weighted images.

F. MR urography. An experimental procedure, MR urography relies on the presence of urine-filled ureters. T2-weighted sequences with very long echo times are best for accentuating the urine-filled ureters against the background of other abdominal–pelvic structures. Challenges to the development of this technique include artifacts caused by bowel motion and breathing, which can be reduced by injecting 0.5 mg of glucagon IM before the examination and by obtaining rapid breath-hold images.

SUGGESTED READING

Bosniak MA. The current radiologic approach to renal cysts. *Radiology* 1986;158:1–10.

Cohan RH. Detection and characterization of renal masses and staging of renal cancers: new considerations in the era of helical computed tomography. *Semin Urol Oncol* 2002;20:166–173.

Einstein DM, Herts BR, Weaver R, et al. Evaluation of renal masses detected by excretory urography: cost-effectiveness of sonography versus CT. *AJR Am J Roentgenol* 1995;164:371–375.

Ellis JH, Cohan RH, Sonnad SS, et al. Selective use of radiographic low-osmolality contrast media in the 1990s. *Radiology* 1996;200:297–311.

Farres MT, Gattegno B, Ronco P, et al. Nonnephrotoxic, dynamic, contrast enhanced magnetic resonance urography: use in nephrology and urology. *J Urol* 2000;163:1191–1196.

Fielding JR, Silverman SG, Rubin GD. Helical CT of the urinary tract. *AJR Am J Roentgenol* 1999;172:1199–1206.

Katzberg RW. Urography into the 21st century: new contrast media, renal handling, imaging characteristic, and nephrotoxicity. *Radiology* 1997;204:297–312.

Lee F, Torp-Pedersen ST, Siders DD, et al. Transrectal ultrasound in the diagnosis and staging of prostatic carcinoma. *Radiology* 1989;170:609–615.

Melchior SW, Brawer MK. Role of transrectal ultrasound and prostate biopsy. *J Clin Ultrasound* 1996;24:463–471.

Rothpearl A, Frager D, Subramanian A, et al. MR urography: technique and application. *Radiology* 1995;194:125–130.

Sung JC, Kabalin JN, Terris MK. Prostate cancer detection, characterization, and clinical outcomes in men aged 70 years and older referred for transrectal ultrasound and prostate biopsies. *Urology* 2000;56:295–301.

Wefer AE, Wefer J, Frericks B, et al. Advances in uroradiological imaging. *Br J Urol Int* 2002;89:477–487.

Zagoria RJ, Bechtold RE, Dyer RB, et al. Staging of renal adenocarcinoma: role of various imaging procedures. *AJR Am J Roentgenol* 1995;164:363–370.

Radionuclide Imaging

Rachel A. Powsner and Dean J. Rodman

Nuclear imaging of the genitourinary tract has the advantage of being essentially noninvasive, providing physiologic as well as anatomic information and subjecting the patient to minimal radiation exposure. Allergic reactions are virtually unknown following the injection of radiopharmaceuticals. The ability to provide functional and quantitative information is fundamentally unique to nuclear imaging and can be extremely useful in the assessment of renal function, renal blood flow, and obstructive uropathy.

I. Renal imaging
A. Evaluation of flow and function

1. **Radiopharmaceuticals** are composed of a radioisotope bound to a carrier with physiologic properties. The radioisotope used in renal imaging is metastable technetium-99 (^{99m}Tc), which is a readily available, low-cost isotope that is extracted from a molybdenum-99 generator. Radiopharmaceuticals based on ^{99m}Tc that are used to assess flow and function are as follows:

   a. **^{99m}Tc-DTPA** (^{99m}Tc-diethylenetriaminepentaacetic acid) is handled primarily by glomerular filtration (80%), and the remainder is subject to tubular secretion.

   b. **^{99m}Tc-MAG3** (^{99m}Tc-mercaptoacetyltriglycine) is handled by tubular secretion (approximately 90%). As a result, it has a higher rate of extraction than DTPA.

   c. **^{99m}Tc-Glucoheptonate** is handled by a combination of glomerular filtration and tubular secretion (approximately 40% is excreted within 1 hour) and peritubular cell deposition (12% of the dose is present in the kidneys at 1 hour).

2. **Imaging and analysis.** After injection of any of the above radiopharmaceuticals, sequential images (frames) are obtained every 1 to 2 seconds for 60 seconds, then every 10 to 60 seconds for 20 to 30 minutes. These digital images are compressed into longer frames for interpretation (Fig. 3.1). Images from the first minute reflect renal blood flow; images from the subsequent 30 minutes reflect parenchymal and excretory function. Counts derived from these images are plotted over time; the plot is called a renogram. The renogram is commonly divided into three phases (Fig. 3.2A):

   a. **Phase I:** evaluation of renal blood flow. The plot of the first minute of data reflects renal blood flow (Fig. 3.2B,C). The aortic flow is plotted as well. Attention is given to the time delay between peak counts in the aorta and peak counts in the kidney; this value should be ≤6 seconds. Because of rapid extraction, the ^{99m}Tc-MAG3 flow curve does not have a clearly defined peak, but rather an inflection point (Fig. 3.2C).

   b. **Phase II:** parenchymal function (extraction and transit of nuclide). After the initial flow of nuclide into the kidney,

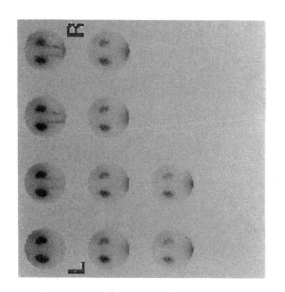

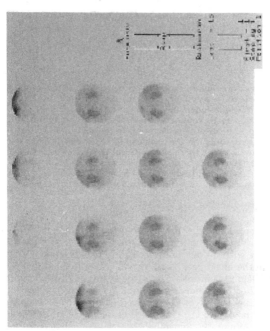

Fig. 3.1. Normal ^{99m}Tc-MAG3 (^{99m}Tc-mercaptoacetyltriglycine) study. Left: Flow images (4 s/frame) obtained for the first 60 seconds following injection. Right: The subsequent 30 minutes of information displayed in sequential 3-minute frames.

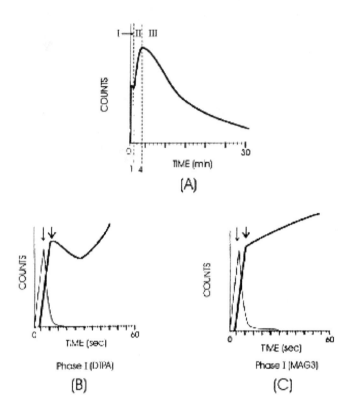

Fig. 3.2.   Normal renogram. A: A plot of counts in the kidney over 31 minutes. The three phases (I, II, III) are marked. B: Phase I 99mTc-DTPA (99mTc-diethylenetriaminepentaacetic acid) blood flow curve. Renal and aortic counts for the first minute are plotted. The thinner arrow indicates the peak counts in the aortic curve, and the thicker arrow indicates the peak counts in the renal curve. The time difference between these peaks should be 6 seconds. C: Phase I 99mTc-MAG3 (99mTc-mercaptoacetyltriglycine) blood flow curve. Because of the more rapid extraction of 99mTc-MAG3 from the blood pool, there is no clear peak in this curve, only an inflection point (*arrow*).

renal uptake depends on parenchymal function. In a normally functioning kidney, counts will at first steadily increase within the kidney secondary to extraction of nuclide from the blood pool. Nuclide will traverse the parenchyma and begin to enter the collecting system. Within 5 minutes, excretion of nuclide into the renal collecting system will exceed the uptake of nuclide from the steadily diminishing blood pool, and the curve will enter phase III down-slope. Peak uptake (the time of reversal of up-slope to down-slope) on a normal renogram should occur within 5 minutes after injection.

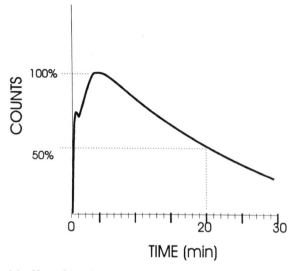

Fig. 3.3. Normal 30-minute 99mTc-DTPA (99mTc-diethylenetri-
aminepentaacetic acid) renogram, demonstrating 50% excretion in
20 minutes.

c. **Phase III:** excretion. This phase in the normal kidney
is characterized by a rapid component of emptying (when
the concentration of radiopharmaceutical in the parenchymal and blood pool is relatively greater), followed by a more
gradual down-slope as the supply of nuclide available for
excretion decreases. A normal DTPA renogram will demonstrate 50% emptying of nuclide from the kidney within
20 minutes (Fig. 3.3).
B. **Evaluation of focal and relative renal function with
cortical agents**
1. Substances that are taken up and retained within the
renal tubular cells may be used for static renal imaging, to
evaluate relative renal function and function of renal masses.
Typical agents available for this use are as follows:
a. During the first 30 minutes, **99mTc-glucoheptonate** is
used as a flow and function agent, as described above. After
excretion is complete at 1 hour, 12% of the injected dose is
retained in the tubular cells.
b. **99mTc-DMSA** (99mTc-dimercaptosuccinic acid) is commonly used for evaluation of renal morphology. It is
extracted from the peritubular extracellular fluid and de-
posited in the tubular cells; 50% of the injected dose is
present in the kidneys at 1 hour.
2. **Acquisition and analysis.** Patients receive an intravenous injection of one of the above nuclides. Images of renal
parenchymal retention are obtained after excretion of the
agent is mostly complete. Images following the administration
of glucoheptonate are obtained 1 to 2 hours after injection,

whereas ^{99m}Tc-DMSA images are obtained 3 to 4 hours after injection. Normal ^{99m}Tc-DMSA images are shown in Fig. 3.4.

C. Imaging of renal infection. Agents used specifically to image infectious or inflammatory processes include the following:

1. **White blood cells labeled with ^{111}In.** Indium-111 is a moderately expensive radionuclide produced by cyclotron. A very careful technique is used to separate white blood cells from a 30- to 60-mL aliquot of whole blood drawn from the patient with a 16-gauge needle. These white blood cells are labeled with ^{111}In, resuspended in the patient's plasma, and reinjected into the patient through another large-bore access. Imaging is performed 24 hours later. The white cells retain their function and localize at sites of infection. White blood cells labeled with ^{99m}Tc are not recommended for imaging the genitourinary system, as the ^{99m}Tc that dissociates is excreted through the renal system.

2. **[^{67}Ga]Gallium citrate.** Gallium-67 is produced by cyclotron. It is an iron analog and attaches to serum proteins including lactoferrin and ferritin. It localizes at sites of infection and inflammation (e.g., interstitial nephritis) and in a limited number of tumor types. ^{67}Ga is normally seen in renal parenchyma up to 72 hours after injection. After this time, accumulation is abnormal and suggestive of infection, inflammation, or certain tumors.

3. **^{99m}Tc-DMSA** is currently recommended as the agent of choice for diagnosis and follow-up of pyelonephritis (see below).

D. Clinical applications

1. **Vascular abnormalities**

    a. **Renal arterial embolus.** Nonvisualization of a kidney on the flow scan is consistent with renal arterial embolus. Segmental embolus presents on scintigraphic study as a regional peripheral perfusion defect (Fig. 3.5).

    b. **Renal arterial stenosis.** The renal flow scan by itself is relatively insensitive to arterial stenosis. Standard evaluation involves the comparison of renal function following the administration of an angiotensin-converting enzyme inhibitor such as captopril with baseline renal function (Fig. 3.6). This technique is very sensitive for the detection of clinically significant stenoses (>65%). After the administration of an angiotensin-converting enzyme inhibitor, the postglomerular compensatory efferent arteriole stenosis will dilate. The subsequent drop in the glomerular filtration pressure will be seen as a prolonged phase II of the renogram during a ^{99m}Tc-MAG3 study and as reduced accumulation in phase II of a renogram performed with ^{99m}Tc-DTPA. This test is less useful with poorly functioning kidneys.

    c. **Renal vein thrombosis.** Although renal vein thrombosis is generally characterized as reduced perfusion and delayed accumulation, nuclear imaging is not the procedure of choice for this entity.

2. **Parenchymal abnormalities**

    a. **Malformations and anatomic variants.** Static imaging of the kidneys with ^{99m}Tc-DMSA or ^{99m}Tc-glucoheptonate

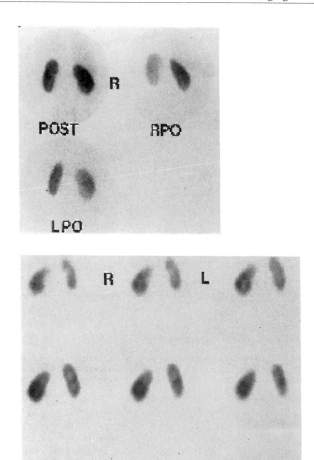

Fig. 3.4.   Normal 99mTc-DMSA (99mTc-dimercaptosuccinic acid) images. The upper images are planar posterior, left posterior oblique, and right posterior oblique. The lower images are coronal tomographic views of the same kidney.

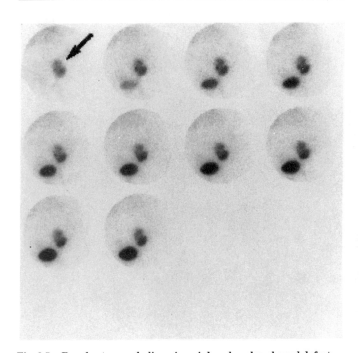

Fig. 3.5. Renal artery embolism. A peripheral wedge-shaped defect consistent with an infarct following embolism (*arrow*) is shown on this 99mTc-MAG3 (99mTc-mercaptoacetyltriglycine) transplant scan.

is an excellent means of determining the size and configuration of functioning renal parenchyma. Polycystic kidneys usually demonstrate multiple bilateral photopenic defects ("cold spots"). Normal renal tissue in aberrant locations (horseshoe kidney, fetal location, hypertrophied column of Bertin) may also be defined by this method. Size and position of even the most atrophic and ectopic renal parenchyma may be assessed if there is a significant amount of functioning tubular mass. With renal duplication, ^{99m}Tc-DMSA or ^{99m}Tc-DTPA scintigraphy can assess regional parenchymal function before corrective surgery. Before nephrectomy, relative renal function can be assessed in the same manner (split function renography).

b. Transplant evaluation: acute tubular necrosis versus rejection. Many transplanted kidneys demonstrate some evidence of acute tubular necrosis postoperatively. Renal scanning with ^{99m}Tc-DTPA demonstrates normal renal perfusion but little or no accumulation or excretion of the tracer. Renal scanning with ^{99m}Tc-MAG3 demonstrates normal renal perfusion and steadily increasing counts in the kidney with reduced excretion. Generally, one can expect gradual improvement in cases of acute tubular necrosis within about 3 weeks (Fig. 3.7), but reso-

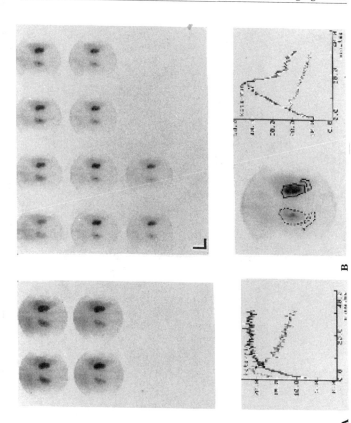

Fig. 3.6.   Renal captopril study. A: Thirty-minute
99mTc-MAG3 (99mTc-mercaptoacetyltriglycine)
functional images (the left kidney is on the left,
the right kidney on the right) and a renogram of
both kidneys following captopril ingestion. The
images and renogram curve for the right kidney
(*darker curve*) demonstrate steadily increasing
counts in the kidney. B: Baseline images and
curves obtained without captopril. The function
of the right kidney is improved because of
restoration of the compensatory efferent arteriolar stenosis.

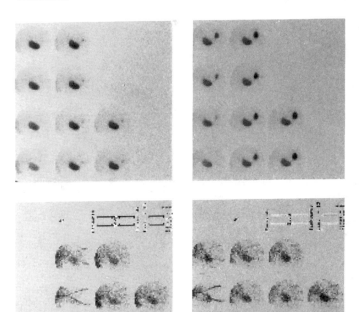

Fig. 3.7.   Resolving acute tubular necrosis. Top left: One day after transplant, the first minute of blood flow is normal. Top right: One day after transplant, the subsequent 30 minutes of imaging demonstrates reduced extraction, clearance, and excretion of nuclide, consistent with acute tubular necrosis. Bottom left and right: Three days later, flow images are still normal, and extraction, clearance, and excretion of nuclide are improved, consistent with resolving acute tubular necrosis.

lution may take several months. Acute rejection is characterized by markedly decreased renal perfusion on scanning with both ^{99m}Tc-DTPA and ^{99m}Tc-MAG3. This is one of the earliest signs of rejection, and it can occur as early as 48 hours before clinical symptoms become apparent. In contrast to the images in acute tubular necrosis, images of parenchymal function are relatively better than the perfusion images. Rejection and acute tubular necrosis may occur simultaneously, however, and differentiation may not be possible. For this reason, many surgeons advocate baseline renal scans at 24 to 48 hours after transplantation, which can be compared with subsequent studies (Fig. 3.8). Cyclosporin A toxicity, particularly in the clinical setting of an ischemic cadaveric renal transplant, can yield images that are indistinguishable from acute rejection.

c.   Acute glomerulonephritis. Scintigraphy has no significant role in the diagnosis or management of this entity.

d.   Acute interstitial nephritis. A characteristic pattern of intensely increased uptake of ^{67}Ga persists >72 hours after injection (Fig. 3.9).

e.   Pyelonephritis. ^{99m}Tc-DMSA is advocated for the diagnosis, assessment, and management of acute pyelonephritis. Photopenic defects indicative of pyelonephritis can be unifocal or multifocal. Defects representing acute infection will resolve on follow-up studies, whereas persistent defects are consistent with permanent scarring (Fig. 3.10). [^{67}Ga]Gallium citrate can be used to diagnose pyelonephritis, but the agent can be visualized for up to 72 hours in the normal kidney, so diagnosis can be delayed. Although white blood cells labeled with ^{111}In are specific for infection, the procedure is relatively more time consuming and costly than a ^{99m}Tc-DMSA study.

3. Postrenal abnormalities

a.   Hydronephrosis and obstruction. Differentiation of obstructive from nonobstructive hydronephrosis may be achieved by furosemide renal scanning. Administration of intravenous furosemide (10 to 40 mg) in the hydronephrotic, nonobstructed kidney initiates a diuresis that clears activity from the kidney and pyelocalyceal system. A normal response to furosemide is characterized by 50% emptying of the kidney and pelvis by 20 minutes after injection (Fig. 3.11). In instances of collecting system obstruction, the tracer activity in the renal pelvis fails to clear or even accumulates further. An indeterminate result (some emptying, but <50% in 20 minutes) will occur in approximately 15% of all cases and is caused by the following:

(1)   Blunting of diuresis by markedly depressed renal function.

(2)   Masking of tracer clearance by grossly distended renal pelvis and ureter.

(3)   Confusion caused by the presence of vesicoureteral reflux, which can be prevented by catheterization of the bladder.

(4)   Marked bladder distention that may result in poor emptying of the upper tracts; it is wise to have the patient void before the study is begun. Occasionally, retention of

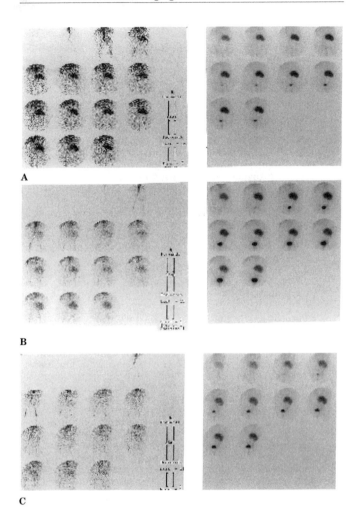

A

B

C

Fig. 3.8.   Transplant rejection. A and B, top left and right: One day
following transplant. The 1-minute blood flow images are relatively
normal, and the 30-minute images demonstrate moderately reduced
function. At this stage, the diagnosis could be acute tubular necrosis
or rejection. A and B, bottom left and right: Sixteen days after transplant, the kidney is not as well seen on flow images, but the functional images demonstrate improved extraction and excretion of
nuclide. C: Twenty-one days following transplant of the same kidney,
there is poor visualization of the kidney on blood flow images and
only mild degradation of function. This is a characteristic pattern
for rejection.

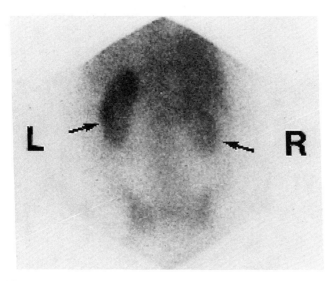

Fig. 3.9. Interstitial nephritis. Intensely increased uptake is seen in the left kidney and moderately increased uptake is seen in the right kidney.

tracer may occur only after furosemide administration, which indicates functional obstruction at high rates of urine flow.

b. Urinary leakage is diagnosed with greater sensitivity by nuclear imaging than by contrast radiography. Depending on the site of the leak, extravasation can be loculated or dispersed throughout the peritoneal cavity (Fig. 3.12). In posttransplant patients, extravasation is generally seen as an area of increased activity in the region of the vesicoureteral anastomosis. When extravasation is suspected but not visualized initially, it is helpful to obtain delayed images before and after emptying of the bladder. A urinoma may present as a photon-deficient area if it represents urine that has accumulated before the injection of the radionuclide tracer.

c. Ureteral reflux studies. Radionuclide cystography (RNC) permits continuous monitoring of the dynamics of bladder filling and emptying. It is more sensitive than radiographic cystography, especially for low-grade reflux. A small dose of tracer, most commonly [99mTc]pertechnetate, is introduced into the bladder through a transurethral catheter. Sequential posterior imaging of the bladder, ureters, and kidneys is performed at 5-second intervals during bladder filling and at 2-second intervals during voiding. Vesicoureteral reflux is easily detected and graded (Fig. 3.13), and bladder volume can readily be calculated. It is recommended that a conventional contrast voiding cystourethrogram (VCUG) be performed as the first study on each

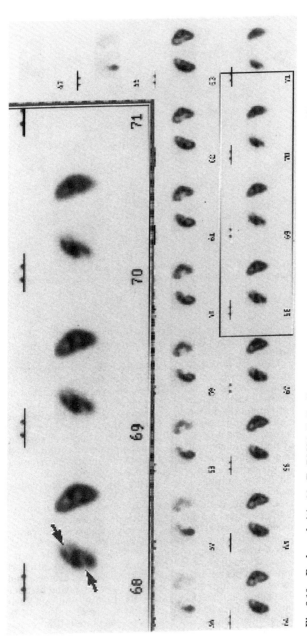

Fig. 3.10. Pyelonephritis: 99mTc-DMSA (⁹⁹ᵐTc-dimercaptosuccinic acid) study. Coronal views from a tomographic study with magnification of select views demonstrate cortical defects (*arrows*) in the right kidney, consistent with known acute pyelonephritis.

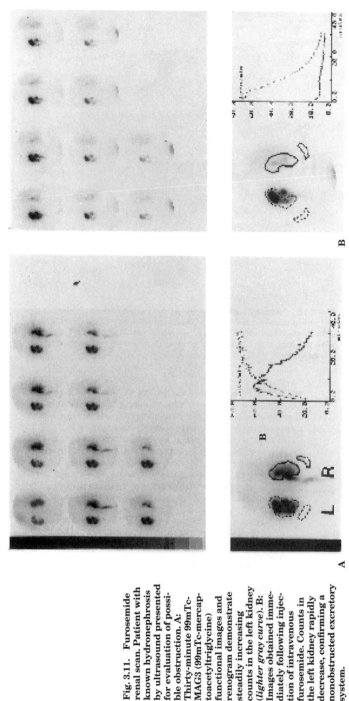

Fig. 3.11. Furosemide renal scan. Patient with known hydronephrosis presented by ultrasound for evaluation of possible obstruction. A: Thirty-minute 99mTc-MAG3 (99mTc-mercaptoacetyltriglycine) functional images and renogram demonstrate steadily increasing counts in the left kidney (*lighter gray curve*). B: Images obtained immediately following injection of intravenous furosemide. Counts in the left kidney rapidly decrease, confirming a nonobstructed excretory system.

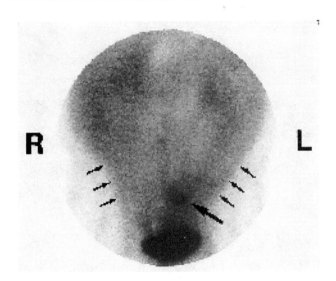

Fig. 3.12. Urinary leakage: postoperative peritoneal urinary ascites following ureteral tear. Throughout the abdomen, 99mTc-MAG3 (99mTc-mercaptoacetyltriglycine) is seen diffusely (*small arrows*), with pooling at the site of the obstructed damaged ureter (*large arrow*).

patient to obtain anatomic information. RNC is then used for subsequent studies and for the screening of siblings. This is because the radiation dose from an RNC study is one-thousandth of the dose from a VCUG study.

d.   Testicular imaging. Testicular scanning is used primarily to differentiate acute testicular torsion from other causes of acute scrotal pain such as acute epididymitis. This distinction is important because acute testicular torsion mandates immediate surgical intervention. The testicle can rarely be saved if surgery is delayed >6 hours after onset of ischemia.

(1)   Technique. Following the intravenous bolus injection of [99mTc]pertechnetate, serial images of the testicles are obtained at 1-second intervals for the first minute as an assessment of testicular blood flow. Static images of the scrotum are obtained immediately following the blood flow images.

(2)   Clinical application. Normally, flow to the testes is equal bilaterally (Fig. 3.14). In acute testicular torsion, the delayed perfusion images show decreased activity over the affected testis (Fig. 3.15). Delayed torsion will demonstrate an intense halo of activity around the infarcted testis (Fig. 3.16). In epididymitis (and/or orchitis), increased perfusion through the spermatic cord vessels is noted, as it is in other inflammatory processes involving the testicle, and increased activity is noted on the involved side (Fig. 3.17). Radionuclide scanning of the scro-

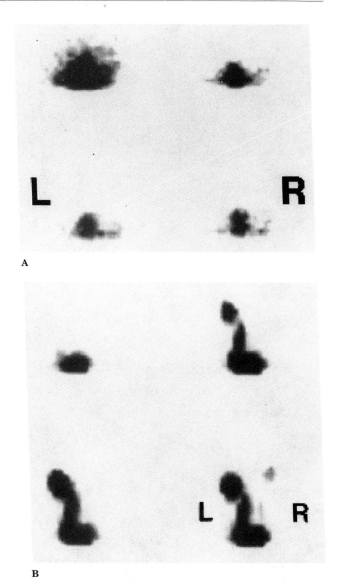

Fig. 3.13.   A: Normal radionuclide cystography: posterior projection.
The lower right image was taken after voiding. B: Vesicoureteral
reflux. Posterior views demonstrate grade III reflux on the left and
grade II reflux on the right. (Courtesy of Dr. Elizabeth Oates,
New England Medical Center, Boston, MA.)

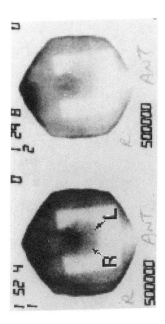

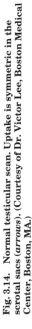

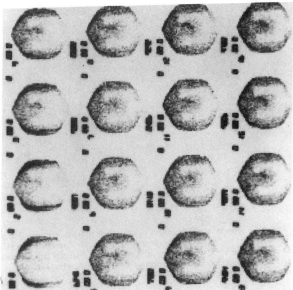

Fig. 3.14.   Normal testicular scan. Uptake is symmetric in the scrotal sacs (*arrows*). (Courtesy of Dr. Victor Lee, Boston Medical Center, Boston, MA.)

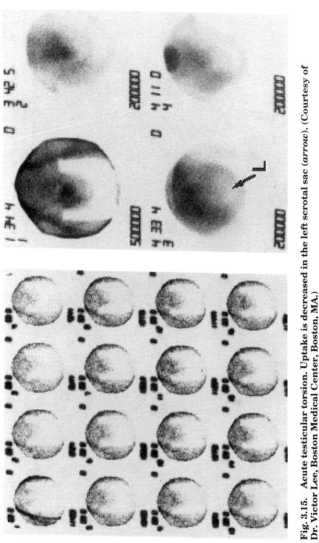

Fig. 3.15. Acute testicular torsion. Uptake is decreased in the left scrotal sac (*arrow*). (Courtesy of Dr. Victor Lee, Boston Medical Center, Boston, MA.)

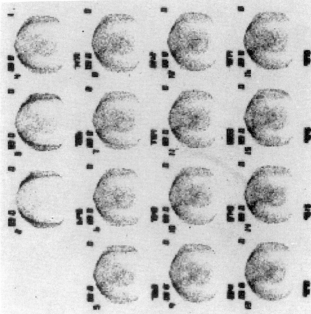

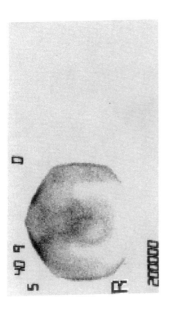

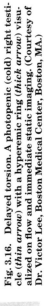

Fig. 3.16.   Delayed torsion. A photopenic (cold) right testicle (*thin arrow*) with a hyperemic ring (*thick arrow*) visualized on flow and immediate static imaging. (Courtesy of Dr. Victor Lee, Boston Medical Center, Boston, MA.)

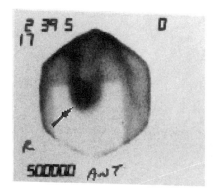

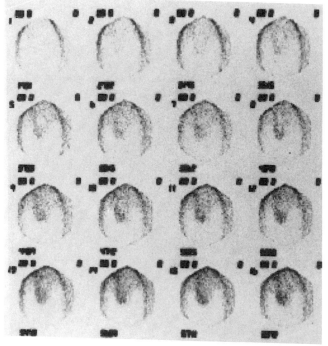

Fig. 3.17.   Epididymitis. Increased flows and immediate uptake in right scrotal sac. (Courtesy of Dr. Victor Lee, Boston Medical Center, Boston, MA.)

tum in trauma, hydrocele, spermatocele, varicocele, testicular tumors, and abscesses produces results of varying specificity and does not have a prominent clinical role at this time.

SUGGESTED READING

Brown ED, Chen MYM, Wolfman NT, et al. Complications of renal transplantation: evaluation with US and radionuclide imaging. *Radiographics* 2000;20:607–622.

Fine EJ. Diuretic renography and angiotensin converting enzyme inhibitor renography. *Radiol Clin North Am* 2001;39:979–995.

Nally JV, Barton DP. Contemporary approach to diagnosis and evaluation of renovascular hypertension. *Urol Clin North Am* 2001;28: 781–791.

Sfakianakis GN, Sfakianaki E. Renal scintigraphy in infants and children. *Urology* 2001;57:1167–1177.

Evaluation of Renal Mass Lesions

Juan P. Litvak and Robert D. Oates

The increased availability of computed tomography (CT) and ultrasonography (US) has dramatically affected the clinical presentation of renal masses. Incidentally found renal masses accounted for 61% of all renal tumors in 1998. Thus, the urologist must now evaluate and manage small renal masses that would otherwise have been undetected. The incidentally detected renal cell carcinoma (RCC) tends to be smaller in size and have lower grade and stage than symptomatic masses.

Many classifications of renal tumors exist, including those based on histologic origin, pathology (benign versus malignant), and radiologic appearance (cystic versus solid). Given the frequency with which renal masses are now diagnosed as incidental findings on radiologic studies, we chose to classify renal masses based on radiologic appearance. We first divide tumors as either solid or cystic and then further categorize between benign or malignant (Table 4.1).

I. Solid renal masses
A. Benign lesions
1. **Angiomyolipoma** (AML) is a rare parenchymal renal mass that accounts for <0.5% of all renal tumors. Histologically, it is composed of angiomatous, adipose, and smooth muscle elements. The adipose tissue component is variable but can constitute up to 80% of the tumor bulk. Approximately 20% of patients with AMLs have **tuberous sclerosis** (TS), an autosomal dominant disease characterized by epilepsy, mental retardation, adenoma sebaceum, retinal phakomas, and hamartomas of the kidneys, brain, and other viscera. However, only 50% of patients with TS develop AMLs. While AMLs associated with TS are more common in men, sporadic cases are more common in women.

   a. **Clinical features and diagnosis.** In patients with TS, AMLs are more likely to be bilateral, multifocal, and large, while in the sporadic form, lesions tend to be unilateral, unifocal, and small. Although thought to be uniformly benign, retroperitoneal lymph nodes, liver, and spleen have been noted to have AMLs identical to the primary renal tumor. However, these have been considered to represent multifocality rather than metastases. Fifty percent of AMLs are discovered incidentally on radiographic studies. However, presentation with clinical symptoms is not uncommon and occurs most frequently in patients with TS. Common presenting symptoms include flank pain or fullness, palpable mass, and hematuria. Hypertension and anemia are also common symptoms. Pain from AML is usually associated with spontaneous hemorrhage into the tumor. Extreme

Table 4.1.   Renal mass lesions

Solid renal masses
  Benign lesions
    Angiomyolipoma
    Oncocytoma
    Xanthogranulomatous pyelonephritis
    Benign mesenchymal tumors
  Malignant lesions
    Renal adenocarcinoma
    Sarcoma
    Metastatic lesions
    Lymphoma/leukemia

Cystic renal masses
  Benign lesions
    Simple cyst
    Multilocular cystic nephroma
    Calyceal diverticulum
  Malignant lesions
    Cystadenocarcinoma
    Cystic necrosis of renal carcinoma
    Renal carcinoma arising in simple cyst

cases of massive retroperitoneal hemorrhage are rare and are referred to as **Wunderlich's syndrome.**

b.   Radiologic diagnosis is often helpful and definitive in AML. The presence of fat within the tumor allows for distinction from other tumors by CT scan, US, and magnetic resonance imaging (MRI). CT is currently the most accurate means of diagnosing AMLs. The large amount of fat within an AML produces areas of low radiographic density characterized by a negative CT attenuation coefficient as measured in Hounsfield units. A Hounsfield unit value of <10 is considered diagnostic of AML. False-negative results of CT may occur if nonadipose tissue or denser, "immature" adipose tissue elements predominate. AMLs are the most echogenic tumors seen on renal US. This is a result of the fat–nonfat interfaces seen throughout the tumor. In addition, shadowing is a common finding seen with AMLs that can help distinguish them from RCC, which tend not to shadow. Intravenous urogram (IVU) will show unilateral or bilateral space-occupying lesions, occasionally distorting the collecting system. Renal arteriography yields a characteristic "onion peel" appearance, although the test cannot reliably distinguish AML from renal adenocarcinoma. In both, there may be a hypervascular mass, tortuous vessels, microaneurysms, and arteriovenous fistulas. T1-weighted MRI will show high signal intensity because of the adipose tissue within the tumor.

c.   Treatment of AML is dependent on lesion size and symptomatology. Tumors <4 cm in diameter are less likely to be either symptomatic or associated with hemorrhage or other complications. The risk of life-threatening hemorrhage is much greater in tumors larger than 4 cm. Based on these patterns, the general recommendation for asymptomatic AMLs <4 cm is observation with either serial US or CT scans every 6 to 12 months. Tumors that are larger than 4 cm should be considered for intervention with either nephron-sparing surgery or selective angioembolization. However, in considering management options, one must consider concomitant factors such as age, comorbidities, and renal function. It should also be considered that patients with TS tend to have bilateral disease and tumors that tend to grow at a faster rate. Patients with significant acute hemorrhage should be explored and usually require total nephrectomy.

2. Renal oncocytoma is an epithelial neoplasm that originates from the intercalated cells of the collecting duct. It accounts for approximately 3% to 7% of all solid renal masses. On gross appearance, the tumor is tan or light brown and is well circumscribed with a pseudocapsule. A central scar is commonly seen on gross examination. Histologically, the cells are characterized by uniformity in size and color, a round to polygonal shape, and finely granular eosinophilic cytoplasm (oncocytes). Ultrastructural analysis demonstrates an overwhelming abundance of mitochondria within each cell, which cause the granular appearance microscopically. Genetic alterations that are commonly seen are deletion of chromosome 1 or the sex chromosome and translocation at 11q13. Up to 12% of oncocytomas are multifocal or bilateral. Multifocal renal oncocytomas can be seen in patients with familial renal oncocytoma and the **Birt–Hogg–Dube syndrome.**

    a. Clinical diagnosis. Nearly 80% of renal oncocytomas are asymptomatic and found incidentally. Symptoms resulting from oncocytoma are not different from those caused by RCC and include hematuria, palpable mass, and flank and/or abdominal pain. It is not possible to conclusively differentiate oncocytoma from RCC by clinical diagnosis. Renal biopsy is often not diagnostic because of the inability to reliably differentiate between RCC and the possibility of the concomitant presence of oncocytoma and RCC within the same tumor.

    b. Radiologic diagnosis. Although there are radiologic signs that are suggestive of oncocytoma, it is not possible to firmly differentiate oncocytoma from RCC by radiologic modalities. Angiographically, a "spoke wheel" pattern in which vessels radiate toward the center of the tumor is suggestive of oncocytoma. CT of large oncocytomas may demonstrate an area of low attenuation that can represent the central scar.

    c. Treatment for renal oncocytoma is guided by the fact that oncocytoma cannot be distinguished preoperatively from RCC. Therefore, surgical management follows that of a putative RCC and is dependent on the size and location of the tumor.

3. Xanthogranulomatous pyelonephritis (XGP) is an atypical chronic bacterial pyelonephritis that can mimic renal carcinoma radiographically. Microscopically, lipid-laden macrophages are the predominant cell in this reactive tissue lesion. In 50% to 80% of instances, obstructing renal or ureteral calculi are found. Positive urine cultures for *Escherichia coli* (40%) and *Proteus mirabilis* (29%) are present in up to 70% of patients. *Klebsiella, Pseudomonas,* and *Bacteroides* may also be implicated. The disease not infrequently is also associated with diabetes mellitus and previous urologic surgery. Women, typically middle aged, are affected three times as frequently as men. Infection proximal to an obstructing calculus presumably stimulates this bizarre inflammatory process. Grossly, diffuse replacement of the entire kidney by lobulated yellow masses occurs, although only focal involvement is found in 17% of instances. Occasionally, XGP penetrates Gerota's fascia into the perinephric space.

   a. Diagnosis. It should be noted that patients with XGP may have constitutional symptoms such as weight loss and anorexia. A syndrome of liver dysfunction may occur in XGP as well as in renal adenocarcinoma. The differential diagnosis rests on the presence of irritative symptoms of the lower tract, leukocytosis, pyuria, and infection in XGP. IVU demonstrates a poorly functioning or nonfunctioning kidney with hydronephrosis in 75% of patients and calculi in 50% to 80%. Focal lesions may show calyceal distortion only. US shows diffusely enlarged kidneys with obstruction of the collecting system; calculi and purulent collections may be imaged as well. CT with contrast demonstrates an enlarged, nonfunctioning, hydronephrotic kidney with stones and sometimes abscess cavities. Areas of lipid concentration may manifest as a negative attenuation coefficient. The extent of local perinephric extension can be assessed by CT. Angiographically, XGP may mimic many of the features of renal adenocarcinoma, including neovascularity and vessel encasement.

   b. Treatment in instances of diffuse involvement requires nephrectomy with excision of any perinephric tissue involved by XGP. Focal disease may be successfully treated by partial nephrectomy in selected patients. Recently, there have been reports of focal XGP being successfully treated nonoperatively.

   4. Benign mesenchymal tumors, including fibromas, lipomas, leiomyomas, and hemangiomas, are extremely rare and usually asymptomatic. Treatment is usually the same as that for renal adenocarcinoma because the diagnosis is unknown preoperatively. Another rarely reported tumor is the **juxtaglomerular tumor,** which is considered benign but causes hypertension as a result of renin secretion.

B. Malignant lesions

   1. RCC, also known as renal adenocarcinoma, accounts for approximately 3% of all malignancies in the United States (Fig. 4.1). The incidence has greatly increased over the last several decades, most certainly owing to the widespread use of imaging modalities such as abdominal US and CT. This has led to early diagnosis of smaller tumors, or "incidentalomas," which may otherwise have been undiagnosed. However, it is

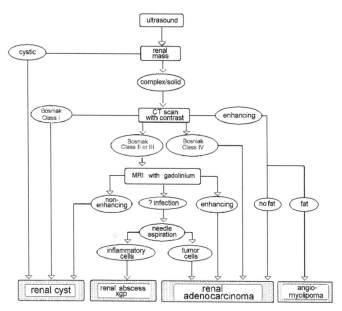

Fig. 4.1. Diagnostic decision tree for evaluation of a renal mass. For masses found to be solid on ultrasonography, computed tomography is indicated for evaluation of metastatic disease but not necessarily for diagnosis. Other possibilities not shown in the diagram should be considered, including transitional cell carcinoma, metastatic lesions to the kidney, and retroperitoneal and adrenal tumors.

also important to note that the number of advanced cases has also increased. Currently, there are approximately 30,000 new cases diagnosed per year in the United States. The incidence is thought to be >100% increased since 1950. The peak incidence is in the fifth to sixth decades of life, although the tumor is known to occur rarely in children and adolescents.

The **etiology** of RCC is unclear. Although many agents have been implicated as a putative cause, only tobacco has been shown to cause an increase in the relative risk. **Von Hippel–Lindau disease** is an autosomal dominant disorder that is strongly associated with RCC. In addition to renal tumors, other manifestations of the disease include cerebellar hemangioblastomas, retinal angiomas, renal cysts, pheochromocytomas, pancreatic cysts, and epididymal cystadenomas. The Von Hippel–Lindau gene (*VHL*) is a known tumor suppressor gene. In families afflicted with this disorder, gene analysis has shown loss of heterozygosity at 3p25-26, the site of the *VHL* gene. In the sporadic form of RCC, tumor cells may demonstrate an allelic loss at the 3p12-14 chromosome. RCC in VHL is more likely to be bilateral and multifocal and presents earlier in life. More recently, a second hereditary form of RCC, the hereditary papillary RCC, has been described. This is also an autosomal dominant disease, and the gene has been localized to chromosome 7.

Histologically, RCCs arise from renal tubular epithelium. The most common subtypes are clear cell and tubulopapillary, which account for 70% and 10%, respectively. Clear cell tumors are the most common form in sporadic RCC, and this is also the form associated with Von Hippel–Lindau disease. They are usually hypervascular. Tubulopapillary tumors are often hypovascular and are more likely to be multicentric. Less common subtypes of RCC are chromophobe, collecting duct, and renal medullary. Chromophobe accounts for approximately 5% of RCCs, and the collecting duct and renal medullary subtypes are quite rare. The renal medullary subtype is almost exclusively associated with African Americans with sickle cell trait or disease and carries an ominous diagnosis with survival measured in weeks. Previously, it was believed that there was a sarcomatoid subtype, which is now recognized as a poorly differentiated region of other tumor subtypes.

   a.   **Clinical diagnosis.** More than 60% of tumors are now discovered incidentally by noninvasive radiologic imaging. Therefore, the "classic triad" of hematuria, flank pain, and abdominal mass is now a rare finding, occurring in <5% of cases (Fig. 4.2). Hematuria remains a common presenting

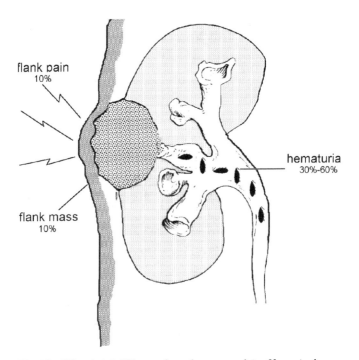

Fig. 4.2. "Classic triad" in renal carcinoma consists of hematuria, flank pain, and flank mass.

symptom and occurs in 30% to 60% of cases, depending on the series (Fig. 4.2). RCC has been described as the "internist's tumor" owing to the frequency of nonspecific symptoms such as anemia as well as associated paraneoplastic syndromes. Hypercalcemia, the most common paraneoplastic syndrome, can occur in up to 15% of patients and is caused by tumor secretion of parathyroid hormone. Tumor production of renin and polycythemia can lead to hypertension or polycythemia.

b. Radiologic diagnosis

(1)   CT scan is currently the most accurate and efficient means of diagnosing renal masses. Images obtained before and after administration of intravenous contrast medium can delineate solid enhancing renal lesions that are highly suggestive of malignant renal tumors. Cystic RCC, discussed later in this chapter, can be graded using the Bosniak classification system to predict likelihood of malignancy. Based on this system, radiologic factors such as contrast enhancement, presence of septations, and appearance of the cyst wall can aid in predicting the likelihood of malignancy. CT scan also provides valuable information for clinical staging of renal tumors. Local extension, intraabdominal metastasis, and tumor thrombi in the renal vein or vena cava can be identified. CT angiogram can also be used to delineate renal vascular anatomy when the possibility of partial nephrectomy is entertained in the treatment of RCC.

(2)   MRI may also be used to diagnose and stage RCC. Patients who have contraindications to contrast-enhanced CT, such as patients with renal insufficiency or contrast sensitivity, are good candidates for this modality. MRI may also be helpful in evaluating complex cysts and abscesses as well as to assess the extent of local tumor involvement. Currently, it is also considered the best means to evaluate involvement of the vena cava or renal vein by tumor thrombi.

(3)   US has come to play an important role in diagnosis of lesions by virtue of its safety, accuracy, and relatively low cost. Renal US can determine whether a mass is solid or cystic, the patency of the renal vein and inferior vena cava, and the presence of enlarged retroperitoneal lymph nodes. US is also useful as an imaging modality for fine-needle aspiration (FNA) of cystic renal lesions.

(4)   Angiography. Since the advent of CT, the use of arteriography has become quite limited in RCC. Classic findings with arteriography in RCC include hypervascularity, microaneurysms, arteriovenous shunting, and venous pooling of contrast agent within the tumor.

(5)   Renal biopsy or FNA. Three-dimensional imaging with CT or MRI has greatly reduced the utility of biopsy or FNA. The high likelihood of malignancy with solid masses identified by CT or MRI, along with the inherent risk of sampling error by biopsy or FNA, have limited the usefulness of this modality. Patients with suspected metastatic disease to the kidney or lymphoma may be candidates for biopsy or FNA. In addition, FNA may aid in diagnosing renal abscess by identifying the presence of inflammatory cells.

c.   Treatment is based on stage, size, and location of the tumor in the kidney. The medical condition of the patient is also an important factor. Although treatment options are evolving in RCC, radical nephrectomy remains the treatment of choice in patients with adequate renal function in the remaining kidney. Historically, radical nephrectomy included excision of Gerota's fascia and the ipsilateral adrenal gland and an extensive regional lymph node dissection. However, with the ability of CT and MRI to detect adrenal pathology with nearly 100% sensitivity, the adrenal can be spared in the majority of patients. The need for a regional lymphadenectomy remains a controversial topic. Removing the perinephric fat with the tumor remains a surgical goal.

In selected patients, partial nephrectomy is a viable treatment option. Initially, it was recommended only in patients with solitary kidney, bilateral tumors, or renal medical disease. However, recent literature suggests that in patients with normal contralateral kidneys and small tumors <4 cm, survival and recurrence data are similar to those for radical nephrectomy. In patients with Von Hippel–Lindau disease, the mainstay of treatment is partial nephrectomy due to the high rate of contralateral involvement. Recurrence in these patients is frequent, and therefore they must have a strict and frequent follow-up protocol.

In selected cases, laparoscopic radical nephrectomy has become available. Disease-free and disease-specific survival are similar to those for open radical nephrectomy. Significant benefit with regard to patient recovery and comfort can be seen with both the hand-assisted and the standard laparoscopic techniques. Surgeon experience determines the ability to perform laparoscopic procedures in larger tumors, inflammatory kidneys, previously operated kidneys, or patients with prior abdominal surgery. Laparoscopic nephrectomy is contraindicated in tumors with extensive local extension or caval thrombi.

New minimally invasive therapeutic modalities such as renal cryosurgery and radiofrequency ablation are under investigation. These techniques, which can be applied via open, percutaneous, or laparoscopic approaches, are minimally invasive and provide the possibility of maximal preservation of renal parenchyma. Further studies will elucidate the long-term efficacy of these newer modalities.

Metastatic RCC is not responsive to traditional chemotherapeutic agents or radiation therapy. There has been a long-standing enthusiasm for management of RCC with immunotherapy. Most recently, there have been promising results with recombinant human interleukin-2 with partial response rates of up to 15%. Factors that predict response to immunotherapy include nephrectomy prior to initiation of treatment, good functional status, and lack of bulky pulmonary or soft tissue metastases.

2. **Sarcomas** of the kidney are rare, making up 1% to 3% of all renal tumors. These include leiomyosarcoma, liposarcoma, rhabdomyosarcoma, fibrosarcoma, malignant fibrous histiocytoma, neural sarcoma, and hemangiopericytoma. Leiomyosarcoma is the most common and accounts for up to 60% of renal sarcomas. Large, rapidly growing tumors without the presence of lymphadenopathy are suggestive of renal sarcomas. However, the preoperative diagnosis of sarcoma is difficult since the symptoms and signs are similar to those of renal adenocarcinoma. The treatment of localized renal sarcoma is nephrectomy, although the rate of local recurrence is high and the prognosis is extremely poor.

3. **Metastatic lesions** in the kidney are the most common renal malignancy. The most common primary site is lung followed by breast, stomach, pancreas, colon, and cervix. These tumors, which are often clinically silent, can present with flank pain or hematuria. Any patient with a history of prior malignancy or with multiple renal masses should be suspected of having metastatic lesions rather than an RCC. In these cases, biopsy should be considered.

4. **Renal lymphoma and leukemia.** Renal involvement is common with these hematologic malignancies but is usually asymptomatic. Primary renal lymphoma is exceedingly rare owing to the paucity of lymphoid cells within the kidney. Secondary lymphoma should be suspected in patients with renal mass and significant retroperitoneal lymphadenopathy or lymphadenopathy elsewhere in the body. It is of primary importance to distinguish these renal malignancies from RCC as the treatment is extirpative only in the rare situation where intractable hemorrhage occurs.

II. Cystic renal masses
A. Benign lesions

1. **Simple renal cysts** are the most common renal masses and are present in 50% of autopsy specimens from patients above 50 years of age. CT studies demonstrate that the prevalence and size increase with age. They are composed of fibrous tissue and are lined by flattened cuboidal epithelium. Simple cysts are usually asymptomatic and are incidental findings on radiologic studies. However, they can become symptomatic when they reach larger sizes or when spontaneous hemorrhage occurs into the cyst.

    a. **Radiologic diagnosis** of a simple cyst can usually be made confidently by US or CT. A confident diagnosis of a benign cyst can be made by US when the lesion is homogeneous and thin and smooth walled, has increased through-transmission, and has an anechoic internal component. If these criteria are not met, further imaging with CT or MRI is necessary. CT criteria for simple cyst are met when they have thin walls, a CT density similar to water, and lack of enhancement with intravenous contrast agent administration. Thin septations or thin mural calcifications are also acceptable features for classification of benign simple cyst. The criteria by MRI are similar to those for CT. In addition, simple cysts exhibit low signal intensity by T1-weighted images and high signal intensity on T2-weighted images.

b.   Treatment. Simple cysts are usually asymptomatic and therefore rarely require intervention. Treatment options for symptomatic simple cysts include aspiration and sclerosis or surgical resection via laparoscopy or open surgery. Although aspiration and sclerosis are less invasive, recurrence rates have been noted to reach up to 90%.

2.   Complicated cysts are those cysts that do not meet the radiologic criteria for simple cysts. Features of complicated cysts include septations, calcifications, thick walls, or enhancement by CT with administration of intravenous contrast medium. These findings are of concern because of the possibility of malignancy in these cysts. Bosniak first proposed a classification of renal cysts in 1986 to clarify the need for further evaluation of complicated cystic lesions (Table 4.2). Class I lesions are presumed to be uncomplicated and do not require further evaluation. Class II lesions have some atypical features and should be followed radiographically. Class III lesions cannot be distinguished from malignant lesions and carry up to a 50% chance of malignancy. They require surgical exploration. Class IV lesions are strongly suggestive of malignancy and are presumed to be RCCs.

a.   Multilocular cystic nephroma is a Bosniak class III lesion that is thought to be benign. It is a well-circumscribed lesion composed of multiple noncommunicating cysts separated by thick fibrous septa. The lesion is well circumscribed by a thick fibrous capsule and compresses adjacent renal parenchyma. There is a bimodal distribution with the first peak occurring most commonly in young boys under the age of 4 years. These account for approximately 70% of all cases. A second peak occurs in women ages 40 to 70. In children, the presentation is usually as a palpable abdominal mass, while in adults, it can be an incidental finding or can be related to pain, hematuria, or urinary tract infection. US will

Table 4.2.   **Bosniak classification of cystic renal masses**

Category	Description	Clinical Examples
I	Uncomplicated cyst	Simple cyst
II	Wall calcification	Simple cyst
	Thin internal septa	Renal abscess
	Nonenhancing components	
III	Thick, irregular calcification	Multilocular cystic nephroma
	Multiloculated lesions	Necrotic renal carcinoma
		Cystic renal carcinoma
		Renal abscess
IV	Thick walls	Renal cell carcinoma
	Solid elements	Xanthogranulomatous pyelonephritis
	Enhancing components	Renal abscess

show a large cluster of fluid-filled cysts (most between 5 and 10 cm in diameter) with highly echogenic stroma between them. CT will confirm the US findings, with the septa showing contrast enhancement. In adults, differential diagnosis should include cystic renal carcinoma and chronic renal abscess. As many as 5% of RCCs may resemble multilocular cystic nephromas. In children, the differential diagnosis should also include cystic Wilms' tumor. In most cases, it will not be possible to exclude clinically a cystic Wilms' tumor, cystic or necrotic RCC, or cystic forms of sarcoma. Therefore, surgical exploration and excision are usually required.

b. Calyceal diverticula, occurring in 0.5% of the population, are small diverticula arising from the tip of the calyx. They are lined with transitional epithelium and communicate with the collecting system. They are usually asymptomatic, but the patient may present with hematuria, pain, infection, or stone within the diverticulum. IVU or CT will show a contrast-filled mass that arises from the tip of a calyx or less commonly the renal pelvis. US can demonstrate a cystic structure with or without debris or calculi. Treatment depends on the size, location, and symptoms associated with the lesion.

B. Malignant lesions. Approximately 5% to 10% of instances of renal adenocarcinoma have a cystic appearance (Bosniak class III or IV). Reasons for this include (a) cystic growth pattern (multilocular or unilocular), (b) cystic necrosis of a renal adenocarcinoma, (c) tumor arising in a benign renal cyst, and (d) cyst arising from ductal obstruction by tumor. The most common reason (70%) is an intrinsically cystic growth pattern, sometimes termed **papillary cystadenocarcinoma.** The diagnosis of a malignant cystic lesion must be considered when a cyst does not meet the criteria for a simple cyst. The radiologic criteria that should raise suspicion for malignancy are discussed earlier. If a combination of US and three-dimensional imaging by CT or MRI is unable to make the distinction, then exploration and either radical nephrectomy or partial nephrectomy are necessary.

SUGGESTED READING

Bechtold RE, Zagoria RJ. Imaging approach to staging of renal cell carcinoma. *Urol Clin North Am* 1997;24:507–522.

Bosniak MA. The use of the Bosniak classification system for renal cysts and cystic tumors. *J Urol* 1997;157:1852–1853.

Cadeddu JA, Ono Y, Clayman RV, et al. Laparoscopic nephrectomy for renal cell cancer: evaluation of efficacy and safety—a multi-center experience. *Urology* 1998;52:773–777.

Chao DH, Zisman AH, Pantuck AJ, et al. Changing concepts in the management of renal oncocytoma. *Urology* 2002;59:635–642.

Clark PE, Novick A. Exophytic noninvasive growth pattern of renal angiomyolipomas: implications for nephron sparing surgery. *J Urol* 2001;52:577–583.

Couch MS, Lindor NM, Karnes PS, et al. Von Hippel–Lindau disease. *Mayo Clin Proc* 2000;75:265–272.

Fazeli-Matin S, Novick A. Nephron-sparing surgery for renal angiomyolipoma. *Urology* 1998;52:577–583.

Fergany AF, Hafez KS, Novick AC. Long-term results of nephron sparing surgery for localized renal cell carcinoma: 10 year follow up. *J Urol* 2000;163:442.

Gill IS, Schweizer D, Hobart MG, et al. Retroperitoneal laparoscopic radical nephrectomy: the Cleveland Clinic experience. *J Urol* 2000;163:1665–1670.

Herring JC, Enquist EG, Chernoff A, et al. Parenchymal sparing surgery in patients with hereditary renal cell carcinoma: 10-year experience. *J Urol* 2001;165:777–781.

Masood J, Lane T, Koye B, et al. Renal cell carcinoma: incidental detection during routine ultrasonography in men presenting with lower urinary tract symptoms. *Br J Urol Int* 2001;88:671–674.

Pantuck AJ, Zisman A, Belldegrun AS. The changing natural history of renal cell carcinoma. *J Urol* 2001;166:1611–1623.

Instrumentation of the Lower Urinary Tract

C. Charles Wen and Richard K. Babayan

The central role of endoscopy requires the practitioner to gain a thorough understanding of urologic instrumentation. Technologic advances such as flexible endoscopes and improved optics continue to effect gradual changes in the design of urologic instruments. Today's instruments provide an excellent image displayed on color monitors combined with much greater safety and comfort for the patient. The following sections review some of the catheters, instruments, and techniques commonly used by urologists to visualize and manipulate the lower urinary tract.

I. Urologic catheters and instruments

A. Catheters. Catheters are hollow tubes used to relieve urinary retention, irrigate the bladder, instill medication or radiographic contrast agent, obtain urine for examination, and measure residual urine volume. Catheters are most commonly calibrated according to the French (F) scale, in which each unit equals 0.33 mm in diameter. A catheter designated 30F, for example, has a diameter of roughly 10 mm.

1. The **Robinson catheter** (Fig. 5.1) is a straight catheter used for short-term catheterization, as in measurement of residual urine and instillation of medication, chemotherapeutic agents, or contrast material into the urinary bladder. The tip of the Robinson catheter is rounded, with one or two drainage ports along the side. If a Robinson catheter is left indwelling, it must be secured to the glans penis by suture or tape.

2. The **Foley catheter** (Fig. 5.2) is a straight catheter with a retention balloon near the tip. Several varieties are available. Foley catheters may have short- or long-nose tips, the retention balloon ranges in size from 5 to 50 mL, the diameter of the catheter ranges from 12 to 30F, and there may be two or three lumina. Two-lumen catheters have one channel for drainage and one for inflating the balloon. Three-lumen catheters have an additional channel that allows for irrigation to be infused into the bladder. Three-lumen catheters are used most commonly when ongoing hematuria is expected, such as after transurethral resection of the prostate (TURP). The balloons can be overinflated, if necessary, to at least twice their stated capacity without breakage. Silicon or silicon-coated catheters are said to produce less tissue reaction and less encrustation than rubber catheters. They also have a larger lumen diameter than catheters made of rubber and thus are preferred by some for long-term indwelling catheterization.

3. The **coude catheter** (Fig. 5.2) is curved at the tip (hence the name, the French word for "elbow"). A straight catheter cannot always pass through a hypertrophied or high bladder

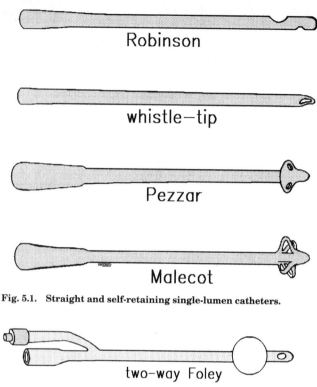

Fig. 5.1. **Straight and self-retaining single-lumen catheters.**

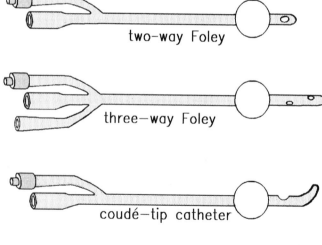

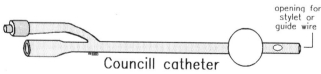

Fig. 5.2. **Examples of self-retaining balloon catheters.**

neck. The curved shape of the coude catheter is designed to guide it over the bladder neck. In addition, this specialized catheter is slightly stiffer than the Robinson catheter. Coude catheters are manufactured with and without retention balloons.

4. The **Pezzar catheter** (Fig. 5.1) is self-retaining with a mushroom-shaped tip. It is most commonly used for suprapubic cystostomy drainage. To avoid dislodgement, the catheter should be secured to the skin by suture or tape.

5. The **Malecot catheter** (Fig. 5.1) is similar to the Pezzar except that the drainage ports at the tip are wider. This may be particularly useful when bloody fluids, such as from a nephrostomy, are drained.

6. The **whistle-tip catheter** (Fig. 5.1) is a straight catheter with a beveled opening at the tip and another opening in the side. It provides better irrigation and drainage than the Robinson catheter.

7. **Councill catheters** (Fig. 5.2) are similar to Foley catheters, except that they have an opening at the end to allow for use with a screw-tip (Councill) stylet or guide wire. This type of catheter is most commonly used in bypassing a urethral stricture or false passage. Councill catheters are especially useful when passage of any other type of catheter is difficult. They are not used to dilate the urethra. The catheter is passed into position over a previously placed guide wire, or it can be used with a Councill stylet, which has a male screw tip that fits through the perforation to engage a filiform. After a stricture is dilated with filiforms and followers, the Councill catheter and stylet are attached to the filiform and guided into the bladder. The stylet and filiform (or guide wire) are then removed through the lumen of the Councill catheter.

8. **Catheter stylets** are malleable metal guides that, when placed into a Foley or other type of catheter, can be used to provide stiffness and shape. There are two type of stylets: one with a blunt tip, used with a Foley catheter, and one with a screw tip, used with a Councill catheter and filiforms. This procedure is useful to accomplish passage through a urethral stricture or tight bladder neck. Catheter stylets also may be used following TURP to avoid undermining the bladder neck. When a catheter stylet is used, the bladder should always be full to avoid injuring the posterior bladder wall.

B. **Dilators and bougies.** Dilators and bougies are used to calibrate or stretch the urethra to aid passage of large-caliber instruments or in the treatment of urethral strictures. A large variety of dilators are available, and the most common are described below.

1. **Van Buren sounds** are solid metal sounds curved in the shape of the male urethra (Fig. 5.3). Ranging in size from 16 to 40F, they are most commonly used for dilating urethral strictures and for stretching the normal urethra to accommodate larger instruments.

2. **Filiforms and followers** are specialized instruments for dilating urethral strictures. Filiforms are very thin, very

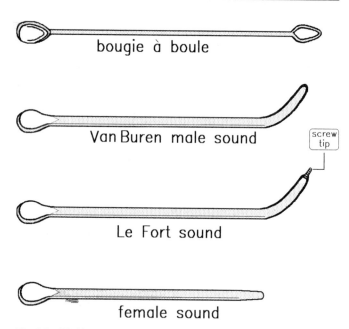

bougie à boule

Van Buren male sound

screw tip

Le Fort sound

female sound

Fig. 5.3. **Rigid metal urethral sounds and dilators. Top to bottom:**
Bougie à boule **for calibrating the urethra, Van Buren sound for**
dilating the male urethra, Le Fort sound for use with a filiform,
and straight sound for dilating the female urethra.

pliable solid catheters ranging in size from 1 to 6F (Fig. 5.4).
They are made of solid plastic or have a woven fiber core with
smooth-coated surfaces. Filiform tips may be straight, pig-
tailed, or of the coude type. They have a female screw tip on
the proximal end to allow attachment of followers or a stylet.
The follower (Fig. 5.4) is made of material similar to that of
the filiform but of a larger caliber (12 to 30F), and it may be
solid or hollow. After introduction of the filiform into the
bladder, the follower is screwed onto the end of the filiform.
Both are advanced through the urethra into the bladder and
withdrawn to permit changing of the follower to a larger size.
The filiform always remains in the urethra as a guide for the
followers.
3.   **Coaxial dilators** are based on the principle of using a
guide wire instead of a filiform for passage through a urethral stricture. A flexible wire is passed into the bladder, and
progressively larger dilators are advanced into the bladder
over the wire. When passing dilators over a guide wire, it is
important to keep the wire taut to prevent the wire from
bending and the dilator from perforating the lumen. A variation is the balloon dilator, which is passed over a guide wire
and inflated at the area of the stricture.

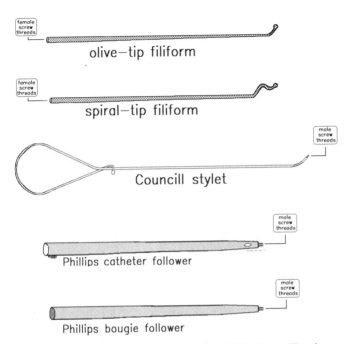

female screw threads

olive—tip filiform

female screw threads

spiral—tip filiform

male screw threads

Councill stylet

male screw threads

Phillips catheter follower

male screw threads

Phillips bougie follower

Fig. 5.4. Filiforms and various followers, including Councill and Phillips types.

4. *Bougies à boules* (Fig. 5.3) are acorn-tipped calibrators used to determine urethral and meatal size. They are available in sizes ranging from 8 to 40F.

5. **Female sounds** are similar to Van Buren sounds but are shorter in length and less curved or straight. Sizes range from 14 to 40F (Fig. 5.3).

C. **Diagnostic and operating instruments**

1. **Rigid cystourethroscopes** (Fig. 5.5) are hollow metal instruments designed for endoscopic observation and surgery. Their sheaths range in size from approximately 8 to 26F. These instruments have **obturators** that are inserted into the sheath to aid passage into the bladder. Obturators can be either solid or (preferred) direct vision types. Interchangeable **telescopes** have fiberoptic lenses that allow a view ranging from 0 to 120 degrees (Fig. 5.6).

The 0-degree (forward) lens is best for intraurethral work, and the 30-degree (forward oblique) lens allows visualization of either the urethra or the bladder (panendoscopy). The 70-degree (lateral) lens is used frequently for inspecting the interior of the bladder, whereas the 120-degree (retrograde) lens provides retrograde viewing of the bladder neck. The telescope contains a fiberoptic light bundle; when connected to a light

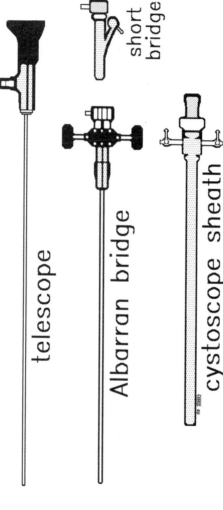

Fig. 5.5.   Top to bottom: Cystoscopic telescope, Albarran deflecting and short bridges, and cystoscope sheath.

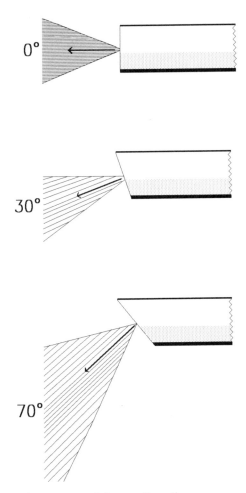

Fig. 5.6. **Various cystoscopic lens configurations.**

source, this allows for illumination. Visualization is aided by irrigating with fluid (usually sterile saline solution or water) through special ports on the cystourethroscope sheath. Operating instruments such as biopsy forceps, cautery (Bugbee) electrodes, laser fibers, and ureteral catheters can be passed through the sheath. The **Albarran (deflecting) bridge** allows for manipulation by deflection of flexible instruments such as flexible biopsy forceps, guide wires, or laser fibers (Fig. 5.7). It utilizes a lever or wheel near the eyepiece to manipulate a small bar at the end of the device (Fig. 5.5).

2. Flexible instruments (Fig. 5.8) have been developed over the last decade for cystoscopy, ureteroscopy, and nephros-

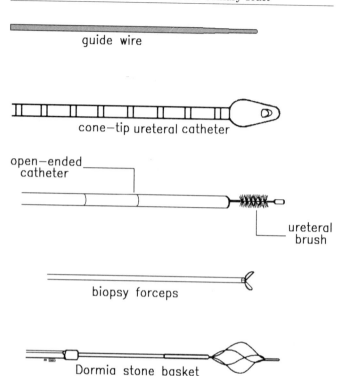

guide wire

cone—tip ureteral catheter

open—ended catheter

ureteral brush

biopsy forceps

Dormia stone basket

Fig. 5.7. **Instruments and catheters that can be directed by the Albarran bridge.**

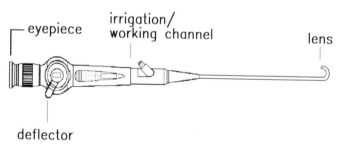

eyepiece

irrigation/ working channel

lens

deflector

Fig. 5.8. **Flexible cystoscope.**

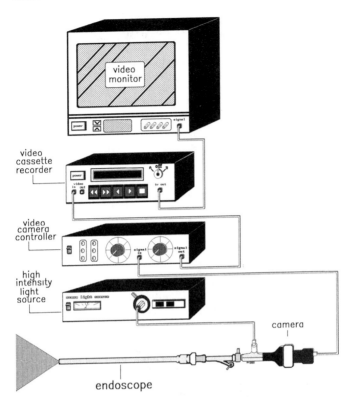

Fig. 5.9. Typical video setup for endoscopy of the lower urinary tract.

copy. Their main advantage is that they are small in caliber and can be used easily under local anesthesia in an outpatient or office setting. Flexible instruments do not provide as clear a view as rigid instruments do. Moreover, operative and diagnostic procedures are limited with the use of flexible instruments by the capacity of the irrigating and working channels, which is smaller than those in rigid instruments. The flexible cystoscope is used most commonly in the office setting for routine diagnostic viewing of the bladder and urethra.

   Video monitoring of endoscopic procedures has now become commonplace (Fig. 5.9). Small, high-resolution color cameras attach to the eyepiece of the endoscopes and allow real-time projection on large television monitors in the operating room. This is invaluable for both teaching and allowing an assistant to share the operator's view. Video monitoring of endoscopic procedures offers several distinct advantages: (a) a standing, comfortable position; (b) magnified, binocular vision; and (c) greater eye protection from blood and irrigating fluid.

D. Percutaneous cystostomy trocars. If the bladder cannot be entered through the urethra, a percutaneous cystostomy tube can be placed into the distended bladder. The technique of percutaneous cystostomy is described later. The following types are available:

1. The **Hurwitz type of trocar** consists of a large-bore metal sheath around a sharp, solid obturator. This permits placement of a standard Foley type of catheter into the bladder.
2. The **Stamey trocar** places a Malecot catheter into the bladder (Fig. 5.10).
3. The **Argyle catheter** uses a Foley-type balloon catheter, which also has an irrigating port.
4. The **Cystocath** is an 8 or 12F simple tube retained in the bladder by means of a flange glued and sutured to the suprapubic skin.
5. The **Rusch trocar** has a peel-away sheath that allows placement of a Foley catheter through it. After the trocar and sheath are inserted into the bladder, the trocar is removed and replaced by a Foley catheter. After the balloon is inflated, the outer sheath can be peeled away, leaving only the catheter.

II.   Clinical applications

  A.   Catheterization technique. Catheterization kits generally contain sterile gloves, sterile paper towels, sterilizing solution, lubricating jelly, a syringe filled with 10 mL of water, and a container for bacteriologic specimens packed in a large plastic basin. Some kits also provide a catheter (Robinson or Foley type) as well as an irrigating syringe. A drainage bag, generally not provided, must be obtained before the procedure is begun if long-term catheterization is expected.

   1.   Male patients. With the patient supine, legs partially abducted, the catheterization kit is opened and the gloves put on. The sterile towels are used to drape the penis. The sterilizing solution, lubricating jelly, and catheter should be prepared before the patient is touched with the gloves. The penis is grasped gently behind the glans with one hand, and slight upward traction is applied to straighten the urethra. The glans and penile shaft are cleansed around the meatus with the opposite hand. If desired, urethral anesthesia may be obtained by instilling 10 mL of 1% to 2% lidocaine jelly through the meatus. Lack of patient allergy to lidocaine should be confirmed first, and 5 minutes should be allowed for the anesthetic effect. The catheter, well lubricated, is inserted into the urethral meatus and gently advanced until almost the entire catheter is inside the urethra. If the patient is uncircumcised, care should be taken to replace the foreskin over the glans to prevent paraphimosis. Force should never be used in urethral catheterization. If the catheter does not enter the bladder easily, the most likely cause is spasm of the external sphincter, followed by urethral stricture or bladder neck obstruction. Prostatic enlargement rarely prevents the passage of a catheter. If urine is not obtained or there is doubt regarding the position of the catheter, the catheter balloon must not be inflated because this may cause severe urethral trauma or rupture.

    a.   External sphincter spasm may be overcome by reassuring the patient, using large amounts of lubricant, telling

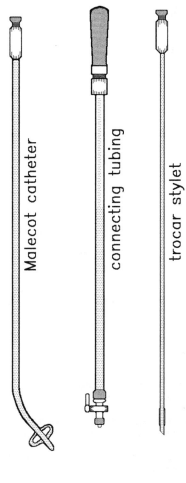

Malecot catheter

connecting tubing

trocar stylet

Fig. 5.10.   Stamey-type suprapubic catheter introducer.

the patient to take a deep breath, and applying minimal steady pressure against the sphincter with the catheter until sphincter fatigue occurs. If a patient is particularly anxious, between 5 and 7 mL of 1% to 2% viscous lidocaine can be introduced into the urethra. Intravenous or oral sedation with diazepam is very rarely required.

b. If difficult catheterization is encountered in a patient known or suspected to have urethral stricture, retrograde urethrography should be carried out to assess the urethra (see Chapter 2). In clearly impassable strictures, percutaneous suprapubic cystotomy is indicated for temporary relief of urinary retention.

c.   Bladder neck obstruction is often the cause of difficulty in passing a urethral catheter. The coude catheter or catheter stylet is especially useful to guide the catheter over an enlarged median lobe, for example, and the risk for traumatizing the urethra with a straight catheter is avoided.

2.   Female patients. Catheterization of female patients is usually quite simple. With the patient supine, legs abducted, and knees flexed, the catheterization kit is prepared as described previously. After the sterile gloves are put on, the left hand is used to spread the labia majora to expose the urethral meatus. The meatus and introitus are cleansed with sterilizing solution, and the lubricated catheter is introduced into the urethra. Once urine is obtained from the bladder, the Foley balloon is inflated. If the urethral meatus is not obvious on initial examination, it can usually be easily exposed by placing a finger in the vagina and depressing the posterior wall of the vagina posteriorly.

3.   Children. Catheterization in female children is similar to that in female adults except that the catheters used are in the 8 to 12F range. In male children, some prefer to use an 8F feeding tube rather than a Foley catheter because the Foley catheter balloon is somewhat larger than the catheter itself, making it difficult to pass. Also, the lumen of the feeding tube is larger than that of the Foley, making drainage more efficient.

B.   Endoscopic diagnosis

1.   Cystourethroscopy, also called panendoscopy, is the endoscopic examination of the urethra and bladder.

a.   Indications and contraindications. Indications for cystourethroscopy include (a) hematuria; (b) follow-up of lower urinary tract cancer; (c) need to obtain anatomic information regarding the bladder, prostate, or urethra; or (d) need to obtain access to the lower or upper urinary tract. The major contraindication is genitourinary infection, especially acute cystitis and prostatitis, as instrumentation in this setting may precipitate urosepsis.

b.   Precautions. Patients with valvular cardiac disease or artificial heart valves should be protected from bacteremia with antibiotic prophylaxis. The American Heart Association recommends the following regimen: 1 hour before instrumentation, 2 g of ampicillin and 1.5 mg of gentamicin/kg of body wt are given, both agents either intramuscularly or intravenously. Eight hours after instrumentation, the dose is repeated. If penicillin allergy is present, vancomycin is started at 1 hour before instrumentation; 1 g IV is given over 60 minutes, and 1.5 mg of gentamicin/kg IV or IM is given. Eight to 12 hours after instrumentation, administration of both antibiotics is repeated. Adequate renal function should be confirmed by determination of creatinine clearance before antibiotics are administered.

c. Sterilization of instruments. Sterilization of endoscopic equipment cannot be achieved by heat or steam because these methods damage the optical systems. Alternative methods commonly used include soaking in 2% glutaraldehyde ("cold" sterilization) or exposing the equipment to ethylene oxide ("gas" sterilization). Twenty minutes of exposure to glutaraldehyde solution kills all bacterial organisms, spores, fungi, and viruses. The glutaraldehyde solution is rinsed from the instruments with sterile saline solution or water before the patient undergoes instrumentation. Ethylene oxide sterilization is equally effective but requires 24 hours of aeration to remove the agent before the instrument is used. Recently, automated sterilizing systems employing exposure to warm peracetic acid (e.g., Steris) have become popular as well.

d. Technique. Most lower tract endoscopies in adults can be carried out using 1% to 2% intraurethral lidocaine (Xylocaine) for local anesthesia in an office or outpatient surgical setting. Pediatric cystoscopy requires general anesthesia. The smallest instrument consistent with the objectives of the procedure should be selected.

(1) Rigid instruments. In both male and female patients, the cystourethroscope may be passed blindly into the bladder with the solid obturator or, preferably, under direct vision with the visual obturator and a 0-degree lens. Urine obtained when the bladder is entered should be sent for bacteriologic culture. If the patient has a history of genitourinary malignancy, urine should be sent for cytologic examination. In male patients, the 30-degree lens provides good visualization of the pendulous, bulbous, and prostatic portions of the urethra. With the instrument located at the verumontanum, the extent of prostatic enlargement and the patency of the bladder neck can be assessed. In female patients, the 30-degree lens permits visualization of the urethral mucosa. After the instrument is passed through the bladder neck, the trigone and ureteral orifices can be visualized. Examination of the bladder interior is facilitated by exchanging the 30-degree lens for the 70-degree lens. Systematically examining the entire surface of the bladder mucosa, the endoscopist notes any tumors, stones, trabeculation, or diverticula. Inflammatory changes and bladder capacity should also be noted. In fact, the results of endoscopic procedures should never be described as "normal," as this provides no information to subsequent examiners. All aspects of the procedure should be noted in detail in the operative report. At the conclusion of the examination, the bladder should be emptied and the cystoscope removed.

(2) **Flexible cystoscopy.** The flexible cystoscope is passed in the same way as a Foley catheter while the lumen is observed through the instrument. The instrument is torqued to obtain a view of the entire bladder mucosa, trigone, and ureteral orifices. The view of the prostatic urethra is not as clear as with rigid instruments, but a general impression of the prostatic size can be obtained.

2. A **mucosal biopsy** is indicated for any mucosal lesion within the bladder or urethra in which tumor is suspected. This procedure can be accomplished endoscopically by using either rigid or flexible biopsy forceps. The rigid biopsy forceps cleanly removes tissue samples of up to 5 mm in diameter; however, some areas of the bladder are difficult to reach with the rigid forceps, such as the dome and anterior wall. The flexible biopsy forceps are available in sizes ranging from 5 to 9F. Although the size of the tissue fragment obtained usually is ≤2 mm with the flexible forceps, all areas of the bladder are accessible. Fulguration can be achieved by using flexible Bugbee electrodes. The electrodes are manipulated with the Albarran bridge to control minor bleeding from biopsy sites or destroy small bladder tumors.

3. **Ureteral catheterization** is a basic technique used for retrograde pyelography, intubation of the ureter for short-term or long-term drainage of the upper urinary tract, and brush biopsy. Ureteral catheters range in size from 4 to 10F and have various tips such as the whistle tip, cone tip, and spiral tip (Fig. 5.6). Ureteral catheters designed for long-term drainage, called ureteral stents, incorporate some method of fixation within the ureter (e.g., the "double-J" stent). The whistle tip is used primarily for short-term drainage but can be used for contrast studies as well. The cone or bulb tip is ideally suited for retrograde pyelography. The spiral tip is designed to intubate an angulated orifice. The ureteral orifice is located by reference to the interureteric ridge.

C. **Miscellaneous procedures**

1. **Percutaneous cystostomy** is a useful method of draining the bladder when intraurethral access is not available. The various types of cystostomy trocars were described previously. The skin is anesthetized with 1% to 2% intradermal and subcutaneous lidocaine. With a no. 11 blade, a small incision is made in the skin and anterior rectus fascia. The location of the full bladder is then confirmed by aspirating urine through a long spinal needle or by ultrasound (US). The trocar is then advanced between the rectus muscles in a slightly caudal direction and into the distended bladder. When urine is obtained, the stylet can be removed. If the cystostomy tube does not irrigate freely, a cystogram should be obtained to confirm its location within the bladder. Percutaneous cystostomy is contraindicated in the presence of surgical scars in the suprapubic area because small bowel may be interposed in the retropubic space. If necessary, the procedure may be performed under US guidance. If the bladder is not distended sufficiently to permit blind trocar cystostomy, the long spinal needle may be used to fill the bladder with saline solution be-

fore trocar cystostomy is performed. After successful percutaneous cystostomy, the tube is connected to a urinary drainage bag and secured to the skin with a flange, tape, or suture.

2. Needle biopsy of the prostate is indicated in the evaluation of any prostatic nodule or indurated area or in cases of an unexplained elevation of the serum prostate-specific antigen level. Access to the prostate is most commonly via the transrectal route using US guidance. If using the perineal approach, the use of local anesthesia in the perineal skin is required. The tip of the biopsy needle is guided into the prostate by the examiner's finger in the rectum or by transrectal US. At least six cores of tissue from different parts of the gland should be taken for examination. Patients should receive broad-spectrum antibiotics within 4 hours of the procedure and for 24 hours afterward. The quinolone antibiotics may be useful in this setting.

3. Perineal urethrostomy is sometimes required for transurethral access to the prostate when the caliber of the urethra is inadequate or occasionally if the patient has had a penile prosthesis placed in the past. With the patient under general or spinal anesthesia in the dorsal lithotomy position, a Van Buren sound is placed in the urethra with the tip in the bladder. The handle of the sound is moved toward the patient's abdomen to place the bulbous urethra on tension. With a surgical blade, the perineal skin is incised vertically for 2 to 3 cm over the bulbous urethra. The incision is deepened until the sound is encountered. The urethral mucosa is fixed to the perineal skin with sutures, and the transurethral instruments are passed through the urethrostomy into the bladder.

D. Complications of endoscopic procedures include bleeding, perforation, infection, urinary retention, and urethral stricture.

1. Minimal bleeding or hematuria is quite common following instrumentation in male patients and usually clears spontaneously within the first 24 hours. The patient should be advised to maintain a high fluid intake to promote diuresis and prevent formation of obstructing clots. Endoscopy and evacuation of clot are indicated to control bleeding that does not clear within 24 hours.

2. Perforation of the urethra or bladder can occur, especially when excessive or poorly directed force is used to introduce a urethral instrument. The diagnosis is made by retrograde urethrography. If minimal extravasation is present, antibiotic coverage and urinary drainage for 1 or 2 days are usually sufficient treatment. If major extravasation into the perineum or scrotum has occurred, drainage of the fluid collection may be necessary. Perforation of the bladder is rare but can occur. The most common location of bladder perforations is at its weakest point, the dome. A cystogram should be obtained to determine whether the perforation is intraperitoneal or extraperitoneal. Extraperitoneal perforations generally can be managed by bladder drainage (urethral or suprapubic). Intraperitoneal perforations can be managed with surgical exploration to rule out injury to the bowel or other organs, closure of the perforation, and suprapubic diversion. Some intraperitoneal perforations occurring after transurethral surgery may be managed nonoperatively with 1 week of broad-spectrum antibiotics and 2 weeks of urethral catheterization, provided that the urine remains clear and uninfected and the patient remains stable.

3.   Infection is a well-known complication of urethral instrumentation. Bacteriuria occurs in approximately 2% of patients after cystoscopy. Bacteremia and sepsis ("urethral chill") occur rarely following routine cystoscopy and urethral dilation, but they should be anticipated if purulent urine or an abscess is encountered. Patients at risk for endocarditis should receive prophylaxis as previously described.

4.   Acute urinary retention may develop following instrumentation of men with prostatic enlargement. Following short-term catheter drainage, many patients resume the voiding pattern they had before instrumentation.

5.   Urethral strictures may develop as a late complication after instrumentation, most commonly at the meatus or bulbous urethra.

SUGGESTED READING

Bloom DA, McGuire EJ, Lapides J. A brief history of urethral catheterization. *J Urol* 1994;151:317–325.

Candela JV, Bellman GC. Ureteral stents: impact of diameter and composition on patient symptoms. *J Endourol* 1997;11:45–47.

Harry W, Herr S, Machele D, et al. Correlation of cystoscopy with histology of recurrent papillary tumors of the bladder. *J Urol* 2002; 168:978–980.

Hofbauer J, Hobarth K, Marberger M, et al. Lithoclast: new and inexpensive mode of intracorporeal lithotripsy. *J Endourol* 1992;6: 429–432.

Matthias A, Reuter HJ. The development of the cystoscope. *J Urol* 1998;159:638–640.

Pansadoro V, Emiliozzi P. Internal urethrotomy in the management of anterior urethral strictures: long-term follow-up. *J Urol* 1996; 156:73–75.

Razvi HA, Song TY, Denstedt JD, et al. Management of vesical calculi: comparison of lithotripsy devices. *J Endourol* 1996;10:559–563.

Te AE, Santarosa R, Kaplan SA, et al. Electrovaporization of the prostate: electrosurgical modification of standard transurethral resection in 93 patients with benign prostatic hyperplasia. *J Endourol* 1997;11:71–75.

Upper Tract Instrumentation and Visualization

Luke M. O'Connell and Richard K. Babayan

Miniaturization in optics and electronics has led to the development of instruments that can be used to access the upper urinary tract in retrograde or antegrade fashion. Ureteroscopy can now be performed with minimal trauma to the ureter, and upper tract pathology such as stones, tumors, or strictures can be treated endoscopically. The following chapter will give a brief overview of the tools used in upper tract instrumentation. A detailed description of specific techniques is beyond the scope of this manual, but some basic techniques will be discussed.

I.   Retrograde ureterography involves opacification of the ureters and renal collecting system with radiologic contrast and visualization by fluoroscopy. Retrograde ureterograms are always performed prior to upper tract instrumentation to define the anatomy of the collecting system and provide a roadmap for the urologic surgeon. Filling defects within the ureters or the collecting system of the kidney may represent stones or tumor. Strictures can be identified by a narrowing of the normal caliber of the collecting system. Contrast agent is injected into the collecting system through various catheters designed to intubate the ureter.

A.   Open-ended and whistle-tip catheters (Fig. 6.1) come in various sizes, usually 5 or 6F in diameter, and have a blunt tip. They are passed through the cystoscope and into the ureteral orifice. Contrast agent is then injected through the catheter to opacify the ureter. Urine specimens can be obtained from the upper tract for cytologic examination by gently instilling saline through the catheter and allowing the urine to drip out through the catheter into a collection container. A brush biopsy can also be passed to obtain material for cytology. Guide wires can be passed through the open-ended catheter and left within the ureter. The open-ended catheter can also be passed over a guide wire to the level of the renal pelvis and left in place if desired.

B.   Cone-tip catheters (Fig. 6.1) have a conical bulb at the most distal end, which can be placed just within the ureteral orifice. The cone-tipped end occludes the orifice and allows contrast to be injected up the ureter without flowing back into the bladder. Placement of the catheter just within the ureteral orifice ensures that the entire ureter will be visualized, including the short intramural portion adjacent to the bladder.

C.   Spiral-tip catheters (Fig. 6.1) catheters may be useful in various circumstances such as bypassing a false passage or ureteral stone.

II.   Intubating or accessing the ureter requires the coordinated use of multiple instruments and techniques.

A.   Guide wires are fundamental to many techniques and instruments. They are available in many varieties, but all have

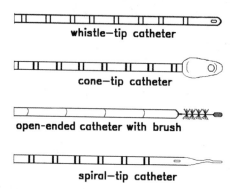

Fig. 6.1. Various ureteral catheters for retrograde pyelography and brush biopsy.

the same basic principle: They have a soft, flexible tip followed by a stiffer body. The flexible tip allows for atraumatic passage through the ureteral orifice and the ureter. The flexible tip can be maneuvered around kinks or obstructions within the ureter without perforating. Gentle introduction is still required as even the most flexible tipped wires can perforate the ureteral wall if not carefully introduced. The stiffer body of the wires will serve to straighten the ureter and ease instrumentation of the upper tract. The most commonly used guide wires are **0.035** and **0.038 inches** in diameter. These sizes can be passed through the working ports of adult-sized cystoscopes and ureteroscopes.

B.   Glide wires have a specialized coating that, when wet, makes them very slippery. While this slick coating can make them more difficult to handle, they oftentimes will slide by obstructions in the ureter more easily. Once a glide wire has been passed up to the renal pelvis, an open-ended catheter can be introduced over the glide wire, the glide wire removed, and a regular guide wire passed up the open-ended catheter and curled within the pelvis. The open-ended catheter is then removed while the guide wire remains in place as a safety wire during any further manipulation. The regular guide wire is easier to work with and less likely to slip out during manipulation. Some wires have **angled tips,** which can facilitate accessing a difficult ureteral orifice or bypassing a ureteral obstruction such as a stone.

C.   Ureteral access sheaths have seen a resurgence in recent years. The sheath offers the advantage of continuous access to the ureter. The uteroscope can be inserted and withdrawn at will without the bother of finding and accessing the ureteral orifice. This results in less trauma to the orifice and the scope. Another advantage is continuous flow of irrigant down the sheath, which prevents overdistension of the upper tract and bladder and allows outflow of fragments when dealing with stones.

  1.   Characteristics. The first-generation sheaths were somewhat bulky, stiff, and often difficult to pass. They also had a tendency to kink. The new-generation sheaths have a lubricious coating much like a glide wire that makes them very slick and easier to pass. The bodies are flexible but resistant to kinking, and this allows them to be passed though the prostatic urethra or bladder neck or over the iliac vessels while maintaining an open lumen though which instruments can be passed. The obturator within the sheath has a tapered end that will gently dilate the ureteral orifice and obviate the need for balloon dilatation of the orifice. The inner cannula of the sheath tapers up to 12F, and the sheath itself is 14F in diameter.

2. Technique of introduction. After introducing the guide wire into the ureter, the cystoscope is removed and the wire left in place. Under fluoroscopic guidance, the ureteral access sheath is passed over the wire and up the ureter. The progress of the sheath must be monitored by fluoroscopy to ensure that it does not coil within the bladder but instead travels up the ureter. Once within the ureter, the inner cannula of the sheath is removed and instrumentation can ensue. The guide wire can be left in place and instruments passed alongside it through the access sheath. The proper length sheath should be selected (20, 28, 35, and 55 cm) depending on the level of the upper tract that one needs to access (Fig. 6.2).

D. Balloon dilators are used to dilate the ureteral orifice for subsequent ureteroscopic instrumentation or to dilate strictures within the ureter. They are dual-lumen ureteral catheters that can be passed over a guide wire into the appropriate position in the ureter. The second channel is then used to inflate the balloon at the catheter tip. Contrast material is injected into the balloon under fluoroscopic guidance, and the area to be dilated is seen as a waist in the filling balloon. When the waist expands, the balloon is deflated and the catheter removed. Instruments can then be passed readily through the dilated ureteral orifice.

E. Ureteroscopes are semirigid or flexible.

1. Semirigid ureteroscopes are usually 7.5F in diameter (but vary from 6 to 12F) and have two channels: 2.5 and 3.5F in size. Different lengths (34 to 43 cm) are available depending on the level of the ureter. The shaft of the ureteroscope is solid but has some flex to it to allow manipulation up the ureter. Some flex is required to get over the bladder neck and

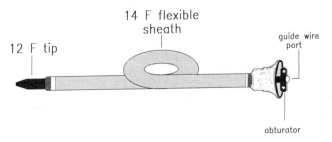

12 F tip

14 F flexible
sheath

guide wire
port

obturator

Fig. 6.2. Ureteral access sheath with 14F sheath and obturator.

into the ureteral orifice and then to maneuver over the iliac vessels. The channels are used for irrigation and instrumentation through the scope. Initially, it is better to run the irrigation through the 3F channel to allow for better visualization. When the area of interest is reached, the irrigant can be switched to the 2F channel, thus freeing the 3F channel for the necessary instruments. Irrigant flow can be increased by using a **pressure bag** or by connecting a **single-action pumping system,** which allows the operator to withdraw fluid into a syringe and then pump that fluid through the ureteroscope in one single maneuver. Given the narrow channel through which the irrigant is flowing, these delivery systems are sometimes necessary to provide the flow required for visualization. The semirigid ureteroscopes are useful for pathology from the renal pelvis down to the ureterovesical junction. These regions can be reached without significant angulation of the tip of the scope.

2.   Flexible ureteroscopes are useful when access to the calyces of the kidney is required or the semirigid scopes cannot be passed over the iliac vessels or through a particular angulation in the ureter. The flexible ureteroscope is similar to the flexible cystoscope but narrower. The flexible ureteroscope generally has a 7.5F diameter like the semirigid (also varying from 7.5 to 12F), but the tip can be angled with manipulation of the thumb lever. Typically, the tip can be deflected in the range of 120 degrees posteriorly and 180 degrees anteriorly. This allows the operator to manipulate the scope into any of the renal calyces to fragment and extract stones or ablate a tumor. The flexible tip can be used to bypass an excessively angulated ureter through which the semirigid scope cannot be passed. The flexible scopes are about 70 cm long, allowing plenty of length to operate up in the kidney. They have a 3.5-cm working channel through which instrumentation can be passed, but this is also the channel through which the irrigant flows, so visualization is often decreased when instruments are passed (Fig. 6.3).

3.   Ureteroscopic instruments of many different types have been developed.

   a.   A stone basket is a long wire from 1.5 to 3.5F that can be passed through the working channel of the ureteroscope. The handle of the instrument slides back and forth to open and close the basket. The baskets are available in **spiral** or **helical** arrangements. The baskets can be manipulated around a stone or stone fragment and then closed, captur-

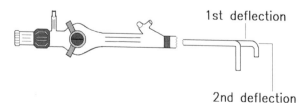

1st deflection

2nd deflection

Fig. 6.3.   Double-deflecting flexible ureteroscope.

ing the stone within the basket. The entire ureteroscope is then removed, with the basket held in the closed position to remove the stone. Care must be taken on withdrawing the stone or fragment to ensure that it is not too large to pass through the ureter. If too much force is applied, the ureter can be stripped. If the stone cannot be extracted easily, it should be released and further fragmented into smaller pieces that can then be removed safely. **Tipless baskets** can be opened within the calyces themselves and allow stones within the calyces to be removed.

b.   Ureteroscopic biopsy forceps and grasping forceps are also available. These can be useful for obtaining tissue from the ureter or renal pelvis for pathologic examination.

c.   Laser fibers are thin, fairly flexible fibers that can be easily passed through the ureteroscope. The **holmium laser** is becoming the main instrument for stone fragmentation or tissue ablation in the upper urinary tract. The laser fiber is available in several different sizes, but for upper tract work, the 365-μm fibers are the most commonly used. The laser fiber is placed directly on the stone to be fragmented or the tissue to be ablated, and the laser is activated. When a stone has been broken into small pieces, these can be removed with a basket. The laser can also be used to incise strictures within the ureter.

d.   Electrohydraulic lithotripsy uses a spark to generate a shock wave that can fragment stones. This technique has a greater potential for ureteral injury as the shock wave can easily disrupt the ureteral mucosa if care is not taken. The probes for electrohydraulic lithotripsy come in various sizes, but the 1.6 to 3.0F sizes are commonly used with the ureteroscopes.

e.   Ultrasonic lithotripsy is most often used in percutaneous procedures to deal with large renal stones through a nephroscope. However, there are probes that have been designed for use through a ureteroscope. Ultrasound produces high-frequency vibration of the probe, a thin, hollow tube. The probe is placed against the stone, and the vibrations break up the stone. Suction is generally applied to the end of the probe, and fragments can be extracted through the hollow core.

F.   A ureteral stent is any catheter that allows urine to drain from the renal pelvis into the bladder. Ureteral stents are generally placed to allow for continued drainage of the upper tract should there be some edema of the ureter after manipulation. Stents can also be used to promote drainage during ureteral healing if a perforation occurred during the procedure. In the case of obstruction by a stone or an extrinsic ureteral process impinging on the ureteral lumen, stents can be used for decompression of the upper tract. Ureteral catheters described above can be used to divert the urine, but these are very prone to downward migration. Also, they exit through the meatus, a situation that can be cumbersome if they need to be left indwelling for any period of time. Indwelling ureteral stents have the advantage of being fully within the body so they are not troublesome to the patient. The most common stent is the **double-J** ureteral stent. This stent curls proximally within the renal pelvis to hold it in proper position and then curls at its distal end within the urinary bladder to prevent proximal migration. The stents come in various diameters from 5 to 8F and various lengths from 20 to 28 cm. Different lengths are used depending on the size of the patient. Newer stents have been developed recently that are basically one-size-fits-all. These stents have extra coils proximally that can unwind as needed for longer ureteral lengths.

III. Ureteroscopy is performed for either diagnostic or therapeutic purposes. The ureteroscope allows direct visualization of the urothelium of the upper urinary tract and may be used to resolve questions such as a radiologic filling defect or an abnormal urinary cytology localized to one ureter. Therapeutically, the ureteroscope may be used to deal with problems such as stone, tumor, or stricture within the upper tract. Ureteroscopy entails risk, and ureteroscopic procedures should be done in a manner that ensures maximum protection to the ureter.

A. Placing the safety guide wire. The initial step is to perform cystoscopy and retrograde ureterography. Once the upper tract has been evaluated by retrograde pyelogram, a guide wire is passed through the cystoscope and up the ureter to the renal pelvis. This is done under direct cystoscopic vision within the bladder and fluoroscopic guidance to follow the progress of the guide wire as it traverses the ureter. The cystoscope is positioned in close proximity to the ureteral orifice to be cannulated. The guide wire is passed through the cystoscope until the tip is visible through the cystoscope lens. With the cystoscope angled so that the wire will follow the approximate direction of the intramural ureter, the guide wire is gently advanced. With use of fluoroscopy, the wire can be followed as it travels up the ureter to the renal pelvis. The cystoscope should be kept in close proximity to the orifice so the wire does not coil within the bladder. If difficulty is encountered in aiming the wire toward the ureteral orifice, an open-ended ureteral catheter can be passed through the scope and the wire through the open-ended catheter. This often gives the wire more stability and eases introduction into the orifice. Once the wire is curled within the renal pelvis, the cystoscope can be removed, leaving the wire in place. Taking apart the cystoscope and removing the lens while leaving the sheath in place allow the operator to hold the wire in place and avoid pulling the wire out as the cystoscope is withdrawn. The sheath can then be removed while advancing the wire and observing the wire in the pelvis with fluoroscopy to ensure it is not pulled out. This wire is now snapped to the drapes and will remain throughout the procedure as the safety wire.

B. Accessing the ureter. If a ureteral access sheath is to be used, this is now passed over the wire as previously described. If no sheath is to be used, a balloon dilator can be passed over the wire, if necessary, to dilate the ureteral orifice.

C. Passing the ureteroscope. The ureteroscope is now connected to the light source, and, if desired, the camera and the irrigant are attached. The ureteroscope should be properly focused prior to its introduction into the genitourinary tract as focusing after passing the scope is often difficult. The ureteroscope is passed gently under direct vision through the urethra and into the bladder. Once within the bladder, the ureteral orifice is located. This can be facilitated by following the safety wire that is already in position. The wire is best located as it traverses the bladder neck and then simply followed to the ureteral orifice. The ureteroscope is then passed into the orifice, and the wire is followed up the ureter. If there is some difficulty in cannulating the ureter with the ureteroscope, it can be helpful to pass a second wire through the ureteroscope and into the ureter. This wire can then be followed directly up the ureter.

D.   Removing the ureteroscope. At the end of the ureteroscopic procedure, the ureteroscope is removed from the ureter under direct vision. Care should be taken not to drag the safety wire out of the ureter with the ureteroscope.

E.   Placing the ureteral stent. The safety wire is still in position and may be used to place a ureteral stent. The stent can be passed directly over the guide wire without cystoscopic guidance, or the cystoscope can passed back over the wire into the bladder by backloading the wire through the cystoscope. If the stent is to be passed without the cystoscope, the progress of the proximal end of the stent is followed under fluoroscopy. As the stent is advanced, the surgeon must make sure that it passes into the ureteral orifice and up the ureter without coiling within the bladder. As the stent is passed up into the renal pelvis, countertraction is held on the wire so that it remains in position and does not advance with the stent. Once the proximal end of the stent is within the renal pelvis, the guide wire can be withdrawn partially to allow the proximal end of the stent to curl within the pelvis. The fluoroscopy unit is now moved down to the bladder to properly position the distal end of the stent. The distal end of the stent is pushed up to the symphysis pubis with the pusher. The radiopaque band on the end of the pusher indicates where the end of the stent is located. In men, the end of the stent is advanced to the level of the upper border of the pubic symphysis, and in women to the lower border of the symphysis. The stent is then held in this position with the pusher as the guide wire is withdrawn. When the floppy tip of the wire is withdrawn into the bladder, the distal end of the stent will start to curl. The wire and the pusher are then removed. For uncomplicated ureteral procedures, the stent can be removed in 24 to 72 hours. If a ureteral perforation occurred, the stent should be left for 2 weeks and an imaging study obtained prior to removal to confirm healing. This can be either an intravenous pyelogram or a retrograde ureterogram done at the time of stent removal.

Urodynamic Studies

C. Charles Wen and Mike B. Siroky

Urodynamic studies include any objective assessment of lower urinary tract function that provides clinically useful information. Such studies include measurements of pressure, flow, and electromyographic potentials and may or may not include radiographic examinations. It is ideal if the patient's symptoms can be reproduced during the urodynamic examination, but this is not always possible. It is also useful to ask patients whether the function observed during urodynamic examination approximates their usual voiding pattern. Urodynamic testing is most useful when used in conjunction with a proper history, physical examination, and other tests to arrive at an accurate diagnosis.

I. The **cystometrogram** measures intravesical pressure during passive filling and active contraction (Fig. 7.1). Ideally, three pressures are measured: the intravesical pressure, the abdominal pressure, and the detrusor pressure, which is the difference between the first two pressures. This allows for differentiation between abdominal and detrusor events. The filling fluid may be either saline solution, water, radiographic contrast medium, or carbon dioxide. Cystometry may be considered a provocative test of bladder function wherein filling (stretch) is the stimulus and detrusor contraction is the evoked response. During cystometry, observations are made regarding bladder capacity, sensation, compliance (the slope of the filling curve), and detrusor contraction and stability.

A. Technique of cystometrography

1. The patient should be in the supine position.
2. The patient's meatus and perimeatal area are prepped in the usual fashion and a 14 or 16F Foley urethral catheter introduced. A rectal balloon catheter is inserted if abdominal pressure is to be measured.
3. Pressure transducers are aligned vertically with the patient's pubic symphysis, the lines flushed free of air bubbles with normal saline, and the transducers zeroed to atmospheric pressure. The transducers should be tested with a cough that should relay a pressure spike to both the abdominal and the vesical pressure channels nearly equally.
4. Filling should proceed at a rate of 50 mL/min (medium fill).
5. The patient should be asked to relay the following sensory information during filling: the first sensation of filling, the first urge to void, a strong urge to void, and maximum capacity.
6. When a contraction occurs, infusion should be stopped. If leakage occurs around the catheter, gentle traction on the Foley catheter or manual occlusion of the penile urethra will allow maximum intravesical pressure to develop. Once peak pressure develops, the patient should be asked to inhibit the contraction to test for detrusor instability of hyperreflexia. The catheter is then opened to the atmosphere, and the bladder is drained.

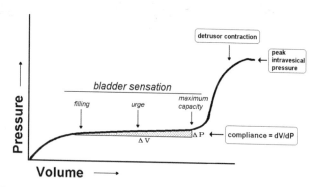

Fig. 7.1.   Idealized cystometric curve showing important parameters, including sensation reported by patient, detrusor contraction, and definition of compliance.

7.   The cystometrogram may be part of radiologic studies such as a voiding cystourethrogram or other urodynamic tests such as uroflowmetry and postvoid residual measurement.

B.   **Characteristics of the cystometrogram**

  1.   **Filling phase.** The normal cystometrogram during the filling phase is nearly flat, demonstrating little increase in pressure with increasing bladder volume. The characteristics of this portion of the cystometrographic curve depend primarily on the physical properties (**compliance**) of the bladder wall. Increased bladder compliance may reveal itself as a large-capacity bladder with little or no increase in pressure with filling. It can be seen after chronic urinary retention due to any cause. With decreased bladder compliance, pressure rises steadily with filling. Possible causes include chronic inflammation, radiation cystitis, interstitial cystitis, and bladder carcinoma. A steep filling curve may be due to a low-grade contraction or poor compliance. These can be differentiated by stopping bladder filling. If the pressure stops rising or dips slightly, this likely represents a poorly compliant bladder.

  2.   **Bladder sensation.** The great majority of normal persons report a sensation of filling at a bladder volume between 100 and 300 mL. This sensation is followed by an urge to void that is distinct from the filling sensation. Sensory abnormalities include absence of filling sensation and urge to void. Discomfort and urgency at low volumes are typical of inflammatory conditions such as lower urinary tract infections, radiation cystitis, and interstitial cystitis.

  3.   **Contraction phase.** Detrusor activity during cystometry represents an isovolumetric contraction because little or no leakage is permitted. The normal contraction is a relatively rapid and sustained rise in pressure to a peak of 60 to 120 cm H_2O. Normal persons are aware of an urge to void before the contraction and can suppress the detrusor contraction completely or partially if asked to do so.

a. Detrusor overactivity, whether from neurogenic causes or not, is usually (but not always) characterized by cystometric capacity of ≤200 mL. *More important than the capacity, however, is the inability to inhibit the detrusor contraction.* The term **detrusor hyperreflexia** is usually reserved for instances caused by a known neurologic lesion, whereas **detrusor instability** is commonly used to denote cases with nonneurogenic or idiopathic causes.

b. Acontractile detrusor is characterized by lack of a detrusor contraction on filling of the bladder. The term **detrusor areflexia** should be reserved for cases in which a clearly defined neurologic condition is the cause; all other instances are more accurately termed acontractile detrusor. It is important to remember that approximately 10% of men and 50% of women without a voiding abnormality demonstrate no detrusor contraction during the cystometrogram because of psychological inhibition. This is one of the most common reasons for overinterpretation of cystometrographic tracings.

(1) **Bethanechol supersensitivity testing** may be used in acontractile bladder to determine whether the cause is neurogenic. This test is based on **Cannon's law,** which states that an exaggerated response to its natural neurotransmitter develops in a denervated organ (**denervation supersensitivity**).

(2) **Use of bethanechol chloride.** As originally described by Lapides, 2.5 mg of bethanechol chloride was used as the test agent, and an increase of 15 cm H_2O in bladder pressure was the test criterion. We have found improved sensitivity and specificity by using a dose of 5 mg in patients weighing >75 kg and a test criterion of 20 cm H_2O. Alternatively, one can use a weight-adjusted dose of 0.03 mg/kg. Bethanechol is contraindicated in patients with gastrointestinal obstruction, bronchial asthma, peptic ulcer, bradycardia, hypotension, or parkinsonism. Atropine (0.4 mg IM) should always be available to reverse any adverse effects of the drug.

(3) **Cystometric pressure measurement.** After the bladder is filled slowly to 100 mL, the intravesical pressure is measured. The appropriate dose of bethanechol chloride is administered subcutaneously (not intradermally or intramuscularly, and never intravenously). The onset of cholinergic effect occurs after about 15 minutes and is indicated by flushing and increased salivation. Cystometry is repeated up to a volume of 100 mL.

(4) **Interpretation.** An increase of 20 cm H_2O in comparison with the baseline value is indicative of supersensitivity and suggests bladder denervation. **False-positive results** may occur in patients with inflammatory bladder disease or acute urinary tract infection. **False-negative results** may occur if the test is performed within the first 8 weeks after denervation, when the supersensitive response may not be fully developed. A

supersensitive response to bethanechol does not imply a therapeutic benefit from oral use of the agent.

(5)   Ice water test. Instillation of 50 to 100 mL of ice-cold water will provoke a bladder contraction in many patients with spinal cord injury, demonstrating that the sacral reflex arc is intact.

c.   Impaired detrusor contractility is characterized by a weak or short-lived detrusor contraction. This is a not uncommon finding in elderly patients of both sexes and may be caused by replacement of smooth muscle by collagen.

II.   Uroflowmetry is among the most useful of all urodynamic studies (Fig. 7.2). The test requires only that the patient void an adequate amount into the flowmeter to permit measurement of the flow rate. The most important determinant of the normal flow rate is the initial bladder volume. The urinary flow increases as initial bladder volume increases. Table 7.1 lists minimal peak flow values for various patient groups. The parameters used in uroflowmetry are shown in Fig. 7.2. To compare flow rates before and after therapy or over a period of time, it is useful to refer to a flow rate nomogram (Fig. 7.3). The shape of the uroflow curve may also provide useful information; for example, an irregular flow curve may indicate abdominal straining or vesicosphincter dyssynergia.

III.   Electromyography of the striated perineal musculature provides two kinds of information: (a) contractile activity and (b) state of innervation. Surface electrodes readily provide the first kind of information and are used widely in children because they are noninvasive. Surface electrodes may also be used in adult patients, either as surface patch or in the form of anal–vaginal plugs.

For more detailed studies of innervation, needle electrodes must be used. In male patients, a 50-mm concentric electrode is placed into the bulbocavernosus muscle or the external urethral sphincter (Fig. 7.4). In female patients, a 30-mm electrode is placed into the external anal sphincter or the periurethral striated muscle (Fig. 7.5). In normal persons, the electromyogram will show no evidence of denervation, normal sacral reflexes will be present, and the patient will be able to contract the perineal muscles voluntarily. With bladder filling, a gradual increase in electromyographic activity is noted, referred to as the **guarding reflex** (Fig. 7.6). With the onset of bladder contraction, electromyographic activity decreases or ceases for the entire voiding process. Failure of the perineal muscles to relax during a detrusor contraction is **vesicosphincter dyssynergia** (Fig. 7.6). In some patients who use abdominal straining to void in the absence of a detrusor contraction, electromyographic activity may persist during straining; this is called **pseudodyssynergia.**

IV.   Urethral pressure may be measured by several different techniques. The primary indications for this examination are in the diagnosis of stress urinary incontinence, evaluation of obstruction, assessment of drug actions, and monitoring of antiincontinence devices.

A. In the **Brown–Wickham technique,** a pressure-measuring catheter is withdrawn from the bladder through the urethra, providing a profile of the urethral pressure at each point. The examination is most commonly performed with

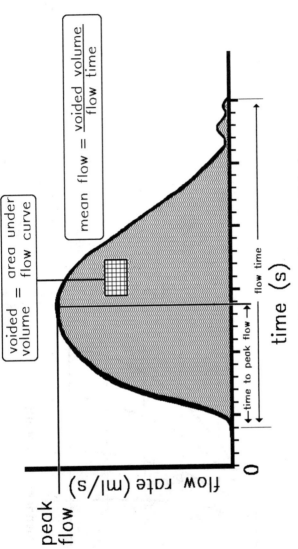

Fig. 7.2. Idealized uroflow curve showing peak flow, mean flow, and voided volume.

Table 7.1. Normal uroflow values for voided volumes of >150 mL

Patient Group	Age (y)	Normal Peak Flow Rate (mL/s)
Men	<40	>22
	40–60	>18
	>60	>13
Women	<50	>25
	>50	>18
Children, adolescents	<10	>15
	10–20	>20

a side-hole catheter, which is perfused with saline solution at a rate of about 2 mL/min while being withdrawn at 0.5 cm/s. An idealized curve showing the parameters of urethral profilometry is depicted in Fig. 7.7. The two most important parameters are the maximal urethral pressure (peak pressure) and the functional urethra length (Table 7.2). In women, maximal pressure tends to fall with age, whereas in men, the functional length tends to increase with age. One can observe from Table 7.2 that the normal range is wide and overlaps considerably with abnormal values, which reduces the usefulness of profilometry as a diagnostic tool.

B. Abdominal leak point pressure, measured during a fluoroscopic cystogram, is useful in determining the minimum pres-

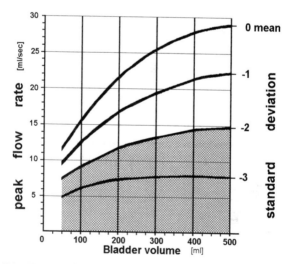

Fig. 7.3. Flow rate nomogram relating maximum flow rate to initial bladder volume.

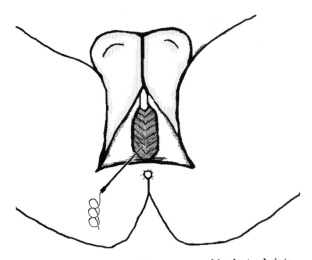

Fig. 7.4. Placement of needle electromyographic electrode into bulbocavernosus muscle in male.

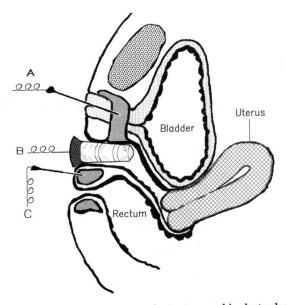

Fig. 7.5. Examples of placement of electromyographic electrodes in female. A: Needle electrode in urethral sphincter. B: Vaginal surface electrode. C: Needle electrode in external anal sphincter.

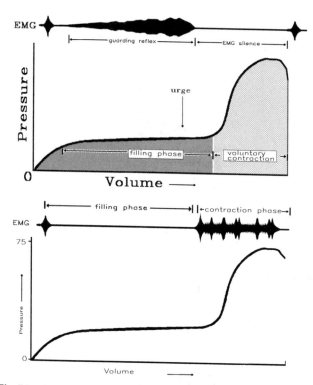

Fig. 7.6.   **Combined cystometrogram and perineal electromyogram showing normal coordinated voiding pattern (top) and vesicosphincter dyssynergia (bottom).**

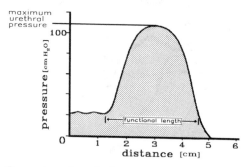

Fig. 7.7.   **Parameters of urethral pressure profile.**

Table 7.2.   Normal values for Brown–Wickham urethral pressure profile

Patient Group	Age (y)	Peak Pressure (cm H$_2$O)	Functional Length (cm)
Men	<50	65–105	3.5–4.5
	>50	65–105	4.0–5.5
Women	<50	60–90	2.0–3.5
	>50	50–80	2.0–3.5

sure required to cause leakage. The bladder is gradually filled with contrast agent and monitored fluoroscopically. After a volume of at least 200 mL has been reached, the patient is placed in a sitting or upright position and asked to perform the Valsalva maneuver gradually. The lowest total bladder pressure at which leakage is detected is the abdominal leak point pressure. If no leakage occurs with the Valsalva maneuver, the patient is asked to cough several times, and fluoroscopic examination for the presence of leakage is repeated. Patients with a competent urethra typically have an abdominal leak point pressure above 120 cm H$_2$O; those with urethral incompetence have an abdominal leak point pressure below 60 cm H$_2$O.

V.   Pressure–flow studies and video urodynamics are especially useful in the diagnosis and localization of outflow obstruction; however, they may be used in all types of voiding dysfunction (Fig. 7.8).

A.   Technique. The study is performed by filling the bladder via a two- or three-lumen 4 to 7F catheter in the urethra. A rectal balloon catheter is placed for measurement of abdominal pressure. The transducers are zeroed to the atmospheric pressure and placed at the level of the patient's symphysis pubis. All air bubbles should be flushed from the pressure lines to prevent damping of the response. The patient should be asked to cough to test the response and accuracy of the measurement. Although some self-retaining catheters are available, most urodynamic catheters are straight catheters that must be taped or otherwise fixed to the penis. In female patients, the catheter is taped carefully to the inner thigh. A two-lumen urodynamic catheter provides for filling through one channel and measurement of bladder pressure through the second lumen. A three-lumen catheter provides for measurement of urethral pressure as well. The bladder is filled at a rate of 20 to 50 mL/min, and a cystometrogram is performed. When the male patient reports the urge to void, he is asked to stand and micturate into the flow meter around the urodynamic catheter in the urethra. In the case of a female patient, a urodynamic chair is used to permit voiding in the sitting position. The entire process may be filmed fluoroscopically and recorded on videotape (video urodynamics). The addition of video capability may permit more accurate localization of the site of outflow obstruction and is also very useful in patients with incontinence.

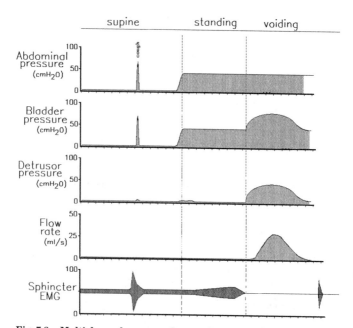

Fig. 7.8.   Multichannel pressure flow study showing abdominal pressure, bladder pressure, detrusor pressure, flow rate, and electromyography.

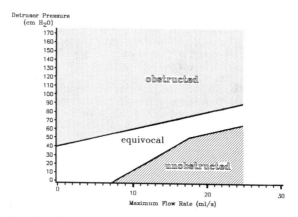

Fig. 7.9.   The Abrams–Griffiths nomogram.

B. Interpretation. High intravesical voiding pressures (typically >50 cm H_2O) associated with low flow rates (below 10 mL/s) are indicative of outflow obstruction. A more accurate assessment of outflow obstruction can be obtained by using the Abrams—Griffiths nomogram (Fig. 7.9). An approximation of the nomogram reading can be obtained by calculating the Abrams–Griffiths number (AG number), which equals P_{det} Q_{max} – $2Q_{max}$, where P_{det} is subtracted bladder pressure and Q_{max} is peak urinary flow. An AG number of >40 is indicative of obstruction, whereas a value of <20 indicates no obstruction; between 20 and 40 is considered equivocal. A variety of other pressure–flow nomograms, such as that of Schafer, exist to classify patients into obstructed or nonobstructed categories. Many times, nomograms are included in software packages that control urodynamic testing equipment. This software can automatically plot patient results on a nomogram to help in making a diagnosis of outlet obstruction.

SUGGESTED READING

Eckhardt MD, van Venrooij GE, Boon TA. Urethral resistance factor (URA) versus Schäfer's obstruction grade and Abrams–Griffiths (AG) number in the diagnosis of obstructive benign prostatic hyperplasia. *Neurourol Urodyn* 2001;20:175–185.

Khourym JM, Marson L, Carson CC III. A comparative study of the Abrams–Griffiths nomogram and the linear passive urethral resistance relation to determine bladder outlet obstruction. *J Urol* 1998;159:758–760.

Klingele CJ, Carley ME, Hill RFC. Patient characteristics that are associated with urodynamically diagnosed detrusor instability and genuine stress incontinence. *Am J Obstet Gynecol* 2002;186: 866–868.

Rosario DJ, Chapple CR, Tophill PR, et al. Urodynamic assessment of the bashful bladder. *J Urol* 2000;163:215.

Siroky MB. Interpretation of urinary flow rates. *Urol Clin North Am* 1990;17:537–541.

Siroky MB. Electromyography of the perineal floor. *Urol Clin North Am* 1996;23:299–302.

Van Venrooij GEPM, Van Melick HHE, Eckhardt MD, et al. Correlations of urodynamic changes with changes in symptoms and well-being after transurethral resection of the prostate. *J Urol* 2002; 168:605–609.

Walker RMH, Romano G, Davies AH, et al. Pressure flow study data in a group of asymptomatic male control patients 45 years old or older. *J Urol* 2001;165:683–687.

Lower Urinary Tract Symptoms

Peter A. Zeman, Mike B. Siroky,
and Richard K. Babayan

I. Pathogenesis of lower urinary tract symptoms

Almost all lower urinary tract symptoms (LUTS) manifest themselves via the bladder. An obstructive process such as benign enlargement of the prostate rarely causes symptoms in its own right. Rather, symptoms are due almost exclusively to secondary bladder dysfunction, either bladder overactivity or underactivity. In general, LUTS are not in themselves diagnostic, and terms such as "obstructive symptoms" should be avoided. Symptoms should be elicited from the patient in great detail, focusing on their onset, characteristics, duration, intensity, and amelioration. Management requires an understanding of the relevant pathophysiology and an orderly approach to diagnosis and therapy.

II. Definitions

The most common **LUTS** are urinary frequency, urgency, and hesitancy, weak stream, and nocturia. This symptom complex was previously referred to as "prostatism," but this has been replaced by the term "LUTS." The reason for this change is that the term "prostatism" implies that these symptoms are caused by the prostate, *which is most often not the case.* For example, bladder instability may exist in the absence of outflow obstruction and can produce the same symptoms as prostatic obstruction. **Voiding symptoms,** previously called "obstructive symptoms," refer to symptoms associated with voiding such as hesitancy, intermittency, weak stream, postvoid dribbling, double voiding, and use of abdominal straining to void. A weak stream is characterized by diminished force, diminished caliber, and prolonged voiding time. Patients may also complain of incomplete emptying. **Storage symptoms,** previously called "irritative symptoms," include daytime frequency, urgency, urge incontinence, nocturia, dysuria, and sometimes enuresis. Urinary frequency is the subjective complaint that voiding occurs at "too frequent" intervals, usually <2 hours apart. Voiding of large volumes of urine is **polyuria** and may be confused with urinary frequency. Urinary frequency is often associated with **urgency,** which is the sudden desire for urination that is difficult or impossible to postpone. **Nocturia** refers to urinary urgency that awakens the patient from sleep, and it should be distinguished from other reasons for voiding during sleep, such as insomnia. **Nocturnal enuresis** is incontinence of urine during sleep. **Acute retention** refers to the sudden onset of complete inability to void in a patient who may or may not have had urinary symptoms previously. **Chronic retention** refers to the presence of postvoiding residual urine in the bladder of a patient who is able to void, albeit poorly. **Sensory symptoms** include bladder hypersensitivity, reduced desire to void, and absence of sensation of bladder fullness.

Table 8.1. Some common causes of lower urinary tract symptoms in adults

Outflow obstruction
  Benign prostatic enlargement
  Vesical neck obstruction
  Urethral stricture
  Meatal stenosis
  Cystocele in females

Impaired detrusor function
  Neuromuscular dysfunction
  Detrusor instability
  Impaired detrusor contractility
  Psychogenic voiding dysfunction

Infection
  Cystitis
  Bacterial prostatitis
  Prostatic abscess
  Urethral diverticulum

Neoplastic
  Prostate cancer
  Bladder cancer, including carcinoma in situ

Other
  Bladder diverticulum
  Bladder stone
  Interstitial cystitis

III. Differential diagnosis

LUTS may result from a wide variety of conditions (Table 8.1), some of which are obstructive, some nonobstructive. These conditions may be classified anatomically as follows:

A. Anterior urethra. Meatal stenosis presents commonly in newborns or during infancy; it may be congenital or secondary to ammonia dermatitis. In male adults, the condition may be secondary to inflammation of the prepuce (posthitis) or of the glans penis (balanitis or balanitis xerotica obliterans). **Urethral** or **meatal stenosis** in female adults is very uncommon. **Urethral strictures** in male adults most commonly result from trauma sustained during instrumentation, catheterization, or endoscopic surgery. Inflammatory strictures, whether caused by gonorrhea or nonspecific urethritis, occur most commonly in the bulbous urethra.

B. Posterior urethra. In male infants and newborns, **posterior urethral valves** are the most common obstructing lesion. These are congenital mucosal folds in the region of the membranous urethra that often obstruct the flow of urine. In adults, **sphincter spasm** may result in obstruction when the striated urethral sphincter fails to relax during micturition; this may be due to neurologic disease (spinal cord injury, multiple sclerosis) or psychogenic voiding dysfunction. When caused by neurologic dysfunction, it is termed **vesicosphincter dyssynergia.**

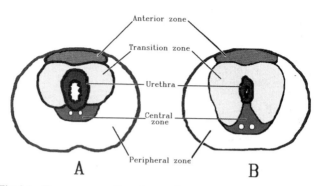

A   B

Fig. 8.1.   Transverse section of normal prostate (A) and prostate with benign hypertrophy (B).

C.   The prostate. The term **benign prostatic hyperplasia** (BPH) refers to well-defined histologic changes characterized by slowly progressive nodular hyperplasia of the periurethral (transitional) zone of the prostate (Fig. 8.1). At autopsy, >75% of men over the age of 80 have histologic evidence of BPH. However, BPH is a histologic diagnosis and does not necessarily imply prostatic enlargement or symptoms (Fig. 8.2). **Benign prostatic enlargement** is a clinical diagnosis of prostatic enlargement. Because we rarely know the precise histologic findings in the prostate, "benign prostatic enlargement" is a preferable term for clinical use. There is only a weak correlation between the presence of LUTS, bladder outflow obstruction, and benign prostatic enlargement. **Prostate adenocarcinoma,** although a common neoplasm, rarely causes obstruction until the disease is quite advanced. **Acute prostatitis** or **prostatic abscess** may rarely cause obstruction or even urinary retention as well as frequency, urgency, and dysuria.

D.   The bladder

1.   Bladder neck obstruction may occur when the bladder neck fails to open as a result of either neurologic disease (very rare), idiopathic dysfunction (not uncommon), or contracture (common). Bladder neck contracture is most often a result of trauma or surgery. Functional bladder neck obstruction is characterized by failure of the vesical neck to open completely during voiding without evident structural cause. This type of obstruction often masquerades as benign prostatic enlargement but typically occurs in a younger age group (30 to 45 years). **Cystocele** in female patients may cause obstruction by creating an acute angulation at the vesical neck.

2.   Bladder neuromuscular dysfunction may present as urinary retention, voiding, or storage symptoms. **Detrusor overactivity** may be associated with neurologic disease (**detrusor hyperreflexia**) or with nonneurologic causes (**detrusor instability**). Detrusor overactivity is characterized by the sudden onset of severe urinary urgency. In some cases, voiding occurs almost immediately after the onset of urgency, leading to urge incontinence. **Impaired detrusor contractility** is usually idiopathic and is common in elderly patients

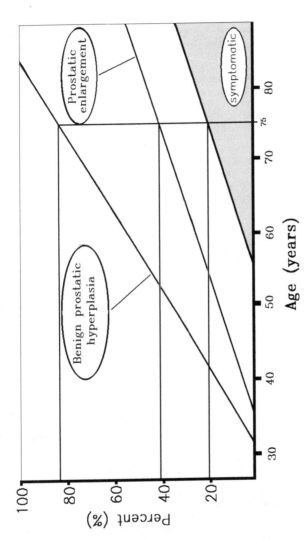

Fig. 8.2. At age 75, >80% of men demonstrate histologic evidence of nodular hyperplasia, but only half of them have prostatic enlargement and even fewer are symptomatic.

of either sex. It may occur after prolonged overdistension of the bladder wall. Patients with impaired contractility may have significant postvoiding residual urine, which does not necessarily indicate the presence of outflow obstruction. **Peripheral neuropathy** may involve the autonomic fibers supplying the detrusor muscle; common causes include diabetes mellitus, alcoholism, uremia, and surgical trauma. **Pharmacologic agents,** including nonprescription drugs, may have antimuscarinic properties and precipitate urinary retention or impaired voiding. Among these are phenothiazines, antihistamines, and α-adrenergic agonists such as pseudoephedrine, ephedrine, and phenylpropanolamine that are contained in many over-the-counter "cold" remedies. **Psychogenic voiding dysfunction** is characterized by lifelong detrusor instability or pelvic floor spasm leading to urge incontinence, impaired voiding, or discomfort in the suprapubic area or perineum.

3. Bladder response to outflow obstruction. The response of the detrusor muscle to the increased work load associated with outflow obstruction varies over time.

a. Early obstruction. At this stage, the detrusor undergoes hyperplasia, and bladder contractility may be normal or slightly impaired. The bladder is able to empty completely or nearly completely; however, **bladder instability** is likely to develop in 60% to 80% of patients. Unstable bladder contractions are involuntary contractions that are difficult to inhibit. Such contractions produce the sensation of urgency even at low volumes and account for symptoms such as urinary frequency and urgency and nocturia.

b. Late obstruction. The bladder is unable to empty completely, and postvoiding residual urine is present. Detrusor muscle contractility is significantly impaired. At this stage, residual urine results as much from poorly sustained bladder contractions as from inadequate detrusor pressure. The patient notes urinary hesitancy and intermittency and a weak stream and may complain of a sensation of incomplete voiding. With severe obstruction, the patient may use abdominal straining to void, and many male patients will sit to void to increase abdominal voiding pressure.

c. Decompensation. The ability of the detrusor muscle to contract is severely impaired to the point that little effective pressure is generated. The bladder may empty by frequent, ineffective voiding or by dribbling (overflow or paradoxical incontinence).

4. Secondary effects of obstruction. Over time, outflow obstruction leads to characteristic changes in the bladder and upper urinary tract. These changes may be observed cystoscopically and radiologically.

a. Bladder trabeculation. Prominence of the submucosal bladder tissue observed through a cystoscope is termed "trabeculation." It is a manifestation of increased collagen deposition in the bladder wall. This finding is often associated with outflow obstruction but may also be seen in unobstructed bladders (e.g., enuresis, neurogenic bladder dysfunction, idiopathic bladder instability). The interureteric ridge (Bell's muscle) becomes prominent, and the bladder neck is also hypertrophied. Hypertrophy of the vesical neck causes an acute angulation between the trigone and prostatic urethra, which is described cystoscopically as a *basfond* deformity.

b. Cellule formation. Extreme degrees of trabeculation allow the vesical mucosa to be pushed between the collagen and muscle fibers of the bladder wall to form small pockets called cellules.

c. Diverticulum formation. Herniation of the vesical mucosa through the detrusor muscle constitutes a bladder diverticulum. Acquired bladder diverticula contain no muscular components and are therefore prone to poor emptying even if the bladder is emptied by catheterization. Because of stasis of urine within the diverticulum, they are likely to harbor infection, stones, and urothelial cancer. A diverticulum near the ureteric orifice (Hutch diverticulum) may cause vesicoureteral reflux.

d. Bladder calculi. In developed countries, bladder calculi form most commonly as a result of outflow obstruction, residual urine, stasis, and infection. The presence of a bladder calculus is strong evidence of long-standing bladder outflow obstruction. The most common mineral constituent of these stones is calcium oxalate. Stones also may occur within bladder diverticula.

e. Hydroureteronephrosis. With hypertrophy and fibrosis of the detrusor wall, increased work is required to transport the urinary bolus from the ureter into the bladder. In the early stages, the condition appears radiologically as mild dilatation of the distal segment and elongation and some tortuosity of the ureter. Later, more marked dilatation of the entire ureter, marked elongation and tortuosity, and attenuation of the ureteral wall are seen.

IV. Diagnostic approach

The patient with LUTS needs a well-planned assessment to determine (a) the nature and severity of symptoms, (b) whether there is objective evidence of obstruction, (c) whether there is objective evidence of detrusor dysfunction, and (d) the effect of the obstruction on the upper urinary tract.

A. Symptoms. The nature and severity of symptoms are important criteria in determining therapy. Symptoms should be quantified with standardized symptom scores such as that developed by the American Urological Association (AUA) (see Appendix I, page 508). The questionnaire consists of seven questions to quantify symptoms and sections to determine how bothersome symptoms are and assess quality of life. The symptom score appears to separate symptomatic patients from control patients fairly well (Table 8.2). Although treatment should be individualized, as a general rule, patients with a score of ≤7 are considered to have mild symptoms that probably do not require immediate treatment unless hydronephrosis or uremia is present. Patients with moderate symptoms (AUA score of 8 to 20) probably are in need of some therapy. Patients with severe symptoms (AUA score above 20) frequently require treatment to avoid development of complications. An eighth question frequently asked in conjunction with the AUA symptom scale is the bothersome index. This categorizes just how bothered a patient

Table 8.2. Distribution of scores on the American Urological Association (AUA) symptom index

AUA Score	BPE Patients (%)	Control Subjects (%)
Mild (0–7 points)	20	83
Moderate (8–19 points)	57	15
Severe (20–35 points)	23	2

BPE, benign prostatic enlargement.

is by his voiding symptoms and the impact it has on his lifestyle.

B. History. A detailed urologic history should be taken, assessing prior surgery, infections, strictures, stones, tumors, or bleeding in the urinary tract. The general medical history should especially focus on vascular disease (cardiac, cerebral, and peripheral), pulmonary disease (asthma, chronic obstructive pulmonary disease), and habits (alcohol consumption, smoking). A detailed list of all medications (prescription and nonprescription) should be developed.

C. Physical examination

1.   In female patients, a **pelvic examination** is required to assess the presence of cystocele, urethral stenosis, or urethral diverticulum.

2.   Flank and abdomen. In thin patients, the bladder can be palpated or percussed when distended to >200 mL. In severe chronic retention, the dome of the bladder may reach almost to the umbilicus. Pressing on the distended bladder may cause discomfort or urgency or both. The flank area should be palpated and percussed for evidence of mass or tenderness.

3.   Male genitalia. The male genitalia are best examined with the patient standing and facing the seated examiner. If this is not feasible, the patient may be supine. The glans and foreskin should be examined for signs of phimosis, infection, and meatal stenosis. The testes should be examined for size, consistency, and mass or tenderness. The spermatic cord may reveal varicocele or inguinal hernia.

4.   Examination of the prostate is best performed with patients bent over the examining table, supported on their elbows. An alternative and less desirable position is the lateral decubitus position with one leg drawn up toward the abdomen. The examiner's gloved, generously lubricated index finger is inserted slowly into the rectum. The purpose of the examination is to assess prostatic size, symmetry, and consistency; to assess anal tone; and to determine the presence of rectal masses. A lax anal sphincter that the patient cannot contract may be indicative of peripheral neuropathy or lower spinal cord lesion. In some patients, the seminal vesicles are easily palpable as thickened cords extending cephalad from the base of the prostate. An inexperienced examiner can confuse the seminal vesicles with prostate cancer. In young adult male patients, the prostate is usually described as about the size of a chestnut. The earliest change in benign prostatic enlargement is loss of the median depression or furrow. With increasing size, the prostate extends laterally and cephalad until the examining finger cannot reach the base of the gland. It is important to remember that only the posterior lobe of the prostate is palpable through the rectal wall. This lobe, however, gives rise to most prostate carcinomas. Early, treatable prostate cancer is most commonly found on prostate examination as an area of induration within the substance of the prostate and not as a nodule extending above the surface of the gland. For this reason, the examiner must assess the consistency of the prostate by firm palpation, which is somewhat uncomfortable for most patients and may produce urinary urgency. The normal prostate has a weight of approximately 20 g, and its consistency is approximated by the tensed adductor pollicis muscle at the base of the thumb. If any areas are more firm than this, the examiner should suspect prostate carcinoma and consider biopsy. The differential diagnosis of a prostate nodule includes prostate cancer, asymmetric BPH growth, prostatic calculi, and granulomatous prostatitis. Approximately 50% of prostate nodules discovered on rectal examination prove to be carcinoma on biopsy.

5.   The **focused neurologic examination** should include perineal sensation and assessment of bulbocavernosus reflex. The bulbocavernosus reflex may be tested during the rectal examination by gently squeezing the glans penis to assess the presence of anal sphincter contraction.

D.   Laboratory tests should include urinalysis, urine culture, complete blood count, and determination of serum creatinine, blood urea nitrogen, blood sugar, and serum electrolytes for most patients. For male patients over age 50 (and even younger if there is a family history of prostate cancer or if the patient is African American), a test for prostate-specific antigen (PSA) is highly recommended to screen for prostate cancer.

E.   Assessment of upper tracts. Routine assessment of the upper tracts is not recommended for the patient with LUTS unless hematuria, recurrent urinary tract infection, azotemia, prior urinary tract surgery, or a history of urinary stones is present. Ultrasonography (US) of the kidneys and bladder is the preferred means of initial radiologic assessment, unless hematuria is detected (see Chapter 2). US is preferred because it offers rapid, accurate assessment of hydroureteronephrosis, prostatic size, and bladder residual. It is safer and less expensive than computed tomography (CT) urography or intravenous urography (IVU). This is especially true in uremic or dehydrated patients because it does not involve contrast agent injection or radiation. However, the presence of hematuria (gross or microscopic) is a strong indication for CT urography and for IVU because they offer more complete visualization of the upper tract urothelial surfaces than does US.

F.   Assessment of the lower tract may include a variety of radiologic and other procedures. These tests are optional and should be selected based on the patient's history and other findings.

1.   Retrograde urethrogram. Retrograde urethrogram (RUG) is performed by retrograde instillation of radiographic contrast medium into the male urethra. RUG is most useful in visualizing lesions of the anterior urethra such as strictures, diverticula, and urethral perforations. Lesions of the posterior urethra (proximal to the genitourinary diaphragm) are poorly visualized by this technique because the striated urethral sphincter often prevents contrast agent from completely filling the posterior urethra or bladder.

2.   Voiding cystourethrogram. The voiding cystourethrogram (VCUG) is performed by filling the bladder with radiographic contrast agent through a urethral catheter or suprapubic tube. The entire process of filling and voiding is monitored by fluoroscopy. Static films are obtained with the bladder full, during micturition, and after voiding. VCUG is an excellent method of diagnosing vesical neck obstruction, vesicosphincter dyssynergia, and vesicoureteral reflux. It is also useful in assessing the presence of cystocele in female patients.

3.   Cystourethroscopy. Endoscopy permits direct visualization of the entire lower urinary tract (see Chapter 5) and contributes to the diagnosis of most obstructive lesions such as prostatic enlargement, vesical neck contracture, and urethral stricture. Changes in the bladder are indicated by the presence of trabeculation, cellules, and diverticula, which provide indirect evidence of obstruction.

4.   Uroflowmetry. An electronic flowmeter can provide a recording of urinary flow rate versus time (Fig. 8.3). The peak flow rate is a sensitive indicator of outflow obstruction. The bladder volume at the start of micturition has an important effect on the peak flow rate and may be accounted for by the use of flow rate nomograms (Fig. 7.3). Other useful parameters are the **time to peak flow** and the shape of the flow curve (see Chapter 7). Uroflowmetry should always be performed in conjunction with estimation of **postvoiding residual urine volume.** This may be done by catheterization or by US examination (preferred). The normal peak flow should be >12 mL/s in normal male adults voiding >150 mL.

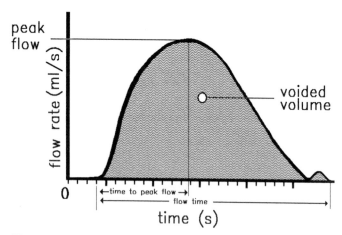

Fig. 8.3.   Important parameters of uroflowmetry include the peak flow, voided volume, and time to peak flow.

5. Cystometry. The cystometrogram (Fig. 8.1) is a continuous recording of bladder pressure during gradual filling and during contraction. The examination is indicated in any patient with LUTS when detrusor instability, neurologic disease, or myogenic bladder failure is suspected. The finding of detrusor instability, even in asymptomatic volunteers, is common and should be interpreted carefully in light of the patient's clinical picture. **Ambulatory cystometry** may be used in cases in which one needs a long-term view of bladder activity (24 to 72 hours). See Chapter 7 for a discussion of cystometrogram technique and interpretation.

6. Pressure–flow studies allow simultaneous measurement of voiding pressure and flow rate and are usually combined with fluoroscopy. These studies are indicated in cases such as incontinence after prostatectomy, failed incontinence surgery, LUTS refractory to standard treatment, and LUTS associated with neurologic disease.

V. Treatment
A. Distal urethra

1. Meatal stenosis of minor degree may simply be dilated. Recurrent or severe meatal stenosis is best managed by surgical meatotomy rather than dilation.

2. Urethral strictures occur most often in male patients after urethral infection or trauma.

    a. Dilation may be accomplished by means of van Buren sounds or filiforms and followers. Dilation of a stricture is generally not curative, as there is a high recurrence rate.

    b. Visual urethrotomy. With an optical urethrotome, the stricture can be visualized and incised with a movable knife blade. This is a safe and effective procedure, with a 1-year patency rate of 60%. Visual urethrotomy may be repeated multiple times as required. The neodymium-YAG (yttrium–aluminum–garnet) and holmium laser can also be used to incise strictures in the urethra and is becoming the procedure of choice where available.

    c. Transurethral balloon dilation catheter. Balloon dilation has been found by one group to offer similar short-term efficacy as rigid dilation and internal urethrotomy. It was found to be associated with minimal complications.

    d. Urethroplasty. The visual urethrotomy has eliminated the need for urethroplasty in many cases. A urethroplasty should be considered in the face of rapid stricture recurrence following visual urethrotomy or difficult dilatation.

B. Benign prostatic enlargement.
The treatment of benign prostatic enlargement is highly individualized and depends on the severity of symptoms and presence of complications (Fig. 8.4). Refractory urinary retention, upper tract deterioration, recurrent infection, hematuria, and bladder stones are strong indications for intervention. For patients without these findings, the level of symptoms is the main determinant of the type and timing of therapy.

1. Watchful waiting involves careful follow-up of symptoms and signs without active intervention and is recommended for the majority of patients with mild symptoms (AUA score of 0 to 7). Approximately 30% of patients will experience improvement with watchful waiting. On the other hand, the risk for symptom progression is low (1% to 5%).

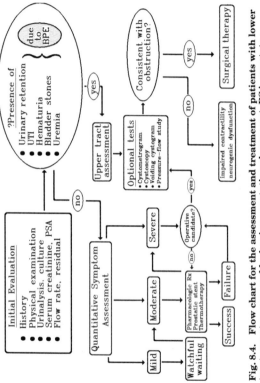

Fig. 8.4.   Flow chart for the assessment and treatment of patients with lower tract symptoms caused by benign prostatic enlargement. PSA, prostate-specific antigen; UTI, urinary tract infection; BPE, benign prostatic enlargement.

2. **Pharmacologic therapy**
  a. **α-Adrenergic blocking agents.** The prostate contains smooth muscle that is controlled by α_1-adrenoceptors (Table 8.3), and blockade of these receptors has been proposed as the mechanism of symptom relief due to α-adrenergic blocking agents. Recently, it has been proposed that α-adrenergic blocking agents with a quinazoline chemical structure (doxazosin, prazosin, terazosin, but not tamsulosin) induce prostatic apoptosis that also contributes to their relief of symptoms due to benign prostatic enlargement. Side effects of α-adrenergic blocking agents include dizziness, light-headedness, and asthenia and are related to their antihypertensive actions. Other side effects include nasal congestion, tachycardia, palpitations, nervousness, and retrograde ejaculation. Less selective α-adrenergic blocking agents such as terazosin tend to be associated with a greater incidence of side effects. Tamsulosin, a superselective α_{1a} blocker, provides even lower potential for drug–drug interactions and fewer vasodilatory effects. About 50% to 75% of patients experience rapid improvement in symptoms with any of the α-adrenergic blocking agents.
  b. **Finasteride,** a 5α-reductase inhibitor, blocks the conversion of testosterone to dihydrotestosterone. Clinical experience has shown that finasteride reduces prostatic size by about 20%, improves urinary flow rate by about 2 mL/s, and reduces AUA symptom scores by 3.6 points. The dose is 5 mg by mouth daily. Side effects are minimal and include headache, minimal loss of libido, and occasional impotence. One important consequence is that finasteride lowers serum PSA by about 50% after 6 months of therapy.
  c. **Phytotherapy.** Pharmaceuticals derived from plant extracts are widely used outside the United States and increasingly within the United States. Although these compounds do not require a prescription, it is important for the urologist to be familiar with self-administered medications.

Table 8.3. α-Adrenergic blocking agents used in benign prostatic enlargement

Generic Name	Brand Name	Dose Forms	Dose	
			Initial	Maximum
Doxazosin	Cardura	1-, 2-, 4-, 8-mg tablets	1 mg qd	8 mg qd
Terazosin	Hytrin	1-, 2-, 5-, 10-mg capsules	1 mg hs	20 mg hs
Prazosin	Minipress	1-, 2-, 5-mg capsules	1 mg tid	20 mg qd
Tamsulosin	Flomax	0.4-mg capsules	0.4 mg qd	0.8 mg qd

The mechanism of action of many of these compounds is unknown or poorly understood. However, there is some evidence that they may inhibit 5α-reductase, aromatase, or growth factors.

(1) Saw palmetto, an extract from the berry of the American dwarf palm tree, is thought to act as a 5α-reductase inhibitor. However, there is doubt about this, as saw palmetto does not lower PSA levels. Nevertheless, saw palmetto does seem to alleviate symptoms, increase peak urine flow, and reduce prostate volume in a manner similar to that of finasteride.

(2) *Pygeum africanum,* an extract of the bark of an African evergreen tree, is thought to inhibit prostaglandins E_2 and $F_{2\alpha}$ as well as fibroblast growth factors. Whether the compound acts on the prostate or has a protective effect on the bladder is unclear. Clinical studies have shown the compound to be more effective than placebo in reducing frequency, urgency, hesitancy, and incomplete emptying.

(3) South African star grass contains phytosterols, the most important of which is β-sitosterol. Clinical effects are similar to those of saw palmetto.

(4) Cernilton, prepared from the rye-grass pollen, has been suggested by some to modestly improve overall LUTS.

3. Prostatic stents. Two essentially similar types of permanent intraurethral stents are available that differ in material and delivery system (Fig. 8.5). Stents are not indicated in the treatment of median lobe enlargement. Stents are useful for high-risk patients because they can be placed under topical urethral lidocaine with intravenous sedation, local prostatic block, or light general anesthesia. If the patient is unable to void immediately after placement of a urethral stent, a temporary suprapubic catheter should be placed because a urethral catheter may displace the stent.

a. The **cobalt–chromium stent** (UroLume; American Medical Systems) is a somewhat flexible stent that expands to a size of 42F. This stent device, placed with a transurethral insertion device (Fig. 8.5), is available in

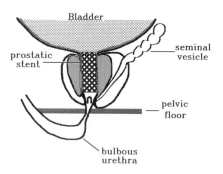

Fig. 8.5. Stent placed in prostatic urethra.

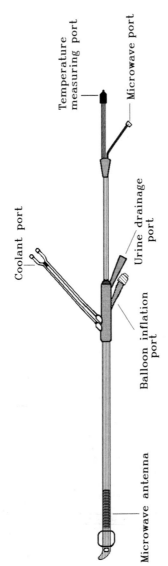

Fig. 8.6. Components of a typical microwave catheter.

three lengths: 2.0, 2.5, and 3.0 cm. The proper size must be selected to prevent the stent from protruding past the verumontanum. Removing the stent after it has been ingrown by urothelium can be difficult.

b.   The **titanium–nickel stent** (Memokath, Horizon, and others) is a self-expanding stent that responds to temperature and can be placed with a flexible cystoscope. Some stents respond to body temperature, whereas others require flushing with water at 45°C to expand. When cooled with cold water ($\leq$10°C), the stents soften and can be easily removed.

4.   Microwave therapy. The development of focused microwave technology has permitted the safe and effective application of controlled heat to the prostate. **Microwaves** are electromagnetic waves with wavelengths in the 300- to 3,000-MHz range. Tissue penetration leads to electromagnetic oscillations of molecules and release of kinetic energy; thus, heat is produced as these waves pass through tissue. Higher frequencies are associated with more energy but lower tissue penetration.

a.   Effects of heat on the prostate. Prostate cells undergo coagulation necrosis when exposed to temperatures of >45°C for $\geq$30 minutes. The prostate cells slough away over a period of weeks to months. However, the urethral pain threshold was found to be about 45°C, making this temperature a practical limit unless urethral cooling was utilized. Cell necrosis does not occur in techniques that heat the prostate to temperatures under 45°C, yet symptom relief is observed. The mechanism is not well understood but is thought to involve changes in the sensory nerve receptors in the prostatic urethra. The term **hyperthermia** is used for treatment at temperatures of <45°C, whereas **thermotherapy** is used for treatment at higher temperatures.

b.   Transurethral microwave thermotherapy. Microwave energy (Fig. 8.6), applied to the prostate by specialized transurethral catheters (Fig. 8.6), may be used to heat the prostate, usually to temperatures above 45°C. In transurethral microwave thermotherapy (TUMT), microwaves are emitted at a frequency of 900 to 1,100 MHz. The urethral antenna is directed toward the lateral lobes of the prostate, and the distribution of the energy corresponds approximately to the transition zone (Fig. 8.7). Most systems currently available use microwave heating along with a cooling system to maintain urethral temperatures at or below 45°C to reduce pain and protect the prostatic urethral mucosa. Clinical experience indicates that >60% of patients experience an improvement of symptoms and 75% have improvement in flow rate (about 3 mL/s). TUMT may be performed in an outpatient setting with only oral analgesics and takes about 30 to 60 minutes. Preprocedure sedation may involve lorazepam 1 mg PO and Percocet 1 tablet PO given 1 hour prior to the procedure. Further pain control may be achieved with a mixture of 15 mL of Xylocaine 2%/15 mL of 0.5% bupivacaine/oxybutynin 10 mg given intravesically just before starting the heating procedure. The oxybutynin tablet should be dissolved in the local anesthetic solution before in-

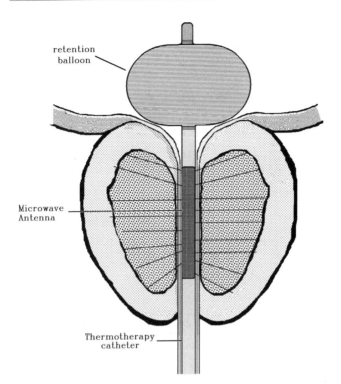

retention
balloon

Microwave
Antenna

Thermotherapy
catheter

Fig. 8.7. Microwave catheter in place, showing the approximate heat field produced.

jecting the solution into the bladder. Xylocaine jelly 2% is used to anesthetize the urethra prior to passing the catheter. Transrectal US assessment of the prostate or cystoscopy should show a prostatic length of at least 3.0 cm to accommodate the prostatic probe. The presence of a significant median lobe is a relative contraindication to TUMT. Thus, patients with smaller prostates are not good candidates for TUMT. Contraindications to TUMT include prior transurethral resection of the prostate (TURP), metallic implants, penile prosthesis, severe urethral stricture disease, severe peripheral vascular disease, or an artificial urinary sphincter. Patients with pacemakers need clearance from their cardiologists concerning turning their pacemakers off during therapy. Up to one-third of patients may have urinary retention after treatment that requires temporary catheterization, intermittent catheterization, or temporary urethral stenting. The posttreatment swelling and irritation from the thermal effect may last 3 to 6 weeks. Most patients will achieve maximal symptomatic relief and flow rate improvement by 6 weeks. Other complications include hematuria, urethral bleeding, and/or hematospermia; these are usually mild and self-limited. TUMT may be performed in patients who are poor operative risks, especially those on anticoagulation therapy. Patients have achieved durable responses for >5 years with TUMT.

c.   Transurethral needle ablation. Transurethral needle ablation (TUNA) involves the transurethral application of microwaves at 490 kHz to the prostate lobes (Fig. 8.8). This is accomplished under direct vision via cystoscopy and produces small areas of thermal injury that eventually produce changes in subjective symptoms, although the mechanism is unclear. TUNA heats a small area of the prostate to temperatures of 80° to 100°C within 3 to 5 minutes. Although there is no significant shrinkage of the prostate, TUNA produces small areas of necrosis of around 2-mm diameter around the tip of each treatment needle. TUNA is associated with a statistically significant improvement in symptom scores, quality of life, urinary flow rate, and postvoid residual after 1 year of follow-up. About one-third of patients experience short-term urinary retention after TUNA. Symptomatic improvement is much more prominent than objective improvement, and long-term durability of the response is unclear. Unlike with TUMT, small prostates can be treated with TUNA. The procedure is well tolerated and can be performed under conscious sedation.

5.   High-intensity focused US. US energy can be focused with a parabolic reflector and is capable of producing significant thermal tissue injury. Current equipment consists of a rectal probe that can image the prostate as well as emit high-intensity focused US. Because the patient must remain still during the treatment, general anesthesia is often required. Clinical efficacy is moderate, with flow increasing to an average of 13 mL/s at 1 year, but symptomatic improvement is significant. Most patients require some period of postoperative catheterization.

6.   Laser prostatectomy offers several potential advantages over transurethral electrocautery resection of the prostate, including (a) lower morbidity and mortality rates and (b) cost savings through the ability to perform the procedure on an outpatient basis. The lower morbidity and mortality are a consequence of the sealing of blood vessels by the laser, which significantly reduces absorption of irrigating fluid as well as blood loss. To be effective, laser energy must be applied with sufficient energy to destroy prostatic tissue, but not so much as to produce charring of tissue. Except for holmium laser enucleation, many of the laser-based procedures have proven to be disappointing over time.

a.   Free-beam laser energy may be delivered through a variety of side-firing laser delivery fibers. These fibers may be passed through a 22F cystoscope. The neodymium-YAG laser produces light at 1,064 nm, which produces excellent coagulation and hemostasis. Neodymium-YAG laser prostatectomy is usually performed under regional, spinal, or general anesthesia. Local anesthesia with periprostatic infiltration of bupivacaine and lidocaine may also be used. Like most less invasive techniques, free-beam laser prostatectomy may produce objective improvement in flow rate and postvoid residual, but not to the same extent as TURP.

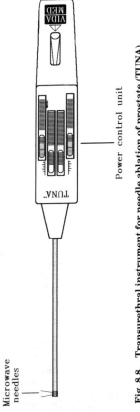

Microwave needles

Power control unit

Fig. 8.8. Transurethral instrument for needle ablation of prostate (TUNA).

Laser prostatectomy produces significant prostatic edema that may actually increase bladder outlet obstruction immediately postoperatively. Long-term results have been disappointing, and the technique is now seldom utilized.

b. Contact laser systems utilize neodymium-YAG or diode laser sources to heat a flexible contact fiber that is used to cut and coagulate tissue. There is no interaction between the laser and tissue. The contact laser can be used to perform bladder neck incision or prostatic ablation. Objective and symptomatic improvement has been similar to that obtained with free-beam lasers, and disappointing long-term outcomes have limited its usefulness.

c. Interstitial laser systems utilize diode-source end-firing delivery fibers that are inserted directly into the prostatic adenoma to produce small spherical areas of tissue destruction. Applying laser heating for 3 to 5 minutes can produce areas of necrosis of 1.5 to 2 cm. Like free-beam lasers, interstitial lasers produce significant prostatic edema and may result in postoperative retention. Urethral catheterization for the first 5 days postoperatively is usually required. Objective and symptomatic results are similar to those obtained with other laser techniques.

d. Holmium laser enucleation of prostate (HOLEP) involves the use of a large ($1,000$-μm) quartz fiber to deliver holmium laser energy through a cystoscope. The aim is to enucleate the median and lateral lobes of the prostate down to the surgical capsule and release them into the bladder. Unlike open surgical enucleation of hyperplastic BPH, the holmium laser energy allows this to be performed in a virtually bloodless field with saline rather than sorbitol irrigation. A problem with this enucleation process is the difficulty in removing the adenoma once it has been released into the bladder. This generally requires the use of an electrical morcellator, which is time consuming, potentially dangerous, and often fraught with mechanical difficulty. The most dramatic advantage of HOLEP is in those patients on anticoagulant therapy who can achieve excellent relief of their bladder outlet obstruction without compromising their anticoagulation status. Although the learning curve is steep, the results can be quite dramatic.

7. Open prostatectomy. Legitimate indications for open prostatectomy still exist, including prostatic enlargement beyond the capability of the surgeon to resect safely (generally >100 g), presence of **bladder calculi** not amenable to transurethral lithotripsy, and presence of **bladder diverticula** requiring excision. As in TURP, only the hyperplastic adenoma, and not the entire prostate, is removed. The choice of operative approach depends on the surgeon's preference, although there are also other considerations that apply:

a. Suprapubic prostatectomy is performed through a suprapubic transvesical approach and is well suited to dealing with concomitant bladder pathology such as diverticula and bladder stones. Postoperatively, a suprapubic tube is necessary until the bladder incision heals (5 to 7 days).

b. Retropubic prostatectomy differs from suprapubic prostatectomy in that the prostate capsule rather than the bladder wall is incised to expose the prostate adenoma. Thus, there is usually no need for suprapubic bladder drainage postoperatively. The operation is poorly suited for glands that are not particularly large.

c. **Simple perineal prostatectomy** is similar to the retropubic operation except the prostatic capsule is approached posteriorly through a perineal incision. Although little used today, it remains a valuable operative approach for patients who are obese or have pulmonary problems. Perineal prostatectomy is extremely well tolerated and avoids the postoperative complications associated with an abdominal incision.

8. **Catheters.** When patients cannot undergo surgery or refuse surgical treatment, temporizing measures should be considered.

a. **Intermittent self-catheterization** is an excellent option in patients who are motivated, have good manual dexterity, and must await surgical treatment of benign prostatic enlargement.

b. **Indwelling catheterization** is indicated in the short-term treatment (2 to 3 days) of acute urinary retention but is best avoided as a long-term solution. An indwelling catheter is associated with a high rate of bacteriuria and carries an increased risk for epididymitis, periurethral abscess, and generalized sepsis.

c. **Suprapubic catheter drainage** as a temporizing measure may be accomplished by means of a Stamey cystotomy catheter.

C. **Detrusor overactivity**

1. **Pharmacologic therapy** remains the most commonly used therapy for detrusor overactivity (Table 8.4). Response rates vary from 25% to 80%, depending on how one defines a successful response. Decreasing urinary frequency and urgency is relatively easy, but complete cure of incontinence is much more difficult. Intolerance of side effects is a common limiting factor in the pharmacologic treatment of detrusor overactivity.

a. **Antimuscarinic/anticholinergic agents** include oxybutynin, tolterodine, hyoscyamine, and dicyclomine. Side effects such as dry mouth, blurring of vision, constipation, and drowsiness occur in >50% of patients receiving antimuscarinic agents. Indeed, patient dropout and noncompliance are major reasons for therapeutic failure. These agents are contraindicated in patients with angle-closure glaucoma. Tolterodine provides efficacy similar to that of other agents but is much less frequently associated with dry mouth. The advent of once-daily extended-release formulations has greatly improved patient compliance.

b. **Antispasmodic agents.** Flavoxate is usually termed a spasmolytic agent, although its precise mode of action is unknown. Its adverse effect profile is similar to that of the antimuscarinic agents, including increased ocular tension.

c. **Imipramine** is a tricyclic antidepressant found to have anticholinergic and sympathomimetic actions peripherally and serotoninergic effects centrally. It has long been used in the treatment of childhood enuresis but also has considerable efficacy in adult detrusor overactivity. The drug may be

Table 8.4.   Agents used in detrusor overactivity

Generic Name	Brand Name	Dose Forms	Dose	
			Initial	Maximum
Oxybutynin chloride	Ditropan	5-mg tabs	1 tab tid	4 tabs qd
	Ditropan syrup	5 mg/5 mL	1 tspn tid (adult)	4 tspn qd (adult)
	Ditropan syrup	5 mg/mL	1 tspn bid (ped)	3 tspn qd (ped)
Oxybutynin (extended release)	Ditropan XL	5-, 10-, 15-mg tabs	5 mg hs	15 mg hs
Tolterodine tartrate	Detrol	1-, 2-mg tabs	2 mg bid	2 mg bid
Tolterodine tartrate (long acting)	Detrol LA	2-, 4-mg tabs	4 mg hs	4 mg hs
Hyoscyamine sulfate	Levsin	0.125-mg tabs	1 tab q4h	12 tabs/24 h
Flavoxate HCl	Urispas	100-mg tab	1 tab tid	2 tabs qid
Dicylomine HCl	Bentyl	10-mg caps	20 mg qid	40 mg qid
Imipramine HCl	Tofranil	10-, 25-, 50-mg tabs	10 mg qid	50 mg qid

used as first-line therapy or in combination with antimuscarinic agents. Imipramine is contraindicated in patients who are receiving monoamine oxidase inhibitors or who have severe hypertension.

2. Biofeedback therapy may be used alone or in conjunction with pharmacologic therapy. One simple biofeedback technique is the use of a voiding diary to record time and amount voided. The patient is rewarded with encouragement for increasing the time between voidings (Frewen regimen or "bladder drill"). More complex methods involve using urodynamic monitoring to provide auditory or visual feedback to the patient when bladder contractions occur. This enables the patient to learn techniques to suppress contractile activity. Success rates with biofeedback techniques vary from 30% to 80%, but there is a significant dropout rate of 40%.

3. Electrical stimulation of sacral nerves may be accomplished by intravaginal or intrarectal stimulating electrodes as well as implantable stimulators. The mechanism of electrical stimulation in modulating detrusor overactivity is unclear. It may promote urine storage by causing perineal muscle contraction, inhibiting detrusor activity, or blocking sensory input to the spinal cord. An implantable neuromodulator (Interstim) has been introduced that delivers low-level electrical stimulation to the S3 nerve root and has demonstrated good efficacy in suppressing detrusor instability.

D. Detrusor underactivity

1. Intermittent catheterization is the best option for most patients with impaired voiding caused by detrusor underactivity. The patient must have some degree of manual dexterity and be motivated to carry out this form of treatment. See Chapter 5 for a discussion of catheterization technique.

    a. Clean intermittent catheterization does not require the use of sterile gloves or catheters. In male patients, the head of the penis is cleansed with povidone–iodine, hexachlorophene, or soap, and a lubricated 14F straight catheter is inserted gently until urine flow is obtained (Fig. 8.9). In female patients, a short 12 or 14F catheter is used (Fig. 8.10). Any water-soluble lubricant can be used. The catheters may be cleaned with soap and water and reused many times. For most patients, clean intermittent catheterization is the most convenient and cost-effective method of emptying the bladder.

    b. Sterile intermittent catheterization differs from the clean technique in that sterile gloves are used during preparation of the skin and handling of the catheter, and a new catheter is used each time. This technique is indicated only in patients who are immune compromised or who have had serious urosepsis while using the clean technique.

2. Pharmacologic therapy of detrusor underactivity is generally unsuccessful. Bethanechol chloride in oral doses of 50 to 100 mg four times daily is capable of increasing bladder wall tension, but the ability of this agent to produce effective bladder contractions has never been shown. However, it may be useful in selected cases as an adjunct to Valsalva or straining, especially in patients with intact bladder sensation. Side effects include flushing, sweating, headache, diarrhea, gastrointestinal cramps, and bronchospasm.

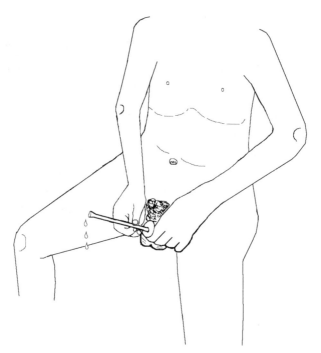

Fig. 8.9. **Technique of clean intermittent catheterization in the male patient.**

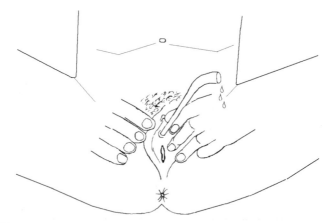

Fig. 8.10. **Technique of clean intermittent catheterization in the female patient.**

SUGGESTED READING

Abrams P. New words for old: lower urinary tract symptoms for "prostatism." *Br Med J* 1994;308:929–930.

Appel R. Clinical efficacy and safety of tolterodine in the treatment of overactive bladder: a pooled analysis. *Urology* 1997;50(suppl 6a):90–96.

Barry MJ, Fowler FJ Jr, O'Leary MP, et al. The American Urological Association Symptom Index for benign prostatic hyperplasia. *J Urol* 1992;148:1549–1557.

Barry MJ, Fowler FJ Jr, O'Leary MP, et al. Correlation of the AUA Symptom Index with self-administered versions of the Madsen–Iversen, Boyarsky and Maine Medical Assessment Program Symptom Indexes. *J Urol* 1992;148:1558–1562.

Cummings JM, Parra RO, Boullier JA. Laser prostatectomy: initial experience and urodynamic follow-up. *Urology* 1995;45:414–420.

Defalco A, Oesterling JE, Epstein H, et al. The North American experience with the UroLume endourethral prosthesis as a treatment for BPH: three-year results. *J Urol* 1995;153:436A(abst).

Kabalin JN. Laser prostatectomy—what we have accomplished and future directions. *J Urol* 1995;154:2093–2095.

Kaplan SA, Chiou RK, Morton WJ, et al. Long-term experience utilizing a new balloon-expandable prostatic endoprosthesis: the Titan stent. *Urology* 1995;45:234–240.

Kirby RS. A randomized, double-blind crossover study of tamsulosin and controlled-release doxazosin in patients with benign prostatic hyperplasia. *Br J Urol Int* 2003;91:41–44.

Kyprianou N. Doxazosin and terazosin suppress prostate growth by inducing apoptosis: clinical significance. *J Urol* 2003;169:1520–1525.

Lam JS, Romas NA, Lowe FC. Long-term treatment with finasteride in men with symptomatic benign prostatic hyperplasia: 10-year follow-up. *Urology* 2003;61:354–358.

Lepor H. Phase III multicenter placebo-controlled study of tamsulosin in benign prostatic hyperplasia. *Urology* 1998;51:892–900.

Lepor H. Long-term evaluation of tamsulosin in benign prostatic hyperplasia: placebo-controlled, double-blind extension of phase III trial. *Urology* 1998;51:901–906.

Madersbacher S, Kratzik C, Susani M, et al. Tissue ablation in benign prostatic hyperplasia with high-intensity focused ultrasound. *J Urol* 1994;152:1956–1961.

Norby B, Nielsen HV, Frimodt-Moller PC. Transurethral interstitial laser coagulation of the prostate and transurethral microwave thermotherapy vs. transurethral resection or incision of the prostate: results of a randomized, controlled study in patients with symptomatic benign prostatic hyperplasia. *Br J Urol Int* 2002;90:853–862.

Osman Y, Wadie B, El-Diasty T, et al. High-energy transurethral microwave thermotherapy: symptomatic vs. urodynamic success. *Br J Urol Int* 2003;91:365–370.

Perry MJA, Roodhouse AJ, Gidlow AB, et al. Thermo-expandable intraprostatic stents in bladder outlet obstruction: an 8-year study. *Br J Urol Int* 2002;90:216.

Resnick NM, Yalla SV. Detrusor hyperactivity with impaired contractile function: an unrecognized but common cause of incontinence in elderly patients. *JAMA* 1987;257:3076.

Wilt TJ, et al. Phytotherapy for benign prostatic hyperplasia. *Public Health Nutr* 2000;3:459–472.

Urinary Incontinence

Elise De and Tracey Wilson

I. Introduction

A. Definition. Urinary incontinence is a symptom—"the complaint of any involuntary leakage of urine"—as well as a sign—"urine leakage seen during examination." In order to serve as a diagnosis, incontinence must be conceptualized with regard to its underlying pathophysiology.

B. Risk factors for urinary incontinence include female gender, Caucasian race, parity, neurologic disease, pelvic trauma, surgery or radiation, nutritional deficit, obesity, tobacco or alcohol abuse, excessive fluid intake, advanced age, and cognitive difficulty.

C. Differential diagnosis. Incontinence may involve fluids other than urine and egress other than the urethra.

  1. Nonurinary wetness refers to loss of bodily fluids that may easily be confused with urine.

    a. Sources of nonurinary wetness include:

      (1) Gastrointestinal tract: diarrhea, fistula, or leakage from a colostomy or ileostomy.

      (2) Vagina: vaginal discharge, exudate, transudate, or pus.

      (3) Infection: serous or purulent drainage from skin infection or hidradenitis.

      (4) Perspiration.

      (5) Subjective wetness: a complaint of wetness when no wetness is demonstrated.

    b. Diagnosis. Since urine contains very high levels of creatinine, the creatinine level of the fluid should be measured. Agents that color the urine such as indigo carmine or phenazopyridine can also be used to identify the fluid as urine. Similarly, feces can be identified using ingested activated charcoal. A perineal pad is helpful in collecting the perineal fluid, and it can be weighed to quantify the leakage. A tampon can be used in the vagina to determine whether the fluid is vaginal fluid or urine.

  2. Nonurethral urinary incontinence involves the leakage of urine via a route other than the urethra.

    a. A **fistula** is an epithelialized connection between two bodily cavities (or between a cavity and the body exterior) and is usually due to trauma, surgery, or tissue injury. Incontinence caused by urinary fistulas may follow pelvic surgery, radiation to the pelvis (sometimes years after the fact), or birth trauma. Incontinence due to a fistula will be described as constant. The fistula can be diagnosed on physical examination, cystoscopy, or imaging studies (voiding cystourethrogram or computed tomography scan). The most common type of fistula in the female urinary tract is vesicovaginal. Vesicovaginal and urethrovaginal fistulas may be repaired by a transvaginal or transvesical approach, depending on the location of the fistula and the experience and preference of the surgeon. Ureterovaginal fistulas require an abdominal approach because reimplantation of the ureter into the bladder is usually necessary.

b. Ureteral ectopia is congenital insertion of the ureter into a location other than its normal location and is almost always discovered in childhood. If the insertion is distal to the external urethral sphincter (an embryologic event that occurs only in female patients), the ectopic ureter may cause continuous incontinence. Concurrent normal voiding is preserved in such circumstances owing to the presence of one or more ureters inserting into the bladder. Male patients with ureteral ectopia are generally not incontinent because ureteral insertion will always be proximal to the external sphincter. However, they may present with epididymitis when the ectopic ureter inserts in the epididymis. Ureteral ectopia is usually associated with ureteral duplication.

c. Vaginal reflux of urine during voiding may result in postvoid wetness. This condition may occur with vaginal stenosis or atrophy, congenital urethral "female hypospadias," or repositioning of the urethra intravaginally following antiincontinence surgery.

d. Urinary diversion may also cause incontinence. Patients who have had placement of a suprapubic catheter, creation of a urostomy (e.g., ileal loop), or creation of a catheterizable stoma can leak urine at these sites.

II. Physiology of continence

The lower urinary tract performs two seemingly simple tasks: storage and emptying of urine. Urinary continence requires that the bladder be able to store an adequate volume of urine at low pressure, that the urethral sphincters be competent, and that the neurologic mechanisms coordinating storage and emptying be intact. The bladder neck must remain closed at all times except during voiding and must be able to withstand momentary increases in intraabdominal pressure.

A. Bladder

1. Viscoelastic properties. The normal bladder will allow expansion during filling with little increase in intravesical pressure. This property is known as compliance, defined as change in volume divided by change in pressure ($C = \Delta V/\Delta P$). Compliance is determined primarily by the viscoelastic properties of the bladder. Radiation, infection, and chronic obstruction commonly affect the compliance of the bladder by causing an increase in type III collagen deposition. As a result, the bladder is less distensible, compliance decreases, and pressure increases.

2. Detrusor muscle is normally relaxed owing to inhibition of its parasympathetic nerves. Neurologic disease as well as obstruction may cause detrusor overactivity (termed hyperreflexia or instability). The coordination between the detrusor muscle and striated sphincter is often lost in neurologic disorders. Impaired contractility may coexist with detrusor overactivity.

B.   Outlet. The anatomic support and innervation of the bladder outlet as well as the intrinsic tone of the bladder neck and urethra all contribute to continence. The prostatic and membranous portions of the male urethra act as the primary continence mechanism, whereas in the female, the entire urethra performs this function. **Urethral hypermobility** and **intrinsic sphincter deficiency** (ISD) are the most common "outlet" causes of incontinence in women.

1.   Urethral support in women derives from the two leaves of the levator ani (endopelvic fascia and pubocervical fascia). This "hammock" supports the urethra and compresses it when intraabdominal pressure increases. In addition, the pubourethral ligament and arcus tendineus provide support to the urethra. When these supporting structures are weakened, **urethral hypermobility** results. Urethral hypermobility involves rotational descent of a poorly supported proximal urethra and bladder neck into the vagina during episodes of increased intraabdominal pressure. During stress maneuvers, urethral hypermobility can be identified by "eyeballing" the urethra or by placing a cotton swab in the urethra and observing the degree of deflection of the swab (the "Q-tip" test). Urethral hypermobility may also be diagnosed with the help of imaging studies: voiding cystourethrogram, magnetic resonance imaging, or video urodynamics. For historical reasons, stress urinary incontinence due to urethral hypermobility is referred to as type II stress urinary incontinence. Pure urethral hypermobility is not seen in men.

2.   Intrinsic sphincteric deficiency refers to impaired sphincter function not related to urethral position or support. The etiology can include neurologic conditions, prior pelvic surgeries, pelvic radiation, or, in women, aging and hypoestrogenic states. In men, ISD is commonly iatrogenic, for example, following a radical prostatectomy or transurethral resection of the prostate. Incontinence due to ISD has historically been referred to as type III stress incontinence. *Urethral hypermobility and ISD may occur in the same patient.* A unifying theory known as the **hammock hypothesis** suggests that a poor muscular backing to the posterior aspect of the urethra results in failure of effective urethral coaptation, excessive urethral mobility, and urinary leakage.

C.   Neural control of the bladder and sphincter is essential for both continence and emptying. The pontine micturition center is central in coordinating these functions. During storage of urine, the detrusor muscle is inhibited and the sphincter active. During normal urination, the spinal reflex arc is allowed to fire and the sphincter relaxes, followed by contraction of the detrusor. Further discussion of these complex neural pathways is found in Chapter 18.

III.   Classification of incontinence

A.   Stress urinary incontinence is the complaint of involuntary leakage on effort or exertion, sneezing, or coughing.

B.   Urge urinary incontinence is the complaint of involuntary leakage accompanied by or immediately preceded by urgency.

C.   Mixed urinary incontinence is the complaint of involuntary leakage associated with urgency and also with exertion, effort, sneezing, or coughing.

D.   Overflow incontinence is urinary leakage in combination with urinary retention. This is demonstrable clinically by measuring high postvoid residuals in conjunction with observable incontinence.

E.   Continuous incontinence is the complaint of continuous urinary leakage.

F.   Nocturnal enuresis is urinary loss that occurs only during sleep.

IV.   Assessment of incontinence

A.   History can provide important information regarding the onset, duration, and severity of incontinence as well as the degree of bother. In combination with the physical examination, the history is crucial in determining whether invasive testing is indicated. For example, one might suspect overflow incontinence in a patient who has little sensation of bladder fullness, weak urinary stream, continuous incontinence worsened by stress, and little or no urgency. However, the diagnosis cannot be made on history alone, and treatment decisions must be based on objective findings. A full review of systems and medical, surgical, medication, allergy, social, and family histories should be obtained. The comprehensive history of urinary incontinence should include the following:

1.   Identification of the **type** of incontinence: stress, urge, overflow, etc.

2.   Duration of symptoms.

3.   Prior therapies attempted, both medical and surgical, and response to those therapies.

4.   Inciting event: surgery, injury, childbirth, and neurologic insult.

5.   Severity. This is often described by pad use: number, type, threshold for changing. It may also be described in terms of degree of bother. Ancillary tools may also be used to assess severity:

  a.   Micturition or bladder diary (Appendix 1).

  b.   Incontinence Impact Questionnaire (Appendix 2).

  c.   Urogenital Distress Inventory (Appendix 3).

  d.   Quality-of-Life Index (Appendix 4).

  e.   American Urological Association symptom score.

6.   Medications can cause or worsen incontinence.

  a.   Sympatholytics (e.g., clonidine, terazosin) can weaken sphincter tone.

  b.   Sympathomimetics (e.g., pseudoephedrine, imipramine) can cause urinary retention and overflow incontinence

  c.   Diuretics can unmask or worsen pathology.

7.   Associated **lower urinary tract symptoms.** Urgency, frequency, nocturia, hesitancy, straining, decreased force of stream, intermittency, pain with urination, suprapubic pain or pressure, and sensation of incomplete void should be evaluated.

8.   Symptoms associated with **pelvic organ prolapse** should also be discussed during the interview and include any introital bulge or mass, pelvic pressure, back pain, heaviness, inability to retain a tampon, and constipation requiring vaginal evacuation.

9.   Associated histories

  a.   Obstetric and gynecologic history

  (1)   Gravity, parity, outcomes, and complications.

  (2)   Vaginal delivery versus cesarean section, prolonged second stage.

  (3)   Hysterectomy: vaginal versus abdominal incision, oophorectomy, indication for surgery.

  (4)   Sexual activity, pain or leakage with intercourse.

  (5)   Menopause and hypoestrogenic state.

  b.   Past surgical history

  (1)   Pelvic surgery (e.g., abdominoperineal resection).

  (2)   Prior antiincontinence surgery, prostate surgery, bladder surgery.

  c.   Neurologic history

  (1)   Back surgery or injuries (e.g., herniating or bulging discs).

  (2)   Spinal cord injury.

  (3)   Cerebrovascular accident.

  (4)   Parkinson's disease.

  (5)   Multiple sclerosis.

  (6)   Diabetes.

  (7)   Myelodysplasia.

  d.   Gastrointestinal history

  (1)   Diarrhea.

  (2)   Constipation (suspicious for rectocele).

  (3)   Fecal incontinence (suspicious for neurologic lesion).

  e.   Other genitourinary history

  (1)   Urinary tract infection.

  (2)   Hematuria.

  (3)   Kidney stones.

  (4)   Prior urinary retention.

  (5)   Pediatric genitourinary history (e.g., ureteral reimplantation).

  (6)   In men: prostate surgery, urethral stricture, bladder stones.

  (7)   In women: prior antiincontinence or pelvic surgery (risk of ISD).

B.   Physical exam should focus on the abdomen and pelvis.

  1.   Abdominal examination may reveal presence of tenderness, palpable masses, suprapubic fullness (distended bladder), and hernias. The patient should also be evaluated for costovertebral angle tenderness. Careful note should be made of all surgical scars, which should be correlated with the history.

  2.   Female pelvis

  a.   External genitalia are examined for signs of chronic wetness (erythema, skin breakdown), atrophy (pale, shiny mucosa), and labial adhesions.

  b.   Internal pelvic organs

  (1)   Urethral examination may demonstrate recess, stenosis, masses, or tenderness. Urethral hypermobility and stress incontinence, if present, will be exhibited on Valsalva or cough maneuvers.

(2)   Vaginal examination may reveal atrophic vaginitis or discharge. Bimanual examination can reveal vaginal narrowing or palpable scars (e.g., episiotomy or prior surgery). For diagnosis of **pelvic organ prolapse,** half of a lubricated translucent vaginal speculum should be inserted and examination of the anterior and posterior vaginal walls should be performed both at rest and during Valsalva maneuvers. Cystocele, enterocele, and rectocele are defined as follows:

(a)   Cystocele: herniation of the bladder into the anterior vaginal wall. Anterior vaginal wall deficiency leads to either an anterior cystocele (weakness of lateral supports) or a posterior cystocele (central defect) (Fig. 9.1).

(b)   Enterocele: herniation of small bowel or omentum into the vagina. Apical vaginal wall weakness leads to an enterocele.

(c)   Rectocele: herniation of rectum into the vagina. Posterior vaginal wall weakness can lead to a low, midvaginal, or high rectocele.

(d)   Classification of pelvic organ prolapse. A number of classification systems have been developed to provide the basis for objective, reproducible clinical examination. These describe the prolapsed organ in reference to the hymen or the introitus, assigning a grade or degree of prolapse. Baden and Walker (1972) classified grade I (proximal) to grade IV (complete eversion) prolapse based on distance of the organ from the hymeneal ring. More recently, the **Pelvic Organ Prolapse Quantification System** has been developed and is based on the distance of six vaginal reference points from the hymen. This system does not attempt to identify the prolapsed organ. The classification ranges from stage 0 (no prolapse) to stage IV (vaginal eversion).

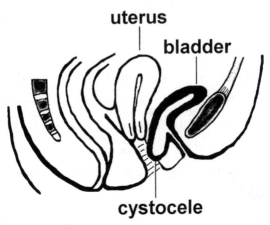

Fig. 9.1.   Anatomic relationship of cystocele and vagina.

3. **Neurologic exam**
   a. The **sensory exam** can help locate the level of sensory deficit. Important reference points include the following:
      (1) T5 = nipple level.
      (2) T10 = umbilicus.
      (3) L3 = knee.
      (4) S3 to S5 = perineum, labia.
   b. **Reflexes**
      (1) Deep tendon reflexes: altered in muscular/peripheral nerve pathology.
         (a) L3 to L4 = quadriceps.
         (b) L5 to S2 = Achilles tendon.
      (2) Cutaneous reflexes: response to stimuli applied to the skin.
         (a) S2 to S4 nerve roots = **Bulbocavernosus (sacral) reflex.** During rectal examination, the glans penis or glans clitoris is squeezed, resulting in reflex contraction of the anal sphincter and bulbocavernosus muscles. This reflex will be absent in approximately 30% of normal women, but absence of the reflex is a reliable indicator of neurologic disease in men.
         (b) L1 to L2 = cremasteric reflex
            (i) T6 to L2 = abdominal reflex.
            (ii) S2 to S5 = anal reflex.
C. **Urodynamic studies** assess lower urinary tract function by measuring physiologic parameters (pressure, volume, flow, leak, and bladder descent). Guided by the patient's history and physical exam, the urodynamic measurements can help determine the underlying pathophysiologic process and aid in making treatment decisions.
   1. **Indications.** It is arguable whether formal urodynamic evaluation is necessary before treatment of urinary incontinence. However, urodynamic evaluation is recommended in the following situations:
      a. Failure of prior treatment.
      b. Mixed incontinence (stress and urge).
      c. Inconsistent history with respect to clinical findings.
      d. Young men with lower urinary tract symptoms.
      e. Neurologic disease.
      f. Prior prostate surgery.
      g. Children with atypical patterns of incontinence.
   2. **Components of the urodynamic examination**
      a. **Uroflowmetry** is a noninvasive recording of the rate of urine flow in milliliters per second. The maximum flow rate and voided volume offer very important data, especially when interpreted in concert with a postvoid residual and the remainder of the urodynamic data. The voided volume must be at least 150 mL to provide a reliable measure of outflow resistance.
      b. **Cystometrogram** involves filling the bladder while recording the pressure–volume relationship. Abnormal bladder sensation, compliance, and detrusor overactivity can be detected.
      c. **Voiding pressure study** records the pressure in the bladder concurrently with the urine flow rate. High void-

ing pressures could indicate abdominal straining or, in its absence, obstruction.

   d.   Assessment of **urethral function**

      (1)   The **detrusor leak point pressure** measures the lowest intravesical pressure that will produce urine leakage in the absence of detrusor contraction.

      (2)   The **Valsalva or abdominal leak point pressure** measures the intraabdominal pressure that will cause leakage of urine in the absence of detrusor contraction. A normal urethra should not leak with increased intra-abdominal pressure.

      (3)   The **urethral pressure profile** is an indication of urethral resistance at various points along the urethra. It is measured by withdrawing a perforated urethral catheter and graphing the pressure at recorded catheter lengths.

   e.   **Electromyogram** measures sphincter activity concurrent with the rest of the exam. Either electrodes are attached to the perineal skin, or needles are placed directly into the urethral sphincter.

   f.   **Videourodynamics** combine cystography with urodynamics to observe for leak point pressures, bladder neck descent, and the physical appearance of the bladder (e.g., diverticula).

D.   Imaging studies

   1.   The **voiding cystourethrogram** (VCUG) allows one to radiographically record urinary incontinence. The patient is asked to strain with a full bladder, at which time leakage, if present, is recorded radiographically. The VCUG may also be used as an objective measure of the degree of a cystocele. The extent of bladder descent below the inferior border of the pubic symphysis is measured. A distance of 0 to 2 cm below the symphysis corresponds to a grade 1 cystocele, 2 to 5 cm below the inferior border of the symphysis to grade 2, and ≥5 cm to a grade 3 cystocele. This radiologic study has proven useful as an objective outcome measure following cystocele repair.

   2.   **Magnetic resonance imaging** may also be used as a radiographic measure of pelvic organ prolapse. This study is useful because it provides detailed anatomic information on the pelvic organs without radiation exposure to the patient. The disadvantage to using this form of imaging is that it must be done in the supine position and may underestimate the degree of prolapse.

V.   Treatment

A.   Nonsurgical

   1.   **Behavioral modification** is an education-based program that teaches patients about their contribution to and control over their urinary symptoms. For example, excessive fluid or caffeine intake and delayed voiding are habits that are modifiable for symptomatic improvement. The program may include a voiding diary (Appendix 1), fluid/dietary management, timed voiding, and urge inhibition.

   2.   **Pelvic floor therapy.** "Kegel exercises" is the widely used term for any type of pelvic floor strengthening. These exercises have proven to be beneficial in treating stress urinary incontinence. However, their efficacy relies heavily upon patient compliance.

3.   Biofeedback is a modification of pelvic floor therapy, incorporating the use of "feedback" in training the patient to gain control of pelvic musculature. The feedback information can be based on physical examination, vaginal cones in women, or other signals (e.g., bladder pressure, electromyography). The therapy can be basic or advanced, ranging from home instruction to regular office visits.

4.   Urethral inserts. The Food and Drug Administration has approved various urethral meatal devices and inserts for women with pure stress urinary incontinence. Each has a mechanism to keep it in place (e.g., a balloon) and acts as a plug to prevent urine escape.

5.   Pessary. Various intravaginal devices are available for support and reduction of pelvic organ prolapse. These devices may also be equipped with a knob for direct urethral pressure when urinary incontinence is present. A physician must fit the devices.

6.   Cunningham clamp. The Cunningham clamp (Fig. 9.2) is an atraumatic clothespin-type device for clamping of the male urethra. It is applied to the penis during social hours and removed in order to void. It is best suited for ISD in men.

7.   Indwelling catheters may be in the form of a urethral Foley catheter or a suprapubic tube. Drainage of urine into a bag is more controllable than random leakage. Indwelling catheters may be responsible for considerable morbidity if used improperly. The incidence of catheter-associated bacteriuria ranges from 3% to 10% per day of catheterization. In addition to bacteriuria, indwelling catheters may produce epididymitis/orchitis, periurethral abscess, and urethral erosion in both male and female patients. Patients with indwelling catheters also have an increased incidence of bladder stones and bladder carcinoma. Catheter fixation is important to prevent trauma to the bladder and urethra resulting from traction on the catheter. All catheters tend to deteriorate over time as they are exposed to urine. When the lumen becomes obstructed, the catheter should be exchanged for one of the same size and type. There are no hard data to support a particular schedule of catheter changes, but once a month is a commonly used schedule.

8.   The **condom catheter** is one of the most effective techniques for managing incontinence in male patients. It consists of a penile sheath, a collecting tube, and a drainage bag (Fig. 9.2). The penile sheath is held in place by an adhesive band or by adhesive inside the sheath. The drainage bag is held in place by belts or straps around the leg. Some men have difficulty keeping the sheath in place because the penis is short or redundant penile skin is present. Such problems may occasionally require circumcision or penile prosthetic implants to increase the shaft length. Another problem is penile skin breakdown or necrosis from overzealous application of the adhesive band.

9.   The **McGuire urinal** consists of a heavy rubber collecting pouch incorporated into an athletic supporter (Fig. 9.2). The patient places the penis into the pouch, obviating the

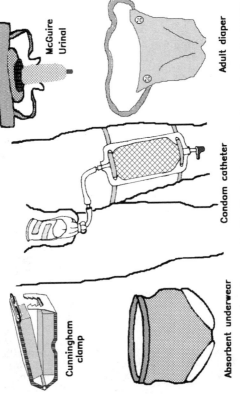

Fig. 9.2. Examples of external collecting devices, occlusion, and absorbent aids.

need for adhesive bands around the penis. The McGuire urinal is best suited for moderately incontinent patients. With severe incontinence, the McGuire urinal can be attached to a leg bag. This device is not intended for nocturnal use.

10.   Absorbent aids are usually made of disposable material with a waterproof backing. **Pads** are commonly used by both women and men for mild to moderate incontinence. The pads can be worn under the patient's usual underwear or under absorbent underwear. **Diapers** for adults are available in both disposable and reusable forms (Fig. 9.2). **Absorbent underpants** can absorb much more urine than pads and are less bulky than diapers (Fig. 9.2). Newer systems lock in fluid in gel form and contain agents to counteract urine odor. Examples are the Tranquility system and Attends disposable briefs.

B.   Pharmacologic agents

   1.   Stress incontinence

   a.   α-Adrenergic agonists are aimed at increasing internal sphincter tone. Pseudoephedrine is the most easily available. Although it has not been well studied for this application, it is nevertheless widely used. The **dose** for the immediate-release form is 30 to 60 mg PO qid. For the extended-release form, the dose is 120 mg q12h. Adverse effects include tachycardia, palpitations, arrhythmias, nervousness, insomnia, dizziness, drowsiness, convulsions, hallucinations, headache, diaphoresis, nausea, and vomiting. The drug should be used cautiously in patients over age 60 and patients with hypertension, hyperthyroidism, diabetes mellitus, cardiovascular disease, ischemic heart disease, and increased intraocular pressure. Overdosage may cause central nervous system depression and death.

   b.   Estrogens have been used in an effort to treat stress urinary incontinence in postmenopausal women. Estrogen is thought to affect adrenergic receptors, improve the urethral mucosal seal, and improve blood supply to the vaginal tissues.

      (1)   Oral estrogen has a first-pass effect on the liver and increases hepatic production of thyroxine-binding globulin, corticosteroid-binding globulin, triglycerides, high-density lipoprotein cholesterol, and clotting factors, whereas their production is only minimally increased by transdermal or vaginal estrogen administration. Thus, oral estrogen should be avoided in women with a tendency to thrombosis or hepatic/gallbladder disease. Many oral preparations of estrogen are available. Some are derived from conjugated equine estrogens (Premarin), whereas others are derived from plant sources (soy and yams). The potency of various preparations differs significantly, and therefore the doses of these estrogen preparations differ. In general, 0.625 mg of conjugated estrogens, esterified estrogens, or estrone sulfate is equivalent to 1 mg of estradiol. The dose is 0.3 to 1.25 mg of Premarin qd or estradiol 1 to 2 mg qd.

      (2)   Vaginal estrogen has the advantage of minimal exposure of other organs. Premarin **vaginal cream** in doses of 0.3 to 0.6 mg/day can normalize vaginal cytology in postmenopausal women and is thus a sufficient dose for stress urinary incontinence. Each gram of Premarin vaginal cream contains 0.625 mg of conjugated estrogens in a nonliquefying base. The cream should be applied once daily in a dose of 0.5 to 2 g for 4 weeks to achieve the desired effect; the frequency can then be decreased to one to two times weekly. At these doses, systemic effects are negligible, and there should be no concern about carcinogenic effects. Similar effects can be obtained with 2 to 4 g/day of estradiol cream intravaginally for 2 weeks, then gradually reducing to one-half the initial dose for 2 weeks, followed by a maintenance dose of 1 g one to three times per week.

Local administration of estrogen to the genitourinary tract can also be accomplished with Estring, a **vaginal ring** that releases 7.5 µg/day of estradiol. It is inserted once every 3 months and does not need to be removed during intercourse or bathing. The use of the Estring is useful in women with significant prolapse. Finally, estrogen is available as **vaginal tablets** (25 µg of estradiol/tablet) that are inserted into the vagina daily for 2 weeks with one to two doses per week thereafter.

2. **Detrusor overactivity**
   a. **Antimuscarinic agents** are used to suppress detrusor overactivity.
   (1) **Oxybutynin chloride** (Ditropan) remains the standard antimuscarinic agent. While considered an antimuscarinic agent, it also has important direct antispasmodic effects on bladder smooth muscle. Onset of action is 30 to 60 minutes after ingestion, with peak effect seen 3 to 6 hours later and total duration of action 6 to 10 hours. Oxybutynin should be used with caution in patients with urinary tract obstruction, angle-closure glaucoma, hyperthyroidism, reflux esophagitis, or heart, hepatic, or renal disease. It may cause confusion in elderly patients. Oxybutynin extended release (Ditropan XL) offers a slow-release form of oxybutynin that, owing to its steady-state level, is thought to avoid the side effects associated with metabolism of the drug to active metabolites in the liver. Immediate-release oxybutynin is supplied as a 5-mg tablet; the **dose** is 1 to 4 tablets spaced out during the day. The extended-release form is supplied in 5-, 10-, and 15-mg tablets. The dose is 1 tablet at bedtime.
   (2) **Tolterodine tartrate** (Detrol) is a newer competitive muscarinic receptor antagonist that demonstrates selectivity for the detrusor muscle over the salivary gland, thus decreasing the incidence of dry mouth. There is an extended-release form (Detrol LA) that allows once-daily dosing. Detrol LA and Ditropan XL have not been directly compared with each other. Tolterodine exhibits antimuscarinic side effects such as dry mouth, constipation, somnolence, headache, blurred vision, dizziness, and dyspepsia.

   The **dose** is 2 mg PO twice daily; the dose may be lowered to 1 mg twice daily based on individual response and tolerability. For the extended-release form, the dose is

2 or 4 mg PO at bedtime. Whereas dose reduction may be needed for renal or hepatic dysfunction, no dose reduction for the elderly is necessary.

(3)   L-Hyoscyamine (Levsin) is an antimuscarinic agent that also antagonizes histamine and serotonin. It is used to treat overactive bladder, but controlled trials demonstrating efficacy are lacking to date. It has rapid onset of action and lasts 4 to 6 hours. The **dose** is 0.125 to 0.25 mg PO q4h prn. An extended-release form is available that should be given at a dose of 0.375 to 0.75 mg PO q12h.

(4)   Imipramine, a tricyclic antidepressant, is sometimes used for its theoretical effects of closing of the bladder neck and relaxing the detrusor. The mechanism of action has been studied extensively without definitive conclusion. Proposals include central anticholinergic or antihistamine effects or an increase in serotonin and norepinephrine concentration in the spinal cord presynaptic nerves. Anticholinergic side effects and cardiotoxicity are possible. The **dose** is 10 to 25 mg PO qid.

C.   Surgical treatment of stress urinary incontinence aims to improve the ability of the bladder outlet to resist increased intraabdominal pressure. Improved urethral support may benefit those with urethral hypermobility as well as those with ISD. Keep in mind that most patients have both conditions. In addition, when assessing cure and improvement rates, it should be noted that there are no accepted outcome measures or definition of cure.

1.   Urethral bulking agents have been used to treat stress urinary incontinence, whether due to ISD, urethral hypermobility, or both. However, they have been more effective in cases due to ISD. The mechanism of action is improvement of urethral coaptation. These agents are also capable of increasing outlet resistance. The biggest disadvantage to their use is poor long-term efficacy.

a.   Glutaraldehyde cross-linked highly purified bovine collagen has an initial success rate (subjective improvement) of 85% to 94%, falling to 26% to 65% at 2 years. Skin testing is required 1 month prior to treatment to screen for allergic reaction (1% to 4%).

b.   Pyrolytic carbon-coated zirconium oxide beads are large (251 to 300 μm) and nonreactive. Improvement in continence in women is reported to be as high as 80% 12 months after injection. Acute retention has been reported in 25% and urgency in 15%.

c.   Autologous fat is inexpensive and nonallergenic. However, resorption rates are high. Short-term success is 50% to 60%, with long-term improvement in 10% to 50% of cases in various series.

d.   Teflon (polytetrafluoroethylene) and **Silicone (polydimethylsiloxane elastomer suspension)** have been used but are not Food and Drug Administration approved for this indication.

2.   Retropubic suspension procedures (colposuspensions) aim to support and restore the bladder neck to its retropubic location. Requiring a lower midline or Pfannenstiel incision, these procedures are somewhat more morbid than intravaginal procedures (see below). They are usually performed if there is an indication for an intraabdominal approach (i.e., in association with an abdominal hysterectomy).

a. The **Marshall–Marchetti–Krantz procedure** fixes and elevates the bladder neck by elevating the paraurethral fascia and submucosal anterior vaginal wall toward the cartilaginous portion of the symphysis pubis. Objective continence of 90% is demonstrated at 3- to 12-month follow-up. Subjective long-term success is 40% after 15 years. A significant risk of osteitis pubis (0.9% to 3.2%) is seen.

b. **Burch colposuspension** elevates the anterior vaginal wall bilaterally toward the iliopectineal (Cooper's) ligaments. Patients must have a mobile vaginal wall. Two to four sutures are placed at 1-cm intervals starting at the bladder neck and moving proximally; each incorporates submucosal vaginal wall and the iliopectineal ligament. Objective continence of 85% is demonstrated at 1 to 60 months of follow-up. Subjective and objective cure is about 80% at 15 years.

3. Transvaginal bladder neck suspensions are somewhat less invasive than retropubic procedures and have become the approach of choice. Initially promising results have deteriorated slightly with time. Overall cure and dry rates have been reported at 65% to 69% after 48 months of follow-up. In general, pubovaginal slings and retropubic suspensions have more durable success than transvaginal needle suspension procedures. As a result, the majority of these procedures have fallen out of favor.

a. **Pereyra needle suspension** was the first transvaginal needle suspension (1959) and utilized steel wires to suspend the pericervical fascia from the abdominal wall fascia. It has undergone a series of modifications to its most recent version (1982), where the pubourethral ligaments are bound to the endopelvic fascia and suspensory ligaments. This multilayered bolster decreased a previously high rate of suture pull-through. Cure or marked improvement rates are reported at 94.5% after 4 to 6 years.

b. **Stamey needle suspension** incorporated the use of cystoscopic guidance to confirm placement of the suspensory sutures at the level of the bladder neck. In addition, Dacron pledgets were used to buttress the suture away from the incision, in an effort to decrease the rate of suture pull-out and erosion.

c. **Gittes needle suspension** is an "incisionless" technique that involves the incorporation of a full-thickness bite of the vaginal wall that is eventually pulled through the vaginal wall as an autologous pledget.

d. **Modified Pereyra–Raz needle suspension** includes the urethropelvic ligament, pubocervical fascia, and vaginal wall (sparing the epithelium) in helical suspensory sutures.

e. **Modified four-corner bladder neck suspension** was developed for patients with a moderate cystocele (grade 2 or lower) due to a central defect. The two distal helical sutures are placed at the level of the bladder neck, incorporating the subepithelial vaginal wall, vesicopelvic fascia, and urethropelvic fascia. Two proximal sutures are placed incorporating either the cardinal ligament complex or the apical scar (in patients who have had a hysterectomy).

f.   The **pubovaginal sling** involves the placement of supporting material under the urethra, which is then attached to a point of fixation, usually by sling sutures or bone anchors, to either the rectus fascia or the pubic bone. The sling is effective in treating stress urinary incontinence due to both ISD and urethral hypermobility by affecting outlet resistance and anatomical position. The optimal degree of sling tension remains unknown. Complications of pubovaginal slings include acute transient urinary retention, which is not uncommon and usually resolves within 4 weeks; long-standing urinary retention, which occurs in 5% to 8%; de novo urgency, developing in up to 25% of patients; and preoperative urgency, which persists in 46%. Genitofemoral nerve entrapment may occur with autologous rectus fascia harvest, and peroneal nerve injury may occur with fascia lata harvest.

(1)   Autologous sling materials include rectus fascia, fascia lata, vaginal wall, round ligament, and dermis. Rectus fascia and fascia lata are the most common. Success rates with autologous rectus fascia vary from 46% to 100%, depending on the definition of success and method of assessment. Preoperative urgency predicts poorer outcome, although 50% to 70% of patients with mixed incontinence have resolution of their urge symptoms after pubovaginal sling.

(2)   Allograft sling materials are those harvested from a human donor. Cadaveric fascia and dermis are sterilized to prevent disease transmission and used as described above. Conflicting reports have arisen with respect to efficacy, as some grafts may undergo autolysis (degradation). There is also a theoretical risk of disease transmission.

(3)   Xenograft sling materials are harvested from nonhuman donors. Porcine dermal and intestinal submucosal grafts are available, however, clinical data regarding safety and efficacy are lacking.

(4)   Synthetic sling materials include monofilament polypropylene mesh, multifilament polyester mesh, polytetrafluoroethylene, silicon elastomer, and collagen-injected woven polyester. Efficacy and complications rates (e.g., urethral erosion) have been debated in the literature and limited the use of some of the products.

g.   The **tension-free transvaginal tape** (TVT) procedure incorporates the use of a polypropylene mesh that is not anchored. Success rates for treatment of urethral hypermobility are reported at 83% to 91%. TVT successfully treats ISD in 61% to 77% of cases. Complications associated with TVT include bladder perforation (0% to 23%), transient urinary retention (3% to 17%), erosion (two reported cases), and, rarely, external iliac vein perforation, hemorrhage, intestinal perforation, and death due to trocar injury.

4.   The **artificial urinary sphincter** (Fig. 9.3) can be used in men and women with incontinence due to a poor urethral

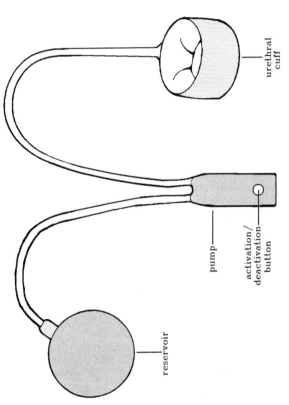

Fig. 9.3. American Medical Systems artificial urinary sphincter.

sphincteric mechanism. It involves placement of a synthetic cuff around the bladder neck/proximal urethra; the cuff remains inflated until intentional deflation by a scrotal or labial pump. The largest series by Costa et al. (2001) found success rates of 89% in patients with nonneurogenic and 82% in those with neurogenic bladders. Complications include erosion, infection, device failure, and intraoperative injury to the urethra, bladder, and/or vagina. In the Costa et al. series, 51 patients experienced intraoperative injuries and 14 required explantation of the device at a median of 11 months post procedure.

5.   Urinary diversion is indicated as a last resort in some patients with stress or urge urinary incontinence that is refractory to the above-mentioned treatment options.

D.   Surgical treatment of urge urinary incontinence

1.   Augmentation cystoplasty using bowel segments can be performed for patients with overactive bladder refractory to medication. Creation of a low-pressure system will decrease stimulation of sensory afferents. Intermittent catheterization will usually be required to completely empty the bladder. If stress incontinence is also present, this procedure may be combined with a pubovaginal sling or artificial urinary sphincter.

2.   Sacral neuromodulation may be used in patients with overactive bladder or urinary retention refractory to medical or conservative management. This involves placement of a surgical electrode permanently stimulating S3 afferent or motor nerves. Pretreatment evaluation includes evaluation of bladder capacity and response to peripheral nerve stimulation.

SUGGESTED READING

Abrams P, Cardozo L, Fall M, et al. The standardization of terminology of lower urinary tract function: report from the Standardization Subcommittee of the International Incontinence Society. *Neurourol Urodynam* 2002;21:167–178.

Baden WF, Walker TA. Genesis of the vaginal profile: a correlated classification of vaginal relaxation. *Clin Obstet Gynecol* 1972;15:1048–1054.

Blaivas JG, Groutz A. Urinary incontinence: pathophysiology, evaluation, and management overview. In: Walsh PC, Retik AB, Vaughan ED, et al., eds. *Campbell's urology.* 8th ed. Philadelphia: Saunders, 2002:1027–1052.

Bump RC, Mattiasson A, Bo K, et al. The standardization of terminology of female pelvic organ prolapse and pelvic floor dysfunction. *Am J Obstet Gynecol* 1996;175:10–17.

Costa P, Mottet N, Rabut B, et al. The use of an artificial urinary sphincter in women with type III incontinence and a negative marshall test. *J Urol* 2001;165:1172.

DeLancey JO. Structural support of the urethra as it relates to stress urinary incontinence: the hammock hypothesis. *Am J Obstet Gynecol* 1994;170:1713–1720.

Hampel C, Wienhold D, Benken N, et al. Definition of overactive bladder and epidemiology of urinary incontinence. *Urology* 1997;50(suppl):4–14.

Herschorn S, Carr L. Vaginal reconstructive surgery for sphincteric incontinence and prolapse. In: Walsh PC, Retik AB, Vaughan ED, et al., eds. *Campbell's urology.* 8th ed. Philadelphia: Saunders, 2002:1092–1139.

Leach GE, Dmochowski RR, Appell RA, et al. Female stress incontinence clinical guidelines: panel summary report on surgical management of female stress urinary incontinence. *J Urol* 1997;158:875–880.

McGuire EJ, Woodside JR, Borden TJ, et al. Prognostic value of urodynamic testing in myelodysplastic patients. *J Urol* 1981;126:205–209.

Nilsson CG, Kuuva N, Falconer C, et al. Long-term results of the tension-free vaginal tape (TVT) procedure for surgical treatment of female stress urinary incontinence. *Int Urogynecol J Pelvic Floor Dysfunc* 2001;2(suppl):S5.

Payne CK. Urinary incontinence: nonsurgical management. In: Walsh PC, Retik AB, Vaughan ED, et al., eds. *Campbell's urology.* 8th ed. Philadelphia: Saunders, 2002:1091.

Webster GD, Guralnick ML. Retropubic suspension surgery for female incontinence. In: Walsh PC, Retik AB, Vaughan ED, et al., eds. *Campbell's urology.* 8th ed. Philadelphia: Saunders, 2002:1140–1150.

Wilson TS, Lemack GE. Transvaginal surgery for stress incontinence. In: Carlin BI, Leong FC, eds. *Female pelvic health and reconstructive surgery.* New York: Marcel Dekker, 2003:137.

Wilson TS, Lemack GE, Zimmern PE. Management of intrinsic sphincteric deficiency in women. *J Urol* 2003;169:1662–1669.

Appendix 1.   Sample Voiding Diary

Date	Time	Volume (mL or oz)	Leakage (Y/N)	Amount Leakage (Large/Small)	No. Pads Used

Appendix 2. Incontinence Impact Questionnaire: Short Form IIQ-7

	Not at All	Less Than Half of the Time	About Half of the Time	More Than Half of the Time	Almost Always
1. Over the past month, has the leakage of urine and/or prolapse affected your ability to do household chores (cooking, housecleaning, laundry)?	0	1	2	3	4
2. Over the past month, has the leakage of urine and/or prolapse affected your physical recreation such as walking, swimming, or other exercise?	0	1	2	3	4
3. Over the past month, has the leakage of urine and/or prolapse affected your ability to attend entertainment activities (movies, concerts, etc.)?	0	1	2	3	4
4. Over the past month, has the leakage of urine and/or prolapse affected your ability to travel by car more than 30 minutes from home?	0	1	2	3	4
5. Over the past month, has the leakage of urine and/or prolapse affected your participation in social activities outside your home?	0	1	2	3	4
6. Over the past month, has the leakage of urine and/or prolapse affected your emotional health (nervousness, depression, etc.)?	0	1	2	3	4
7. Over the past month, how many times has the leakage of urine and/or prolapse made you feel frustrated?	0	1	2	3	4

Appendix 3.   Urogenital Distress Inventory: Short Form UDI-6

Do you experience, and, if so, how much are you bothered by:

	Not at All	Slightly	Moderately	Greatly
1. Frequent urination	0	1	2	3
2. Urine leakage related to the feeling of urgency? (sudden desire to urinate)	0	1	2	3
3. Urine leakage related to physical activity, coughing, or sneezing?	0	1	2	3
4. Small amounts of urine leakage (drops)?	0	1	2	3
5. Difficulty emptying your bladder?	0	1	2	3
6. Pain or discomfort in the lower abdominal or genital area?	0	1	2	3

Appendix 4:   Quality-of-Life Visual Analog Scale

If you were to spend the rest of your life with your urinary condition just the way it is now, how would you feel about that?

Please draw a line across the scale to best reflect your feelings about your urinary problem.

Pleased   Terrible

I———I———I———I———I———I———I———I———I———I———I

Male Sexual Dysfunction

Ronald E. Anglade, Ricardo M. Munnariz, and
Irwin Goldstein

I. Definitions

Male sexual dysfunctions are classified into dysfunctions of libido, problems with emission/ejaculation/orgasm, erectile dysfunction, and priapism.

Erectile dysfunction (ED), defined as the persistent inability to obtain and maintain an erection sufficient for sexual intercourse, affects over 30 million men in the United States. ED is more prevalent among patients with atherosclerotic peripheral vascular disease, hypertension, diabetes mellitus, hypercholesterolemia, and heart disease and among men who smoke cigarettes. ED is an age-dependent disorder (Fig. 10.1) that affects the diabetic male an average of 10 to 15 years earlier than it does his nondiabetic counterpart.

Primary ED refers to ED that is lifelong, whereas **secondary ED** implies the loss of previously normal potency. ED caused exclusively by emotional stress or psychiatric disease is termed **psychogenic ED** and accounts for an estimated 10% to 50% of all cases of ED. **Organic ED,** which is ED caused exclusively by vascular, neurologic, endocrine, or other physical disease, accounts for an estimated 50% to 80% of cases. In the majority of impotent men, erectile impairment has both a psychological and an organic basis, and a complete management program will take this into account. **Priapism** is persistent erection that is not associated with sexual desire; it may be venoocclusive (associated with arterial ischemia and usually painful) or arteriogenic (occurring in high-flow states and painless). Erectile function must be differentiated from libido, ejaculation, orgasm, and fertility. **Libido** is a psychological concept that describes the desire for sexual intercourse. **Ejaculation,** which is neurophysiologically distinct from penile erection, consists of three events: (a) seminal emission (delivery of semen to the posterior urethra), (b) bladder neck closure, and (c) propulsion of semen to the external meatus. **Orgasm** is the cerebral and psychological appreciation of release of sexual tension. **Infertility** is the inability to produce offspring and is usually not due to ED.

II. Physiology of erection

The bulk of the penis is composed of paired erectile bodies (the corpora cavernosa) (Fig. 10.2). The corpus spongiosum surrounds the urethra and distally expands to form the glans penis.

The tunica albuginea, a tough layer of fibrous tissue that surrounds the corpus cavernosum, is composed of wavy collagen and elastin that allow erectile tissue to expand and elongate. Formation of tunical fibrotic plaques (Peyronie's disease) can result in loss of tunical compliance, penile curvature, and venoocclusive dysfunction. The interior of the corpus cavernosum contains specialized, widely communicating, endothelium-lined vascular lacunar

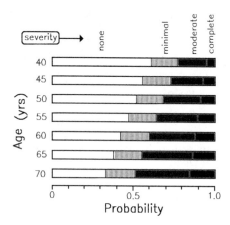

Fig. 10.1.   **Probability of various degrees of erectile dysfunction according to age.** (Adapted from data in Feldman et al. Impotence and its medical and psychosocial correlates: results of the Massachusetts Male Aging Study. *J Urol* 1994;151:54–61.)

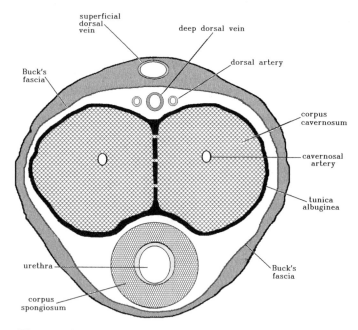

Fig. 10.2.   Cross-sectional view of penile anatomy, showing corpora cavernosa, corpus spongiosum, urethra, and their fascial coverings.

spaces that consist of connective tissue (50% to 55%) and corporal smooth muscle (45% to 50%) (Fig. 10.3).

A. Blood supply to the penis is from the internal pudendal artery, which enters the perineum through Alcock's canal and gives rise to four terminal branches (dorsal artery, cavernosal artery, bulbar artery, and scrotal artery). Within the corpora, the cavernosal artery branches into the helicine arterioles. These arterial resistance vessels open into the lacunar spaces (Fig. 10.3). There are interconnections between the dorsal penile artery and the cavernosal artery. This communication is responsible for the success of microvascular penile bypass surgery between the inferior epigastric artery (donor vessel) and the dorsal artery (recipient vessel) in patients with cavernosal artery occlusion. Last, accessory pudendal arteries provide additional blood flow to the corpora cavernosa. Injury to these arteries during radical retropubic prostatectomy may explain why some patients experience ED following successful nerve-sparing procedures.

B. Venous drainage

1. Intracavernosal drainage from the peripheral lacunar spaces passes into subtunical venules, which lie between the peripheral erectile tissue and the tunica albuginea (Fig. 10.3). A series of subtunical venules coalesce into emissary veins, which pierce the tunica albuginea to join extratunical veins.

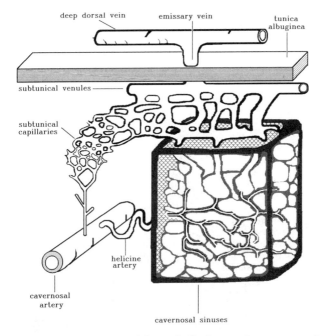

Fig. 10.3. Microcirculation of the penis. During erection, cavernosal expansion compresses the subtunical venules against the rigid tunica albuginea, impeding venous outflow from the cavernosal sinuses.

In the flaccid state, lacunar venous blood passes unimpeded from the subtunical to the emissary to the extratunical veins. In the erect state, however, the subtunical venules become stretched and compressed, thus forming the primary site of resistance to venous outflow during penile erection.

2. Extracavernosal drainage. The three routes of extratunical venous drainage are the (a) deep dorsal veins, (b) cavernosal and crural veins, and (c) superficial dorsal vein. The deep dorsal veins accept most of the venous flow from the distal corpora by way of emissary and circumflex veins. The deep dorsal veins empty into Santorini's vesicoprostatic plexus. The proximal corporal bodies are drained by the cavernosal and crural veins, which drain into both Santorini's vesicoprostatic plexus and the internal pudendal vein. The superficial dorsal vein drains blood from the pendulous penile skin and glans and communicates with the deep dorsal vein.

C. Vascular physiology

1. Nitric oxide. The corporal smooth muscle is contracted in the flaccid state and relaxed in the erect state. Following sexual stimulation, initially contracted helicine arteriolar smooth muscle undergoes relaxation through release of neuronal nitric oxide, arterial inflow increases, and nitric oxide is released from endothelial cells. Nitric oxide is a gas that diffuses into the corporal smooth muscle and induces smooth muscle relaxation. This latter process can occur only if the partial pressure of oxygen in the lacunar spaces is above 50 mm Hg, a situation that occurs only after exposure of the lacunar space to systemic arterial blood.

2. Venous outflow resistance. Filling of the lacunar spaces stretches the subtunical venules to create venous outflow resistance and a further increase in intracavernosal pressure.

3. Detumescence is brought about by neuronally mediated smooth muscle contraction, with restoration of corporal venous drainage. The **sympathetic nerves** (T10 to L2), which are responsible for detumescence and maintenance of flaccidity, project to the corpora as well as to the prostate and bladder neck via the hypogastric nerves. Adrenergic tone is crucial in initiating detumescence and in maintaining the flaccid state of the penis, since the smooth muscle of the arteries and cavernosal trabeculae must remain actively contracted. Contraction of cavernosal trabecular smooth muscle in response to norepinephrine is mediated by α_1-adrenergic receptors.

D. Neurophysiology. Erectile function in the penis is regulated by autonomic (parasympathetic and sympathetic) and somatic (sensory and motor) pathways to the erectile tissues and perineal striated muscles. Three sets of peripheral nerves innervate the penis: the sympathetic nerves (inhibitory), the parasympathetic nerves (excitatory), and the pudendal nerves (sensory).

The **parasympathetic nerves,** originating in the intermediolateral nuclei of the S2 to S4 spinal cord segments, provide the major excitatory input to the penis and are responsible for vasodilation of the penile vasculature and subsequent erection. The efferent pathway is via the pelvic nerves, which are preganglionic parasympathetic nerves originating from S2 through

Table 10.1. **Neurologic pathways of the sexual response**

Response	Afferent	Spinal Cord	Efferent
Erection			
Reflexogenic	Pudendal nerve	S2–4 sacral	Pelvic nerves
Psychogenic	Cerebral	Suprasacral	Pelvic nerves
Emission	Pudendal nerve	Lumbosacral	Sympathetic nerves
Ejaculation	Pudendal nerve	S2–4 sacral	Pudendal nerve

S4. The pelvic nerves join the pelvic plexus, which gives rise to the cavernous nerve of the penis. Stimulation of the pelvic nerves causes a marked increase in flow through the pudendal arteries and entrance of blood into the cavernosal spaces. The afferent limb of the erection response is mediated by the dorsal penile nerve (a branch of the pudendal nerve), which transmits sensory impulses to the spinal cord.

Penile erections are elicited by local sensory stimulation of the genital organs (reflexogenic erections) and by central psychogenic stimuli received by or generated within the brain (psychogenic erections). Most cerebral regulatory functions for erection occur in the hypothalamus and limbic system (Table 10.1). The role of the **sympathetic nervous system** in the initiation of penile erection is not clear, but its activation is generally associated with contraction of corpus cavernosal smooth muscle and penile detumescence.

The **pudendal nerves** comprise motor efferent and sensory afferent fibers innervating the ischiocavernous and bulbocavernous muscles as well as the penile and perineal skin. Pudendal motor neuron cell bodies are located in Onuf's nucleus of the S2 to S4 segments. The pudendal nerve enters the perineum through the lesser sciatic notch at the posterior border of the ischiorectal fossa and runs in Alcock's canal (pudendal canal) toward the posterior aspect of the perineal membrane. At this point, the pudendal nerve gives rise to the perineal nerve, with branches to the scrotum, and the rectal nerve, supplying the inferior rectal region. The dorsal nerve of the penis emerges as the last branch of the pudendal nerve. It then turns distally along the dorsal penile shaft, lateral to the dorsal artery. Multiple fascicles fan out distally, supplying proprioceptive and sensory nerve terminals to the dorsum of the tunica albuginea and the skin of the penile shaft and glans penis.

III. Causes of ED
A. Vasculogenic ED
1. **Arterial disease.** Atherosclerosis is a common cause of organic ED. Arterial ED is characterized clinically by erections that take longer than usual to develop (diminished spontaneity), have diminished rigidity, and demonstrate poor sustainability (Table 10.2). Arterial ED may be associated with general vascular risk factors such as hypertension, cigarette smoking, diabetes mellitus, and hypercholesterolemia. The

Table 10.2. Etiology of erectile dysfunction

I. Psychogenic
II. Organic
   a. **I**nflammatory: prostatitis, urethritis, stricture
   b. **M**echanical: chordee, Peyronie's disease, phimosis
   c. **P**ostoperative: iatrogenic
   d. **O**cclusive: arteriogenic
   e. **T**raumatic: pelvic fracture, urethral rupture
   f. **E**ndurance: chronic and systemic diseases
   g. **N**eurologic: neuropathy, temporal lobe epilepsy,
      multiple sclerosis
   h. **C**hemical: alcohol, marijuana, prescription drugs
   i. **E**ndocrine: testicular failure, pituitary failure,
      hyperprolactinemia

Source: From A. D. Smith, personal communication.

incidence of ED in atheromatous aortoiliac and peripheral vascular disease is about 50%. Blunt trauma to the perineum related to falls, sporting accidents, or bicycle injuries and blunt trauma to the pelvis (pelvic fractures) related to motor vehicle accidents may cause site-specific, nondiffuse arterial-occlusive disease in the common penile or cavernosal artery.

2.   Venoocclusive ED. The venous outflow regulatory mechanism depends on the completeness of trabecular smooth muscle relaxation and the expandability of the erectile tissue, defined as the ability to achieve maximal corporal volumes at low intracavernosal pressures. An increase in corporal smooth muscle tone during stress or anxiety may induce a functional venous leak. An increase in the trabecular connective tissue content, which can be secondary to abnormal collagen metabolism induced by chronic ischemia, plays a central role in the pathogenesis of organic venous leak ED. Ultimately, fibrosis of the erectile tissue causes a decreased expandability of erectile tissue, with subsequent poor stretching of the subtunical venules, poor venous outflow resistance, and failure to maintain erection.

B.   Diabetes mellitus. Diabetes mellitus is a common cause of organic ED, affecting up to 75% of diabetic patients. Patients with insulin-dependent juvenile diabetes commonly have peripheral neuropathic ED. Those with non–insulin-dependent, adult-onset diabetes usually have vasculogenic ED, but a combination of the neuropathic and angiopathic effects of diabetes is probably responsible in most cases. It is hypothesized that cavernosal artery insufficiency, corporal venoocclusive dysfunction, and/or autonomic neuropathy are the major organic pathophysiologic mechanisms leading to persistent erectile impairment in men with diabetes mellitus.

C.   Renal failure. Approximately 50% of dialysis-dependent uremic patients suffer from ED, but improvement after transplantation occurs in many patients—presumably because of reversal of the anemia associated with chronic renal failure or improvement in uremic neuropathy. Correction of abnormalities in zinc metabolism may also contribute to restoration of potency following renal transplantation. Hyperprolactinemia secondary to decreased clearance and increased production seen in end-stage renal disease has also been associated with ED.

D.   Neurologic lesions can affect erectile function at many levels:

1.   Intracerebral (Parkinson's disease, cerebrovascular disease). Efferent pathways from the medial preoptic area may be affected in addition to higher cortical functions, affecting sexual response.

2.   Spinal cord (spinal cord trauma, multiple sclerosis, myelodysplasia). Approximately 80% of patients with cervical spinal cord lesions, 70% with thoracic lesions, and 50% with lumbar lesions are able to have reflex erections. Psychogenic erections may occur in approximately 25% of patients whose spinal cord injury or lesion is below T12. Psychogenic erections are not possible in patients with complete lesions above T12. ED may, in rare cases, be the sole presenting symptom of multiple sclerosis. Sexual dysfunction may be seen in up to 75% of patients with multiple sclerosis.

3.   Peripheral nerves [alcoholic neuropathy, diabetic neuropathy (see above), after surgery or trauma]. Damage to the cavernous nerves during radical pelvic surgery such as radical prostatectomy is not uncommon. Diabetic neuropathy is the most frequent cause of peripheral neurogenic ED.

E.   Endocrine disorders are responsible for fewer than 5% of instances of ED. The etiologic significance of the hypothalamic–pituitary–testicular axis in ED is unclear. Androgens influence the growth and development of the male reproductive tract and secondary sexual characteristics. Their effect on libido and sexual behavior is well established, but the effect of androgens on normal erectile physiology is poorly understood. Isolated testosterone deficiency is rare and is usually accompanied by a marked loss of libido.

1.   Hypogonadotropic hypogonadism (Prader—Willi and Laurence—Moon—Biedl syndromes). These syndromes are rare, and patients usually present to the pediatrician or internist with delayed puberty.

2.   Hypergonadotropic hypogonadism (Klinefelter's syndrome, mumps orchitis, surgical orchiectomy). These conditions are all characterized by excessive pituitary hormone secretion in an attempt to overcome underlying testicular pathology. Potency may persist despite decreased libido.

3.   Hyperprolactinemia (pituitary adenoma, craniopharyngioma, drug therapy). Although prolactin promotes the action of androgens, at pharmacologic doses, it may inhibit luteinizing hormone and testosterone release as well as the peripheral conversion of testosterone to dihydrotestosterone. Hyperprolactinemia is associated with low or low-normal levels of serum testosterone. Androgen replacement therapy without restoration of normal prolactin levels will not restore potency. The effects of hyperprolactinemia on erectile function appear to be centrally mediated. Serum prolactin may be lowered by administering bromocriptine, L-dopa, or cyproheptadine.

Hyperthyroid states are commonly associated with diminished libido and, less frequently, with ED. ED associated with hypothyroid states has been reported and may be secondary to associated low levels of testosterone secretion and elevated levels of prolactin.

F. Trauma

1. Pelvic fracture with ruptured posterior urethra. Damage to the neurovascular bundle or to the internal pudendal or common penile artery at the time of injury is predominantly responsible for most of the ED seen following these injuries. Primary realignment with immediate repair is associated with a high incidence of ED or decreased rigidity, likely secondary to disruption of the cavernous nerves during manipulation of the hematoma. Suprapubic cystotomy with delayed repair of the urethra has a lower incidence of associated ED, ranging from 13% to 56%.

2. Perineal trauma. Many patients previously thought to have primary psychogenic ED are found to have occlusion of the common penile or cavernosal artery secondary to perineal trauma that occurred before puberty. Bicycle accidents and extensive bicycle riding account for a significant portion of these blunt perineal injuries.

G. Postoperative or iatrogenic ED

1. Aortic or peripheral vascular surgery may impair blood flow through the hypogastric arteries and thus cause arterial ED.

2. Renal transplantation may cause ED, especially if a second contralateral transplantation is performed with end-to-end hypogastric artery anastomosis. In most instances, however, renal transplantation improves sexual function by reversing the anemia and uremic neuropathy associated with chronic renal failure.

3. Pelvic irradiation may cause an accelerated occlusive atherosclerosis of the pelvic vessels, leading to ED. Fibrosis of cavernosal erectile tissue secondary to irradiation of the crural region is also likely to contribute to postirradiation ED.

4. Cavernosal–spongiosal shunts performed for the emergency treatment of priapism (Winter, Quackles, and El Ghorab procedures) can rarely produce a permanent corporal leak ED.

5. Neurosurgical procedures. Surgery such as lumbar laminectomy, sacral rhizotomy, and pudendal neurectomy can produce neurogenic ED, especially if the sacral roots at S2, S3, and S4 are injured.

6. Abdominoperineal resection of the rectum. The incidence of ED is higher if this operation is performed for malignant disease.

7. Radical prostatectomy or cystoprostatectomy. The incidence of ED can be lowered to perhaps 40% to 60% if "nerve-sparing" techniques are used.

8. Transurethral sphincterotomy may lead to ED in rare instances. One should avoid incision at the 3 o'clock and 9 o'clock positions to prevent thermal injury to the cavernosal arteries.

H. Drugs. Various medications are associated with ED. Please refer to Table 10.3 for a partial list of these agents.

Table 10.3.   Partial list of medications that can cause erectile dysfunction

Centrally acting agents
  Marijuana
  Reserpine
  Clonidine
  α-Methyldopa
  Tricyclic antidepressants
  Phenothiazines
  Ethanol
  Opioids

Anticholinergic agents
  Antimuscarinic agents
  Antihistamines
  Tricyclic antidepressants
  Phenothiazines

Antiandrogenic agents
  Spironolactone
  Estrogens
  Cyproterone acetate
  Disopyramide
  Ketoconazole
  Cimetidine

Hyperprolactinemic agents
  Estrogen
  Phenothiazines
  Haloperidol
  Metoclopramide
  Opiates
  Imipramine
  Reserpine
  α-Methyldopa

Sympatholytic agents
  α-Adrenergic blockers
  Bretylium
  Reserpine
  Clonidine
  Guanethidine
  β-Adrenergic blockers
  α-Methyldopa

Agents with unknown mechanism
  ε-Aminocaproic acid
  Naproxen
  Thiazides
  Digoxin

IV. Evaluation

A. Sexual history. The onset, duration, and circumstances of the erection problem are all important. One can distinguish three different types of erections: partner induced, nocturnal, and self-induced (masturbation). Three important qualities are hardness, maintenance, and spontaneity. It is useful to ask the patient questions concerning the qualities of all three types of erection. The degree of axial penile rigidity (hardness) can be quantified by using a scale of 1 to 10, in which 1 denotes the rigidity of a marshmallow and 10 the rigidity of a steel rod. Questions about the degree of maintenance should be asked and compared with prior capabilities. Questions concerning the degree of spontaneity should relate to the work, effort, and concentration required to achieve an erection compared with prior capabilities. Other questions include the following: Are there associated abnormalities in ejaculation, libido, or orgasm? Some symptoms suggest psychogenic ED, and others suggest organic disease. A psychogenic cause is suggested by the sudden onset of ED or the presence of ED under some circumstances but complete erection at other times. In contrast, gradual deterioration of erectile quality over months or years with preservation of libido suggests organic disease. Most patients with ED can ejaculate despite poor or absent erections.

B. Medical history. Inquiries should be made about diabetes mellitus, hypertension, smoking, hypercholesterolemia, and hyperlipidemia as well as about liver, renal, vascular, neurologic, psychiatric, and endocrine disease. Is there any history of abdominal, pelvic, or perineal surgery or trauma? The possible use of androgenic substances, whether prescribed or over the counter, mandates inquiries about these agents, as they are associated with decreased serum testosterone levels and decreased libido.

C. Psychological evaluation. Given the personal, interpersonal, social, and occupational implications of sexual problems, a brief psychosocial history is mandatory for every patient. Current psychological state, self-esteem, and history of sexual trauma/abuse, as well as past and present relationships and social and occupational performance, should be addressed.

A psychological interview with a psychologist or sex therapist may be indicated to assess the presence of personality disorders and anxiety. If possible, the couple should be present for the evaluation to assess their expectations from the planned therapy.

D. Physical examination. The general body habitus and status of **secondary sexual characteristics** should be assessed. Gynecomastia may be present in patients with androgen deficiency or estrogen excess. Absence of the peripheral pulses in the lower extremities may indicate vascular insufficiency. The penis should be examined carefully for adequacy of length, fibrotic regions of the tunica albuginea (Peyronie's disease), or deformity of the corporal bodies. It is important to stretch the penis to examine for tunical pathology. The dorsal penile pulse should be easily palpable. The presence, size, and consistency of the testes should be determined by palpation. The sensory function of the pudendal nerve can be assessed by pinprick testing of the penile and perineal skin. The integrity of the sacral reflexes is determined by eliciting the bulbocavernosus reflex.

E.   Laboratory tests. Laboratory testing is strongly recommended. Standard serum chemistries, complete blood cell count, and lipid profiles may elucidate vascular risk factors such as hypercholesterolemia, diabetes, and renal failure. Determinations of serum prostate-specific antigen (PSA) and serum thyroid-stimulating hormone may be indicated in select cases. The integrity of the hypothalamic–pituitary–gonadal axis should be examined in every patient with ED. It is unclear which testosterone assay (total, free, or bioavailable) is best; however, there is a consensus that at least one of these assays should be performed. Although pituitary adenomas are a rare cause of sexual dysfunction, this potentially life-threatening disease and reversible cause of ED should not be forgotten.

F.   Specialized diagnostic tests. The introduction of sildenafil in 1998 dramatically reduced the need for specialized testing. Diagnostic modalities such as duplex Doppler ultrasound, cavernosometry, caversonography, and selective pudendal arteriography expand the physician's and patient's understanding of the pathophysiologic mechanisms, but disadvantages such as invasiveness, cost, and associated risks and complications have reduced the indications for specialized testing.

    1.   Nocturnal penile tumescence (NPT) is the assessment of changes in penile circumference that occur during sleep. Such testing may be used to distinguish organic from psychogenic ED, but its ability to evaluate axial rigidity is poor. The accuracy of NPT in distinguishing organic from psychogenic ED is approximately 80%. In the normal postpubertal male, three to five erections occur each night during rapid eye movement stage sleep. Each erection lasts approximately 30 minutes, and these episodes occur every 90 minutes. The number and duration of tumescence episodes decrease gradually with age. Types of NPT techniques include the following:

        a.   Penile strain gauge. A circular strain gauge is placed at the base and tip of the penis. Penile erection results in stretching of the strain gauge, which is recorded. This technique measures only change in circumference, not rigidity.

        b.   Snap gauge. A disposable band is placed around the penis; the band contains three plastic strips that snap on stretching. Each strip has a different tensile strength (approximately 80, 100, and 120 mm Hg). The snap gauge provides a rough measure of rigidity and circumferential change but not a written record.

        c.   Rigiscan is an ambulatory device consisting of two loops placed around the base and tip of the penis that send information to a microcomputer to measure penile circumference and radial rigidity.

    2.   Neurologic testing. Penile biothesiometry (vibration testing) is used to assess the threshold for vibratory sensation and has proved helpful in the management of diabetic patients with ED. Other specialized tests have been described and include (a) dorsal nerve conduction time for peripheral sensory neuropathy, (b) sacral evoked response for pudendal nerve and sacral cord lesions, and (c) dorsal nerve somatosensory evoked potential testing for peripheral and central nervous system lesions in the sensory (afferent) pudendal pathway.

3. Vascular testing includes office intracavernosal injection testing, duplex Doppler ultrasound, studies of the penile brachial index, penile plethysmography, cavernosal artery systolic occlusion pressure in the erect state, recordings of the change in the diameter of the cavernosal artery in the flaccid and erect state, and selective internal pudendal arteriography in the erect state. The detection rate for suspected vascular pathology has ranged from 33% to 87%.

a. Penile brachial index testing. A Doppler stethoscope and a 1.2-cm penile cuff are used to determine penile artery systolic pressures. This value is expressed as a ratio with the systemic blood pressure measured in the arm, and the result is considered abnormal if the ratio is <0.60. This test is still valuable but has been replaced by ultrasound-based testing.

b. Duplex ultrasonography. B-Mode images and Doppler values are obtained with a 7.5-MHz transducer during a pharmacologically induced penile erection. This test is performed to assess cavernosal artery diameter and flow velocity; simultaneous functional and anatomic information is thereby obtained. Peak flow velocity, acceleration time, diastolic flow velocity, and resistive index are some of the parameters that can be measured to gather information about the relative status of penile inflow and outflow mechanisms in a minimally invasive fashion. This test is performed after the penis has been maximally relaxed using pharmacologic agents.

c. Dynamic infusion cavernosometry and cavernosography. The intracavernosal pressure and volume are measured following injection of intracavernosal vasoactive agents. In healthy persons, the equilibrium intracavernosal pressure is recorded after 10 minutes to approximate the mean systemic arterial blood pressure (90 mm Hg). Subsequently, infusion of saline solution into the corpora is begun through a separate intracavernosal needle. Flow rates for maintenance of various intracavernosal pressures are recorded. Generally, an infusion rate of <5 mL/min is required to maintain a series of intracavernosal pressure values. Once a pressure of 150 mm Hg is reached, the infusion is stopped, and the "pressure decay" is noted after 30 seconds. Normally, the pressure should not drop >45 mm Hg in 30 seconds. Patients suspected of having venous leak ED, based on abnormalities of the flow to maintain and pressure decay studies, undergo infusion of x-ray contrast agent into their corpora to confirm the diagnosis. Radiographic demonstration of contrast agent outside the corpora following administration of intracavernosal papaverine, combined with the inability to sustain intracavernosal pressure, indicates ED caused by "corporal venous leak." Arterial integrity is assessed in this study by recording the cavernosal artery systolic occlusion pressure and comparing this value with the systemic brachial artery systolic occlusion pressure.

d. Selective internal pudendal arteriography. Arteriography is a more invasive test that is indicated if arteriogenic ED is suspected in a candidate for microvascular arterial bypass surgery for ED. Arteriography is usually

performed with intravascular and intracavernosal vasodila-
tors and patient sedation to optimize visualization of the
cavernosal vessels.

V.   Treatment
A.   First-line therapy

1.   **Sex therapy.** For patients with evidence of psychogenic
ED and no discernible organic cause, a short course (6 to
12 weeks) of sex therapy should be prescribed. The details of
this therapy are beyond the scope of this chapter. In organic
ED, behavioral sex therapy may be combined with various
other forms of therapy in selected cases to optimize patient
response. Because performance anxiety may continue to play
a significant role in a couple's sexual life after medical or surgical treatment, behavioral sex therapy may be useful even
in the presence of organic pathology.

2.   The **vacuum erection device** (VED) is one of the main-
stays of noninvasive therapy for ED. It consists of a cylindrical component and a suction device that the patient places
around the penis to create negative pressure and achieve an
erection (Fig. 10.4). Maintenance of erection is then accomplished with an elastic constriction ring placed at the base of
the penis. The advantages of VED include simplicity of use,
low cost, relative safety, and ability to start treatment immediately. Patients with significant peripheral vascular disease,
those receiving anticoagulants, and diabetics are generally
not good candidates for the VED.

   a.   **Efficacy.** Patient acceptance and satisfaction with
vacuum constrictive devices in all types of ED, including
diabetic ED, have been reported to be 68% to 83%. The reasons for discontinuation of this treatment have included

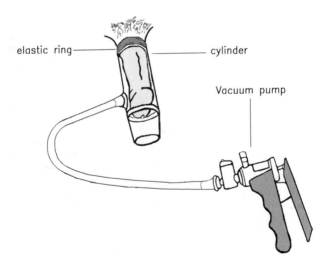

Fig. 10.4.   Hand-operated vacuum erection device.

premature loss of penile tumescence and rigidity, penile pain, pain during ejaculation, and inconvenience.

b.   Complications. Patient compliance with the recommended guidelines for use is mandatory because serious problems may be encountered if the VED is left in place for a long period. To date, the complications from the use of these devices have been minor and self-limited. They have included difficulty with ejaculation, penile pain, ecchymoses, hematomas, and petechiae. Patients taking aspirin or warfarin are more likely to develop complications related to vascular fragility. Many of the devices manufactured have a valve that limits the vacuum pressure (<250 mm Hg), a feature that might decrease these types of complications.

3.   Oral agents. The introduction of **sildenafil citrate** in 1998 revolutionized the management of men with ED. Sildenafil has not only encouraged patients and health care professionals to more openly discuss human sexuality, it has also increased the number of patients using other therapeutic modalities such as intracavernosal injections and penile prostheses.

a.   Sildenafil citrate is a potent and selective inhibitor of phosphodiesterase type 5 (PDE5). The drug blocks the hydrolysis of cyclic GMP, enhancing the accumulation of cyclic GMP and potentiating the relaxant effects of nitric oxide. After oral administration, the drug is rapidly absorbed and 40% bioavailable. Fatty foods decrease the bioavailability of the drug to 29%. Sildenafil is metabolized in the liver by the cytochrome P450 enzyme system and is excreted in feces (80%) and urine (13%). Sildenafil is effective in treating ED resulting from a variety of organic causes, including diabetes mellitus.

(1)   Dosing. Sildenafil is used on demand (prn). The recommended initial dose is 50 mg taken 1 hour before sexual activity. After the initial dose, it can be adjusted based on efficacy and tolerability. The maximum recommended dose is 100 mg, no more than once per day, independent of the dosage used. The majority of patients (75%) use 100 mg, and only 2% of patients use 25 mg. The initial dose in patients older than 65 years, in patients with renal or liver insufficiency, or in patients receiving drugs that inhibit cytochrome P450 (erythromycin, cimetidine) is 25 mg.

(2)   Contraindications. Sildenafil is contraindicated in patients who require nitroglycerine to treat myocardial ischemia. The American College of Cardiologists and the American Heart Association also recommend that sildenafil be used with caution in patients receiving complex antihypertensive regimens; in patients with coronary artery disease, borderline blood pressure, or renal/liver insufficiency; and in patients who use drugs that inhibit cytochrome P450.

(3)   Adverse effects. The rate of discontinuation of this agent is extremely low (0.4% to 1.2%), most likely because of its low side effect profile and high efficacy. The most common side effects are headaches (16%), facial flushing

(10%), dyspepsia (7%), nasal congestion (4%), and diarrhea (3%). In addition, at the 100-mg dose, 2% to 3% of men may experience transient alterations in color vision.

b.   Yohimbine hydrochloride is a natural product derived from the bark of the yohimbe tree that produces a presynaptic α_2-adrenergic blocking agent. Peripherally, its effect is to increase cholinergic and decrease adrenergic activity. Yohimbine also acts as a mood stimulant. Its efficacy rate is only about 20% to 25% overall, and it seems to be most effective in patients with psychogenic ED. Nevertheless, the drug continues to find use as a safe and low-cost alternative to sildenafil. Standard dose is 5.4 mg PO tid. Adverse effects include dizziness, flushing, nausea, and headache.

c.   Vardenafil, a potent and selective PDE5 inhibitor, is currently in clinical trials and will soon be available in the USA. It offers a slightly quicker onset of action than sildenafil.

d.   Tadalafil is also a potent and selective PDE5 inhibitor with a long half-life (almost 18 hours) that will soon be available in the USA. Because of its long half-life, it will be administered once daily rather than prn as sildenafil is. The most common adverse events were headache, back pain, myalgia, and dyspepsia. Interestingly, no color vision alterations were observed with tadalafil.

4.   Androgen replacement is indicated only in patients with documented androgen deficiency; it should not be used empirically. The cause of androgen deficiency should be thoroughly investigated. Older men should be followed regularly for prostatic enlargement or nodularity while receiving androgen therapy. PSA must be checked annually.

a.   Parenteral testosterone has a long history as reliable treatment of male hypogonadism. Both testosterone enanthate and testosterone cypionate are very lipophilic, resulting in slow release from the adipose tissue at the injection site. The dose is 200 to 400 mg IM every 2 to 4 weeks.

b.   Oral testosterone may be given as 10 to 30 mg of methyltestosterone daily or 5 to 20 mg of fluoxymesterone daily but is generally less effective than parenteral therapy. Oral testosterone therapy is associated with cholestatic jaundice (reversible on withdrawal of drug therapy) and hepatocarcinoma. Liver toxicity is caused by 17α-methyl preparations of testosterone. For these reasons, oral testosterone therapy is not recommended.

c.   Transdermal testosterone therapy that can achieve steady serum levels of testosterone is now available in several forms. Compliance may be significantly improved because of the ease of application.

(1)   Scrotal patch application is based on the observation that genital skin is the only skin across which sufficient natural testosterone can be absorbed to raise the serum testosterone concentration to normal levels. The patch is applied to the scrotal skin once a day and worn continuously except when bathing. Absorption is better with hairless skin.

(2) Body skin patch. A 5-mg patch is applied to the arm, torso, or thigh and delivers 5 mg of testosterone over 24 hours.

(3) Testosterone gel is supplied in 2.5- and 5.0-g packets. These contain 25 and 50 mg of testosterone, respectively. The dose is 50 to 100 mg qd applied to normal skin. It may take a month for the serum testosterone concentration reach the normal male range.

B. Second-line therapy

1. Intracavernous pharmacotherapy. Most patients suffering from ED, both organic and mixed, may potentially be treated with intracavernous pharmacotherapy. Before intracavernosal pharmacotherapy is instituted as a long-term form of therapy, a diagnostic and therapeutic trial must be performed in the office so that the patient is fully comfortable with the technique of injection and the dosage. Patients are usually advised to inject a maximum of three times per week. The initial acceptance rate for intracavernosal pharmacotherapy is between 65% and 85% in most studies, but there is a nearly 50% 1-year dropout rate. Loss of interest in sexual activity and complications of intracavernosal pharmacotherapy (e.g., pain, dislike of self-injection, recovery of spontaneous erections, other medical conditions) are some of the reasons for the high dropout rate. Agents that have been used in this mode include papaverine, phentolamine, prostaglandin E_1, and forskolin in various combinations. Lower doses of vasoactive agents are indicated in spinal cord–injured patients, whereas diabetic individuals usually require higher doses. Onset of erection is usually around 10 minutes from the time of injection, and duration may range from 30 minutes to 6 hours. Intracavernosal pharmacotherapy with vasoactive medications is contraindicated in patients taking monoamine oxidase inhibitors, patients with hypersensitivity to these agents, and those prone to secondary priapism (e.g., sickle cell disease or trait, leukemia, or multiple myeloma).

a. Papaverine hydrochloride is a direct smooth muscle relaxant and vasodilator whose action is unrelated to nerve activity. It is supplied as a solution containing 30 mg/mL. The dose varies from patient to patient and must be individualized. The drug is given alone (rare) or in combination with other agents such as phentolamine or phentolamine and alprostadil (tri-mix) (Table 10.4).

b. Phentolamine mesylate is a short-acting α-adrenergic blocking agent that is most often combined with

Table 10.4.   Vasoactive agents for intracavernous injection

Vasoactive Agent(s)	Typical Dose Range
Papaverine HCl	15–45 mg
Prostaglandin E_1	10–40 µg
Papaverine/phentolamine	30 mg/1 mg
Papaverine/phentolamine/prostaglandin E_1	30 mg/1 mg/10 µg

papaverine or alprostadil. It is supplied in a 1-mL vial containing 5 mg. The intracavernous dose is up to 1 mg.

c. **Alprostadil** alone (usually 10 to 40 µg) or in combination with papaverine and/or phentolamine mesylate may be injected intracavernosally. Most studies show increased efficacy for the three-drug combination regimen compared with monotherapy.

d. **Three-drug regimen solution** consists of 30 mg of papaverine, 1 mg of phentolamine, and 10 µg of prostaglandin E_1 per milliliter of solution. The dose is highly individualized, ranging from 0.05 to 1 mL or sometimes more if required to obtain an adequate response. A safe test dose is 0.25 mL.

e. **Forskolin,** a naturally occurring alkaloid that directly activates the catalytic domain of adenylate cyclase, has demonstrated efficacy as an auxiliary vasoactive agent in patients who had previously failed high-volume, high-concentration injection therapy. Forskolin is especially useful in patients with diabetes or post–radical prostatectomy ED who develop significant corporal pain with the use of intracavernosal prostaglandin E_1.

f. **Technique of injection** is important in obtaining satisfactory results and reducing the risk of complications. The vasoactive solution selected should be drawn up in a 1-cc syringe with a 27G needle. The needle should penetrate the tunica albuginea at the lateral border near the base of the penis but not go so deep as to injure the cavernous artery (Fig. 10.5). Firm pressure should be placed on the injection site for 3 minutes after injection to prevent hematoma.

g. **Complications** of intracavernosal pharmacotherapy may include the following:

(1) **Local hematoma** can be largely prevented by instructing the patient to compress the injection site manually for at least 3 minutes.

(2) **Corporal fibrosis** is the most significant long-term complication of intracavernosal pharmacotherapy and may be related to a number of factors, including drug effect, genetic predisposition, local trauma during intercourse, injection frequency, or a combination of these. It

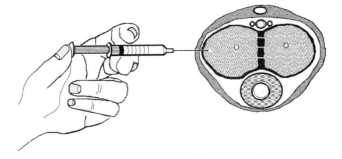

Fig. 10.5. Technique of injecting vasoactive agents into corpus cavernosum.

may resolve spontaneously in 35% of patients, and intracavernosal pharmacotherapy may be reinstituted. Persistence of corporal fibrosis is not necessarily a reason to stop intracavernosal pharmacotherapy if the degree of fibrosis and deformity is not severe and they are not interfering with intercourse. In more severe cases, insertion of a penile prosthesis and penile straightening will be required. Local induration may be reduced by alternating injection sites and limiting the injections to no more than two or three per week.

(3) **Priapism** is a potentially serious complication that can lead to permanent corporal fibrosis. Priapism of <24 hours' duration can usually be managed without surgery by corporal aspiration and intracavernosal injection of α-adrenergic agents.

(4) **Pain** may be reported by the patient on intracavernosal pharmacotherapy. The pain may be at the injection site for a short time after injection, but diffuse penile "ache" is more common. Prolonged pain may be experienced in the penile shaft or the perineum in approximately 20% of patients on prostaglandin E_1 monotherapy, but this is rare with papaverine or phentolamine.

2.   **Transurethral alprostadil,** a Food and Drug Administration–approved medication for the treatment of men with ED, is a semisolid pellet inserted intraurethrally with an applicator. This compound is the same as that used for intracavernosal injection, but the doses required are significantly larger (125 to 1,000 μg). From the corpus spongiosum, the agent must pass into the corpus cavernosum to initiate the hemodynamic events leading to erection. The most commonly used initial dose is 500 μg. About 65% of patients using transurethral alprostadil report erections sufficient for intercourse, but only one-third report erections with 100% rigidity. The major advantage is ease of delivery compared with intracavernosal injections. The most common side effect is penile pain (10%), with hypotension-related symptoms the next most common (3%). Priapism or penile fibrosis has not been reported. Recent studies suggest that placement of a penile ring may enhance the effectiveness of this mode of treatment.

C.   **Third-line therapy**

1.   **Surgical prostheses.** Third-line treatment interventions are invasive, irreversible, and associated with many potentially serious complications such as device infection, erosion, and malfunction. Penile prostheses should be viewed only as a last-resort therapy in patients with treatment-refractory ED. Despite their significant cost and potential invasiveness, penile prostheses continue to find application in patients who have failed other forms of therapy.

a.   **Historical notes.** Interest in treating ED developed among urologists following the development of a successful intracorporal noninflatable penile prosthesis by Small and Carrion and an inflatable prosthesis by Scott and Bradley in the 1970s. Over the next two decades, further development of penile prostheses proceeded along these two distinct lines:

the malleable or rigid prosthesis and the multicomponent inflatable prosthesis. More recently, two-component and self-contained inflatable devices have been introduced.

b. Counseling and selection of prosthesis. A variety of prostheses are available (Table 10.5). The ideal penile prosthesis would result in a normal-appearing penis when flaccid while providing increased girth and length when erect. This ideal is rarely achieved, and patients should be counseled that penile prostheses will not restore the full length previously achieved by natural erections. Thus, careful counseling and selection of the device most appropriate for the individual patient are very important to patient satisfaction. Considerations include patient anatomy, physical habitus, cosmetic preference, surgeon's preference, and cost of the device. The advantages of the malleable/ semirigid devices are easier placement, less dependence on patient manual dexterity, lesser chance of component failure, and far lower cost. The disadvantages are somewhat higher risk of erosion, more difficult concealment, and lack of change in girth. The malleable/semirigid devices are preferred in patients who have physical problems such as severe arthritis or abdominal obesity. Younger patients with good hand dexterity will often choose the three-piece prothesis (Fig. 10.6). This device is especially appropriate for those concerned about cosmesis in the flaccid state.

c. Preoperative preparation. The following protocol is recommended prior to implantation of penile prostheses to reduce the risk of device infection:

(1) Scrub genitalia and perineum for 10 minutes each day for 7 days prior to surgery with chlorhexidine digluconate soap (Hibiclens).

Table 10.5. Types of penile prostheses

Type	Manufacturer	Models	Description
Mechanical	Timm Medical	Dura II	Ball-and-socket articulation
Malleable	AMS	600, 650	Wire core
	Mentor	Malleable, Accuform	Silver wire core
Inflatable			
One piece	AMS	Dynaflex	Proximal reservoir activated by pressure on glans
Two piece	AMS	Ambicor	Pump and reservoir combined
	Mentor	Mark II	—
Three piece	AMS	Ultrex	Full fluid transfer during inflation/ deflation
	Mentor	Alpha 1	

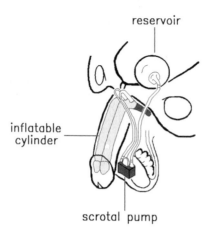

reservoir

inflatable
cylinder

scrotal pump

Fig. 10.6.   Typical three-piece inflatable penile prosthesis.

(2)   Prescribe an oral quinolone (e.g., gatifloxacin 400 mg
PO) for 3 days prior to the surgery.
(3)   Give perioperative antibiotics (vancomycin 1 g and
gentamycin 80 mg IV 1 hour prior to surgery).
(4)   Scrub and prep lower abdomen, genitalia, inguinal
folds, perineum, and thighs with iodine-containing solution for 15 minutes.
(5)   Carefully catheterize the bladder with 16F Foley
catheter. After draining the bladder, plug the Foley
catheter.
(6)   Change gloves after draping, and put on double
gloves.
d. Postoperative care. The Foley catheter can be removed on the morning after surgery. For inflatable prostheses, the patient should be sent home with the device
semiinflated. Oral antibiotics should given for 14 days. Sexual activity is prohibited until after the first office visit at
6 weeks postoperatively.
e. Device infection. The incidence of infection following
penile prosthetic surgery ranges between 0.4% and 9%. Following implantation, the time frame for the presentation of
infection will vary depending on the organism involved. Infections with more virulent and aggressive bacteria will
usually present within the first few postoperative days,
with the patient presenting with fever, pain, and swelling
overlying the prosthesis accompanied by purulent wound
drainage. However, a group of patients will complain of prolonged pain but will not have obvious purulent drainage
from the wound. Prolonged pain, fixation of the pump or
tubing to the overlying scrotal skin, elevated white blood
cell count and sedimentation rate, and hyperglycemia in diabetic patients may all be helpful in suggesting a possible
infection by less virulent organisms. Duplex Doppler ultra-

sound may also be helpful in cases in which clinical findings are not conclusive.

2. Arterial revascularization may be indicated in the rare patient with a focal arterial lesion that can be identified on arteriography. The best candidates for penile revascularization are patients who are young, nondiabetic, and non-smokers and who have no underlying neurologic disease.

3. Venous surgery. At present, the available procedures (crural plication, ligation, or excision of the deep dorsal vein of the penis; ligation of cavernosal veins; spongiolysis; or a combination of the above, including the radiologic administration of coils or sclerosing agents) have not demonstrated long-term success in most impotent patients. Complications reported from the various procedures, especially those involving proximal penile dissection, include diminished penile sensation and shortened penile length.

SUGGESTED READING

Carson CC, Mulcahy JJ, Govier FE. Efficacy, safety and patient satisfaction outcomes of the AMS 700CX inflatable penile prosthesis: results of a long-term multicenter study. AMS 700CX Study Group. *J Urol* 2000;164:376–380.

Feldman HA, Goldstein I, Hatzichristou DG, et al. Impotence and its medical and psychosocial correlates: results of the Massachusetts Male Aging Study. *J Urol* 1994;151:54–61.

Fried FA, Carson CC III. ED—improving patient treatment. *J Urol* 1996;155:1624–1625.

Jarow JP. Risk factors for penile prosthetic infection. *J Urol* 1996; 156:402–404.

Krane RJ, Goldstein I, Saenz de Tejada. ED. *N Engl J Med* 1989;321: 1648–1659.

Lue T. Erectile dysfunction associated with cavernous and neurological disorders. *J Urol* 1994;151:890–891.

Mulcahy JJ. Long-term experience with salvage of infected penile implants. *J Urol* 2000;163:481–482.

Mulhall JP, Jahoda AE, Cairney M, et al. The causes of patient dropout from penile self-injection therapy for impotence. *J Urol* 1000;162:1291–1294.

Rajfer J. ED—the quick workup. *J Urol* 1996;156:1951.

Skolnick AA. Guidelines for treating erectile dysfunction issues. *JAMA* 1997;277:7–8.

Genitourinary Trauma and Emergencies

Meir Daller and Gennaro Carpinito

A urologic emergency arises when a condition requires rapid diagnosis and immediate treatment. This chapter focuses on traumatic and nontraumatic genitourinary (GU) emergencies typically arising in the emergency department, outpatient clinic, or inpatient ward. The evaluation of hematuria is discussed separately in Chapter 1, and Chapter 13 provides a discussion of GU sepsis.

Trauma to the GU organs generally does not result in an immediate threat to life. However, failure to appropriately evaluate and treat these injuries may result in significant long-term patient morbidity. Recent advances in intensive care and radiologic imaging have greatly improved diagnosis and survival in serious trauma. As a member of the trauma team, it is the responsibility of the urologist to provide proper interpretation of urologic imaging and intervene surgically when necessary.

I. General principles of trauma management

Approximately 10% of all trauma involves the GU tract, but only 2% involves the GU tract exclusively. The GU system may be divided into three regions, each with its own pattern of injury. The upper tract includes the renal arteries, the kidneys, and the ureters. The lower tract consists of the bladder, the prostate, and the posterior urethra. The external portion consists of the anterior urethra, penis, scrotum, and testicles in the male. Trauma patients presenting to the emergency room may have (a) unstable vital signs requiring immediate surgical intervention, (b) penetrating trauma with stable vital signs, or (c) blunt trauma with stable vital signs.

A. History. Attempt to obtain a detailed history of the trauma from the patient or from witnesses and emergency personnel. Loss of consciousness is a rough indicator of the force of trauma and the possible presence of head injury. In falls, the height from which the victim has fallen and the nature of the landing surface are important. In motor vehicle accidents, the speed of the vehicle, location of the victim within the automobile, and use of seat belts are important. In gunshot wounds, the type of weapon, caliber of the projectile, and distance from the victim at which the shot was fired can be used to estimate the extent of tissue damage.

B. Physical examination is performed during the generalized trauma evaluation. Hemodynamic instability requires aggressive resuscitation and emergency surgical exploration in many cases. Physical findings of tenderness, ecchymosis, or penetrating injuries in the flank, suprapubic region, pelvis, or external genitalia strongly suggest an underlying urologic injury. Pelvic bony instability indicates a likely pelvic fracture and should alert the trauma team to the possibility of urethral or bladder injury. Likewise, gross blood at the urethral meatus and superior displacement of the prostate on rectal examination are indicative of possible urethral injury.

C. Diagnostic tests begin with routine urinalysis to look for the presence and extent of hematuria and should be performed on all patients. The urethra should be catheterized *unless urethral injury is suspected.* If blood is seen at the urethral meatus *or* a significant pelvic fracture is present, urethral injury must first be ruled out by retrograde urethrography (see below).

D. Radiologic examination

1. Plain films of the abdomen may reveal bony fractures of the pelvis, ribs, or vertebrae. Loss of the perirenal outline, loss of the psoas shadow, or displacement of bowel gas may indicate retroperitoneal hematoma or urinoma. A "ground-glass" appearance on plain film may be caused by intraperitoneal urinary extravasation.

2. Retrograde urethrogram is indicated whenever urethral injury is suggested by the presence of blood at the meatus, superior displacement of the prostate on digital rectal examination, pelvic fracture, or inability to pass a urethral catheter. The study may be performed easily by using either a Brodney clamp that fits onto the glans penis or a 12F Foley catheter inserted into the fossa navicularis. The balloon is inflated only enough to hold the catheter gently in place. After the patient is placed in the 30-degree oblique position, 15 mL of radiographic contrast agent is injected gently. The presence of extravasation is indicative of urethral injury. The posterior portion of the urethra above the pelvic floor is difficult to interpret on retrograde urethrography, as the external sphincter is often closed.

3. Cystography is indicated to rule out bladder injury in all patients with blunt or penetrating trauma that manifest gross or microscopic hematuria. In patients who have penetrating trauma without hematuria, the indications for cystography depend on the nature and location of the wound. Ideally, cystography should be performed in a radiology suite with fluoroscopic capacity to obtain oblique and real-time images. Some centers have advocated computed tomographic (CT) cystogram as their study of choice. Regardless of the technique used, it is essential that the bladder be completely filled with contrast agent to demonstrate small amounts of extravasation. Extravasation from the bladder may be missed on intravenous urogram (IVU) or CT scan if the bladder is incompletely distended. Allow contrast agent to flow through the urethral catheter under gravity until the bladder is full; at least 250 mL is often required. After the bladder is emptied, a postvoid film is vital to assess extravasation located behind the bladder.

4. CT with intravenous contrast agent has become the "gold standard" of trauma evaluation and is our preferred study in the initial assessment of renal trauma. Scanning in the spiral (helical) mode may be done in <5 minutes and provides an excellent assessment of renal parenchymal integrity, injury to other organs in the abdomen, and the presence of hematomas or urinomas. CT can also establish the presence of both kidneys and their excretory function.

5.   IVU is no longer recommended as the initial screening examination in patients with suspected renal injury. IVU may be useful in patients with traumatic hematuria if CT is not available. In the case of the unstable patient who is brought straight to the operating room without radiologic studies, a **"one-shot" IVU** is essential before any exploration of the kidneys to evaluate the contralateral side. After a scout film of the abdomen has been obtained, contrast agent (Renografin-60 in a dose of 1 mL/kg) is injected intravenously by hand during 3 to 5 minutes. A film is taken at 5 to 10 minutes after injection of contrast agent. Adequate visualization of the kidneys may not be obtained on IVU unless the patient has a stable systolic blood pressure above 90 mm Hg.

6.   Renal arteriography may be indicated in instances of renal vascular injury, a diagnosis suggested by nonvisualization of the kidney on CT or IVU. In selected patients, it also may be useful in identifying the source of persistent renal bleeding following trauma. If a source of bleeding is clearly identified, arteriographic embolization may be performed at the same time.

7.   Ultrasonography (US) permits noninvasive assessment of perirenal and subcapsular hematomas and is useful in following patients with renal trauma who are being managed nonsurgically.

8.   Radionuclide studies may be useful in the follow-up care of patients with trauma in whom hypertension develops.

II.   Kidney

A.   Trauma. Located high in the retroperitoneum, the kidneys are relatively well protected by the bony rib cage, lumbar spine, and vertebral muscles. However, trauma sufficient to fracture a rib or vertebral process often is accompanied by trauma to the kidney. Renal trauma accounts for approximately 50% of all cases of GU trauma, and >50% of cases involve patients under the age of 30. There is a male-to-female predominance of 4:1. In children aged 5 to 15, the most common cause of renal injury is bicycle riding.

1.   Blunt trauma to the abdomen, flank, or back accounts for >80% of all renal injuries. The most common causes are motor vehicle accidents, falls, sports accidents, and assaults. Rapid deceleration such as commonly occurs in motor vehicle accidents or falls may cause tears in the renal artery intimal layer or even complete avulsion. In adult patients with blunt trauma, gross hematuria, shock, and direct trauma to the flank are associated with an increased risk of sustaining major renal injury (about 25%). In children, the most common cause of blunt renal trauma is bicycle riding.

2.   Penetrating trauma is most commonly caused by knife and bullet wounds. Approximately 85% of instances of penetrating trauma involving the kidney are associated with injury to other intraabdominal organs (Table 11.1). Children are especially prone to renal injury because of the underdevelopment of the back muscles and rib cage and because the kidneys are relatively larger than in adults. In addition, the kidneys in children are not as well protected by perirenal fat and Gerota's fascia, which can act as a buffer against trauma. Renal injury

Table 11.1. Intraabdominal injuries associated with penetrating renal trauma (% risk)

Liver	45
Stomach	25
Pancreas	25
Small bowel	25
Spleen	20
Right colon	20
Left colon	15
Major vessels	15
Duodenum	15

is more likely in the presence of preexisting conditions such as hydronephrosis or tumors.

3. **Classification of renal injury**
   a. **Grade 1** injury (**renal contusion**) is bruising of the renal parenchyma without true parenchymal disruption (Fig. 11.1). An associated **subcapsular hematoma** may be present, but the kidney is intact. Such injuries account for the majority of cases of blunt renal trauma.
   b. **Grade 2** injury involves ruptures or tears of the renal capsule and parenchyma that are **<1 cm** in length (non-expanding **perirenal hematoma** may be present). The injury does not involve the collecting system or the medulla of the kidney (no urinary extravasation). Grade 1 and 2 injuries are classified as minor injuries and account for 85% of all renal injuries.
   c. **Grade 3** injury is the same as grade 2 injury but extends **>1 cm** (no urinary extravasation).
   d. **Grade 4** injury is a major laceration that extends into the collecting system and produces **extravasation of urine.** Involvement of a segmental vessel also qualifies as a grade 4 injury.
   e. **Grade 5** indicates the most extensive renal injury. Severe multiple lacerations, fracture, **shattering of the kidney,** and avulsion of the renal hilum are all examples of grade 5 injury. Grade 3, 4, and 5 injuries are classified as major injuries. **Renal lacerations** account for approximately 15% of blunt renal injuries and 30% of penetrating injuries. **Renal vascular injury** includes occlusion, thrombosis, or avulsion of the renal artery, renal vein, or one of their branch vessels; it occurs in <1% of instances of blunt renal trauma but in up to 10% of instances of penetrating trauma. Renal vascular injuries are difficult to diagnose quickly enough to prevent renal loss because significant and irreversible renal injury occurs within 1 hour if significant ischemia is present.

4. **Diagnosis**
   a. Patients who are **hemodynamically unstable** will almost always need to be explored quickly. The urologist is often called to the operating room for consultation after the patient has been explored by the general surgeons and must

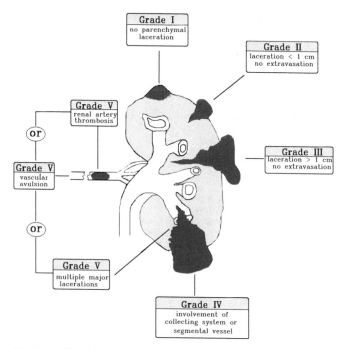

Fig. 11.1.   Classification of renal injury. (Classification system from Moore et al. Organ injury scaling: spleen, liver, and kidney. *J Trauma* **1989;29:1664.)**

determine whether both kidneys are present and functioning. This can be accomplished with a **one-shot IVU** performed on the operating table. If there is no evidence of renal injury, no exploration is indicated. Major injuries or unilateral nonfunction noted on intraoperative IVU should be explored. If only minor injury is noted on the IVU but retroperitoneal bleeding is present, the kidney should be explored and repaired.

b.   In patients who are **hemodynamically stable,** CT is the preferred initial radiologic examination (see Chapter 2).

5.   Treatment of renal injury depends heavily on the nature and severity of injury, determined by the evaluation previously described.

a.   Blunt trauma. In general, the likelihood of significant urinary tract injury in patients with blunt trauma who are hemodynamically stable and have no hematuria is low. Patients with microscopic hematuria who are hemodynamically stable also have a low risk for significant renal injury, but they should be observed more closely if the mechanism of injury warrants it. Patients with hemodynamic instability or gross hematuria are more likely to have a significant injury and should therefore undergo a more aggressive radiologic assessment if time allows. These patients are monitored for signs of bleeding, such as a change in vital signs, decrease in the hematocrit, or expanding flank hematoma. Patients with fractured kidney or renal vascular injuries usually require prompt surgical intervention for repair of the kidney or urgent nephrectomy. The management of **urinary extravasation** in blunt renal injury is controversial; some authorities favor conservative treatment, and others feel that early surgical intervention is preferable. Antibiotic therapy is usually indicated, especially if the urine is infected at time of injury, and serial US can be used to monitor the resolution of the urine collection. If signs of abscess formation or sepsis appear, the urinoma should be drained surgically or percutaneously. The proponents of early surgical exploration in patients with urinary extravasation argue that it results in decreased length of hospital stay and reduced incidence of complications such as infected urinoma; however, the incidence of nephrectomy is increased in patients explored surgically.

b.   Penetrating trauma. All patients with abdominal gunshot wounds and almost all patients with stab wounds should undergo surgical exploration (Table 11.2). The only exception is the patient with a stab wound of the flank, no hematuria, normal CT findings, and no abnormal physical findings. This type of case can be managed nonoperatively. In other instances of penetrating trauma, abdominal exploration is required to repair associated injuries and the urologic injury itself. Surgical management of penetrating renal trauma consists of gaining control of the renal pedicle, obtaining adequate hemostasis, debriding devitalized tissue, repairing the collecting system, and providing adequate drainage. When the severity of the injury makes this treatment impossible, nephrectomy is indicated, which occurs in approximately 10% of patients with stab wounds and in 40% of those with gunshot wounds (Table 11.3).

6.   Complications of renal injury include delayed bleeding, hypertension, formation of arteriovenous fistulas, hydronephrosis, and loss of renal parenchyma. Delayed bleeding may occur during the first month after injury. Persistent hematuria may be an indication of a traumatic arteriovenous

Table 11.2.   Indications for renal exploration

Absolute	Relative
Pulsatile or expanding retroperitoneal mass	Major renal injury
Hemodynamic instability from renal bleeding	Urinary extravasation
Renal vascular injury in solitary kidney	Laparotomy for associated injury
	Nonviable renal tissue needing debridement

Table 11.3.   Results of renal exploration

Surgery	Blunt Trauma (%)	Stab Wound (%)	Gunshot Wound (%)
Debridement and repair	35	60	40
Partial nephrectomy	15	15	20
Nephrectomy	10	7.5	15
Vascular repair	10	7.5	10
Pelvic repair	15	0	0
Exploration only	15	10	15

Source: Modified from McAninch JW. *World J Urol* 1999;17:65.

fistula and should prompt arteriography. The patient's blood pressure should be monitored carefully during the first 6 months after injury. If hypertension develops, CT or renal US should be performed at the end of that period.

B.   Renal vascular emergencies

1.   Renal arterial emboli constitute 2% of arterial emboli. The main renal arteries are most frequently involved by systemic emboli from the left atrium in association with atrial fibrillation, artificial heart valves, the vegetations of endocarditis, or a mural thrombus from a myocardial infarct. Iatrogenic emboli are being increasingly seen because of the widespread use of invasive vascular procedures. The intrarenal arteries are end arteries, so their occlusion leads to a wedge-shaped infarction of the renal parenchyma. These infarcts may be unilateral or bilateral, although they are more common on the left. Clinically, a spectrum ranges from no symptoms in a large number of patients to acute flank pain that may radiate to the groin, nausea, vomiting, and fever when infarction occurs. This picture closely mimics that of a ureteral calculus. Microscopic or gross hematuria is found in 50% of cases. This may be accompanied by proteinuria, leukocytosis, and epithelial cells in the urine. Renal infarction causes a characteristic sharp rise in the serum glutamic–oxaloacetic transaminase level, followed by a prolonged elevation of lactate dehydrogenase.

a.   The **diagnosis** is suspected when CT with contrast agent fails to visualize all or part of the kidney. Although visualization may be poor or delayed with ureteral stone, *some* nephrogram is usually seen. The presence of a cardiac or vascular lesion lends credence to the diagnosis. A dynamic technetium scan demonstrating nonperfusion of the kidney and selective renal arteriography are required to confirm the diagnosis.

b.   The **treatment** of choice is systemic anticoagulation (heparin). Intraarterial fibrinolytic agents (streptokinase), if instituted promptly within 4 to 6 hours, can lead to a significant recovery of renal function. The underlying cardiac disease usually precludes surgical embolectomy in these high-risk patients. Late-onset hypertension, a sequela of renal ischemia, and activation of the renin–angiotensin system may require nephrectomy.

2. Renal vein thrombosis. Rare in adults, it is frequently unilateral and usually associated with membranous glomerulonephritis and nephrotic syndrome, invasion of the renal veins and vena cava by tumor, or retroperitoneal disease. In infants and children, it is more commonly bilateral and associated with severe dehydration resulting from diarrhea or vomiting. In its clinical presentation, renal vein thrombosis closely mimics acute pyelonephritis and ureteral calculus. The patient presents with severe flank pain, hematuria, and fever. Signs of sepsis and shock are variable. A large, tender, smooth mass is usually felt in the flank, which represents the passively congested kidney.

  a. Diagnosis. Gross or microscopic hematuria caused by focal renal infarction is invariably found. Thrombocytopenia is also a consistent finding in the acute setting, and its absence should make one suspect the renal vein thrombosis to be in the resolving stage. Proteinuria is more common in the adult type of thrombosis, where it may be massive. Rising blood urea nitrogen and creatinine are found quite frequently, even in unilateral thrombosis. CT scan shows a large kidney with delayed or absent enhancement of the parenchyma. US usually shows an enlarged hypoechoic kidney with a renal vein or vena caval thrombus. CT and magnetic resonance imaging are sensitive, but selective renal venography remains the definitive test.

  b. Treatment. This depends on the age of the patient. In infants and children with bilateral renal vein thrombosis, the prognosis is dismal; prompt rehydration, antibiotics for infection, and correction of electrolyte imbalance form the mainstay of treatment. In adults, early heparinization and selective intravenous fibrinolysis (streptokinase or urokinase) have yielded promising results. Surgical thrombectomy is reserved for caval thrombosis. Following renal vein thrombosis, renal function usually recovers completely. In a small subset of patients, nonfunction, renal hypertension, or chronic renal infection may necessitate delayed nephrectomy.

III. Ureter

A. Trauma to the ureter is almost always penetrating trauma. Blunt trauma to the ureter is extremely rare and usually involves disruption of the ureteropelvic junction following rapid deceleration, a mechanism seen most commonly in children. The most common cause of ureteral trauma is iatrogenic injury during pelvic surgery, in particular abdominal hysterectomy; however, ureteral injury has occurred in a wide variety of intra-abdominal, pelvic, and retroperitoneal surgical procedures. Ureteroscopy is an increasingly important cause of ureteral perforation or avulsion. The second most common cause of ureteral injury is gunshot wound, most commonly from low-velocity weapons. All portions of the ureter are at equal risk for penetrating trauma from gunshot wounds. Stab wounds involving the ureter are rare.

1. **Diagnosis**
    a. **Iatrogenic injury.** Any patient in whom flank pain, fever, and paralytic ileus develop during the first 10 days following intraabdominal or pelvic surgery should be suspected of having ureteral injury. In female patients, a ureterovaginal fistula may develop after ligation of the ureter during hysterectomy. IVU or CT will demonstrate delayed excretion, hydronephrosis, and sometimes extravasation of contrast material.
    b. **External penetrating injury.** Hematuria is present in approximately 80% of patients with penetrating injury of the ureter. Thus, the absence of hematuria does not rule out penetrating ureteral injury. The diagnosis is usually apparent on IVU. In patients with ureteral transection from penetrating trauma, there is little time for a urinary collection to develop, and the IVU may demonstrate no abnormality except for extravasation at the point of injury. In approximately 10% of patients, IVU findings will be completely normal. The injury can be well delineated with a retrograde pyelogram. To avoid the risk of contaminating the retroperitoneum, however, this study should be performed immediately before surgical exploration.
2. **Treatment** depends on whether the injury is recognized immediately or after some period of delay.
    a. **Immediate recognition.** Injuries diagnosed within a few days should generally be treated with surgical exploration. Sepsis, abscess formation, and other injuries or medical problems may delay surgical exploration. Debridement and primary anastomosis should be performed whenever possible. Injuries involving the lower third of the ureter can generally be managed by reimplantation into the bladder, with or without the use of a bladder flap or psoas hitch. An internal stent should be provided until healing is complete (usually 3 to 4 weeks). At that time, the stent can be removed via cystoscopy.
    b. **Delayed recognition.** In instances of delayed recognition, the presence of infection usually prevents primary reconstruction; urinary diversion by percutaneous nephrostomy and drainage of any urinary collection are the initial steps. Reconstructive surgery is undertaken after the hydronephrosis and infection have resolved.
3. **Complications of ureteral injury** include ureteral stricture, retroperitoneal fibrosis, pyelonephritis, and ureterocutaneous fistula.
B. **Ureteral calculi** may cause semiemergent situations regarding management of ureteral obstruction and pain. These are discussed in Chapter 14.
IV. **Bladder**
A. **Trauma.** The bladder normally is protected from injury by the bony pelvis; however, the bladder and/or the urethra are frequently injured when the pelvis is fractured. Severe blunt trauma to the lower abdomen may result in bladder rupture if the bladder is filled at the time of trauma. Penetrating trauma to the bladder may occur by the same mechanisms as to the ureter (see preceding discussion).

1. **Classification**
    a. **Contusion** involves injury to the bladder wall, resulting in hematuria and perivesical hematoma with no extravasation of urine demonstrated.
    b. **Extraperitoneal rupture.** In this injury, the lateral wall or floor of the bladder is ruptured, leading to extravasation of urine into the pelvis and retroperitoneum. This type of injury accounts for approximately 50% of all bladder ruptures and is almost always associated with pelvic fracture. Conversely, approximately 15% of patients with pelvic fracture have bladder rupture.
    c. **Intraperitoneal rupture** usually involves bladder rupture at the dome, leading to intraperitoneal extravasation of urine. This type of injury is almost always caused by blunt trauma to the lower abdomen and is often seen in intoxicated patients who fall with a full bladder or are involved in a motor vehicle accident.
    d. **Spontaneous rupture.** Rarely, the bladder ruptures without external trauma, usually indicating underlying pathology such as bladder tumor.
2. **Diagnosis.** Acute bladder trauma rarely produces specific symptoms or signs. Extraperitoneal rupture is characterized by the presence of contrast agent outside the bladder in the pelvis and paracolic areas. The bladder may assume a "teardrop" appearance during compression by a pelvic hematoma. Intraperitoneal rupture is characterized by the presence of contrast agent in the peritoneal cavity, outlining loops of small bowel. A small number of patients may have both kinds of injury. Even if bladder trauma is demonstrated by cystography, all trauma patients with hematuria should undergo IVU.
3. **Treatment** in almost all patients with bladder trauma involves exploration, debridement, surgical repair, drainage of the perivesical space, and diversion of urine, usually by a suprapubic catheter. Following repair, a low-pressure cystogram should be obtained to assess the integrity of the bladder before the catheter is removed.
    a. **Extraperitoneal rupture.** Many patients may be successfully treated by **urethral catheter** drainage alone, provided that (a) only a minor degree of extraperitoneal extravasation is present, (b) there is no evidence of infected urine, and (c) the patient is carefully monitored for the development of clot retention and infected pelvic hematoma. However, all patients with significant extraperitoneal extravasation should undergo exploration. Extraperitoneal rupture of the bladder from blunt trauma usually is repaired transvesically.
    b. **Intraperitoneal rupture** requires a transperitoneal approach to rule out associated injuries and to permit removal of extravasated urine from the peritoneal cavity. With penetrating trauma, concomitant injury to the rectum, iliac vessels, or ureters should be ruled out during surgical exploration.
4. **Complications of bladder injury** include cystitis, sepsis, pelvic collection, nephrogenic adenoma, and vesicovaginal fistula.

B.   Urinary retention

1.   Diagnosis. The most common causes are prostatic enlargement or cancer, prostatitis or abscess, prostatic infarction, urethral stricture, blood clots, medications, and neuropathic and psychogenic conditions. The history should include the voiding pattern before retention, past urologic surgery, and medications with anticholinergic side effects, especially common cold remedies containing nasal decongestants and antihistaminic compounds. The physical examination should focus on the suprapubic area to determine whether a distended bladder can be palpated or percussed. In most cases, pressure on the bladder during the examination will produce discomfort or pain. With long-standing chronic retention, the patient feels no discomfort from pressure on the distended bladder. A rectal examination should be performed to determine the size of the prostate and possible presence of prostatic abscess.

2.   Treatment. Placement of a Foley catheter, if possible, is the treatment of choice. In many cases, this can be made difficult by the presence of urethral stricture, prostate enlargement, or prostate cancer. The basic aspects of urethral catheterization are discussed in Chapter 5. **Percutaneous suprapubic cystotomy** should be performed in cases of impassable urethral stricture or prostatic obstruction. *The bladder must be full to perform this safely.* The presence of prior surgical scars in the suprapubic area is a contraindication to blind cystotomy since bowel may be adherent in the space of Retzius. It is much safer in such cases to use US guidance to avoid bowel injury. If in doubt about the bladder location, use a long spinal needle to aspirate urine from the bladder and determine its location. Mark the depth on the spinal needle, and make a mental note of it. Infiltrate local anesthetic (1% or 2% lidocaine) at a spot one finger-breadth above the symphysis pubis. Many different varieties of trocar catheters sets are available (Fig. 11.2). Insert the trocar through a small incision made with a no. 11 knife blade through the skin and the anterior rectus fascia. Keep in the midline, stay perpendicular to the skin, and make a short, quick stab into the bladder. Balloon catheters are the best means of securing the catheter in the bladder. Secure the catheter with a stitch to the skin.

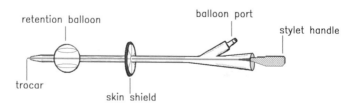

Fig. 11.2. Percutaneous suprapubic cystostomy catheter consisting of a balloon retention catheter and trocar stylet.

V. Urethra

A. Difficult catheterization. The difficult urethral catheterization is a common clinical problem. A frequent cause is spasm
of the external sphincter, followed by urethral stricture and
then bladder neck contracture. Prostatic enlargement rarely
prevents the passage of a catheter, as the prostate lobes are easily pushed aside by the catheter, especially one with a 22F diameter. If the patient is known or suspected to have urethral
stricture, retrograde urethrography should be carried out to assess the urethra (see Chapter 2). If this shows a clearly impassable stricture, percutaneous suprapubic cystotomy should be
performed for temporary relief of urinary retention. If no stricture is evident, a coude catheter should be tried—a maneuver
that is often successful in negotiating a prominent bladder
neck. The coude catheter should be oriented with the tip point-
ing anteriorly during passage.

1. Flexible cystoscopy is the safest maneuver if initial attempts to pass a catheter are unsuccessful. This allows direct
visualization of the urethral lumen. If a stricture is seen and
a lumen through the stricture is visible, a guide wire can usually be passed through the cystoscope into the bladder. Dilators can be passed over the guide wire. After the stricture is
dilated, place a well-lubricated Councill catheter over the
guide wire into the bladder. After irrigating the catheter to be
certain it is in the bladder, inflate the catheter balloon (to at
least 15 mL) and withdraw the guide wire.

2. Filiforms and followers may be used if no flexible cystoscope is available. Filiforms are narrow, solid catheters with
various configurations at the tip (see Chapter 5). They are
sometimes successful in bypassing urethral strictures and
false passages. With adequate lubrication, the filiform is
passed gently until it meets resistance in the urethra. The first
filiform is left in place, and another one is passed adjacent to
it. If it fails to pass, a third or fourth one can be passed. By try-
ing each filiform in turn, one hopes that one of them will enter
the urethral lumen and pass into the bladder. If this happens,
the other filiforms should be removed, and a small 8 or 10F follower should be screwed on. The follower then follows the filiform into the bladder, where it curls upon itself. After passing
the first follower, it is withdrawn to the meatus and unscrewed
from the filiform, and the next size follower is screwed on and
passed into the bladder. This process is repeated until the
stricture or urethra is adequately dilated. A Councill catheter
with screw-tip stylet can be screwed onto the filiform and
passed into the bladder.

B. Periurethral abscess. Periurethral abscess usually results from spontaneous rupture of a urethral abscess caused by
urethral stricture. The purulent collection may present in the
perineum as a warm, tender, erythematous, sometimes fluctuant mass. If the abscess has drained spontaneously, purulent
material can be expressed. Diagnosis consists of retrograde urethrography to demonstrate patency of the urethra and any fis-
tulous connection between the urethra and abscess cavity. The
purulent drainage should be examined for acid-fast bacilli and
cultured. Treatment consists of surgical incision and drainage

with diversion of the urine by Foley catheter or, preferably, by percutaneous cystostomy. Urethral injuries in male patients are usually divided into those involving the anterior portion (penile and bulbous urethra) and those involving the posterior portion (membranous and prostatic urethra).

C.   Urethral trauma

1.   Anterior urethral injury occurs most often as a result of blunt trauma suffered during straddle-type falls in which the urethra is crushed against the pubic bones. If the urethra remains intact, the injury is a urethral contusion, whereas the presence of extravasation implies urethral laceration.

2.   Posterior urethral injuries are usually associated with **pelvic fractures.** Most severe pelvic fractures are associated with motor vehicle accidents, especially a pedestrian being struck by a vehicle. The incidence of urethral injury in pelvic fracture cases is 5% to 10% in males and 1% to 5% in females. The risk of urethral injury associated with a traumatic pelvic fracture is also dependent on the type of fracture. The more severe the fracture of the pelvis, the higher risk of urethral injury exists. Owing to the major force necessary to fracture the pelvis, the prostate is displaced upward and the urethra may be stretched, partially ruptured, or completely ruptured at the bulbomembranous junction. Disruption of the periprostatic venous plexus as well as bleeding from the bony fragments often result in a large pelvic hematoma. **Classification of posterior urethral injuries** in males consists of type I (stretch injury with intact urethra, type II (partial tear but some continuity remains), and type III (complete tear with no evidence of continuity) (Fig. 11.3). Type I is rare. Type II constitutes about 25% of injuries, and Type III constitutes about 75%. In women, partial rupture at the anterior position is the most common urethral injury associated with pelvic fracture.

3.   Diagnosis

a.   Anterior urethral injuries. The patient gives a history of trauma to the perineum followed by perineal pain and inability to void. Almost always, a bloody urethral discharge is present. The bulbous urethra is extremely vascular, and both blood and urine will extravasate if the urethra is lacerated. This injury results in a characteristic ecchymosis, in which the pattern depends on the fascial planes of the genitalia and perineum. If Buck's fascia is not ruptured, the ecchymosis is limited to the penis. If Buck's fascia is ruptured, the extent of the ecchymosis is limited by Colles' fascia in the perineum and by Scarpa's fascia in the abdomen. This injury results in a "butterfly" ecchymosis in the perineum with possible extension along the anterior abdominal wall up to the clavicles.

b.   Posterior urethral injuries

(1)   Symptoms. The patient presents with suspected pelvic fracture and inability to void. Most patients have bloody urethral discharge. Inability to void may, of course, be caused by pain or hypovolemia. With partial rupture, voiding may be normal, but the urine is usually bloody. Although blood at the meatus or gross hematuria is the most reliable indicator of urethral injury, the amount of

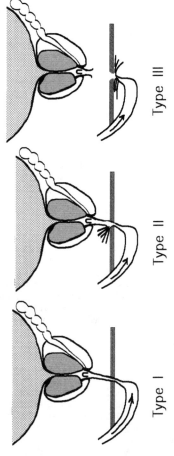

Fig. 11.3.   Classification of posterior urethral injuries.

urethral bleeding correlates poorly with the severity of injury. In women, urethral injury should be suspected when pelvic fracture, vaginal bleeding, and inability to void are present. Labial edema after pelvic trauma may represent urinary extravasation.

(2)   Physical examination may reveal malrotation of the hemipelvis or shortening of a leg without long bone fracture. Abdominal examination may reveal suprapubic fullness or dullness due to a pelvic hematoma. In contrast to anterior urethral injuries, posterior urethral injuries in men are not characterized by perineal ecchymosis. There may be hematoma or swelling in the perianal area if the pelvic hematoma enters the ischiorectal fossa. Rectal examination is mandatory to determine the presence of rectal injury. The finding of a boggy, indistinct mass on digital rectal examination is often assumed to indicate that the prostate has been displaced upward. This can be misleading because of obliteration of perirectal planes by the pelvic hematoma. Diagnosis of a "high-riding" prostate is difficult by physical examination and is best appreciated by CT scan or other x-ray study. The gland is still not far from its normal position. Displacement of the prostate may indicate complete transection of the posterior urethra. In women, vaginal examination should be performed using a clear plastic speculum to look for any vaginal laceration or tear.

(3)   Radiologic studies. Regardless of the presence or absence of bloody urethral discharge, retrograde urethrography (Chapter 2) should be the initial study in all male patients with pelvic fracture (Fig. 11.4). Retrograde urethrography is usually performed with the patient in the 45-degree oblique position and the penis stretched perpendicular to the femur. However, in trauma patients, it may not be feasible to situate the patient obliquely, and urethrography may need to be performed with the patient supine and the penis stretched to one side. Retrograde urethrography is quite accurate in diagnosing the presence and type of urethral disruption. Extravasation of contrast medium with no contrast agent visible in the bladder and proximal urethra is diagnostic of complete urethral disruption (although lack of proximal filling may be due to external sphincter spasm). Extravasation with partial filling of the proximal urethra and bladder is diagnostic of partial disruption. Lack of extravasation with displacement of the prostate upward is diagnostic of stretch injury to the posterior urethra. In women, urethrography is less reliable than endoscopy as a means of diagnosing urethral injury.

(4)   Instrumentation of the urethra may convert a partial urethral tear into a complete transection and may introduce infection into the pelvic hematoma. This is especially true if a Foley-type catheter is used and the balloon is distended at the site of the rupture. Catheterization should not be attempted until after a negative retrograde urethrogram is obtained.

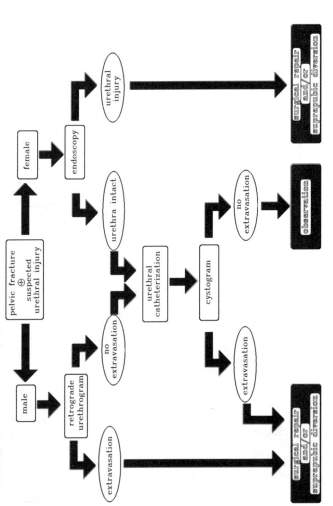

Fig. 11.4. Evaluation of the patient with pelvic fracture and suspected urethral injury.

4.   **Treatment**

a.   Anterior urethral contusion may be treated non-operatively. If the patient is able to void without significant hematuria, no treatment is needed. If there is significant bleeding, urethral catheterization for several days is usually sufficient.

b.   Anterior urethral laceration is best treated by diverting the urine by suprapubic cystotomy (open or percutaneous). In the absence of significant extravasation, conservative treatment will result in spontaneous healing in most cases, although surgical repair may be considered in the acute setting or if warranted by the clinical situation. In patients in whom a urethral stricture develops, this complication can almost always be treated in a delayed fashion successfully by endoscopic means. In the presence of perineal or scrotal hematoma, drainage of the extravasated urine and blood may be indicated in addition to suprapubic drainage.

c.   Posterior urethral injury in the male. Stretch injury (type I) and incomplete urethral tears (type II) are best treated by stenting with a urethral catheter. The case with complete rupture remains a difficult problem because the patient is at varying risk of urethral stricture, urinary incontinence, and erectile dysfunction (ED) (Table 11.4).

(1)   Historically, **primary anastomosis** at the time of injury was the earliest treatment modality attempted in posterior urethral rupture. Exploration of the injury site may release the pelvic hematoma, resulting in significant blood loss and making repair difficult. Dissection in the area of the prostatic apex increases the risk of injuring the neurovascular bundles and producing ED. Some have advocated initial management with suprapubic cystotomy and attempting primary repair at 7 to 10 days after injury. This modality results in a stricture rate of about 50% but the highest rate of ED.

(2)   **Primary realignment** involves opposing the torn ends of the urethra over a catheter with concomitant suprapubic cystostomy. Various techniques have been used to manipulate the catheter across the urethral gap during repair, including catheter placement under direct vision and sound-to-sound techniques. The urethral catheter is left indwelling for 6 to 8 weeks. Follow-up

Table 11.4.   Complication rate (%) according to treatment of urethral injury

Complication	Suprapubic Cystotomy	Primary Realignment	Primary Repair
Stricture	95	50	50
Incontinence	5	5	20
Erectile dysfunction	20	35	55

Source: Modified from Koraitim MM. *J Urol* 1999;161:1433–1441.

studies may be obtained through the suprapubic tube. The major disadvantage of primary realignment is the increased risk of ED.

(3) **Suprapubic diversion with delayed repair** carries the lowest risk of ED but the highest risk of stricture (Table 11.4). Because stricture is considered to have less of an impact on quality of life than ED, most practitioners favor this approach. With this method, no attempt is made to explore or manipulate the urethra at the time of injury. The urine is diverted with a suprapubic tube introduced through a small suprapubic incision or by trocar. This modality accepts the inevitability of stricture formation following complete urethral rupture, which can be repaired electively. If the injury is overstaged and is actually a partial tear, spontaneous voiding through the urethra may be noted 1 to 2 weeks after injury.

(4) **Endourologic techniques** may allow primary alignment without the risk of surgical exploration of the disrupted urethra. A flexible cystoscope is passed through the suprapubic tract to visualize and enter the vesical neck. A guide wire or 4F ureteral catheter is passed antegrade through the cystoscope; it is hoped that the urethral gap can be bridged and the wire or catheter will exit through the meatus. An indwelling catheter can be passed into the bladder over the guide wire. Endoscopic alignment may be performed anytime during the first 2 weeks after injury. Although encouraging, experience with these techniques is still limited.

d. **Urethral injury in the female.** The level of injury (proximal or distal) has major implications for treatment. **Rupture of the distal urethra** is not associated with increased risk of incontinence. Thus, transvaginal surgery to reconstruct the external meatus is recommended. Because **proximal urethral injury** in the female has major implications for continence, diversion and delayed repair as performed in the male patient are not advised. The patient should undergo immediate retropubic exploration with realignment of the urethra and end-to-end anastomosis over a stenting urethral catheter. Any vaginal laceration should be repaired to reduce the risk of urethrovaginal fistula.

VI. Penile trauma and emergencies

A. **Trauma to the penis** may occur from gunshot wounds, stab wounds, machinery accidents, animal attacks, and self-mutilation. Penetrating injury to the penis is managed by debridement, hemostasis, and repair of the injured tissue along with systemic antibiotic therapy. Machinery accidents may result in partial or total avulsion of the genital skin. Such injuries require careful debridement and skin grafting. Urethral continuity may need to be assessed by retrograde urethrography.

B. Spontaneous **penile fracture** may occur during intercourse and result in rupture of the tunica albuginea of the corpora. Penile fracture typically occurs in young men (average age 30 years). The clinical signs and symptoms of penile fracture consist of sudden onset of sharp pain, swelling, ecchymosis, bloody urethral discharge, deviation of the penis away from the side of the injury, and spontaneous loss of erection during sexual intercourse. Penile fracture can occur anywhere on the shaft or at the base of the penis. Delayed presentation of penile fracture may mimic Peyronie's disease. Injury to the urethra may occur concomitantly and should be ruled out with a retrograde urethrogram. Sexual trauma may concomitantly produce rupture of the urethra or rupture of the testicles or suspensory ligaments of the penis. Injuries to the penile ligaments may present with abnormal angulation, deviation, or dislocation or as an unstable erect penis. Most cases of penile fracture will require surgical exploration of the injury to debride devitalized tissue, evacuate hematoma, and close the defect in the tunica albuginea. We advocate a penoscrotal incision with eversion of the corporal bodies to gain access to the injury site.

C.   Penile vascular injuries. Sexual trauma to the superficial dorsal vein of the penis may result in thrombosis of the vein and present as painful erections, ecchymosis, and palpable thrombosed veins on the dorsal surface of the penis. Rupture of the deep dorsal vein of the penis may mimic fracture of the penis. **Traumatic lymphangitis** after intercourse may present as nodular, firm, circumferential swelling of the coronal sulcus. Patients with coagulopathy of any etiology are more prone to vascular injuries of the penis. **Frenular artery laceration** may occur during intercourse. For patients with tears in the frenular artery, the artery should be surgically ligated, and, if indicated, a circumcision should be performed.

D.   Phimosis is the inability to retract the foreskin of the penis. Chronic low-grade infection eventually leads to loss of elasticity and scarring of the foreskin. The patient usually complains of erythema, itching, or pain on intercourse. Most commonly, there is a mild associated infection (balanoposthitis), which should be treated with a broad-spectrum antibiotic such as tetracycline (250 mg four times daily by mouth). The phimosis is then treated electively by dorsal slit or circumcision. Rarely, the patient presents with tight phimosis and severe balanitis. Under these circumstances, semiemergent dorsal slit is indicated to promote drainage. Once the infection is controlled, elective circumcision can be performed. Very rarely, tight phimosis may present as a cause of urinary obstruction.

E.   Paraphimosis is a condition in which the foreskin becomes trapped in a retracted position behind the glans. Most commonly, this occurs in a patient with preexisting phimosis. With time, the entrapped foreskin becomes edematous, and the glans itself becomes engorged. Rarely, vascular insufficiency of the glans can occur. Treatment consists of firm compression of the glans to decrease edema and continuous traction on the foreskin, combined with counterpressure on the glans. Field block of the penis with 1% lidocaine (Xylocaine) is sometimes helpful. When this treatment is unsuccessful, incision of the constricting ring under local anesthesia should be performed. Once the inflammation and edema have subsided (3 to 4 days), elective circumcision is indicated.

F.   Priapism is characterized by persistent erection unrelated to sexual activity. It is discussed in Chapter 21.

VII. Scrotum

A. Trauma to the scrotum is relatively rare. The peak incidence occurs in the 10- to 30-year age range. Embarrassment associated with the injury or its mechanism often results in delayed presentation. Physical examination should assess corporal integrity and look for blood at the meatus that may indicate urethral injury. Retrograde urethrography is warranted in suspected urethral injury. Color Doppler US imaging of the testes should be performed to assess integrity of the blood supply and the tunical coverings of the testes.

1. **Antibiotic therapy** is indicated in injuries acquired in the field (e.g., farm, hunting, military related) and must be treated with clindamycin (900 mg IV/IM q8h) and penicillin (nafcillin 1 to 2 g IV q4h) to cover *Clostridium perfringens* and tetanus. Treatment of animal bites should cover *Streptococcus* sp and *Pasteurella multocida*. The antibiotic of choice is amoxicillin/clavulanate (500 to 875 mg PO bid).

2. **Surgical therapy**

   a. **Scrotal avulsion** is managed by debridement and primary closure with absorbable sutures. The vascularity and elasticity of the scrotum allow closure of relatively large defects. Complete scrotal loss requires skin grafting.

   b. **Blunt trauma** to the scrotum often involves testis injury as well. Dislocation of the testis can occur in blunt trauma and should be approached inguinally to obtain control of the spermatic cord. Testis tumors may present as scrotal hemorrhage after minor trauma.

   c. **Penetrating trauma.** Low-velocity bullets and stab wounds to the scrotum require surgical exploration to determine testis viability. High-velocity missiles imply a higher risk of subsequent vascular thrombosis and tissue loss. Skin should be extensively debrided and drains used. With late necrosis, further debridement and wound care will be necessary.

B. Fournier's gangrene. Described in 1883 by Jean-Alfred Fournier, a French venereologist, Fournier's gangrene is the sudden onset of fulminant gangrene of the external genitalia and perineum in an apparently healthy person. A form of necrotizing fasciitis, it usually begins in the scrotum or penis and may spread along fascial planes (beneath Scarpa's fascia) to the perineum and abdominal wall up to the axillas. Originally, the term "Fournier's gangrene" meant idiopathic gangrene of the genitalia; in modern usage, it has been applied to nonidiopathic cases of genital gangrene as well. A source can now be identified in 80% of cases (Table 11.5). It is common for patients to have predisposing systemic conditions such as alcoholism (50%) or diabetes (33%) (Table 11.6). The common denominator seems to be a depressed immune state, as both diabetes and alcoholism are known to impair the immune system.

1. **Diagnosis.** Fournier's gangrene presents suddenly with marked swelling and erythema of the genitalia, fever, chills, and malaise. There may be a prodrome lasting 2 to 5 days. The mean duration of symptoms is 5 days. Physical examination is the cornerstone of diagnosis. Blistering of the scrotal or penile

Table 11.5.   Etiology of Fournier's gangrene

Colorectal source (30%)
  Perianal gland infection
  Ischiorectal abscess
  Colonic diverticulitis
  Appendicitis

Urogenital source (50%)
  Bulbourethral gland infection
  Periurethral abscess
  Urethral stricture
  Urinary tract infection

Skin source (20%)
  Hidradenitis suppuritiva
  Scrotal ulcer or lesion
  Scrotal trauma

skin overlying a cellulitic area with yellow–brown fluid is pathognomonic of underlying necrotizing fasciitis. Crepitus may be elicited at this stage, and a feculent odor caused by anaerobes is usually present. If untreated, gangrenous sloughing soon ensues. The testes and spermatic cord are almost always spared.

   a.   Radiology. Plain film imaging may show moderate to large amounts of soft tissue gas or foreign bodies. US is sensitive for gas, but the need for pressure on the skin to perform the examination is a drawback. CT is very sensitive for gas in tissue and fluid collections. If a urethral source is suspected from a history of stricture or urethral instrumentation, a retrograde urethrogram is indicated.

   b.   Physical examination. Fever and tachycardia may be present. The skin may be erythematous, edematous, cyanotic, blistered, or frankly gangrenous. A feculent odor is quite characteristic secondary to infection with anaerobic bacteria. Crepitus may be present, but its absence does not exclude the presence of tissue gas. A thorough genital and perianal examination is required to detect potential

Table 11.6.   Comorbidity associated with Fournier's gangrene

Diabetes mellitus
Morbid obesity
Cirrhosis of the liver
Malignancies
Drug and/or alcohol abuse
Malnutrition
HIV infection
Chronic steroid use

portals of entry. If the rectal examination suggests a bowel source, proctoscopy should be performed.

c.   Microbiology. Cultures reveal polymicrobial flora with gram-negative rods (*Escherichia coli, Pseudomonas* sp, and *Klebsiella* sp), gram-positive cocci (β-hemolytic streptococci, *Staphylococcus aureus,* and *Enterococcus*), and anaerobes (*Bacteroides fragilis, C. perfringens*).

2.   Treatment. The basic tenets of management include the following:

a.   Radical debridement of all necrotic and gangrenous tissue must be performed emergently. The testicles are often spared from necrosis. The exposed testicles may be placed in a subcutaneous pocket in the thigh to protect them. If a testicle is involved, orchiectomy should be performed.

b.   Blisters and abscess cavities not included in the initial debridement are **incised and drained.**

c.   Intravenous broad-spectrum antibiotics designe to cover both aerobic and anaerobic organisms are adm istered, followed by more specific therapy once t' sults of culture are obtained. We use a regimen o' piperacillin/1.5 g of tazobactam IV for 7 to 10 vided doses of 3.375 g q6h, 80 mg of gentamicir 600 to 1,200 mg/day divided q6–8h of clind As an alternative to clindamycin, 500 mg IV can be given every 8 hours.

d.   Supportive measures

(1)   Hyperbaric oxygen therar extensive anaerobic infection has t results.

(2)   Cystostomy or colostomy may temporary diversion in patients with p\ perirectal suppuration.

(3)   Systemic corticosteroids have been found to be useful in isolated cases unresponsive to standard measures.

(4)   Wound care following debridement involves application of wet-to-dry saline dressings for local debridement.

(5)   Delayed split-thickness skin grafting of denuded genitals is sometimes required. In most cases, remaining scrotal skin can be mobilized to cover the testicles.

(6)   Prognosis. Despite extensive therapeutic measures, the overall mortality approaches 30%, which stresses the need for prompt diagnosis and early treatment of this condition. Common postoperative complications include prolonged sepsis, coagulopathy, and pulmonary insufficiency.

VIII. Testis trauma and emergencies

A.   Trauma. Injuries to the testes typically occur in young men, usually aged 15 to 40 years. Blunt trauma accounts for about 85% of cases. The most common cause of blunt trauma is sports injuries, followed by kicks to the groin. Less common etiologies of blunt testicular trauma include motor vehicle accidents, falls, and straddle injuries. The most common cause of penetrating testicular injuries is a gunshot wound. Severe blunt trauma to the testis may result in testicular rupture. The testis may also rupture spontaneously or with minimal trauma if underlying pathology, especially carcinoma, is present. Following rupture of the tunica albuginea, there is considerable bleeding into the space around the testis, resulting in a hematoma.

1. **Diagnosis.** The patient usually presents with a fairly clear history of blunt trauma to the scrotum often associated with nausea and vomiting. For penetrating injuries, determine the entrance and exit sites of the projectile. Carefully examine the contralateral side, the perineum, the rectum, and the femoral vessels. On physical examination, there is a tender, swollen scrotal mass that does not transilluminate. Scrotal or perineal ecchymosis may be present. US should be performed to delineate the injury.

2. **Treatment** depends on the degree of trauma and extent of the hematoma. When there is little or no trauma, an underlying carcinoma should be suspected, and the patient should undergo testis exploration by the inguinal approach. Patients with severe trauma and bleeding should undergo scrotal exploration and repair of the testis, if possible. Shattered testis is best treated with orchiectomy. Patients in whom there is a clear history of trauma but minimal hematoma formation may be treated conservatively with analgesics, elevation, and ice packs applied to the scrotum.

SUGGESTED READING

Aihara R. Fracture locations influence the likelihood of rectal and lower urinary tract injuries in patients sustaining pelvic fractures. *J Trauma* 2002;52:205–208.

Cass AS, Luxenberg M. Testicular injuries. *Urology* 1999;37:528–530.

Corman JM, Moody JA, Aronson WJ. Fournier's gangrene in a modern surgical setting: improved survival with aggressive management. *Br J Urol Int* 1999;84:85–88.

Dobrowolski ZF. Treatment of posterior and anterior urethral trauma. *Br J Urol Int* 2002;89:752–754.

Dreitlein DA. Genitourinary trauma. *Emerg Med Clin North Am* 2001;19:569–590.

Eke N. Fournier's gangrene: a review of 1,726 cases. *Br J Surg* 2000; 87:718–728.

Fishman EK. CT evaluation of bladder trauma: a critical look. *Acad Radiol* 2000;7:309–310.

Hejase MJ, Simonin JE, Bihrle R, et al. Genital Fournier's gangrene: experience with 38 patients. *Urology* 1996;47:734–739.

Koraitim MM. Pelvic fracture urethral injuries: the unresolved controversy. *J Urol* 1999;161:1433–1441.

Koya MP, Rice ML, List A. Blunt bladder trauma—is conservative management appropriate in all extraperitoneal ruptures? *Aust NZ J Surg* 1999;69(suppl):A90.

Losanoff JE. Penile injury. *J Urol* 2001;166:1388–1389.

McAninch JW. Genitourinary trauma. *World J Urol* 1999;17:65.

Moore EE, Shackford SR, Pachter HL, et al. Organ injury scaling: spleen, liver, and kidney. *J Trauma* 1989;29:1664.

Morey AF, Iverson AJ, Swan A, et al. Bladder rupture after blunt trauma: guidelines for diagnostic imaging. *J Trauma* 2001;51: 683–686.

Munter DW, Faleski EJ. Blunt scrotal trauma: emergency department evaluation and management. *Am J Emerg Med* 1989;7:227–234.

Mydlo JH. Blunt, penetrating, and ischemic injuries to the penis. *J Urol* 2002;168:1433–1435.

Palmer LS. Penetrating ureteral trauma at an urban trauma center: 10-year experience. *Urology* 1999;54:34–36.

Safir MH, McAninch JW. Diagnosis and management of trauma to the kidney. *Curr Opin Urol* 1999;9:227–281.

Shenfeld OZ, Kiselgorf D, Gofrit ON, et al. The incidence and causes of erectile dysfunction after pelvic fractures associated with posterior urethral disruption. *J Urol* 2003;169:2173–2176.

Wessells H, McAninch JW, Meyer A, et al. Criteria for nonoperative treatment of significant penetrating renal lacerations. *J Urol* 1997; 157:24–27.

Endoscopic Surgery of the Lower Urinary Tract and Laparoscopy

C. Charles Wen, Juan P. Litvak, and
Richard K. Babayan

Endoscopic surgery utilizes instruments that permit the surgeon to operate within the genitourinary tract without making a skin incision. Major endoscopic surgery can be accomplished safely with adequate light, adequate irrigating capacity, and proper use of the electrosurgical unit and other sources of energy. In addition, the endoscopic surgeon needs a proper understanding of optics and the application of energy to living tissues. Prior to passing any instrument into the patient, it should be checked for proper vision, function, and alignment. **Cystourethroscopy,** the endoscopic examination of the urethra and bladder, has been described in Chapter 5.

I. General principles of electrosurgery

Electrosurgery refers to the application of high-frequency alternating current of various waveforms to cut, coagulate, fulgurate, or vaporize tissue. It should not be confused with "cautery," which refers to the application of physical heat to tissue. Electrocautery refers to an electrically heated wire used to transfer heat to the patient; current does not enter the patient's body. In electrosurgery, the patient is included in the circuit, and high-frequency (above 300 kHz) alternating current enters the patient's body. Modern electrosurgical units (sometimes called "the Bovie" after the original model) provide a variety of current types and power levels.

A. Cutting and coagulating current. High-frequency, low-voltage, undamped current cuts or vaporizes tissue, whereas lower-frequency, high-voltage, damped current tends to heat tissue and produce coagulation. This is obviously useful for hemostasis during endoscopic surgery. A third type of current, produced by blending cutting and hemostatic currents in varying proportions, is useful in resecting vascular tissues with minimal bleeding (Fig. 12.1). The most important variable is the rate at which heat is produced. High heat produced rapidly causes vaporization. Low heat produced more slowly produces coagulation.

B. Monopolar and bipolar electrodes are available in a variety of configurations (Fig. 12.2). By far the most commonly used type is a monopolar electrode in which the electric current is returned to the electrosurgical unit via a broad, highly conductive grounding plate. The function of the patient return electrode is to provide an exit for current leaving the patient's body. Careless application of the grounding plate can result in electric burns to the patient or to personnel in contact with the patient. In contrast, a bipolar electrode requires no grounding pad and returns

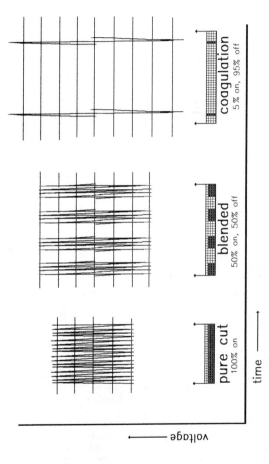

Fig. 12.1. Different types of electrosurgical current.

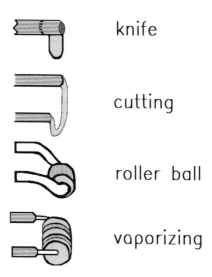

knife

cutting

roller ball

vaporizing

Fig. 12.2.   Various types of electrodes for endoscopic surgery.

the current to itself. Bipolar electrodes are safer but less efficient in cutting than monopolar electrodes. Bipolar electrodes can be used safely with isotonic sodium chloride solution irrigation, thus practically eliminating the risk of dilutional hyponatremia. A further advantage is the elimination of inadvertent stimulation of the obturator nerve with potentially dangerous spasm of the obturator muscle.

C. Irrigating solutions. For monopolar electrodes, saline cannot be used as an irrigating solution because as an excellent conductor, it diffuses the current and prevents it from cutting or cauterizing tissue. To solve this problem, various nonconductive solutions such as sterile water, glucose, urea, glycine, and sorbitol/mannitol have been used. Sterile water should never be used because it causes intravascular hemolysis when absorbed. Therefore, nonhemolyzing solutions of sorbitol/mannitol or glycine are used today. Dilutional hyponatremia may still occur when these solutions are absorbed. Glycine, one of the most popular irrigants, has an osmolality of approximately 200 mOsm/kg compared with normal serum (290 mOsm/kg) and is thus hypotonic rather than isotonic. The metabolism of glycine into ammonia has been postulated as a contributing factor to transurethral resection (TUR) syndrome. Glycine inhibits neurotransmission and may rarely cause visual disturbances if absorbed in large amounts. Thus, solutions containing sorbitol/mannitol come closest to addressing the requirements for safe endoscopic surgery using monopolar electrodes.

D. Patient body temperature may be substantially decreased during endoscopic surgery owing to cooling by the irrigant solution. Ambient temperature in the operating room is another important factor. Cooling leads to bradycardia, reduced cardiac output, higher mean arterial pressure, increased vascular resistance, and increased oxygen demand.

Therefore, using irrigating fluid warmed to body temperature is highly recommended. A commercial fluid warmer is available.

II.   Transurethral/endoscopic procedures

A.   Preoperative preparation in patients undergoing endoscopic surgery involves several important considerations.

1.   Patients who are **uremic** (serum creatinine level >1.5 mg/dL) have considerably increased postoperative morbidity and mortality rates. For these patients, surgery should be delayed until urinary drainage permits improvement of their uremic state.

2.   Specific antibiotic treatment is indicated in patients who have bacteriuria or pyuria before endoscopic surgery. Whenever possible, obtain culture evidence of urinary sterilization before proceeding with prostatectomy. Patients with indwelling Foley catheters are presumed to be infected and should be given antibiotic coverage perioperatively before surgery.

3.   Anticoagulants. Warfarin (Coumadin) should be stopped 3 to 4 days preoperatively. For patients who must remain anticoagulated right up to the operative day, in-hospital heparinization will be needed. Aspirin and nonsteroidal anti-inflammatory agents should be stopped 7 full days prior to surgery. For patients on clopidogrel (Plavix), 14 days off the medication prior to surgery is recommended. Warfarin may be resumed 24 hours after the urine has turned grossly clear. For aspirin and clopidogrel, 48 hours of clear urine is recommended.

4.   An **enema** should be ordered the evening before surgery to ensure an empty rectum during the procedure and for the first few days postoperatively.

5.   Sleeping medication or an antianxiety agent may be needed the evening before surgery.

6.   For patients undergoing transurethral resection of the prostate (TURP), the use of preoperative finasteride (Proscar) has been demonstrated to help reduce bleeding during and after TURP. A 2-week course of finasteride 5 mg hs preoperatively is recommended.

B.   General principles of transurethral surgery. Passing large instruments through the urethra requires attention to several points of technique.

1.   Resectoscopes (Fig. 12.2) are instruments designed for resecting tissue in the lower urinary tract under direct vision. A large variety of electrodes can be fitted to the mechanism of the resectoscope, depending on the particular operative need (Fig. 12.3). Continuous-flow models, with small drainage holes at the tip of the sheet, eliminate the necessity of intermittent emptying. Constant suction or gravity is used to achieve continuous inflow and outflow, permitting more efficient resection and greater safety. When used properly, continuous-flow resectoscopes prevent excessive distention of the bladder and allow for better visualization.

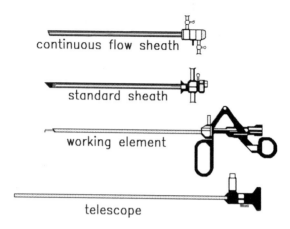

Fig. 12.3.   **Continuous-flow resectoscope with Iglesias working element.**

2.   Excellent visualization is obtained using endoscopic cameras fitted to the resectoscope. The image is displayed on a large monitor placed at a convenient location. The image can be recorded on videotape or printed for permanent records. Video imaging for endoscopic surgery results in better visualization and less strain on the surgeon.

3.   The larger the sheath size selected, the larger the resecting ability of the instrument; however, the risk for urethral trauma and stricture is increased by use of too large a sheath. A 26F sheath is a good compromise for both prostatic and bladder tumor resection.

4.   With liberal use of lubricating jelly, the urethra should be dilated carefully with Van Buren sounds until it is at least 2F larger than the selected sheath.

5.   If stricture or meatal stenosis prevents passage of an adequate-sized sheath, the problem should be surgically corrected. A meatotomy may be needed. Alternatively, transurethral surgery can be accomplished through a perineal urethrostomy.

6.   Careful observation endoscopy of the anterior urethra, prostate, and bladder with a standard cystoscope should be completed before the endoscopic surgery is begun. This provides information on the location of important landmarks such as the ureteral orifices, bladder neck, verumontanum, and external (striated muscle) sphincter.

7.   The choice of irrigating fluid has already been discussed. Irrigating fluid should be kept at the lowest (pressure) level possible to maintain an adequate flow. A fluid height of 60 cm is usually sufficient. Irrigating fluid should be warmed to body temperature to avoid lowering the patient's body temperature. Body temperature should be routinely monitored during endoscopic surgery.

   8. Priapism occurs in approximately 5% of patients undergoing TURP, especially in those younger than 50 years. Treatment is usually by inhaling amyl nitrate. Alternatively, one can give an intracavernosal injection of phenylephrine (1 to 2 mL of a solution containing 10 mg of phenylephrine in 49 mL of normal sodium chloride for injection). Whereas amyl nitrate may cause mild hypotension, phenylephrine may cause a transitory rise in blood pressure.
   9. At the completion of the procedure, it is important to obtain the maximum degree of hemostasis possible. In the case of prostatic resection, all prostate chips should be removed from the bladder using an Ellik evacuator. Either blood clots or chips can obstruct the catheter postoperatively.
   10. If there is difficulty in passing a Foley catheter at the completion of the procedure, use of a coude catheter or catheter stylet is advisable. The bladder should be full to prevent injury to the posterior bladder wall. Ordinarily, a 22F continuously irrigating three-way Foley catheter with a 30-mL balloon is used after endoscopic prostatic resection. It may be necessary to overfill the balloon to 60 mL to prevent the Foley balloon from slipping into the prostatic fossa. Mild traction on the Foley catheter may be necessary to control postoperative bleeding. Irrigation should be minimized after resection of bladder tumor to reduce risk of extravasation through the resection site.

C. Urethral strictures may be congenital or acquired. With the advent of modern antibiotic therapy, postgonococcal strictures are becoming much less common. At the same time, traumatic strictures are being seen more frequently. Most strictures can be managed at the time of diagnosis by endoscopic means. For short strictures confirmed by a retrograde urethrogram, a filiform may be placed through the lumen of the stricture under direct vision and followers used to gently dilate the stricture. Alternatively, a guide wire can be passed through the stricture under direct vision, and a dilator passed over the wire. Blind passage of Van Buren sounds in the face of urethral stricture, even in the best of hands, can cause urethral perforation and should be avoided. For strictures, visualization with a 0-degree lens is recommended. A guide wire, ureteral catheter, or filiform is placed through the stricture under direct vision, and the stricture is incised, usually at the 12 o'clock position, with a urethrotome (Fig. 12.4). If the lumen of the stricture is not obvious under direct vision, a suprapubic tube can be placed for temporary urinary diversion. Longer, complex strictures may require open urethroplasty.

D. External sphincterotomy is occasionally indicated for relief of obstruction due to vesicosphincter dyssynergia in patients with neurogenic bladder dysfunction, although other therapeutic choices, such as intermittent catheterization and urethral stenting, have reduced the need for this procedure. In vesicosphincter dyssynergia, the striated sphincter contracts when the bladder contracts, thus obstructing normal voiding. The striated urethral sphincter is incised with either a standard resecting loop or a knife electrode at the 12 o'clock position.

E. Benign prostatic hyperplasia (BPH) is the most common cause of urinary retention in elderly male patients and is a major

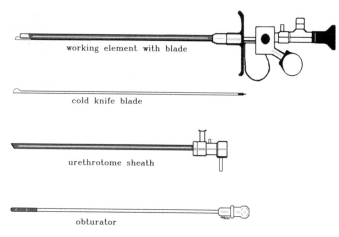

Fig. 12.4. Components of optical urethrotome.

contributor to the prevalence of lower urinary tract symptoms. Indications for surgery in BPH are given in Table 12.1. Determining whether an enlarged gland is resectable endoscopically or requires open surgery is based largely on the ability and experience of the surgeon. In general, however, the smaller the gland, the more difficult is an open procedure and the easier is an endoscopic procedure.

1. TURP remains one of the most effective treatments for long-term control of adenomatous hyperplasia of the prostate. It was the first successful minimally invasive surgical procedure of the modern era. The prostate is resected by removing chips using a cutting electrode. The prostatic chips float into the bladder and are then evacuated through the resectoscope. The average amount of tissue resected is 22 g. Arterial blood flow to the prostate is cauterized either by using coagulating current or by utilizing vaporization techniques with specialized loops and solid-state electrosurgical generators. Use of

Table 12.1. Accepted indications for surgical intervention in BPH

Refractory urinary retention

Recurrent urinary tract infections due to prostatic hypertrophy

Recurrent gross hematuria

Renal insufficiency secondary to bladder outlet obstruction

Bladder calculi

Decompensated detrusor function

Large bladder diverticula that do not empty well owing to prostatic hypertrophy

ℵↃ **Table 12.2.** **Indications for laparoscopic pelvic lymph node dissection in prostate cancer**

Serum prostate-specific antigen >20
Gleason sum ≥8
Number of positive biopsies ≥5
Clinical stage T3 or T4
Positive seminal vesicle biopsy
Suspicious pelvic CT scan

3% sorbitol is recommended as irrigant during the procedure. Resection technique varies widely among experienced urologic surgeons. Some surgeons prefer to resect or vaporize the bladder neck at the 5 and 7 o'clock positions and remove the median lobe (if any) first. Others prefer the classic Nesbit technique of resecting first at the roof of the prostate and proceeding in the capsular plane. The decision can be based on preference and experience. The end result is a cavity surrounding the prostatic urethra.

a. **Perioperative complications** include sepsis and shock, hemorrhage (may require return to the operating room if severe), excessive absorption of irrigant, and perforation of the bladder or urethra. Pulmonary embolus may occur in the early postoperative period. Significant amounts of irrigating fluid may be absorbed into the extravascular and intravascular space through the prostatic capsule during TURP (**post-TURP syndrome**). Contributing factors are resection weight over 45 g and resection time of >90 minutes. Because the irrigating fluid is isotonic but electrolyte-free, the fluid absorption is manifested biochemically as hyponatremia, hypochloremia, and, in the case of glycine, hyperammonemia (see Chapter 24). Clinically, the patient may complain of dyspnea and chest discomfort. Accompanying hypertension, tachycardia, and mental confusion or obtundation are also seen. Although referred to as the post-TURP syndrome, these symptoms often begin during the procedure. See Chapter 24 for a discussion of treatment. The use of solid-state generators and modified TUR loops that vaporize as well as resect prostate tissue has significantly contributed to reduced fluid absorption and bleeding in TURPs. Overall mortality rate following TURP is 0.5%.

b. **Delayed complications** include retrograde ejaculation (50% to 90%), urethral stricture (10%), vesical neck contracture (10%), epididymitis or orchitis (2%), severe permanent incontinence (1%), and erectile dysfunction (5%).

(1) **Incontinence.** Some degree of incontinence is common following TURP, usually caused by inflammation and detrusor instability. This type of incontinence usually resolves completely within 6 weeks of surgery. Persistent incontinence from sphincteric insufficiency, however, occurs in about 0.5% of cases and does not resolve spontaneously.

(2)   **Impotence.** Although the mechanism of this complication is not understood, it occurs in a tiny fraction of patients following TURP.

(3)   **Retrograde ejaculation** is a common result of TURP and bladder neck resection, occurring in up to 90% of patients.

(4)   **Bleeding.** Significant hematuria may occur immediately after TURP or may be delayed until 10 days to 2 weeks after TURP. Immediate bleeding is caused by poor hemostatic technique during surgery, whereas delayed bleeding is thought to result from sloughing of necrotic tissue and eschar in the prostatic fossa, often caused by patient straining.

(5)   **Epididymoorchitis** may occur after instrumentation or surgery, either in conjunction with a urinary tract infection or alone. If diagnosed, it should be treated with appropriate antibiotics.

(6)   **Urethral stricture and bladder neck contracture** can result from injury to urethral epithelium or the surrounding corpus spongiosum, which leads to fibrosis, scarring, or stricture.

2.   **Transurethral incision of the prostate** (TUIP) is performed by making deep incisions through the bladder neck and prostate to the level of the verumontanum. Orandi's original description included incisions at 5 and 7 o'clock, but other locations appear to work as well. Success seems to depend on adequate depth of the incisions, to the prostatic capsule, and not their location. In addition, prostate size should not exceed 30 g, and a significant median lobe should be absent. The main advantage of TUIP in comparison with TURP is shortened operating time, diminished blood loss, and diminished fluid absorption. TUIP has a much lower incidence of retrograde ejaculation than does TURP. For the smaller gland, TUIP is at least as efficacious a treatment as TURP with lesser morbidity.

3.   **Transurethral vaporization of the prostate** is a modified TURP in which a high-energy cutting current, from a solid-state generator, instantly heats and vaporizes prostatic tissue. Its main advantage is that fluid absorption and blood loss are reduced in comparison with TURP. It is difficult to perform on very large glands because of the slower rate of tissue removal. Little or no tissue is produced for pathologic examination. The original "vaportrode" design has been modified into a number of variations, and many of the vaporizing principles have been adapted for modified TURP electrodes, as well.

4.   **Bipolar electrode prostatic resection** uses a bipolar electrode rather than the monopolar one used in TURP. When cutting current is applied, an ionization field is formed around the bipolar loop that effectively cuts the tissue.

Because electrical current does not enter the patient, tissue damage is much more limited, there is less coagulation artifact produced, and good hemostasis is achievable. Saline may be used as irrigation in bipolar surgery, which virtually eliminates post-TUR syndrome and dilutional hyponatremia. A special bipolar electrical generator is required.

5.   Laser vaporization of the prostate may utilize potassium–titanyl–phosphate (KTP), holmium, or other types of laser energy. KTP laser energy at 532 nm is highly absorbed by oxyhemoglobin and penetrates only 1 to 2 mm into the prostatic tissue. The limited tissue penetration, compared with neodymium-YAG (yttrium–aluminum–garnet) lasers, minimizes the irritative symptoms often seen with prostate laser vaporization.

6.   Holmium enucleation of the prostate uses holmium laser energy to carve out the lateral and median lobes of the prostate in an endoscopic version of an open enucleation. This technique allows a virtually bloodless field, and saline rather than sorbitol irrigation can be used. Removing the adenoma once it has been released into the bladder generally requires the use of an electric morcellator, which is time consuming, potentially dangerous, and often fraught with mechanical difficulty. The most dramatic advantage of holmium enucleation of the prostate is in those patients on anticoagulant therapy who can achieve excellent relief of their bladder outlet obstruction without compromising their anticoagulation status.

F.   Prostate cancer that has advanced to cause urinary obstruction may be resected in a manner similar to that described for BPH if there are no plans to attempt cure. The endoscopic landmarks may be obliterated by the growth of the tumor, however, making resection of prostate cancer difficult.

G.   Bladder neck obstruction may result from dysfunction of the smooth muscle or from scarring secondary to trauma or surgery. The condition may be surgically managed either by incision with the urethrotome or by electrocautery (knife electrode). Alternatively, bladder neck obstruction may be treated by resection and removal of obstructing tissue; however, some say this method leads to further scarring. Laser vaporization of bladder neck tissue may obviate this problem.

H.   Bladder calculi may be endemic in some countries owing to nutritional deficiencies or secondary to obstruction or foreign bodies. Most bladder calculi can be managed endoscopically, obviating the need for open cystolithotomy. Small calculi of <5 mm can be washed out through the cystoscope sheath or removed with foreign body cystoscopic forceps.

1.   Mechanical lithotripsy. Larger calculi may be difficult to fragment by means of ultrasound (US) or electrohydraulic lithotripsy. Occasionally, it may be necessary to crush such stones under direct vision with the Hendrickson lithotrite. This instrument is passed into the bladder in a blind fashion, similar to the method of cystourethroscopy. A fiberoptic telescope is placed through the instrument, allowing visualization of the area between the jaws. Once the stone is grasped under direct vision, the jaws are closed to crush the stone. Stones larger than 3 cm are generally too large to fit within the jaws of the lithotrite. This instrument must be used with extreme care to avoid bladder perforation.

2.   US lithotripsy. By means of a rigid US transducer passed through an endoscope, vibrations are generated that can fragment bladder calculi. The transducer incorporates suction to remove fragments and provide cooling. The transducer must be in contact with the stone to transmit the US energy. With larger stones, US lithotripsy can be time consuming. This method is also quite useful for renal calculi when the instrument is passed through a nephroscope.

3. In **electrohydraulic lithotripsy,** a spark discharge within a liquid produces shock waves that fragment the stone. Under endoscopic control, the tip of the flexible transducer probe is placed very near, but not touching, the stone. Bursts of repetitive sparks from a generator, lasting 1 to 2 seconds, are used to fragment the stone, and irrigation is used to wash the fragments out of the bladder. Power is proportional to the diameter of the probe.

4. In **pneumohydraulic lithotripsy,** a probe similar to a jackhammer delivers 12 to 15 ballistic shocks per second directly to the stone. It appears to be quite effective and costs much less than laser lithotripsy.

5. Laser lithotripsy. Laser fibers may be delivered through rigid or flexible scopes. A variety of laser types may be used. The properties of each type vary, depending on the wavelength and power generated. Larger-diameter fibers deliver more energy, resulting in faster stone fragmentation rates.

I.   Bladder tumors and urethral tumors can be managed endoscopically in most instances. Specimens are obtained with flexible or rigid biopsy forceps, as discussed previously. Occasionally, the biopsy removes the entire tumor. The base and any remaining tumor can then be fulgurated with a laser or a Bugbee or roller ball electrode. Larger tumors require resection under general or spinal anesthesia. Careful endoscopy under anesthesia should be performed to determine whether any tumors were missed during the initial cystoscopy. Care must be taken in applying cutting current because perforation of the bladder wall can occur during the resection in up to 5% of instances. Intraperitoneal perforation requires abdominal exploration owing to the possibility of bowel injury when using electric current. Resection of larger tumors is currently most often done with a resectoscope.

III. Laparoscopy

The earliest laparoscopic procedures in urology were done for exploration of undescended testes in children during the 1970s. Laparoscopic pelvic lymph node dissection for staging of prostate cancer was the first procedure to be performed extensively by urologists (1989). Starting with the first laparoscopic nephrectomy in 1991, the list of laparoscopic procedures performed in urology has grown dramatically and now includes cancer staging, diagnostic, extirpative, and reconstructive operations. The procedures that are most frequently performed include laparoscopic nephrectomy (LRN) and adrenalectomy. Laparoscopic adrenalectomy is accepted as the standard of care for most adrenal masses except for large adrenal cancers. Laparoscopic nephrectomy is rapidly achieving the same status. Laparoscopic radical prostatectomy is in the early stages of development.

A. Preoperative preparation. The preoperative evaluation of the patient undergoing laparoscopy is similar to that for open procedures. The requirements for bowel preparation do not differ from those for traditional open surgery. A full mechanical prep is necessary only when the bowel will be intentionally opened or when there is a high likelihood of inadvertent enterotomy. A bowel prep is not necessary for retroperitoneoscopy.

B. Contraindications specific to laparoscopy include intestinal obstruction, abdominal ascites, and chronic obstructive pulmonary disease with CO_2 retention. Consent forms should include the same risks as the corresponding open procedure. The possibility of conversion to an open procedure should always be included in the consent. Current laparoscopic vascular control limits application of LRN to patients without renal vein or inferior vena cava tumor thrombi. Cautiously approach patients with T3a (tumor involving perinephric tissue inside the Gerota fascia) and T4 (tumor beyond the Gerota fascia) tumors because no large series with long-term safety and efficacy data exist for these. Consider a history of prior renal or abdominal surgery a relative contraindication, and individualize each patient's treatment based on surgeon experience. Systemic conditions that must be considered include chronic obstructive pulmonary disease with hypercarbia, bleeding diatheses, ascites, and bowel obstruction.

C. Patient preparation and positioning. Proper patient positioning is essential. The patient is initially placed in the supine position for induction of anesthesia. At this point, a Foley catheter and a nasogastric tube should be placed to decompress the bladder and stomach and minimize chances of injuring them. For renal surgery, retroperitoneal or transperitoneal, the patient is placed in a flank position similar to open surgery. The patient is secured to allow for rotation during the procedure. If the approach is transperitoneal, it is essential to position the patient close to the edge of the table to permit a wide range of motion with the camera. The table can be flexed and unflexed as needed during the procedure. Care is taken to cushion pressure points, and an axillary roll is placed to prevent a brachial plexus injury. A wide prep is always performed, keeping in mind the possibility of conversion to open surgery.

D. Basic laparoscopic techniques

1. Pneumoperitoneum can be established either by a closed technique via the Veress needle or by an open technique (Hasson). Although the technique chosen is essentially dependent on surgeon preference, the Hasson technique may minimize the risk of injury and is the preferred method when multiple adhesions are expected. The Veress needle is a 14-gauge needle that is 12 to 15 cm in length. It has a sharp beveled tip and a spring-loaded inner blunt tip. When the needle enters the peritoneal cavity, the blunt tip is activated to protect the peritoneal contents. It is usually placed above the umbilicus, where the distance to the peritoneum is usually the shortest, but can be placed lateral to the umbilicus. The Hasson technique allows for entrance into the peritoneum under direct vision through a small 2- to 3-cm incision. Once the peritoneum is entered, a blunt tip port can be inserted. The location of the incision is dependent on the procedure to be performed. Placement of the initial trocar is performed blindly if the Veress needle (Fig. 12.5) is used and under direct vision if the Hasson technique is used. A pneumoperitoneum of no less than 15 mm Hg should be obtained prior to placement of trocars.

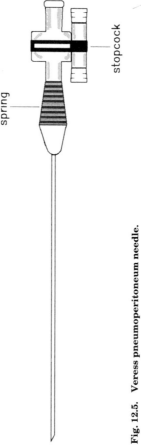

Fig. 12.5. Veress pneumoperitoneum needle.

2. Trocars and cannulas. Trocars have either a pyramidal or a conical tip to permit penetrating the abdominal wall. Most trocars are constructed with a hollow channel with openings at the tip and at the top of the instrument. This creates a rush of gas when the peritoneal cavity is penetrated by the trocar; the instrument does not need to be passed into the abdomen beyond this point. It is essential to make the skin incision of sufficient length to accommodate the trocar in order to minimize the downward pressure needed to place the trocar. The trocar should be inserted with steady downward pressure and a subtle twisting motion. The majority of trocar injuries can be minimized by ensuring an adequate skin incision (i.e., 10 mm for a 10-mm port). In the event of a leak around the trocar, a towel clip can be placed on the skin to prevent loss of pneumoperitoneum. Subsequent trocars should all be placed under direct vision. Cannulas are available in diameters from 3 to 12 mm to accommodate laparoscopes and instrumentation of all sizes (Fig. 12.6). They are equipped with valves to prevent gas leakage.

E. Physiologic effects of pneumoperitoneum. The most common insufflant used in laparoscopy is carbon dioxide. Although CO_2 is readily absorbed into the blood from the peritoneum, it is highly diffusible, allowing for expulsion of CO_2 via the lungs. It is important to monitor patients after prolonged laparoscopic procedures for hypercarbia and acidosis. This is particularly important in patients with respiratory compromise, as the acidosis may predispose to cardiac arrhythmias. Increased intraabdominal pressure resulting from pneumoperitoneum has been shown to cause a decrease in urine production. Although it has been postulated that this is due to ureteral compression, placement of ureteral stents during laparoscopy did not improve urine output. The most likely cause of decreased urine output is a decrease in glomerular filtration rate resulting from renal parenchymal compression and reduced renal blood flow.

F. Laparoscopic approaches include transperitoneal, retroperitoneal, and hand assisted.

1. Transperitoneal approach provides several advantages. A larger workspace allows for increased maneuverability of instruments intracorporeally and facilitates the

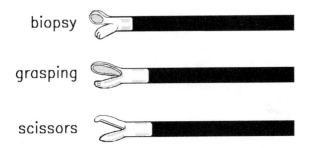

biopsy

grasping

scissors

Fig. 12.6. Various laparoscopic instruments for biopsy, grasping, and cutting.

manipulation and entrapment of extracted organs. The increased workspace also allows the surgeon to place trocars further apart, which facilitates use of the instruments. Orientation during transperitoneal procedures is facilitated by the presence of other intraperitoneal structures. Disadvantages of the intraperitoneal approach include increased incidence of bowel injury when compared with the retroperitoneal approach. Furthermore, urine leaks or hematomas are not contained within the retroperitoneal cavity.

2. **Retroperitoneal approaches** also have notable advantages and disadvantages. There is decreased incidence of both paralytic ileus and bowel injury. Furthermore, urine leaks or hematomas are contained and therefore are quicker to resolve and also less likely to result in prolonged ileus. Disadvantages include the need for creation of workspace with balloon dilatation and a decreased workspace. In addition, lack of anatomic landmarks makes orientation more difficult.

3. **Hand-assisted laparoscopy.** Many procedures are amenable to placement of a hand into the peritoneum for assistance with laparoscopic procedures. This is accomplished by using a pneumo-preserving device such as the GelPort (Applied Medical Resources), LapDisc (Ethicon), or PneumoSleeve (Dexterity). These can be inserted with a small muscle-splitting incision between 6 and 7 cm in length. The greatest advantage to this approach is the added benefit of tactile sensation, which the surgeon can use for dissection. This is thought to decrease the learning curve for surgeons inexperienced with laparoscopy. Furthermore, in procedures that require removal of intact specimens, such as living donor nephrectomies, this may be the preferred approach.

G. **LRN** has been shown to result in shorter hospital stays, less pain, and an earlier return to normal activities compared with open nephrectomy. Cancer control appears to compare favorably with open radical nephrectomy. Conversion to open nephrectomy is necessary in about 5% of cases.

1. **Indications.** LRN should be considered for T1 or T2 cystic or solid renal masses. The laparoscopic approach may also be considered in patients with symptomatic metastatic disease to the kidney.

2. **Contraindications.** LRN is not indicated in patients with renal vein or inferior vena cava tumor thrombi. There is insufficient experience to recommend LRN for T3a or T4 tumors. A history of prior renal or abdominal surgery is a relative contraindication. LRN is more risky in patients with chronic obstructive pulmonary disease with hypercarbia, bleeding diatheses, ascites, and bowel obstruction.

3. **Approach (Fig. 12.7).** One of three approaches may be taken, based on patient anatomy and surgeon preference: transperitoneal, retroperitoneal, and hand assisted. Retroperitoneal LRN may allow quicker access to the renal hilum and may be technically easier in obese patients. Disadvantages include a more difficult learning curve due to restricted working space. The transperitoneal approach has the advantages of familiar anatomy and a much larger working space. However, longer operative times and the possibility of bowel injury are disadvantages. The hand-assisted approach offers the advantage of removing the specimen intact. This is obviously critical in donor nephrectomy. The disadvantage of the hand-assisted approach is a larger incision, more postoperative pain, and a slower recovery. Adrenalectomy should be performed for T2 or larger renal tumors and for upper pole tumors.

4. Postoperative care. A blood gas determination is typically performed soon after extubation to check for hypercarbia. The nasogastric tube may be removed soon after extubation. Patient-controlled analgesia with morphine is useful for immediate postoperative pain control. On the first postoperative day, the patient usually will tolerate a liquid diet, the urinary catheter may be removed, and oral analgesic agents may be provided. Patients are typically discharged on the second or third postoperative day.

5. Complications occur at a rate of 10% to 15% following LRN, which is comparable with the rates following open radical nephrectomy. Postoperative complications such as pulmonary embolus, myocardial infarction, and deep venous thrombosis occur at rates similar to open surgery. Bowel injuries can occur either during trocar placement or from electrocautery. A small bowel perforation can be managed laparoscopically. Cautery injuries to the bowel can be missed during the procedure and may result in serious sequelae if not dealt with early. Severe pain at one of the trocar sites should suggest the possibility of bowel injury. Another common injury during LRN is splenic or liver laceration. Both of these will often require conversion to open laparotomy for management.

H. Laparoscopic pelvic lymph node dissection (LPLND) provides a means of excluding high-risk patients from noncurative therapy for prostate and other cancers. Imaging studies such as computed tomography, magnetic resonance imaging, and positron emission tomography cannot reliably diagnose small-volume pelvic lymph node involvement. LPLND offers the means to obtain adequate tissue for pathologic examination and diagnosis in such cases.

1. Indications for pelvic lymphadenectomy include those cases of prostate cancer involving a high likelihood of pelvic lymph node involvement and are summarized in Table 12.2. Bladder cancer patients with enlarged lymph nodes on pelvic imaging may also be candidates for laparoscopic staging prior to radical cystoprostatectomy. Other cancers in which LPLND may have a role include penile cancer and urethral cancer.

2. Contraindications for LPLND include severe cardiopulmonary disease, bowel obstruction, and morbid obesity. Prior abdominal surgery, history of pelvic fracture, and hip replacement may be considered relative contraindications.

3. Approach. Patients are started on clear liquids the afternoon prior to the procedure, and enemas are administered the evening prior to surgery to decompress the colon. Broadspectrum antibiotics are administered parenterally 1 hour prior to surgery. After induction, a nasogastric tube is placed. The patient is placed in the supine position, and the skin is prepped from the xiphoid process to the pubis and from the right to the left anterior axillary lines. The penis and scrotum are prepped and draped into the sterile field, and a Foley catheter is passed into the bladder. A sterile gauze bandage is wrapped around the penis, scrotum, and catheter to prevent carbon dioxide accumulation in the penis and scrotum.

4.   Postoperative care. Patients should be observed overnight and a complete blood count obtained the morning after surgery to rule out any occult hemorrhage. The bladder catheter is removed, and a clear liquid diet is ordered. Patients can be sent home on oral analgesics on the first postoperative day.

5.   Complications may include hemorrhage, bowel perforation, hypercarbia, obturator nerve injury, wound infection/dehiscence, lymphocele, and conversion to the open procedure. The risk of bowel perforation can be minimized by avoiding the use of electrosurgical current in the area of the intestine. The obturator nerve is injured most commonly during the dissection of the obturator node packet. Conversion to open surgery occurs most commonly after an injury has occurred to the iliac vessels.

I.   Laparoscopic donor nephrectomy has been increasingly accepted in the harvesting of kidneys from living related donors. The mortality rate (approximately 0.04%) appears similar to that for open donor nephrectomy. Also, in comparison with open donor nephrectomy, there has been no difference in renal function when measured 1 month after transplantation. One-year graft survival has also been comparable.

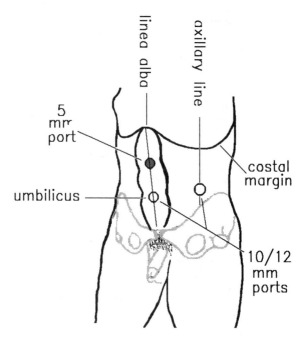

Fig. 12.7.   Typical port placement for laparoscopic left nephrectomy.

SUGGESTED READING

Berry A, Barratt A. Prophylactic antibiotic use in transurethral prostatic resection: a meta-analysis. *J Urol* 2002;167:571–577.

Bosch J. Urodynamic effects of various treatment modalities for benign prostatic hyperplasia. *J Urol* 1997;158:2034–2044.

Chiu AW, Azadzoi KM, Hatzichristou DG, et al. Effects of intraabdominal pressure on renal tissue perfusion during laparoscopy. *J Endourol* 1994;8:99–103.

Fahlenkamp D, Rassweiler J, Fornara P, et al. Complications of laparoscopic procedures in urology: experience with 2,407 procedures at 4 German centers. *J Urol* 1999;152:765–771.

Flanigan RC, Reda DJ, Wasson JH, et al. Five-year outcome of surgical resection and watchful waiting for men with moderately symptomatic benign prostatic hyperplasia: a Department of Veterans Affairs Cooperative Study. *J Urol* 1998;160:12–16.

Flowers JL, Jacobs S, Cho E, et al. Comparison of open and laparoscopic live donor nephrectomy. *Ann Surg* 1997;226:483.

Gill IS. Retroperitoneal laparoscopic nephrectomy. *Urol Clin North Am* 1998;25:343–360.

Gilling P, Mackey M, Cresswell M, et al. Holmium laser versus transurethral resection of the prostate: a randomized prospective trial with 1-year followup. *J Urol* 1999;162:1640–1644.

Hahn RG. Cooling effect from absorption of prewarmed irrigating fluid in transurethral prostatic resection. *Int Urol Nephrol* 1993; 25:265–270.

Hahn RG, Sandfeldt L, Nyman CR. Double-blind randomized study of symptoms associated with absorption of glycine 1.5% or mannitol 3% during transurethral resection of the prostate. *J Urol* 1998; 160:397–401.

Jacobs SC, Cho E, Dunkin BJ, et al. Laparoscopic live donor nephrectomy: the University of Maryland 3-year experience. *J Urol* 2000; 164:1494.

Jarrett TW. The present and future of laparoscopic renal and adrenal surgery. *J Urol* 2001;165:1882–1883.

Medina JJ, Parra RO, Moore RG. Benign prostatic hyperplasia (the aging prostate). *Med Clin North Am* 1999;83:1213–1229.

Nakada SY. Hand-assisted laparoscopic nephrectomy. *J Endourol* 1999;13:9–14.

Sofer M, Vilos GA, Borg P, et al. Stray radiofrequency current as a cause of urethral strictures after transurethral resection of the prostate. *J Endourol* 2001;15:221–225.

Van Melick HH, Van Venrooij GE, Eckhardt MD, et al. A randomized controlled trial comparing transurethral resection of the prostate, contact laser prostatectomy and electrovaporization in men with benign prostatic hyperplasia: urodynamic effects. *J Urol* 2002;168: 1058–1062.

Zheng W, Denstedt JD. Intracorporeal lithotripsy: update on technology. *Urol Clin North Am* 2000;27:301–313.

Genitourinary Infection

Joseph Alukal, Julita Mir, and Colm Bergin

I. **General principles**
Infections of the genitourinary tract are common clinical problems in urology. Most patients with these problems do not have underlying anatomic, metabolic, or functional abnormalities. General factors that may affect the clinical approach include patient age, sex, state of immunocompetence, comorbidities, site of infection, and the infectious agent. Local factors, including blood supply and presence of obstruction, are also important considerations.

II. **Classification of urinary tract infections**
   A. **Bacteriuria** should be distinguished from **urinary tract infection,** which implies invasion of genitourinary tissue.
   B. **First infection** is the first documented episode of clinically significant or symptomatic bacteriuria.
   C. **Unresolved bacteriuria** refers to failure to eradicate the infecting organism. Causes of unresolved bacteriuria include the following:
      1. **Bacterial resistance** to the antibiotic used is noted in approximately 5% of patients on antimicrobial therapy. Tetracyclines, penicillins, sulfonamides, cephalosporins, and trimethoprim are capable of transferring R-factors that make bacteria simultaneously resistant to multiple agents, including ampicillin, cephalosporins, and others. The fluoroquinolones and nitrofurantoin are not associated with R-factor resistance.
      2. **Multiple-organism bacteriuria** may fail to resolve when different bacterial species have mutually exclusive sensitivities.
      3. **Rapid reinfection** with a new resistant species during initial treatment for the original sensitive organism may occur.
      4. **Azotemia** may lead to poor excretion of antibiotic into the urine.
      5. **Papillary necrosis** may prevent adequate concentration of antibiotic in the urine.
      6. **Infected calculi, bladder tumors, or foreign bodies** may act to protect sensitive bacteria from antimicrobial inhibition.
      7. **Patient noncompliance** should be suspected when the urine culture during therapy reveals the same organism and sensitivity that were identified on initial culture.
   D. **Recurrent infection** refers to repeated infection interrupted by periods of sterile urine. It is caused by either persistence of bacteria within the urinary tract or reinfection by a new organism from a source outside the urinary tract.
      1. **Bacterial persistence** refers to cases in which urine is sterilized by therapy, but a persistent source of infection remains. Examples include infected stones and foreign bodies, chronic bacterial prostatitis, urethral or bladder diverticula,

and renal abscess. The formation of **biofilm** has recently been suggested as a mechanism by which bacteria may form protective capsules that adhere to the urinary tract. This protects bacteria from antibiotics as well as host defenses. Urine cultures may be negative in the presence of biofilm-encapsulated bacteria.

2. Reinfection accounts for 80% of recurrent infections. Most cases represent new infections with a new organism after initial therapy has sterilized the urine. Reinfections tend to occur >2 weeks after completion of therapy and are more frequent after cases of cystitis. Most recurrent infections in female patients are reinfections of the urinary tract caused by bacteria that ascend from the rectum to the vaginal introitus and then into the bladder. Reinfections in men are usually associated with an anatomic or functional abnormality of urine transport. The possibility of a vesicoenteric or vesicovaginal fistula should be considered when there is a history of pneumaturia, fecaluria, diverticulitis, previous gynecologic surgery, or radiation therapy.

III. Laboratory diagnosis

Although colony counts below 100,000 do not necessarily rule out infection, counts in excess of this number are always considered significant. Diagnosis depends on proper specimen collection to avoid contamination, prompt culturing, and quantitative bacteriologic techniques. If prompt culturing is not possible, containers should be transported in iced water and stored at 4°C. Cooling stops bacterial growth, but bacteria may still grow on media the following day. The urinary white cell count will be affected.

A. Specimen collection. Urine collected in a normal patient by suprapubic aspiration is sterile and represents the gold standard of diagnosis of urinary tract infection (Table 13.1). It is best to examine urine collected under supervision in the clinic or hospital rather than samples taken at home. In men, the specimen should be collected before prostatic examination to prevent contamination by prostatic secretions. Collection of urine from a drainage bag is not a reliable technique for urine culture.

Table 13.1. Probability of infection based on single-specimen colony counts

| Colony Count (CFU/mL) | Method of Collection | | |
	Clean Catch (%)	Catheterization (%)	Suprapubic Aspiration (%)
<10,000	2	2	100
10,000–100,000	5[a]	50	100
>100,000	80[b]	95	100

CFU, colony-forming units.

[a] Probably higher in male patients.

[b] If obtained from two consecutive specimens, 95%.

1.   Men. Urine should be collected with the midstream clean-catch method. In uncircumcised men, the foreskin should be retracted and the meatus cleansed with antiseptic. The first 25 mL of urine is passed without collection. The sterile container is then placed into the urinary stream, and 50 to 100 mL is collected. The urine should be cultured as soon as possible after collection.

2.   Women. After the labia are separated with one hand, the urethral meatus is cleansed with an antiseptic. A wiping motion toward the perineum should be used (to avoid contamination). After the first 25 mL is passed, the next 50 to 100 mL is collected in a sterile container. If a satisfactory specimen cannot be obtained, urine should be collected by a single straight catheterization of the bladder. A single catheterization causes urinary tract infection in 1% of ambulatory patients and in 5% to 10% of hospitalized patients.

3.   Children. In very young children, urine is usually collected by cleansing the meatus and placing a sterile plastic bag over the penis or vulva. Suprapubic needle aspiration of the bladder may be required to obtain a reliable urine specimen and is easily accomplished in young children because the bladder is located in a more intraabdominal position than in adults.

4.   Catheterized patients. In patients with indwelling catheters attached to closed drainage systems, urine for culture may be obtained from the needle port by using a sterile needle and a syringe to aspirate the urine. A closed drainage system should never be opened to collect urine for culture.

5.   Upper urinary tract. Neither history nor physical examination can reliably distinguish infection limited to the lower tract from infection affecting the upper tract. Noninvasive tests, including antibody-coated bacteria, have not proved sensitive or specific enough to be used in clinical practice. The only reliable methods involve invasive procedures (cystoscopy and collection of urine from both catheterized ureters or the bladder washout of Fairley).

6.   Prostatic secretions. In men with relapsing urinary infection, the most common source is the prostate gland. To make the diagnosis of bacterial prostatitis, the bacteriologic status of the prostate gland may be assessed either by semen culture or by expressing prostatic secretions with prostatic massage. Firm massage per rectum from side to midline bilaterally causes the contents of the prostatic ducts to be expressed. Vertical strokes in the midline will then project the secretions into the urethra and permit counting of leukocytes. Segmented cultures of the lower urinary tract may be obtained (Fig. 13.1) and interpreted as follows (Table 13.2):

   a.   The first 10 mL of voided urine (VB1) represents the urethral flora.

   b.   The midstream specimen (VB2) represents the bladder flora.

   c.   The expressed prostatic secretions (EPS) obtained by massage represent the prostatic flora.

   d.   The final specimen is the first 10 mL of urine voided immediately after prostatic massage (VB3) and represents the combined flora of the bladder and prostate.

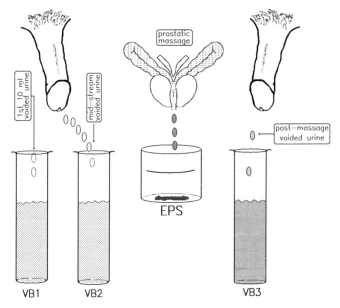

Fig. 13.1. Segmented urine cultures to localize lower tract infection in men.

B. Microscopic examination of urine

1. **Unspun urine.** Examination of fresh unspun urine is useful when one or more bacteria or one or more leukocytes per oil-immersion field are observed.

2. **Centrifuged urine** should be examined under high power (×400).

   a. **Pyuria** is defined as the presence of at least 5 leukocytes/high-power field in men and >20 leukocytes/high-power field in women. Ten or more leukocytes/high-power field are observed in 60% to 80% of patients with positive urine cultures. However, 25% of patients with negative

Table 13.2. Interpretation of segmented urine cultures

Culture Result	Interpretation
VB1 > VB2 or EPS or VB3	Urethral source
EPS and VB3 > VB1 or VB2	Prostatic source
VB2 > VB1 or EPS	UTI without prostatic source
VB1 = VB2 = EPS = VB3	UTI with prostatic source

VB, voided urine; EPS, expressed prostatic secretions; UTI, urinary tract infection.

urine cultures may also have pyuria. The differential diagnosis of sterile pyuria includes antibiotic effect, atypical organisms (*Mycobacterium tuberculosis, Chlamydia, Ureaplasma*), chronic interstitial nephritis, uroepithelial tumor, or nephrolithiasis.

   b. Bacilluria correlates well with culture results. Only 10% of patients with negative cultures have bacteria in the centrifuged urine specimen. Gram stain should be performed on specimens demonstrating bacilli.

C. Dipstick detects the presence of leukocyte esterase and nitrite; the former corresponds to significant pyuria and the latter to the presence of *Enterobacteriaceae,* which convert urinary nitrate to nitrite. Dipstick has a sensitivity of 75% to 95% and a specificity of 65% to 95%. The positive predictive value is relatively low at 30% to 40%, and the negative predictive value is 99%. Thus, these tests may be an alternative means of ruling out urinary tract infection when microscopy is not available.

D. Interpretation of urine culture. Results depend on method of collection, type of organisms, the patient's clinical symptoms, and number of colony-forming units per milliliter of urine.

   1. Organisms. *Escherichia coli* is cultured from >80% of urine specimens in patients with uncomplicated cystitis or pyelonephritis. *E. coli* is cultured in the vast majority of community-acquired infections; *Klebsiella* sp and *Enterobacter* sp are more likely to be hospital acquired. Infections with *Pseudomonas* sp and *Candida albicans* usually occur in patients with poor resistance who have received multiple courses of antibiotics. *Staphylococcus* sp may be true pathogens, especially in the setting of obstruction. *Proteus* infections are often associated with struvite or "infection" calculi. Most urinary pathogens are incapable of producing infection calculi, as they lack the enzyme urease, which alkalinizes the urine by converting urea to ammonia. This leads to supersaturation, a decrease in solubility of magnesium and calcium phosphate, and formation of stones composed of struvite and apatite. *Proteus* sp, *Klebsiella* sp, occasionally *Pseudomonas* sp, and *Staphylococcus* sp possess this enzyme. Multiple organisms are isolated in only 5% of true infections.

   2. The **colony count in midstream voided urine** has been compared with that in urine obtained by suprapubic bladder aspiration or bladder catheterization. Based on studies in asymptomatic women, Kass proposed the criterion of 100,000 colonies/mL as a positive test result for urinary infection. In an asymptomatic woman, a finding of >100,000 colonies/mL has an 80% positive predictive value, whereas in a symptomatic woman, such a finding has a 95% positive predictive value. However, the usefulness of this cutoff point depends on the method of collection and the clinical situation.

   a. False-negative results

      (1) Of acutely symptomatic women demonstrated to have bladder bacteriuria on suprapubic aspiration, fewer than 50% had >100,000 colonies/mL in the midstream specimen.

(2)   With markedly dilute urine or very frequent voiding, the colony count may be artificially reduced.
(3)   Antibiotic therapy may suppress counts.
(4)   Soaps or detergents used in specimen collection may suppress counts.
   b.   False-positive results may be caused by contamination during collection or more commonly by delay in specimen culturing.

IV.   Indications for evaluation of urinary tract infection
   A first presentation or history of urinary tract infection in male patients warrants evaluation. In female patients, recurrent, relapsing, or persistent urinary tract infection warrants investigation. In either sex, sepsis, fever, urinary tract infection lasting >7 days, gross hematuria, evidence of obstruction, and a history of stones are all indications for further evaluation. Risk factors such as pregnancy, diabetes, immunosuppression, and other debilitating disease should also be taken into account.

V.   Treatment of asymptomatic bacteriuria is indicated in   *N.B* certain clinical situations:
   A.   During **pregnancy:** A 3-day regimen of amoxicillin, oral cephalosporin, or trimethoprim–sulfamethoxazole (TMP/SMX) should be given (except in the third trimester).
   B.   Before **urologic instrumentation, endoscopy, or surgery.**
   C.   After **removal of a long-term indwelling catheter.**
   D.   In **renal transplant recipients** or other immunosuppressed patients.
   E.   In **children.**

VI.   Bacteremia and septic shock
   Gram-negative bacteremia arises from the urinary tract in about one-third of cases. Most commonly, it occurs in a hospitalized patient following instrumentation or develops from a primary focus in the genitourinary tract.
   A.   Etiology. Genitourinary bacteremia is most commonly caused by aerobic gram-negative bacteria such as *E. coli* and *Klebsiella, Enterobacter, Serratia, Pseudomonas,* or *Proteus* sp. Following transrectal prostatic biopsy, anaerobic bacteria (*Bacteroides fragilis*) may be causative. Gram-positive bacteria, particularly enterococci, are occasionally the causative organisms. Patients with bacteriuria before instrumentation or with urinary tract obstruction are at particular risk.
   B.   Diagnosis
      1.   Fever, especially with chills, should be considered evidence of bacteremia in any patient who has recently undergone genitourinary instrumentation. Fever may be absent at the onset of sepsis, as approximately 10% of patients may be hypothermic and another 5% may be unable to mount a fever in response to infection.
      2.   Other symptoms and signs include tachycardia, tachypnea, hypotension, and oliguria. A change in mental status such as confusion or agitation may also occur. Later, the patient may become lethargic and stuporous; the skin may become cold and moist.
      3.   Laboratory findings. Leukocytosis is common. Thrombocytopenia occurs in 50% of patients with early sepsis. Ad-

vanced or fulminant sepsis may be accompanied by liver function abnormalities, azotemia, and disseminated intravascular coagulation.

C. Septic shock may occur in up to 25% of bacteremic patients. Generally, shock develops rapidly and early (within 12 hours) after the onset of bacteremia. Early or "warm" shock is characterized by intense vasodilatation, increased cardiac output, and little or no hypotension. Late or "cold" shock is characterized by severe systemic hypotension (systolic pressure <90 mm Hg) accompanied by intense peripheral vasoconstriction (clammy skin), decreased cardiac output, and anuria or oliguria.

D. Treatment

   1. Initial measures. Patients need to be assessed hemodynamically (pulse, blood pressure, respiration rate), and cultures of blood and urine are required. A gram stain of the urine is essential in determining whether gram-positive or gram-negative organisms are present. A complete blood cell count, renal function tests, coagulation screen, and liver function tests should be ordered. Determination of arterial blood gases may also be necessary.

   2. Antibiotics. If one or more organisms have been cultured previously and sensitivity to antibiotics determined, the appropriate antibiotics should be administered immediately. More often, the causative organism is unknown, and empiric antibiotic treatment is indicated until the causative organism has been identified (see below for a discussion of antibiotic therapy). To cover possible gram-positive (especially enterococcal) infection, ampicillin or one of the cephalosporins should be added to the empiric regimen. If anaerobic bacteria are suspected (following transrectal biopsy), antimicrobial coverage will need to be broadened accordingly (e.g., clindamycin, metronidazole, or a second-generation cephalosporin, depending on other antimicrobial agents used and patient history of drug allergy).

   3. Cardiovascular support requires placement of a central venous pressure line or Swan–Ganz catheter in most instances. If the patient is hypotensive, administer crystalloids and colloids and correct acidosis and hypoxemia, if present. Volume expansion is continued as long as the venous pressure remains below 15 cm H_2O or pulmonary wedge pressure remains below 22 mm Hg. If hypotension is not corrected by these measures, a dopamine infusion should be initiated at 2 to 5 mg/kg/min and then titrated to maintain blood pressure at near-normal levels and urine output at 30 to 50 mL/h.

   4. Pulmonary support includes administration of 5 L of oxygen/min by face mask. If respiration is inadequate as indicated by blood gas determination, intubation is indicated with mechanical ventilation to maintain the oxygen tension above 70 mm Hg and carbon dioxide tension below 40 mm Hg.

   5. Corticosteroids have been advocated in septic shock for many years, but the rationale for their use remains controversial. Large-scale multicenter trials have demonstrated an increase in morbidity and mortality among septic patients given large doses of corticosteroids.

VII.   Infection of the upper urinary tract

A.   Acute pyelonephritis is acute bacterial infection of the kidney. Symptoms of lower urinary tract infection may be noted 1 to 2 days before or concurrently with an episode of upper urinary tract infection.

  1.   Etiology and pathogenesis. The most common cause is aerobic gram-negative bacteria (*E. coli* most often). Gram-positive organisms such as staphylococci and enterococci rarely cause pyelonephritis. Infection with urea-splitting organisms, such as *Proteus mirabilis* and some strains of *Klebsiella,* leads to a highly alkaline urine secondary to liberation of ammonia. This promotes the precipitation of struvite stones in the collecting system of the kidney.

   a.   Ascent from the lower tract is the most common mechanism of infection.

   b.   Vesicoureteral reflux is absent in most patients with pyelonephritis, and not all patients with reflux have clinical evidence of pyelonephritis, but reflux is associated with an increased risk for infection.

   c.   Obstruction increases the risk for pyelonephritis through stasis of urine. Obstruction may be congenital or acquired. Pyelonephritis is more common in patients with neurogenic bladder dysfunction, which leads to a high intravesical pressure that is transmitted to the upper urinary tract.

   d.   Hematogenous spread is often associated with staphylococci from the skin or gram-negative bacteria from the gastrointestinal tract.

   e.   Anatomic factors. Acute pyelonephritis is more common in female patients (the shorter urethra may predispose to colonization of the lower tract). The prostate secretes antibacterial factors that may provide some protection from infection.

   f.   Diabetes mellitus may predispose to infection by causing obstruction by sloughed renal papillae, bladder dysfunction, and decreased host resistance. A rare form of pyelonephritis caused by gas-forming organisms—"emphysematous pyelonephritis"—is seen almost exclusively in diabetic patients.

  2.   Clinical findings include fever, chills, flank pain, and dysuria. Constitutional symptoms are common. Examination reveals tenderness of the costovertebral angle, abdominal tenderness, and systemic signs of infection. Urinalysis shows pyuria, bacteriuria, and sometimes microscopic hematuria. Urine culture reveals growth of the causative organism to >100,000 colonies/mL.

  3.   Radiologic findings. Roentgenographic examination of the kidneys, ureter, and bladder may show calcifications overlying the kidney or ureter, indicating possible obstruction. Ultrasonography (US) is the preferred examination and may provide information regarding obstruction, stones, or abscess without exposing the patient to radiation. Focal infection of the kidney may be visualized with US; this has been termed "lobar nephronia." Intravenous urogram (IVU) or computed tomography (CT) usually shows some degree of renal enlargement and a decreased nephrogram. Occasionally, there may be complete nonvisualization of the infected kidney.

4.   Differential diagnosis includes acute cholecystitis, acute appendicitis, and acute pancreatitis. In women, gynecologic diagnoses may mimic acute pyelonephritis.

5.   Treatment. It is important to diagnose and treat complicating factors, such as obstructive uropathy or stones, in addition to addressing the acute pyelonephritis itself. If these factors are not present, therapy consists of specific antibiotics determined by culture and sensitivity. In most cases, however, empiric therapy is necessary pending culture data (Table 13.3). For mild to moderate disease treated in the outpatient setting, therapy with oral TMP/SMX or quinolone is recommended for 14 days. Document success with urine culture obtained 1 to 2 weeks after completion of therapy. For severe illness or possible urosepsis when hospitalization is required, use parenteral quinolone, ceftriaxone, or ampicillin and gentamicin until fever resolves for 2 days, and then complete a 14-day course with oral antibiotics. If the clinical response is poor after 48 to 72 hours despite appropriate antibiotics, the presence of an intrarenal abscess, perinephric abscess, or obstructive pyonephrosis must be ruled out. Nitrofurantoin should not be used for the treatment of pyelonephritis because it does not achieve reliable tissue levels. If obstruction of the upper tract is identified, begin antibiotic therapy and establish drainage either with a ureteric stent placed cystoscopically or via percutaneous nephrostomy. Complete removal of calculi is generally required for bacteriologic cure and to prevent further renal damage.

B.   Chronic pyelonephritis is a term that most commonly refers to radiologic findings of renal scarring, fibrosis, and calyceal deformities presumed to be caused by previous infection. A more appropriate term is **chronic interstitial nephritis.** Differential diagnosis includes analgesic nephropathy, renal tuberculosis, and renovascular disease. Chronic bacterial infection of the kidney in adults is rare. Renal scarring is thought to be the result of infection in childhood, especially when accompanied by vesicoureteral reflux. Renal scarring almost always begins by age 4 and rarely develops in later years. The adult patient with bilateral chronic pyelonephritis usually presents with azotemia and hypertension rather than signs of urinary infection. Radiologic findings include characteristic polar renal scarring with underlying dilated calyces. In bilateral disease, both kidneys are small, but in unilateral disease, compensatory hypertrophy of the normal kidney occurs.

1.   Xanthogranulomatous pyelonephritis is a form of unilateral chronic pyelonephritis characterized by multiple parenchymal abscesses, pyonephrosis, and poor renal function. The inflammatory response includes the formation of granulomas with lipid-laden macrophages (xanthogranulomas). These cells may be difficult to differentiate from clear cells of renal carcinoma. Although its exact cause is unclear, xanthogranulomatous pyelonephritis seems to be related to a combination of renal obstruction and chronic urinary tract infection. **Predisposing factors** include renal calculi, urinary

Table 13.3. Empiric antibiotic therapy of genitourinary infection

Clinical Situation	Suspected Organisms	Therapy — Recommended	Therapy — Alternative
Uncomplicated pyelonephritis (outpatient)	E. coli S. faecalis	TMP/SMX DS 1 tab PO bid × 14 d Ciprofloxacin 500 mg PO bid × 14 d Norfloxacin 400 mg PO bid × 14 d	Amoxicillin 875 mg/clavulanate 125 mg PO q12h × 14 d
Complicated pyelonephritis (inpatient)	E. coli	Ciprofloxacin 400 mg IV q12h[a]	Ticarcillin 3 g/clavulanate 0.1 IV q4–6h[a]
	P. aeruginosa	Ampicillin 1 g IV q6h/gentamicin 1 mg/kg IV q8h[a]	Ampicillin 2 g/sulbactam 1 g IV q6h[a]
	S. faecalis Proteus sp. K. pneumoniae	Ceftriaxone 500 mg IM/IV q12h[a]	Piperacillin 3 g/tazobactam 0.375 IV q6h[a]
Renal or perinephric abscess	S. aureus	Nafcillin 2 g IV q4h[a] × 2–6 wk or cefazoline 1 g IV q6h[a] × 2–6 wk	Vancomycin 15 mg/kg IV q12h[a] × 2–6 wk
Renal or perinephric abscess	E. coli	Ampicillin 1 g IV q6h or ciprofloxacin 400 mg IV q12h with gentamicin 1 mg/kg IV q8h[b]	

continued

Table 13.3. Continued

Clinical Situation	Suspected Organisms	Therapy	
		Recommended	Alternative
Uncomplicated cystitis	E. coli S. aureus	TMP/SMX DS 1 tab PO bid × 3 d Ciprofloxacin 250 mg PO bid × 3 d Norfloxacin 400 mg PO bid × 3 d	Nitrofurantoin 50–100 mg PO bid × 3 d Doxycycline 100 mg PO bid × 3 d
Acute prostatitis	E. coli	Ampicillin 1 g IV q6h/gentamicin 1 mg/kg IV q8h[b]	TMP/SMX DS 1 tab PO bid × 42 d Ciprofloxacin 500 mg PO bid × 42 d
Chronic bacterial prostatitis	E. coli	TMP/SMX DS 1 tab PO bid × 42 d Ciprofloxacin 500 mg PO bid × 42 d	
Chronic nonbacterial prostatitis	M. hominis C. trachomatis or U. urealyticum	Erythromycin 500 mg PO qid × 7 d Doxycycline 100 mg PO bid × 7 d Azithromycin 1 g PO qd × 7 d	
Chronic nonbacterial prostatitis	T. vaginalis	Metronidazole 2 g PO qd × 5 d	

TMP/SMX, trimethoprim/sulfamethoxazole; DS, double strength.
[a]Switch to oral therapy as soon as patient is afebrile for 48 h.
[b]Give aminoglycoside for 2 wk and ampicillin or ciprofloxacin for total of 6 wk.

obstruction, partially treated urosepsis, renal ischemia, altered lipid metabolism, abnormal immune responses, diabetes, and primary hyperparathyroidism. Bacteriuria and pyuria are almost always present. Because of the chronic nature of the disease, two-thirds of patients are anemic and only 50% manifest leukocytosis.

   a.   Radiologic findings on IVU or contrast CT typically include a nonvisualized kidney (80%) with calculi in the collecting system (70%). Parenchymal calcifications may also be present.

   b.   Treatment. Patients are generally not cured with antibiotics alone, and surgical intervention is usually required. In many cases, nephrectomy is indicated because the disease cannot be differentiated from renal cell carcinoma.

   2.   Papillary necrosis may result from bacterial infection of the kidney or other causes (chronic abuse of analgesics, diabetes mellitus, sickle cell disease, renal vascular disease, chronic obstruction, hypertension, disseminated intravascular coagulation, lead nephropathy, Balkan nephropathy, hypercalcemia, potassium depletion, radiation nephritis). It is most commonly seen in female diabetic patients. The pathophysiology is vascular insufficiency leading to necrosis and sloughing of renal papillae. Although the disease is usually bilateral, the symptoms are usually unilateral as the ureter becomes obstructed by one or more necrotic papillae.

   a.   Radiologic findings are determined by the stage of the disease. The papillae may be calcified with radiolucent centers, or they may be absent. If they are still in the collecting system, they appear as triangular filling defects.

   b.   Treatment involves control of infection, adequate hydration, and removal of inciting causes. Because the disease is usually bilateral, nephrectomy is recommended only as a lifesaving measure.

C.   Renal and perirenal abscess. Renal abscess may be secondary to hematogenous spread from a distant site or to direct spread from ascending infection. Perirenal abscesses usually result from rupture of a renal abscess into the perinephric space. Fungi and mycobacterial species have also been implicated. Twenty-five percent of cases may be polymicrobial. Results of urine culture often correlate with abscess cultures, but in some patients, the urine culture is positive for bacteria different from those isolated from the abscess. About one-third of patients will have positive blood cultures. Anemia is present in 40% and azotemia in 25%. Pyuria and proteinuria are common, although results of urinalysis may be normal in up to one-third of patients and 40% have sterile urine.

   1.   Pathogenesis. The organism most commonly involved in hematogenous spread is *S. aureus* from a skin lesion, osteomyelitis, or endovascular infection. This form of renal abscess is now rare, as staphylococcal infections are generally treated early in their course. Conditions associated with an increased risk for staphylococcal bacteremia include intravenous drug abuse, hemodialysis, and diabetes mellitus. A solitary renal abscess that involves the cortex of the kidney is termed a **renal carbuncle.** The urine may remain sterile if the abscess does not communicate with the collecting system. Intrarenal abscesses secondary to ascending infection, **medullary abscesses,** account for >75% of renal and perinephric abscesses. They are often associated with obstruction by calculi, involve the medulla as well as the cortex, and are multifocal. The cause is almost always gram-negative uropathogens.

2. **Clinical findings** are determined by the cause of the abscess. A hematogenous abscess will characteristically present with acute onset of fever, chills, and flank pain. There is usually no history of previous urinary tract infection, and the urine may be sterile. In contrast, patients with medullary abscess have a well-defined history of previous urinary tract infection, calculi, obstruction, or surgery. In these patients, the clinical presentation does not differ greatly from that of acute pyelonephritis. Persistence of fever and leukocytosis despite apparent appropriate antimicrobial therapy suggests that simple pyelonephritis is not the diagnosis. Usually, pyuria and bacteriuria are present.

3. **Radiologic findings.** A renal carbuncle may appear as a space-occupying lesion on IVU. CT is considered the diagnostic modality of choice, as it will identify the abscess and define its extension beyond the renal capsule and surrounding structures. Medullary abscesses are generally small and multifocal and may manifest only as a poorly functioning kidney. In the presence of a perinephric abscess, the renal outline and the psoas shadow may be obliterated.

4. **Treatment.** Prompt intervention is required to preserve renal function (Table 13.3).

a. **Renal carbuncle** caused by *S. aureus* should be treated with 12 g of naficillin/24 h (if the strain is methicillin sensitive). Antibiotic therapy alone may be sufficient if initiated early enough. Parenteral antibiotics should be continued for a minimum of 6 weeks. Typically, fever resolves 5 to 6 days after the initiation of antimicrobial therapy and flank pain improves within 24 hours. A different clinical course suggests an incorrect diagnosis, uncontrolled infection, or resistant bacteria.

b. **Medullary abscesses** are usually caused by gram-negative organisms. Previously untreated patients should receive a parenteral aminoglycoside with a penicillin or fluoroquinolone. If the abscess develops while the patient is being treated for pyelonephritis, aspiration of the abscess should be carried out to obtain culture material. If the abscess is sterile or grows the same organisms as does the urine, continue the same antibiotic therapy. The aminoglycoside is generally administered for 2 weeks, and the penicillin or fluoroquinolone is continued for >2 weeks (duration guided by radiographic resolution; resolution of pain, fever, and malaise; normalization of the erythrocyte sedimentation rate; disappearance of the abscess cavity on CT). Any obstruction of the urinary tract must be relieved. If the abscess is localized, drainage by percutaneous or surgical means may be required. In cases of multiple abscesses involving the entire kidney, nephrectomy may be necessary.

VIII. Infection of the lower urinary tract

A. **Dysuria** is a common complaint and accounts for a significant proportion of clinic visits per year.

    1. In **male patients,** acute dysuria may be caused by sexually transmitted disease, foreign body in the urethra, urethral stricture/periurethral abscess, bacterial cystitis, and carcinoma of the bladder in situ.

    2. **Female patients.** Dysuria may or may not be caused by bacterial infection (Table 13.4). Only one-third of women with acute dysuria will have bacterial infection as indicated by the finding of >100,00 colonies/mL in voided urine. Conversely, of women with acute dysuria and <100,000 colonies/mL in voided urine, 15% will have bacterial infection on suprapubic aspiration. **Urethral syndrome** refers to chronic dysuria of unknown cause in female patients. Urinary infection is usually ruled out by no or low colony counts on culture. However, low bacterial counts in symptomatic patients may be significant and warrant antibacterial therapy. If no clinical response is observed, sexually transmitted disease or vaginitis should be ruled out.

    a. **Sexually transmitted disease** should be suspected in young, sexually active women, especially those with multiple partners or a new partner in recent months. Among women with acute dysuria, *Chlamydia trachomatis* is found in 7% and *Neisseria gonorrhoeae* in 2%. Rare causes include herpes infection and condyloma acuminata. **Diagnosis** requires a thorough clinical examination to detect pelvic inflammatory disease and obtain material from the cervix and urethra for gram stain, culture, or polymerase chain reaction testing.

    b. **Vaginitis** is characterized by vaginal discharge, pruritus, and dysuria. The most common organisms are *Trichomonas vaginalis* and *C. albicans.* Nonspecific vaginitis is usually caused by *Haemophilus vaginalis* in combination with anaerobic bacteria. **Diagnosis** is made on the basis of gram stain and culture of the discharge. For **treatment,** trichomonal vaginitis responds to 2 g of oral metronidazole as a single dose (contraindicated in first trimester of pregnancy), and partners should also be treated. Vaginitis caused by *C. albicans* responds well to topical antifungal

Table 13.4. Differentiation of acute dysuria in women

	Bacterial Cystitis	STD	Vaginitis
Onset	Acute	Acute	Gradual
Associated symptoms	Suprapubic pain	Nonspecific	Pruritis
Examination	Nonspecific	Vaginal discharge	Vaginal discharge
Urinalysis	Pyuria in >90% Hematuria in 50%	Pyuria No hematuria	No pyuria No hematuria

therapy (e.g., clotrimazole vaginal cream or miconazole nitrate 2% vaginal cream for 7 to 14 days). Nonspecific vaginitis including bacterial vaginosis is treated with 500 mg of oral metronidazole twice daily for 7 days or with topical metronidazole (MetroGel) for 5 days.

c. Noninfectious conditions include interstitial cystitis, carcinoma in situ or bladder cancer, foreign body, chemical irritation, atrophic changes, neurogenic bladder dysfunction, and perineal muscle spasm or tension.

B. Acute bacterial cystitis occurs in the vast majority of women as a result of ascending infection after colonization of the perineum and vaginal introitus. In male patients, bacterial cystitis may be caused by foci of infection in the prostate, outflow obstruction, urinary stone, or bladder cancer. In ambulatory patients, bacterial cystitis is caused by *E. coli* in 80% of cases. *Staphylococcus saprophyticus* and *Enterococcus* sp may account for another 10%. The remainder are caused by *Klebsiella, Enterobacter, Proteus,* and anaerobic bacteria. On the other hand, *Pseudomonas, Serratia marcescens,* and *C. albicans* account for a large portion of hospital-acquired infections. Patients on broad-spectrum antibiotics and those who are immunocompromised are particularly at risk.

1. Clinical findings include abrupt onset of dysuria, frequency, urgency, and suprapubic pain. Fever and costovertebral pain are indicative of involvement of the upper tract. See Table 13.4 for clinical findings that may help differentiate acute bacterial cystitis from vaginitis and sexually transmitted diseases in female patients.

2. Laboratory findings. Urinalysis reveals pyuria in almost all cases of bacterial infection. Microscopic hematuria is found in 50% of women with acute cystitis.

3. Radiologic findings. Investigations are warranted only in cases of bacterial persistence or unresolved bacteriuria, patients infected with unusual organisms, or patients with symptoms and signs suggestive of disease of the upper tract. Screening should include renal US and a voiding cystourethrogram to detect reflux.

4. Endoscopy is indicated in the presence of gross or microscopic hematuria that persists after the infection is treated. Cystoscopy should be delayed until the acute infection has been treated.

5. Treatment. Please see Fig. 13.2.

a. First infection is very likely caused by *E. coli.* Antibiotic therapy options include TMP/SMX or one of the fluoroquinolones. These agents have little effect on the normal anaerobic and microaerophilic vaginal flora such as *Lactobacillus.* At the same time, they eradicate the infecting *E. coli* strain from the vaginal and fecal reservoir, thus reducing the risk for reinfection. Agents that adversely affect the fecal and vaginal anaerobic flora, such as amoxicillin and first-generation cephalosporins, may enhance the susceptibility to rapid reinfection, particularly if they are not effective in eradicating enteric gram-negative rods from those sites. Resistance to TMP/SMX is well recognized, and risk factors for such resistance include use of TMP/SMX

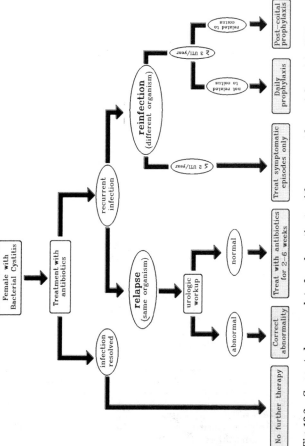

Fig. 13.2.   Suggested approach to female patients with recurrent bacterial cystitis. UTI, urinary tract infection.

within past 6 months, recent hospitalization, and diabetes. Resistance to quinolones remains <5% in most studies. All regimens are given for 3 to 7 days (consider a 7-day regimen in diabetic individuals, those with more severe symptoms or recent urinary tract infection, and patients older than 65 years). Recent controlled trials have demonstrated that single-dose regimens are less effective than 3- to 7-day regimens. Furthermore, single-dose therapy is less likely to be effective in treating infections in which unrecognized complicating factors are present and is also unsuitable for treating occult disease of the upper tract. Urine culture should be obtained if symptoms persist after >72 hours of antimicrobial therapy. It is important to note that even in areas with TMP/SMX resistance of up to 30%, the overall clinical and microbiological cure rates remain high at 80% to 85%.

b.   Relapse or bacterial persistence. The time to relapse is often <2 weeks. A detailed evaluation should be carried out for any possible focus of infection. In instances suggestive of vaginitis or sexually transmitted diseases, appropriate cultures should be collected before therapy is initiated. Provided that no focus of infection is found, treat relapsing or persistent infection for 2 to 6 weeks.

c.   Multiple recurrent infections. Approximately 50% of women will have a second infection within 12 months, almost always with a different organism or a different serotype of the original organism. Such patients are best managed by prophylaxis. Any acute infection should be eradicated by one of the regimens discussed above before any prophylactic regimen is implemented. For women with two or fewer episodes a year, suggest that the patient initiate therapy for symptomatic episodes (3-day regimen). For those women with three or more urinary tract infections per year, determine whether symptoms are temporally related to sexual intercourse. If they are, suggest postcoital prophylaxis with 1 tablet of TMP/SMX, 250 mg of cephalexin, or 50 mg of nitrofurantoin. If there is no discernible relation to coitus, suggest daily or thrice-weekly prophylaxis with the same agents.

C.   *C. albicans,* a normal inhabitant of the gastrointestinal and female genital tract, may become a pathogen in the urinary tract in immunocompromised patients and in those exposed to broad-spectrum antibiotics. Symptoms are generally mild and consist of bladder irritability or flank pain.

1.   Diagnosis is suggested by observing yeast on microscopic examination of the urine and is confirmed by culture. Fungus balls may cause filling defects in the upper urinary tract on IVU or CT.

2.   Treatment

a.   Bladder. Alkalinize the urine by giving 650 mg of sodium bicarbonate orally every 6 hours to keep the pH at ≥7.5. In patients requiring sodium restriction, potassium bicarbonate or potassium citrate may be used instead. In patients unable to take oral medication, sodium bicarbonate may be given intravenously. If this fails to eradicate the infection, irrigate the bladder three times daily with a solution of amphotericin B (50 mg in 1 L of saline solution).

b.   Renal involvement may also be treated with the same amphotericin B solution, administered either through a ureteral catheter or preferably through a nephrostomy catheter.

c.   Candidemia or candidal sepsis may be treated with fluconazole 400 mg PO, then 200 mg/day PO for at least 28 days. For patients unable to take oral medication, the same antifungal dose may be given intravenously. Amphotericin B, the previous drug of choice, is rarely used currently owing to potential nephrotoxicity and need for parenteral therapy.

IX.   Prostatic infection

According to use of the National Institutes of Health (NIH) Chronic Prostatitis Symptom Index (see Appendix 1, page 230), approximately 10% of men experience symptoms consistent with prostatitis. Of patients presenting with complaints that can be referred to the prostate, <5% have evidence of bacterial infection. Although the vast majority of cases are not caused by bacterial infection, it nevertheless must be excluded. Prostatitis may also be caused by gonococcal, tuberculous, fungal, or parasitic infection.

A.   Classification has changed somewhat because of criteria proposed by the NIH for research in prostatitis. In the past, cases with prostatitis symptoms were classified as nonbacterial prostatitis if the patients had leukocytes in the prostatic secretions and as prostatodynia if there was no evidence of inflammation. The new classification changes the term "nonbacterial prostatitis" to "inflammatory chronic prostatitis/pelvic pain syndrome" (CP/CPPS) and the term "prostatodynia" to "noninflammatory chronic prostatitis/pelvic pain syndrome" (Table 13.5). The criteria for diagnosis of inflammatory CP/CPPS are considerable broader as they now include not only expressed prostatic secretions but also post–prostatic massage urine and semen analysis. Whether this new terminology and classification will impact clinical practice remains to be seen.

B.   Mechanism of prostatic infection includes direct reflux of infected urine into prostate ducts, lymphatic spread from the

Table 13.5.   Classification of prostatitis

Stamey–Mears Classification	NIH Consensus Classification
Acute bacterial prostatitis	Type I: acute bacterial prostatitis
Chronic bacterial prostatitis	Type II: chronic bacterial prostatitis
Chronic nonbacterial prostatitis	Type IIIA: inflammatory chronic prostatitis/pelvic pain syndrome
Prostatodynia	Type IIIB: noninflammatory chronic prostatitis/pelvic pain syndrome
	Type IV: asymptomatic inflammatory prostatitis/pelvic pain syndrome

rectum, and hematogenous spread from distant sites. The urine is by far the most likely source of prostatic infection.

C.   Acute prostatitis is acute infection of the prostatic glands characterized by sudden onset of fever, chills, low back and perineal pain, dysuria, and obstructive voiding symptoms. Constitutional symptoms may also be present. Early diagnosis and treatment are important for both symptom control and the prevention of secondary problems such as gram-negative sepsis, prostatic abscess, and metastatic infection. Acute prostatitis is generally caused by coliform bacteria. Most infections (80%) are due to a single organism, most commonly *E. coli, P. mirabilis,* or *Klebsiella* sp. Obligate anaerobic bacteria and gram-positive bacteria, other than enterococci, rarely cause acute bacterial prostatitis. *N. gonorrhoeae* should be suspected in sexually active men younger than 35 years.

1.   The prostate is extremely tender, swollen, and warm to the touch. Vigorous prostatic massage is contraindicated because of concern about resulting bacteremia. Microabscesses occur early in the disease, and they may coalesce into a large abscess as a late complication. Transrectal US or CT will confirm this diagnosis if it is not apparent on clinical examination. Laboratory parameters include leukocytosis and marked pyuria and bacteriuria.

2.   Medical treatment. Hospitalization may be necessary in patients with urinary retention and in those who require intravenous antimicrobial therapy. Limited drug entry into the prostate is less of a problem in the setting of acute prostatitis, in which permeability is increased; thus, a variety of antimicrobials can be used to eradicate infection. Gram stain of the urine (if positive) can be used to guide initial therapy. Until results of urine cultures are known, treatment should consist of an aminoglycoside and penicillin combination for those requiring parenteral therapy or an oral fluoroquinolone or TMP/SMX for less severe cases (Table 13.3). Duration of therapy should be at least 4 to 6 weeks to ensure eradication of the infection. Clinical studies of fluoroquinolones suggest that a negative urine culture at 7 days following initiation of therapy predicts cure at the conclusion of the full 4 to 6 weeks of treatment.

3.   Surgical therapy. Surgical drainage of a prostatic abscess can be accomplished by either transrectal, perineal, or transurethral approach. Because of the potential for systemic infection and bacteremia, urethral instrumentation should be avoided in acute prostatic prostatitis. For acute urinary retention, gentle passage of a Foley catheter may be attempted, as tolerated by the patient. If passing the catheter is difficult or not tolerated, a percutaneous suprapubic cystostomy is indicated.

D.   Prostatic abscess is very commonly (70%) caused by coliform bacteria and occurs more frequently in patients with diabetes mellitus. Examination reveals a tender, fluctuant prostate. Treatment consists of antibiotic therapy as outlined for acute bacterial prostatitis combined with surgical drainage (perineal incision and drainage, transurethral resection, or transrectal drainage).

E.   Chronic prostatitis includes several syndromes, bacterial as well as nonbacterial in etiology.

  1.   Chronic bacterial prostatitis is a generally asymptomatic, indolent bacterial colonization of the prostatic ducts; these may act as a repository of bacteria for colonization of the urine. It is the most common cause of relapsing urinary tract infection in men. Gram-negative rods are the most common etiologic agent, although enterococci, chlamydiae, fungi, and tuberculosis have all been reported. Patients are symptomatic only when bacteriuria is present and complain of irritative voiding symptoms and perigenital pain. Examination of the prostate reveals a normal or minimally tender gland. Urinalysis shows pyuria and bacteriuria during episodes of acute cystitis. When the urine is sterile, segmented urine cultures as described previously should be used to attempt to localize the infection to the prostate. Chronic prostatitis is suspected when VB3 has >12 leukocytes/high-power field; >20 is almost diagnostic unless leukocytes are also present in VB2. Negative cultures do not exclude the diagnosis. **Granulomatous prostatitis** may be caused by *Mycobacterium* sp but more often represents a nonspecific inflammation of unknown cause. A specific form may be seen in patients who received intravesical bacille Calmette-Guérin therapy for superficial bladder cancer. Biopsy is required to exclude carcinoma. **Treatment** is aimed at eradicating the prostatic focus of infection. Fluoroquinolones have significantly improved medical management, with cure rates of 60% to 90% reported. Advantages of quinolones include a broad spectrum of activity, small molecular size, high degree of lipid solubility, and low level of protein binding, all of which enhance prostatic penetration. Apart from TMP/SMX, most antibiotics, including penicillins, cephalosporins, aminoglycosides, sulfonamides, and most tetracyclines, are ineffective. Duration of therapy should be a minimum of 4 to 6 weeks. Men with recalcitrant prostatitis can be treated with radical transurethral resection of the prostate (TURP) (infection is usually harbored in the periphery of the gland, and traditional TURP removes only the central adenoma). This surgery cures approximately 40% but is complicated by an increased risk for incontinence.

  2.   Chronic nonbacterial prostatitis. Many patients with symptoms of dysuria and perineal pain have no evidence of urinary or prostatic infection but have large numbers of inflammatory cells in their prostatic secretions. The presence of large numbers of lipid-laden macrophages is particularly suggestive of prostatic inflammation. A definitive role for *Mycoplasma, Ureaplasma, Chlamydia,* or *Trichomonas* remains to be proved, although empiric antimicrobial therapy is often aimed at these organisms. Empiric therapy with tetracycline, erythromycin, or azithromycin may be warranted. Treatment of infections caused by *C. trachomatis* is 1 week of doxycycline (100 mg twice daily), erythromycin (500 mg four times daily), or azithromycin (1 g daily). Other noninfectious causes, such as autoimmunity and neuromuscular dysfunction, have been suggested. Urinary frequency and urgency may be ameliorated with the use of low-dose antimuscarinic therapy.

F. CPPS. The clinical manifestations of nonbacterial prostatitis (type IIIA) are indistinguishable from those with noninflammatory disease also known as prostatodynia (type IIIB). The process is considered chronic after 3 months' duration, and the predominant symptom is pain localized to the perineum, suprapubic area, and penis but that can also occur in the testes, groin, or low back. Pain during or after ejaculation is also a prominent feature in many patients, as well as urgency, frequency, hesitancy, and poor interrupted flow. Studies haves shown that quality of life is impaired in these patients. Management of patients with the inflammatory form includes antimicrobials, prostatic massage, nonsteroidal antiinflammatory drugs, and α-adrenergic blocking agents. In patients with prostatodynia (type IIIB), urine cultures are negative, and expressed prostatic secretions reveal no inflammatory cells. The condition may be caused by detrusor hyperreflexia or pelvic floor myalgia. Stress seems to play a significant role, whether by cause or effect. Urodynamic studies are required to identify any major abnormalities in the voiding pattern. Treatment with α-adrenergic blockers or biofeedback may help. Significant obstruction of the bladder neck can be relieved by bladder neck incision.

X. Scrotal contents

A. Orchitis usually results from hematogenous spread during bacterial or viral illness. **Mumps orchitis** is less of a risk in prepubertal boys, but 20% of adolescent patients with mumps have mumps orchitis, and it may be bilateral in 10%. Testicular pain and swelling develop 3 to 4 days after onset of parotitis. The scrotum is erythematous and very tender. Approximately 30% of involved testes suffer permanent loss of spermatogenesis because of pressure necrosis.

B. Acute epididymitis initially involves the tail of the epididymis but may spread to involve the entire epididymis, testis (epididymoorchitis), or spermatic cord (funiculitis). Symptoms are usually unilateral, with dull, aching pain radiating to the spermatic cord, lower abdomen, or flank. Pain may be relieved by elevating the testis (Prehn's sign), which may aid in differentiating the condition from acute torsion. Epididymitis is usually caused by one of two types of infection:

1. Sexually transmitted disease is usually secondary to *Chlamydia* (most common) or *N. gonorrhoeae.* Isolation of *Chlamydia* requires specific cell media. Serologic testing is rarely of value. The direct fluorescent antibody test and enzyme-linked immunosorbent assay have sensitivities of 70% to 85% and 70% to 80%, respectively. Ligase chain reaction is at least as sensitive as culture and has the advantage of being rapid and easy to perform. Uncomplicated chlamydial infection can be treated with 1 g of oral azithromycin as a single dose or 100 mg of oral doxycycline twice daily for 7 days. Azithromycin is 98% effective and is now the preferred regimen because of improved compliance. Alternative treatments include fluoroquinolones. All sex partners should be evaluated and treated.

2. Bacterial genitourinary infection is more common than sexually transmitted disease as a cause of epididymitis in men over age 40. Gram-negative pathogens are found in the urine, prostate, or urethra, and antimicrobial therapy is guided by culture data. Nonspecific measures include nonsteroidal antiinflammatory drugs, bed rest, and scrotal support. Injection of the spermatic cord with a local anesthetic may be of symptomatic benefit.

C. **Chronic epididymitis.** Symptoms usually consist of mild pain. The epididymis is exquisitely tender, indurated, and thickened. Antibiotic therapy is the same as for acute epididymitis, extended for another 3 weeks. Epididymectomy may be required in some cases.

XI. Antimicrobial prophylaxis in urologic surgery

To achieve effective antimicrobial prophylaxis, adequate tissue levels must be present at the time of surgical incision. At the same time, there is no benefit to continuing the antibiotic for >24 to 48 hours after surgery. Although antimicrobial prophylaxis is not necessary for most patients who have sterile urine at the time of surgery, many continue to advocate short-term antibiotic prophylaxis for endoscopic procedures. If an active urinary infection is present, it should be cleared before the surgery, whenever possible. If this cannot be done (e.g., indwelling Foley catheter), perioperative antibiotics are indicated to prevent bacteremia. The American Heart Association recommends prophylaxis for prostate surgery, urethral dilatation, and cystoscopy in patients with valvular cardiac disease, artificial heart valves, or other prosthetic devices (see www.americanheart.org for details).

A. **Transrectal prostate needle biopsy.** The patient should receive an enema the evening before the procedure. Prophylactic antibiotics are directed at aerobic and anaerobic bowel flora (Table 13.6).

B. **Colon and small bowel surgery.** Because the distal ileum has the same bacterial flora as the colon, antibiotic prophylaxis for ureteroileal diversion is the same as that for colonic surgery.

   1. On preoperative day 1, give a clear liquid diet; give 4 L of polyethylene glycol–electrolyte solution (GoLYTELY) at 10 A.M. and 1 g of neomycin–erythromycin base PO at 1 P.M., 2 P.M., and 11 P.M.; nothing by mouth after midnight.

   2. On the day of operation, give 2 g of cefoxitin IM or IV 30 minutes before surgery and 0.5 g of metronidazole IV as a single dose.

C. **Prostheses (penile implants, artificial sphincters)**

   1. Administer hexachlorophene or povidone–iodine (Betadine) skin scrubs for 5 to 7 days before surgery.

   2. Give 1 g IV of cefazolin (or equivalent first-generation cephalosporin) 30 minutes to 1 hour before surgery and repeat every 6 hours for 24 hours postoperatively. Depending on the local resistance patterns, intravenous vancomycin plus gentamicin may be more appropriate.

   3. Some prostheses need to be soaked in antibiotic solution before implantation (bacitracin, Aerosporin, neomycin).

   4. Irrigate the wound with antibiotic solution before closure.

D. **Prophylaxis for bacterial endocarditis.** Patients at risk for bacterial endocarditis (Table 13.6) include those with valvular heart disease, prosthetic heart valves, most forms of congenital heart disease, idiopathic subaortic stenosis, mitral

Table 13.6. Antibiotic prophylaxis in urologic surgery

Clinical Situation	Recommendation
Endoscopy	Gatifloxacin 400 mg PO × 3 d
Endoscopic surgery	Cefazolin 1 g IM/IV on call to OR *and* q6h × 24 h *or* gentamicin 1 mg/kg IM/IV on call to OR *and* q8h × 24 h
Transrectal prostatic needle biopsy	Gatifloxacin 400 mg PO × 3 d (start day before procedure)
Colon and small bowel surgery	Cefoxitin 2 g IV and q6h × 24 h *and* metronidazole 0.5 g IV
Artificial prosthesis	Cefazolin 1 g IM/IV on call to OR *and* q6h × 24 h
Valvular cardiac[a] and prosthetic devices	Ampicillin 2 g IM/IV *and* gentamicin 1.5 mg/kg body wt IM/IV 1 h before surgery; repeat dose 8 h after instrumentation If patient is penicillin allergic, use vancomycin 1 g IV over 60 min instead of ampicillin

OR, operating room.
[a]Or other conditions at high risk for endocarditis (see www.americanheart.org).

valve prolapse with regurgitation, history of prior infective endocarditis, and transvenous cardiac pacemakers.

SUGGESTED READING

Anderson KK, McAninch JW. Renal abscesses: classification and review of 40 cases. *Urology* 1980;16:333–338.

Anderson RU. Management of lower urinary tract infections and cystitis. *Urol Clin North Am* 1999;26:729–735.

Berger RE, Alexander ER, Harnish JP, et al. Etiology, manifestations and therapy of acute epididymitis: prospective study of 50 cases. *J Urol* 1979;121:750–754.

Curtis Nickel J, Downey J, Hunter D, et al. Prevalence of prostatitis-like symptoms in a population based study using the National Institutes of Health Chronic Prostatitis Symptom Index. *J Urol* 2001;165:842–845.

Drach GW, Fair WR, Meares EM, et al. Classification of benign diseases associated with prostatic pain: prostatitis or prostatodynia? *J Urol* 1978;120:266.

Fihn SD. Acute uncomplicated urinary tract infection in women. *N Engl J Med* 2003;349:259–265.

Gupta K, Hooton TM, Stamm WE. Increasing resistance and the management of uncomplicated community-acquired urinary tract infections. *Ann Intern Med* 2001;135:41–50.

Hook EW, Holmes KK. Gonococcal infections. *Ann Intern Med* 1985;102:229–243.

Hooten TM, Scholes D, Stapleton AE. A prospective study of asymptomatic bacteriuria in sexually active young women. *N Engl J Med* 2000;343:992–997.

Krieger JN, Jacobs RR, Ross SO. Does the chronic prostatitis/pelvic pain syndrome differ from nonbacterial prostatitis and prostatodynia? *J Urol* 2000;164:1554–1558.

Krieger JN, Nyberg L Jr, Nickel JC. NIH consensus definition and classification of prostatitis. *JAMA* 1999;282:236.

Nazareth I, King M. Decision making by general practitioners in diagnosis and management of urinary tract symptoms in women. *Br Med J* 1993;306:1103–1106.

Nickel JC, Nigro M, Valiquette L. Diagnosis and treatment of prostatitis in Canada. *Urology* 1998;52:797–802.

Parsons CL. Protocol for treatment of typical urinary tract infection: criteria for antimicrobial selection. *Urology* 1988;32(suppl 2): 22–27.

Propp DA, Weber D, Ciesla ML. Reliability of a urine dipstick in emergency department patients. *Ann Emerg Med* 1989;18:560.

Roberts RO, Lieber MM, Rhodes T. Prevalence of a physician-assigned diagnosis of prostatitis: the Olmsted County Study of Urinary Symptoms and Health Status among Men. *Urology* 1998;51: 578–584.

Stamm WE, Counts GW, Running KR, et al. Diagnosis of coliform infection in acutely dysuric women. *N Engl J Med* 1982;307:463–467.

Stamm WE, Horton TM. Management of urinary tract infections in adults. *N Engl J Med* 1993;329:1329–1334.

Stamm WE, Running KR, McKevitt M, et al. Treatment of the acute urethral syndrome. *N Engl J Med* 1981;304:956–958.

Warren JW, Abrutyn E, Hebel JR, et al. Guidelines for antimicrobial treatment of uncomplicated acute bacterial cystitis and acute pyelonephritis in women. *Clin Infect Dis* 1999;29:745–758.

National Institutes of Health (NIH)
Chronic Prostatitis Symptom Index

Pain or Discomfort

1. In the last week, have you experienced any pain or discomfort in the following areas?

	Yes	No
a. Area between rectum and testicles (perineum)	$\square_1$	$\square_0$
b. Testicles	$\square_1$	$\square_0$
c. Tip of the penis (not related to urination)	$\square_1$	$\square_0$
d. Below your waist, in your pubic or bladder area	$\square_1$	$\square_0$

2. In the last week, have you experienced:

	Yes	No
a. Pain or burning during urination?	$\square_1$	$\square_0$
b. Pain or discomfort during or after sexual climax (ejaculation)?	$\square_1$	$\square_0$

3. How often have you had pain or discomfort in any of these areas over the last week?

$\square_0$ Never

$\square_1$ Rarely

$\square_2$ Sometimes

$\square_3$ Often

$\square_4$ Usually

$\square_5$ Always

4. Which number best describes your AVERAGE pain or discomfort on the days that you had it, over the last week?

$\square$	$\square$	$\square$	$\square$	$\square$	$\square$	$\square$	$\square$	$\square$	$\square$	$\square$
0	1	2	3	4	5	6	7	8	9	10
NO PAIN										PAIN AS BAD AS YOU CAN IMAGINE

Urination

5. How often have you had a sensation of not emptying your bladder completely after you finished urinating over the last week?

$\square_0$ Not at all

$\square_1$ Less than 1 time in 5

$\square_2$ Less than half the time

$\square_3$ About half the time

$\square_4$ More than half the time

$\square_5$ Almost always

6. How often have you had to urinate again less than two hours after you finished urinating, over the last week?

   ☐$_0$ Not at all

   ☐$_1$ Less than 1 time in 5

   ☐$_2$ Less than half the time

   ☐$_3$ About half the time

   ☐$_4$ More than half the time

   ☐$_5$ Almost always

Impact of Symptoms

7. How much have your symptoms kept you from doing the kinds of things you would usually do, over the last week?

   ☐$_0$ None

   ☐$_1$ Only a little

   ☐$_2$ Some

   ☐$_3$ A lot

8. How much did you think about your symptoms, over the last week?

   ☐$_0$ None

   ☐$_1$ Only a little

   ☐$_2$ Some

   ☐$_3$ A lot

Quality of Life

9. If you were to spend the rest of your life with your symptoms just the way they have been during the last week, how would you feel about that?

   ☐$_0$ Delighted

   ☐$_1$ Pleased

   ☐$_2$ Mostly satisfied

   ☐$_3$ Mixed [about equally satisfied and dissatisfied]

   ☐$_4$ Mostly dissatisfied

   ☐$_5$ Unhappy

   ☐$_6$ Terrible

Scoring the NIH-Chronic Prostatitis Symptom Index Domains

Pain: Total of items 1a, 1b, 1c, 1d, 2a, 2b, 3, and 4   = _____

Urinary Symptoms: Total of items 5 and 6   = _____

Quality-of-life Impact: Total of items 7, 8, and 9   = _____

Urinary Calculi and Endourology

Ronald E. Anglade, David S. Wang, and
Richard K. Babayan

Urinary stones have plagued humans since the beginning of recorded history. Archaeologists have uncovered urinary stones in the mummified remains of Egyptians estimated to be more than 7,000 years old. Since that time, humans have sought improved methods for dealing with stones. Currently, our understanding of the metabolic pathways that contribute to stone formation has lead to the development of effective medical management strategies for most calculi. The treatment of stones of the urinary tract has dramatically changed over the last 20 years; historically, most renal and ureteral stones required open surgical intervention. Today, the vast majority of stones can be effectively treated with minimally invasive surgical alternatives such as endourologic techniques, and extracorporeal shock wave lithotripsy (ESWL) has eliminated the need for open surgery in the vast majority of patients. Indeed, open surgery for urolithiasis is exceedingly rare.

I. Epidemiology of stones

Stones affect 1% to 5% of adult populations in industrialized nations. In the United States, stone disease accounts for >400,000 hospitalizations annually. The peak incidence is in the third to fifth decades. Men are affected three times as commonly as women and whites four to five times as commonly as blacks. In a patient who has passed one stone, the likelihood of passing another stone is about 15% by 3 years and 30% by 15 years. Urolithiasis is a lifelong disease, with an average of 9 years intervening between episodes.

II. Etiology and pathogenesis

The development of stones in the urinary tract is a complex, multifactorial process. Approximately 75% of urinary stones contain calcium. The remaining 25% are composed of uric acid, struvite, or cystine. Some factors related to stone formation are listed in Tables 14.1 through 14.3.

A. Supersaturation occurs when there is an overabundance of solute in solution. In the supersaturated state, nucleation and aggregation of solute crystals may occur, leading to stone formation. Urine may be intermittently in the supersaturated state, as during dehydration. Supersaturation and crystallization account fairly well for uric acid, xanthine, and cystine stone formation but do not completely explain calcium stone formation. **Epitaxy** is the growth of one type of crystal on a different type of crystal. For example, calcium oxalate stones frequently contain a core of uric acid.

B. Inhibitors are substances in the urine that can block crystallization. Some recurrent stone-formers lack sufficient urinary inhibitors such as citrate, pyrophosphate, magnesium,

Table 14.1.   Factors associated with urolithiasis

Factor	Conditions of Increased Incidence
Genetics/heredity	Cystinuria, autosomal recessive Renal tubular acidosis, type I Medullary sponge kidney
Geography	High temperature/humidity (southeastern United States)
Diet	Increased intake of calcium or oxalate
Occupation	Sedentary jobs

zinc, nephrocalcin, Tamm–Horsfall glycoprotein, uropontin, and macromolecules. It is now believed that the lack of adequate inhibitors of stone formation, especially citrate, in the urine plays a major role in the pathophysiology of urinary calculus formation.

C.   Matrix is a noncrystalline mucoprotein often associated with urinary calculi. In persons who do not form stones, urinary matrix may act as an inhibitor; however, matrix may act as an initiator in some stone-formers and may even provide the framework on which crystal deposition occurs. Pure matrix calculi may be seen in association with *Proteus* infection.

Table 14.2.   Urinary calculi: composition, frequency, and characteristics

Type of Stone	Frequency (%)	Effect of pH on Solubility	Radiographic Density (Bone = 0.0)
Calcium stones	80		
Oxalate (monohydrate and dihydrate)	35	Little effect	0.50
Phosphate	10	Increased at pH <5.5	1.0
Oxalate and phosphate	35	Variable	Variable
Struvite	10	Increased at pH <5.5	0.20
Uric acid	8	Increased at pH >6.8	0.05
Cystine	1	Increased at pH >7.5	0.15
Other types	1		
Triamterene			
Xanthine		Increased at pH >6.8	0.05
Matrix (noncrystalline)			

Table 14.3.   **Types of urinary calculi and etiologic factors**

Type of Stone	Etiologic Factors
Calcium oxalate Calcium phosphate Calcium carbonate	Supersaturation of urine with calcium from (a) renal leak, (b) intestinal absorption, (c) bone resorption; hyperoxaluria
Uric acid	Hyperuricosuria, constantly low urine pH
Cystine	Cystinuria
Magnesium ammonium phosphate (struvite)	Alkaline urine produced by urea-splitting organisms
Matrix	Alkaline urine produced by urea-splitting organisms

D.   Renal tubular dysfunction may be an important factor in stone formation. The initial crystal growth occurs in distal collecting tubules and gradually extrudes into the collecting system to become free urinary calculi.

E.   Exogenous substances may be ingested and become stone components, albeit rarely. **Indinavir** is a protease inhibitor used in the treatment of human immunodeficiency virus infection. Indinavir stones are soft and gelatinous. They are radiolucent on x-ray examination of the kidney, ureter, and bladder (KUB) as well as on computed tomography (CT). *Indinavir stones are virtually the only urinary tract stones not visible on CT scan.* **Triamterene,** a component of Dyazide, may also produce radiolucent stones.

III.   Upper urinary tract stones

A.   Clinical presentation. A renal calculus is generally asymptomatic until the stone moves within the urinary tract and produces either hematuria or some degree of urinary obstruction. Urinary obstruction may be accompanied by pain, urinary tract infection, generalized sepsis, nausea, or vomiting. Chronic obstruction may be asymptomatic. A urinary calculus should be suspected in a patient who presents with the sudden onset of severe, colicky flank or abdominal pain (ureteral colic). Pain may radiate to the groin, testes, or tip of the penis, depending on the location of obstruction. In 25% of cases, patients give a family history of stone disease. Hematuria, gross or microscopic, almost always accompanies an acute episode of stone colic. However, microscopic hematuria may be absent in up to 15% of cases, and absence of hematuria does not exclude urinary calculi. Microscopic inspection of the urinary sediment may reveal crystals that can suggest the type of stone present.

B.   Diagnosis. Initial evaluation (often in the emergency department) should include serum white blood cell count and creatinine level, urinalysis, urine culture, and plain film of the abdomen. More than two-thirds of urinary calculi are radiopaque and can be seen on KUB. The initial radiologic investigation may be a renal ultrasonogram (US), if readily available. This may demonstrate the presence of a stone (US shadowing) in the kidney or ureter as well as any hydronephrosis, if present. Axial or spiral CT (noncontrast) is now the initial study of choice at nearly all centers. CT scan will confirm the presence of calculus in the urinary tract, demonstrate the degree of obstruction, and identify other intraabdominal pathology. The spiral CT is rapid, does not require a bowel preparation, and avoids the use of intravenous contrast agent. With a sensitivity over 95%, it is very accurate in identifying stones in the collecting system and ureter. One type of stone that may not appear on CT scan is the indinavir stone. The intravenous urogram (IVU), once the primary imaging modality to evaluate patients with flank pain, is infrequently used today to evaluate stone patients.

C. Acute treatment of the acute episode depends on the size and location of the stone, the degree of obstruction, and the patient's clinical status.

  1. Ureteral colic. The most important goal in the management of ureteral colic is obtaining adequate pain relief. This can be accomplished with parenteral narcotics or nonsteroidal antiinflammatory drugs. Morphine sulfate is the parenteral narcotic analgesic agent of choice. Ketorolac tromethamine (Toradol) is often effective as well for renal/ureteral colic. Antiemetic agents such as metoclopramide HCl and prochlorperazine should be used as needed. Patients tolerating oral medication may be treated with 1 to 2 oral narcotic/acetaminophen tablets every 4 hours as needed for pain, 600 to 800 mg of ibuprofen every 8 hours, and 30 mg of nifedipine extended-release tablet once daily to induce ureteral smooth muscle relaxation.

  2. Indications for immediate intervention. Most patients who present with ureteral colic can be managed with adequate analgesics and undergo definitive stone management at a later date. However, there are indications for urgent intervention, usually in the form of a ureteral stent or a percutaneous nephrostomy tube. Patients with acute or suspected urinary tract infection in the presence of obstruction generally require prompt intervention; failure to relieve urinary tract obstruction in this setting can lead to life-threatening sepsis. The presence of high-grade obstruction generally necessitates prompt intervention to prevent long-term renal loss. In addition, patients who should be given consideration for immediate intervention include those with a solitary functioning kidney, elevated creatinine, preexisting renal insufficiency, and fever of unclear etiology (suspected urinary tract infection). Finally, patients with pain that is not manageable without parenteral narcotics generally require immediate intervention.

  3. Stenting of the ureter with a temporary internal ureteral catheter may be indicated to relieve obstruction. This may also result in sufficient dilation of the ureter to allow some stones to pass after removal of the stent. Again, a follow-up radiographic study is required to confirm stone passage.

  4. Percutaneous nephrostomy tube insertion is required when stenting is unsuccessful or when a tube larger than 7F is needed.

D.   Definitive management of renal or ureteral calculi.
For most patients, immediate intervention is not necessary, and
definitive management of renal or ureteral calculi can be accomplished on an elective basis. Several management options
exist:

   1.   Expectant treatment. Patients with small stones
   (<5 mm) and minimal hydronephrosis may be treated conservatively as outpatients with oral hydration and analgesics.
   About 90% of ureteral calculi measuring <4 mm in diameter
   pass spontaneously, whereas only 20% of stones >6 mm in diameter pass. Stones are most likely to obstruct the upper urinary tract at one of three locations: (a) the ureteropelvic
   junction; (b) the pelvic brim, where the ureter crosses the iliac
   vessels; and (c) the ureterovesical junction, which is the nar-
   rowest of the three (Fig. 14.1). Stones located in the proximal
   ureter are much less likely to pass than those located at the
   ureterovesical junction.
      Therefore, nonsurgical management may be indicated in
   the asymptomatic, nonobstructed, noninfected patient with
   a stone <5 mm in diameter in the lower third of the ureter.
   The patient is instructed to drink copious quantities of water,
   strain the urine, and save for analysis any stone that may be
   recovered. Plain films of the abdomen should be obtained
   every week to monitor the progress of the stone as it passes
   down the ureter. Four to 6 weeks should be allowed for stone
   passage. *It is important to obtain a follow-up study in the
   form of US or intravenous pyelogram to confirm that stone
   passage has occurred.*
   2.   Extracorporeal shock wave lithotripsy. ESWL is indicated for treatment of most renal calculi <1.5 to 2 cm in size.
   Insertion of a temporary internal stent is recommended for
   stones >1.5 cm in size to prevent *steinstrasse* ("street of
   stones") or ureteral obstruction caused by passage of stone
   fragments. Although its primary use is in the fragmentation
   of renal calculi, ESWL is also advantageous for ureteral
   stones, especially those <8 mm in diameter. Patients are often
   placed in a prone position for distal ureteral stones, to focus
   the stone within the shock path and avoid the bony structures
   of the pelvis.
   3.   Ureteroscopic management may include extraction
   or lithotripsy. Rigid ureteroscopy is primarily utilized in the
   distal ureter, whereas use of the flexible ureteroscope is most
   common above the iliac vessels and for stones within the
   renal pelvis and calyces.
      a.   Access to the ureter for ureteroscopy is greatly facil-
      itated by use of the **ureteral access sheath.** Under fluo-
      roscopy, the sheath is passed over a guide wire into the
      proximal ureter. Passage of the sheath causes ureteral di-
      lation, and the sheath itself provides a continuous working
      channel for the introduction of endoscopes and instruments
      during ureteroscopic procedures. Sheaths are manufac-
      tured with an internal diameter of up to 12F to accommo-
      date stone fragments as well as instruments.
      b.   Lithotripsy techniques include US, electrohydraulic,
      pneumatic, or laser lithotripsy. For ureteroscopic stone frag-

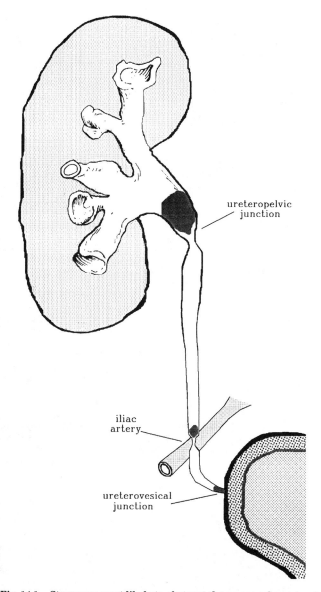

Fig. 14.1. Stones are most likely to obstruct the upper urinary tract at the ureteropelvic junction, iliac vessels, or ureterovesical junction.

mentation, the holmium-YAG (yttrium–aluminum–garnet) laser has become a standard of care, with high efficacy and the widest safety margin. Success rates are approximately 95%. Indications for endoscopic lithotripsy include stone burden of <2 cm, cystine calculi (poor success rates with ESWL), ESWL failure, body habitus precluding ESWL, or associated collecting system abnormalities (ureteral stricture, calyceal diverticulum).

   c.   Stone extraction of small stones may be accomplished by a stone basket. The advent of rigid and more recently flexible ureteroscopy has eliminated the need for blind or radiologically guided basket extraction. *Because of this, blind or fluoroscopically guided basketing of ureteral stones is never recommended and should never be performed.* After passage of a guide wire above the stone, the ureteral orifice seldom requires dilatation if one utilizes the smaller semirigid miniscopes, many of which have an outer diameter of <7F. Once the stone is visualized, several options are available. Small stones may be grasped directly or engaged in a stone basket and extracted. Larger stones should be fragmented, and the basket should not be used. Extreme caution must be exercised when using baskets, and if resistance is met during stone extraction, then the stone should be further fragmented.

4.   Percutaneous nephrostolithotomy (PCNL) is indicated for large stones >2 cm in size or for staghorn calculi. With use of rigid and flexible nephroscopes and a variety of fragmenting tools, approximately 85% of patients can be rendered stone-free at 3 months; long-term results are comparable with those of open surgery, although many large stones will require staged procedures. Even full staghorn calculi can be successfully removed with PCNL.

5.   Open stone surgery is virtually never required today, given the advances in minimally invasive surgery and ESWL. In the past, **ureterolithotomy** and **open nephrolithotomy** (**anatrophic nephrolithotomy**) were common urologic procedures, but today they are rarely performed.

6.   Laparoscopic surgery has been performed in select patients with large (>2 cm) stones in the proximal ureter, though experience is limited.

IV.   Bladder stones

   In the Western world, bladder stones are most often found in male patients and are caused by bladder outlet obstruction or foreign bodies (portions of catheters, sutures, or objects inserted through the urethra). Ureteral stones that reach the bladder can also act as a nidus for bladder stone formation. Bladder stones are composed of variable proportions of calcium oxalate, uric acid, and ammonium urate. If uric acid is a major component, bladder stones may be radiolucent. They vary from extremely hard to quite soft. Patients with long-standing bladder stones are at risk for squamous metaplasia or carcinoma.

   A.   Clinical presentation includes pain felt in the hypogastrium or referred to the penis, intermittent stream, dysuria, and hematuria (Fig. 14.2). Patients may also present with recurrent urinary tract infections.

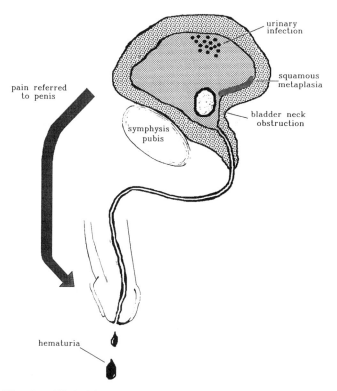

urinary
infection

squamous
metaplasia

pain referred
to penis

bladder neck
obstruction

symphysis
pubis

hematuria

Fig. 14.2. Clinical features of vesical stone.

B. Diagnosis includes plain films of the abdomen, bladder US, and cystoscopy.

C. Treatment. Most bladder stones can be successfully managed by endoscopic techniques.

1. Laser lithotripsy has become one of the most common modalities for the treatment of bladder stones. Laser fibers can be used in both flexible and rigid instruments and are very effective in fragmenting bladder stones. The laser beam can be focused on the stone, and thus risk of bladder injury and bleeding is minimized.

2. Lithotrites are mechanical devices that permit crushing of large, hard bladder stones under direct vision. The lithotrite should be closed only with the bladder partially filled to prevent bladder wall injury. The fragments are then washed out through a resectoscope. This instrument is now rarely used owing to the potential for bladder injury.

3. Electrohydraulic lithotripsy. Based on the principle of underwater spark generation, the electrohydraulic lithotripsy probe produces a hydraulic shock wave near the stone that usually produces fragmentation after delivery of several shocks.

The electrohydraulic lithotripsy probe is flexible and can be passed through both fiberoptic and rigid endoscopes.

4.   US lithotripsy is based on ultrasonic energy delivered through a rigid probe passed through an endoscope. Small fragments are removed by continuous suction attached to the hollow US probe. Larger fragments can be extracted with grasping forceps or stone baskets.

5.   Pneumatic lithotripsy uses a ballistic device that fragments the stone with a "jackhammer" effect.

6.   Cystolithotomy can be performed through a small suprapubic incision or may be combined with open prostatectomy. Cystolithotomy has the advantage of removing the entire stone rather than leaving fragments in the bladder, but the recovery period is extended.

V.   Recurrent stone disease

A.   Diagnosis. A metabolic or environmental etiology of nephrolithiasis can be found in approximately 90% of patients evaluated for stone disease. Passage of a single urinary stone is an indication for screening studies, including determination of serum calcium, phosphorus, and uric acid levels and measurement of 24-hour urinary creatinine, calcium, phosphorus, uric acid, and oxalate levels. Patients found to have any abnormalities on screening studies should have a more extensive evaluation, described below. Patients with "metabolically active" stone disease should also have a metabolic evaluation. Such patients include any with radiologic evidence of new stone formation, an increase in size of a preexisting stone, or passage of stone in the last year. Metabolic evaluation should be performed at a time far removed from the acute stone episode.

B.   Metabolic evaluation

1.   Baseline studies. While on their regular diet, patients collect a 24-hour urine sample for creatinine, calcium, phosphorus, uric acid, oxalate, and citrate (Table 14.4). The pH and volume of the urine are recorded. Blood is drawn for creatinine, calcium, phosphorus, and uric acid.

2.   Dietary restriction. The patient is placed on a diet limited to 400 mg of calcium and 100 mEq of sodium for 1 week. A 24-hour urine specimen is again obtained, and serum studies as described previously are repeated.

3.   Calcium loading. After an overnight fast during which only distilled water is permitted, the patient reports to the office or clinic at 7:00 A.M. After the first urine voided is discarded, a 2-hour pooled specimen is collected from 7:00 A.M. to 9:00 P.M. The patient receives 1 g of calcium gluconate orally at 9:00 A.M. and collects a 4-hour urine specimen from 9:00 A.M. to 1:00 P.M.

C.   Hypercalciuria may be caused by bone resorption (most commonly from hyperparathyroidism), renal leak, or increased absorption from the gastrointestinal tract. Table 14.5 lists the serum and urinary abnormalities in various types of hypercalciuria.

1.   Resorptive hypercalciuria is characterized by constant hypercalciuria regardless of dietary restriction.

a.   Etiology. Hyperparathyroidism accounts for <5% of patients with calcium urolithiasis and is a common cause of

Table 14.4. Normal 24-hour urine values

Biochemical Component	Male Patients (mg)	Female Patients (mg)
Calcium	<300	<250
Uric acid	<800	<750
Oxalate	<50	<50
Citrate	450–600	650–800

the resorptive type of hypercalciuria. Stones occur in approximately 50% of patients with hyperparathyroidism. In instances caused by hyperparathyroidism, serum calcium levels are also frequently elevated, but normocalcemic forms of the disease exist. Other causes of resorptive hypercalciuria are neoplasms metastatic to bone, multiple myeloma, immobilization (e.g., spinal cord injury), Cushing's disease, and hyperthyroidism.

   b. Treatment of resorptive hypercalciuria consists of treatment of the underlying disorder.

2. Absorptive hypercalciuria is the single most common cause of hypercalciuria and is found in >50% of patients with stones.

   a. Etiology. These patients are felt to have an exaggerated intestinal response to vitamin D, leading to hyperabsorption of ingested calcium. This mechanism explains why the urinary calcium may normalize when oral calcium is restricted and will rise to the abnormal range under calcium loading.

   b. Treatment

   (1) Diet and hydration are important in controlling absorptive hypercalciuria. Patients should be placed on a diet restricted to 400 mg of calcium/day and 100 mEq of sodium/day. The addition of bran to the diet is useful because brain binds calcium in the gastrointestinal tract. Patients should be required to drink 3 to 4 L of water daily to reduce urinary concentration of calcium.

   (2) Cellulose phosphate is a calcium-binding resin that exchanges sodium for calcium in the gastrointestinal tract. It must be used in conjunction with a calcium-restricted diet. The usual dose is 5 g three times daily

Table 14.5. Classification of hypercalciuria

Type	Serum Calcium	Urine Calcium	
		Fasting	After Loading
Resorptive	Up	Up	Up
Absorptive	Normal	Normal	Up
Renal leak	Normal	Up	Up

with meals. Because cellulose phosphate lowers serum magnesium and elevates urinary oxalate levels, patients should receive oral magnesium supplementation and should restrict oral intake of oxalate.

(3) **Orthophosphates** act by decreasing urinary excretion of calcium and increasing excretion of citrate and pyrophosphate, both of which act to inhibit calcium stone formation. The usual dose is 3 to 6 g daily. The most frequent side effect is diarrhea.

3. **Renal hypercalciuria** accounts for approximately 10% of instances of hypercalciuria.

   a. **Etiology.** The disorder is thought to be caused by the inability of the kidney to resorb calcium from the tubular fluid. Thus, placing the patient on a calcium-restricted diet will not reduce the loss of calcium in the urine. Calcium loading may increase urinary calcium even further.

   b. **Treatment**

   (1) **Thiazide diuretics** are the drugs of choice in renal hypercalciuria. The mechanism of action involves increased calcium resorption in the distal tubule and contraction of extracellular volume, thus stimulating calcium resorption in the proximal tubule. The usual dose of hydrochlorothiazide is 50 mg twice daily. Potassium supplementation is necessary in most patients.

   (2) **Orthophosphates.** In patients unresponsive to thiazide diuretics alone, orthophosphates may be used in combination with calcium restriction.

D. **Hyperuricosuria.** Pure uric acid stones account for approximately 10% of urinary calculi. The solubility of uric acid is highly pH dependent; uric acid becomes insoluble in urine at a pH of <5.8.

1. **Etiology.** Approximately 25% of patients with uric acid calculi will be found to have gout. Most patients with uric acid calculi, however, have neither hyperuricemia nor hyperuricosuria. The development of these calculi is dependent upon constantly acid urine, low urine output, and uric acid excretion. Hyperuricosuria is also found in 20% of patients with recurrent calcium stones. Some investigators feel that uric acid crystals may act as a nidus for calcium stone formation.

2. **Treatment** is based on hydration, alkalinization of the urine, and reduction of uric acid load presented to the kidney.

   a. **Hydration** is achieved by oral intake of at least 3 L of water daily.

   b. **Alkalinization** of the urine is usually achieved by giving 650 mg of sodium bicarbonate (2 tablets) orally every 6 hours. Urinary pH should be maintained at no less than 6.5. In patients requiring sodium restriction, potassium bicarbonate or potassium citrate may be used instead. In patients unable to take oral medication, intravenous hydration with sodium bicarbonate may be used. Alkalinization is usually effective in dissolving even large uric acid stones over a period of weeks.

   c. **Reduction of uric acid load** may be achieved by dietary restriction and use of allopurinol. Such measures are indicated in patients who are unresponsive to hydration and alkalinization of urine, who have myeloproliferative disorders, or who are receiving cancer chemotherapy. Dietary protein should be restricted to 90 g daily. Allopurinol is a xanthine oxidase inhibitor that is effective in doses of 200 to 600 mg daily. Xanthine stones may form in patients undergoing long-term allopurinol therapy.

E.   Hyperoxaluria. Oxalic acid is an extremely insoluble end product of metabolism. Although the diet may contain large amounts of oxalate, <10% of ingested oxalate is absorbed from the gastrointestinal tract and most is derived from metabolism.

    1.   Primary hyperoxaluria is a rare autosomal recessive disorder characterized by early onset of nephrocalcinosis. There are two types, distinguished by their specific enzymatic defect, but the clinical picture is similar in both. Urinary levels of oxalate may exceed 100 mg/day. Widespread deposition of oxalate in the kidneys and other soft tissues (oxalosis) eventually occurs. Medical treatment with 100 to 400 mg of pyridoxine daily has been reported to reduce oxalate excretion in some patients. General measures should also be employed, including adequate hydration and reduction of dietary oxalate.

    2.   Enteric hyperoxaluria may occur in patients with malabsorption from any cause (inflammatory bowel disease, small bowel bypass surgery). The increased amount of fatty acids in the bowel binds calcium, leaving increased oxalate for absorption. Treatment includes a low-oxalate, low-fat diet, oral fluid hydration, and calcium supplementation. Cholestyramine has been found to bind oxalate and may be useful in patients with malabsorption.

    3.   Exogenous hyperoxaluria occurs when substances metabolized to oxalate are ingested in large quantities, such as ethylene glycol (a component of antifreeze), ascorbic acid in amounts >5 g/day, and the anesthetic methoxyflurane.

F.   Hypocitraturia. Recently, hypocitraturia has been recognized as a major correctable cause of calcium oxalate nephrolithiasis. Often coexisting with other metabolic abnormalities, low urinary citrature levels can be found in up to 50% of patients with calcium stones. Therefore, urinary citrate levels should be routinely checked as part of the metabolic evaluation of recurrent stone-formers. *Citrate therapy in the form of potassium citrate is a new and promising medication for the treatment of recurrent calcium oxalate nephrolithiasis.*

G.   Struvite stones are composed of magnesium ammonium phosphate and carbonate apatite ("triple-phosphate stones"). They may grow to fill the entire renal pelvis and collecting system ("staghorn calculus"). These stones form only when urinary pH is markedly elevated and increased concentrations of ammonia, bicarbonate, and carbonate are present in the urine. Such conditions may be caused by organisms that produce the enzyme urease, which splits urea into ammonia and carbon dioxide. *Proteus* sp are the most common "urea-splitting" organisms and are identified in >75% of patients with struvite stones. Other organisms may produce urease also, including *Klebsiella, Pseudomonas, Providencia,* and *Staphylococcus. Ureaplasma urealyticum* has recently been shown to be a urea-splitting organism. Female patients are affected about twice as often as male patients. Approximately 10% of spinal cord–injured patients have struvite calculi. Other populations at risk are patients with indwelling catheters for many years and persons with ileal conduit or other supravesical diversions.

1. Diagnosis. Struvite stones should be suspected in any patient with high urinary pH caused by infection. The organisms cultured from the urine may not correspond to the organisms within the stone itself. Plain film of the abdomen will usually demonstrate the stones, but they may be poorly mineralized and relatively radiolucent. Spiral CT should be performed to determine whether obstruction is present and causing persistence of infection. Radionuclide studies should be performed to assess renal perfusion and function. Voiding cystourethrogram and urodynamic studies may be indicated if bladder dysfunction is suspected.

2. Treatment. Successful treatment depends on complete elimination of the stones, correction of any obstruction that may be present, and eradication of infection. Selection of the best treatment method is still controversial, and each instance presents unique problems. For example, patients with obstruction or areas of stasis in the upper urinary tract are poor candidates for treatment by ESWL alone. Another consideration is that percutaneous techniques often require multiple treatments.

    a. Surgical techniques. Surgical nephrolithotomy—"anatrophic nephrolithotomy"—can render approximately 80% of patients permanently stone-free. When there is little or no functioning renal tissue, laparoscopic nephrectomy should be performed. In instances of partial staghorn calculi with renal parenchymal damage, partial nephrectomy should be considered.

    b. Percutaneous lithotripsy has replaced open surgery in many patients with dendritic or large staghorn calculi. Approximately 85% of patients can be rendered stone-free at 3 months.

    c. ESWL. As mentioned previously, ESWL alone can be used in patients without obstruction or stasis; however, stone-free rates are in the range of 40% to 60%, and multiple treatments are usually required. One of the most effective techniques is the so-called "sandwich technique," involving percutaneous lithotripsy followed by ESWL, followed by secondary percutaneous lithotripsy, extraction, or chemolysis.

    d. Chemolysis. Chemolysis is generally ineffective in calcium stones but can be used very effectively to dissolve uric acid, cystine, struvite, and carbonate apatite stones.

        (1) Uric acid and cystine stones occasionally require local irrigation through a urethral catheter, ureteral catheter, or nephrostomy tube. These stones are readily soluble in alkaline solutions. Uric acid stones can be treated with a solution of sodium bicarbonate in normal saline solution to bring the pH to 7.5. Oral alkalinizing agents such as potassium citrate may be better tolerated for long-term maintenance of an alkaline pH. Cystine stones may be treated with a solution of 60 mL of 20% acetylcysteine and 300 mg of sodium bicarbonate per liter of normal saline solution. An alternative agent is tromethamine B, an organic buffer with a pH of 10.2.

(2) Struvite and carbonate apatite calculi are amenable to dissolution by acidic solutions with pH of <5.5. The most widely used solution is 10% hemiacidrin (Renacidin), which has a pH of 4.0. The solution is delivered to the stone via nephrostomy tube or ureteral catheter. Normal saline solution should be infused at 30 mL/h initially to determine the response of the collecting system. The saline infusion rate is increased over 24 hours to the maximal rate tolerated without flank pain or rise in pressure above 30 cm H_2O. Hemiacidrin is then infused at half the maximal rate achieved with normal saline solution.

When chemolysis is used, several important precautions must be observed: (a) Care must be taken to avoid excessive pressure in the collecting system. A manometer must be placed in the infusion line to monitor pressure and provide a blow-off valve in case of obstruction. Intrapelvic pressure must be below 30 cm H_2O. Treatment should be discontinued if the patient reports any flank pain. (b) The infusate must have adequate egress, which may be a problem when infusion is through a single ureteral catheter. (c) Chemolysis is contraindicated in the presence of active urinary tract infection. The urine must be cultured daily during chemolysis, and treatment should be stopped if urinary infection is found or a fever develops. (d) Hemiacidrin contains magnesium that can be absorbed to cause hypermagnesemia. Serum magnesium levels should be monitored three times weekly during treatment. Success rates of 85% have been reported for complete dissolution of struvite calculi. Hemiacidrin may be used as primary therapy given through a nephrostomy tube, or as an adjunct to percutaneous lithotripsy, surgical lithotomy, or ESWL.

3. Prevention of struvite calculi depends on elimination of infection with urea-splitting organisms. When chronic infection cannot be eradicated, urease inhibitors such as **acetohydroxamic acid** may be used to decrease urinary pH and ammonia levels. This drug has been shown to be effective in preventing struvite calculi in spinal cord–injured patients, although it may be difficult to tolerate.

H. Renal tubular acidosis is characterized by metabolic acidosis caused by defects of the renal tubule. Although several types of renal tubular acidosis are recognized, urinary lithiasis occurs only in type I, a disorder in which the distal tubule is unable to maintain adequate hydrogen ion gradients. Renal tubular acidosis accounts for approximately 1% of calcium stone-forming patients. Patients with renal tubular acidosis may form calcium phosphate, calcium oxalate, or mixed stones. Treatment involves alkalinizing the urine with sodium bicarbonate or potassium citrate.

I.   Cystinuria. An overabundance of cystine in the urine will result in the formation of stones. Cystine has poor solubility at normal urine pH. Cystinuria is an autosomal recessive disorder characterized by a transepithelial transport defect in the intestine and kidney that manifests as a decrease in renal cystine absorption. The peak incidence of cystine stones is in the second to third decade. A urinary cystine level of >250 mg/24 h is diagnostic of cystinuria.

The treatment of cystinuria requires the dietary restriction of cystine, by avoiding foods rich in methionine (meat, poultry, dairy products). In addition, hydration and alkalinization with sodium bicarbonate or potassium citrate are essential for appropriate therapy. Alkalinizing the urine to a pH >7.0 increases the solubility of cystine to 400 mg/L of urine. When alkalinization and hydration fail, D-penicillamine and α-mercaptopropionyl-glycine are used to bind cystine and form soluble compounds.

VI.   Endourologic techniques

Percutaneous access to the upper urinary tract is the cornerstone of endourologic technique. The first "nephroscopes" were actually cystoscopes modified to avoid trauma to the renal pelvis. In the early 1980s, specially designed rigid nephroscopes were produced with offset lenses and straight instrumentation ports to allow passage of alligator forceps and stone graspers. Flexible fiberoptic endoscopes intended for the biliary and bronchial tracts were used in the upper urinary tract until specially designed instruments became available. Percutaneous stone retrieval was initially limited by the size of the nephrostomy tract. This limitation was addressed by the development of US probes that could be passed through the nephroscope and used to fragment large calculi. The combination of rigid and flexible endoscopes with US or electrohydraulic lithotripsy allows virtually all stones to be treated by percutaneous means. In comparison with open surgery, percutaneous treatment offers a reduction in cost, discomfort, and recovery time.

A.   Percutaneous puncture techniques. The patient is placed on the fluoroscopy table in the prone position, and imaging of the kidney is carried out by fluoroscopy or US. The puncture site is most commonly on the posterior axillary line midway between the 12th rib and the iliac crest. In general, the nephrostomy tube should be placed through a renal pyramid into a posterior calyx. Direct pyelostomy is not recommended because it is difficult to stabilize the nephrostomy tube. Once the collecting system is entered, a 0.038-in guide is inserted through the needle or introducer sheath and advanced into the renal pelvis or down the ureter. The nephrostomy tract can then be dilated with either fascial dilators or a high-pressure balloon. Depending on the clinical indication, one can pass a nephrostomy catheter over the guide wire or introduce a 28 or 30F Amplatz sheath into the kidney for nephroscopic stone manipulation. A second guide wire—"safety" guide wire—is necessary before nephroscopic stone extraction begins to permit reentry should the primary guide wire become dislodged.

B.   US lithotripsy is based on the ability of high-frequency sound waves to fragment stones. The US energy is delivered through a rigid probe passed through the nephroscope. Small fragments are removed by continuous suction attached to the hollow US probe. Larger fragments can be extracted with grasping forceps or stone baskets passed under direct vision through the nephroscope.

C.   Electrohydraulic lithotripsy. Stones resistant to US lithotripsy can be fragmented by means of electrohydraulic lithotripsy. Based on the principle of spark generation, the electrohydraulic lithotripsy probe produces a hydraulic shock wave near the stone that readily leads to fragmentation. Unlike the US probe, the electrohydraulic lithotripsy probe is flexible and can be passed through both fiberoptic and rigid endoscopes. The disadvantage is that the fragments produced by electrohydraulic lithotripsy discharge tend to scatter widely, and retrieval is not as easy as with US lithotripsy.

D.   Pneumatic lithotripsy. The introduction of the Swiss lithoclast has offered yet another alternative to stone fragmentation. This device delivers a "jackhammer" effect; compressed air is used to cause stone fragmentation. It can be passed through all rigid scopes in the kidney, ureter, and bladder.

E.   Laser lithotripsy. The coumarin green pulsed dye laser has largely been replaced by the holmium laser, which is both more efficient and versatile. In addition to excellent stone fragmentation, the holmium laser is an effective incisor of tissue and may be used to cut scars and ureteral strictures.

VII.   ESWL

ESWL was developed in Germany in the early 1980s and has had an enormous impact on the treatment of stones. The treatment is based on the propagation of focused shock waves through the body, which fragment the stones. The shock wave may be produced by discharging a high voltage (spark gap), deforming a piezoelectric crystal, or moving a membrane by electromagnetic energy (Table 14.6). The "third-generation" machines are characterized by more compact designs, with lower pressures and narrower focusing, allowing anesthesia-free lithotripsy. Depending on the en-

Table 14.6.   Characteristics of "third-generation" shock wave lithotriptors

Manufacturer/ Model	Localization	Energy Source	Anesthesia
Mobile			
Dornier Compact S	X-ray and US	Electromagnetic	IV sedation
Medirex Tripter X	Mobile C arm	Spark gap	IV sedation
Medispec Econolith	Mobile C arm	Spark gap	IV sedation
Fixed			
Siemens Lithostar	X-ray, US	Electromagnetic	IV sedation
Medstone STS	X-ray, US	Spark gap	IV sedation
Storz Modulith	X-ray, US	Electromagnetic	IV sedation
Dornier (DoLi)	X-ray ± US	Electromagnetic	IV sedation

ergy source, many of the newer lithotriptors need not be gated to the electrocardiogram, and shocks may be produced at a rate of 2/s; the average patient requires 1,000 to 4,000 shocks to fragment stones completely. The fragments usually pass through the ureter without a problem. In some cases, these fragments may cause obstruction of the ureter (*steinstrasse*). A combination of percutaneous techniques may be required to reduce large staghorn calculi to smaller fragments ("stone debulking") before ESWL is performed. Experimental and clinical work has failed to demonstrate significant long-term tissue damage to the kidney or surrounding tissues by ESWL. There remains, to this date, no evidence to suggest that those stone patients treated with ESWL are at a greater risk of developing hypertension than those managed by other means. The absolute contraindications to ESWL are pregnancy, uncontrolled coagulopathy, and acute urinary tract infection. Relative contraindications include infundibular obstruction and obstruction of the ureter.

SUGGESTED READING

Auge BK, Preminger GM. Update on shock wave lithotripsy technology. *Curr Opin Urol* 2002;12:287–290.

Consensus Conference on the Treatment and Prevention of Kidney Stones. *JAMA* 1988;260:977–981.

Segura JW, Preminger GM, Assimos DG, et al. Nephrolithiasis clinical guidelines: panel summary report on the management of staghorn calculi. *J Urol* 1994;151:1648–1651.

Segura JW, Preminger GM, Assimos DG, et al. Ureteral stones clinical guidelines: panel summary report on the management of ureteral calculi. *J Urol* 1997;158:1915–1921.

Shekarriz B, Stoller ML. Uric acid nephrolithiasis: current concepts and controversies. *J Urol* 2002;168:1307–1314.

Neoplasms of the Genitourinary Tract

Andrew Kramer and Mike B. Siroky

The most common genitourinary neoplasms arise in the prostate, bladder, and kidney, in that order. Testicular cancer is not a common neoplasm but is nevertheless an important disease because it is a highly malignant tumor that affects younger men. Neoplasms of the renal pelvis, ureter, urethra, and penis are rare.

I. **Carcinomas of the kidney parenchyma** arise from the proximal convoluted tubular cell in 85% of cases. The remainder arises from the collecting duct or connective tissues. The term **renal adenoma** is used for tumors <3 cm in diameter; however, there is no way to differentiate renal adenomas histologically from adenocarcinomas, and adenomas most likely represent early carcinomas. Renal adenocarcinoma is also called renal cell carcinoma (RCC), clear cell carcinoma of the kidney, hypernephroma, and Grawitz's tumor.

   A. **Incidence.** Adenocarcinoma of the kidney accounts for 80% to 90% of all renal neoplasms. RCC is the third most common genitourinary neoplasm. In 2002, RCC was diagnosed in 31,000 people in the United States; it is responsible for about 12,000 deaths annually. The incidence of the disease has been rising, probably owing to the increased number of tumors discovered incidentally during imaging. There is a twofold to threefold male predominance, although this disparity appears to be narrowing more recently. No obvious racial predilection has been noted, although some have noted increased risk in people of northern European descent. The peak incidence is in the sixth and seventh decades of life, but the disease is seen occasionally even in adolescents. Thirty percent of patients with RCC have metastatic disease at diagnosis, and in 40% who undergo nephrectomy, disease ultimately recurs (25% distant metastasis, 10% regional nodes, 5% local recurrence). The most common sites of metastases are the lung and bones, followed in decreasing order by regional nodes, liver, adrenal glands, brain, and other adjuvant organs. Patients with pathologic stage T4 and metastatic disease have a median survival of 6 to 10 months and a 2-year survival of 10% to 20%.

   B. **Etiology and risk factors.** Although the etiology of RCC is unknown, several interesting associations have been noted.

      1. **Estrogens.** Administration of exogenous estrogens produced renal carcinoma in hamsters.

      2. **Diet and obesity.** There is a positive correlation between the incidence of renal carcinoma and high consumption of fats, oils, milk, and sugar. Obesity is also a risk factor.

      3. **Renal failure.** About 20 years ago, it was recognized that patients with renal failure who are undergoing hemodialysis are at risk for development of multiple renal cysts, acquired

cystic kidney disease, and occasionally renal carcinoma. Patients undergoing peritoneal dialysis are also at increased risk. The risk is increased in proportion to the number of years of dialysis. Acquired cystic kidney disease develops eventually in 40% to 80% of patients maintained on long-term dialysis, and approximately 20% of patients with acquired cystic kidney disease have renal neoplasms. The risk in all patients undergoing dialysis may be as high as 8%, and it is 50-fold higher than in the general population.

4. Von Hippel–Lindau disease is strongly associated with RCC, which develops in about one-third of patients with von Hippel–Lindau disease. The autopsy incidence is 40% to 60%; multiple and/or bilateral tumors are usually found. Abnormalities of the *VHL* gene have been seen in 50% to 60% of sporadic RCC cases. Inherited syndromes associated with renal tumors are listed in Table 15.1.

5. Smoking. A twofold increased risk for RCC exists in cigarette smokers in comparison with nonsmokers, although the mechanism of this association is unclear.

6. Toxic agents. Exposure to heavy metals such as lead and cadmium has been associated with clinical RCC. Recently, asbestos exposure has been associated with RCC.

C. Tumor classification and histology. Several histologic subtypes of renal adenocarcinoma are now recognized, and the histologic classification has changed.

1. Clear cell tumors are composed mostly of round or polygonal cells with abundant cytoplasm containing glycogen. Clear cell carcinomas have recently been found to have a deletion of either one or both copies of loci on chromosome 3p. Higher nuclear grade or a sarcomatoid pattern are associated with a poorer prognosis.

2. Chromophilic carcinoma also arises from the proximal tubule and is frequently multifocal and bilateral. The tumor is sometimes called papillary RCC. The tumor commonly presents as a small early-stage lesion and thus has a good prognosis in those with localized disease.

3. Chromophobic carcinoma is composed histologically of sheets of cells that are darker than those in clear cell carcinoma. Originating from intercalated cells, the cells lack abundant lipid and glycogen seen in clear cell carcinoma. In general, these tumors are associated with a good to excellent prognosis.

4. Oncocytomas are composed of oncocytes: large, well-differentiated, neoplastic cells with intensely eosinophilic granular cytoplasm due to a large number of mitochondria. This feature may require electron microscopy to be certain that the tumor is an oncocytoma. They appear to originate from collecting duct cells and almost invariably behave in a benign fashion.

5. Collecting duct tumors tend to occur in younger patients and often behave aggressively. Because they arise from the collecting duct, gross hematuria occurs early in their course. Sarcomatoid variants have been described.

D. Diagnosis. RCC may present in a myriad of ways; for this reason, it has been called the "internist's" tumor. The "classic

Table 15.1.   Hereditary syndromes with kidney tumors

Syndrome	Inheritance	Kidney Manifestation	Other Manifestations
Von Hippel–Lindau	AD	RCC in 30–40%	Pheochromocytoma Pancreatic cysts Islet cell tumors Retinal angiomas CNS hemangioblastomas Epididymal cystadenomas
Tuberous sclerosis	AD	Angiomyolipoma Multiple renal cysts RCC in <5%	Skin tumors (adenoma sebaceum) Brain tumors
Hereditary papillary renal carcinoma	AD	Bilateral, multifocal papillary RCC	
Familial renal oncocytoma	AD	Bilateral, multifocal renal oncocytomas	
Birt–Hogg–Dube	AD	RCC	Hair follicle tumors Polyps of colon Pulmonary cysts

AD, autosomal dominant; RCC, renal cell carcinoma.

Table 15.2.   Paraneoplastic syndromes in
renal cell carcinoma

Finding	Incidence (%)
Anemia	30
Hypertension	25
Fever	20
Hypercalcemia	10
Abnormal LFT findings	5
Erythrocytosis	5

LFT, liver function test.

triad" of an abdominal mass, hematuria, and flank pain is noted
in only 10% of those with RCC. Today, the majority of patients
with renal masses present with incidental findings on computed
tomography (CT) scan after investigation of an unrelated entity.
A discussion of symptoms, signs, and differential diagnosis can
be found in Chapter 4. Paraneoplastic syndromes occur in 10%
to 40% of patients as a result of specific hormone production by
the tumor cells or an immune response to the tumor (Table 15.2).
Hepatic dysfunction (Stauffer's syndrome) in the presence of
RCC does not imply metastatic disease to the liver and is reversible on removal of the primary tumor. The presence of this
syndrome, however, does portend a worse prognosis. In addition
to the syndromes listed in Table 15.2, renal carcinoma may secrete gonadotropins, human chorionic gonadotropin (hCG), an
adrenocorticotrophic hormone-like substance, renin, glucagon,
and insulin.

E.   Staging. The staging system of the American Joint Committee on Cancer (AJCC) (Fig. 15.1) has replaced the older
Robson staging system. The 2002 AJCC classification has added
categories T1a and T1b to reflect the better survival in patients
with tumors <4 cm in diameter (Table 15.3).

F.   Treatment. Renal neoplasms are highly resistant to nonsurgical forms of treatment such as chemotherapy, radiation
therapy, hormonal manipulation, and immunotherapy.

   1.   Radical nephrectomy is distinguished from simple
   nephrectomy by early control of the renal pedicle and en bloc
   removal of the kidney, the ipsilateral adrenal gland, and
   Gerota's fascia. The two basic approaches to radical nephrectomy are open and laparoscopic. Recent experience with laparoscopic and hand-assisted laparoscopic nephrectomy has
   shown similar survival, with decreased hospital stay and morbidity for the patient. For stage I and stage II disease, radical
   nephrectomy is the treatment of choice for localized disease.
   For open surgery, an anterior, thoracoabdominal, or modified
   flank incision may be used according to the surgeon's preference. In hand-assisted laparoscopic nephrectomy, the hand incision may be made periumbilically or over McBurney's point.
   Typically, only two other ports are necessary in addition to the

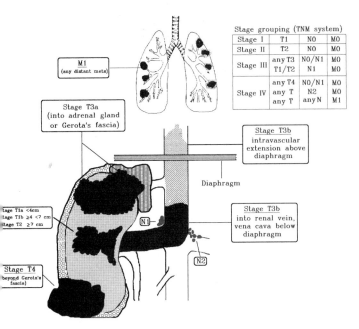

Fig. 15.1. American Joint Committee on Cancer (AJCC) staging system for renal carcinoma.

hand port, but occasionally a third is required for right-sided tumors for retraction of the liver. Laparoscopy is generally limited to tumors <10 cm in diameter. Adrenalectomy is required only in patients with preoperative evidence of adrenal involvement or with large tumors of the upper pole.

a. Renal artery embolization (angioinfarction) can be used to shrink large hypervascular tumors before surgery and to control bleeding and pain in symptomatic patients with inoperable RCC. Following the procedure, most patients experience pain, fever, and nausea for 1 to 3 days.

b. Most authorities feel that **regional lymphadenectomy** adds little, if anything, to survival but may provide useful prognostic information.

c. Vena caval involvement. Almost 20% of patients with RCC have renal vein involvement, and 5% have extension into the vena cava. Because of the shorter renal vein, vena caval involvement is more common in right-sided tumors. Tumors extending into the vena cava but without invasion of the wall of the vena cava and without extension outside the kidney capsule may have a favorable prognosis following surgical excision. Even tumors extending into the atrium of the heart can be removed with reasonable expectation of long-term survival; these patients require cardiopulmonary bypass, profound hypothermia, and temporary cardiac arrest.

Table 15.3.   Current AJCC staging in renal cancer and survival

AJCC Stage	Description	Approximate 5/10-Year Survival (%)
Primary tumor		
T1	Tumor <7 cm, limited to kidney	95/90
T1a	Tumor <4 cm	
T1b	Tumor =4 cm but <7 cm	
T2	Tumor ≥7 cm, limited to kidney	80/70
T3a	Tumor invades adrenal gland/perinephric tissues but not beyond Gerota's fascia	65/50
T3b	Tumor grossly extends into renal vein or inferior vena cava	50/40
T3c	Tumor extends into vena cava above diaphragm	45/40
T4	Tumor invades Gerota's fascia	20
Lymph nodes		
N1	Single regional node involved	
N2	More than one node involved	
Metastases		
M1	Distant metastasis	

AJCC, American Joint Committee on Cancer.
Source: Data modified from Gettman et al. *Cancer* 2001;91:354.

   d.   Metastatic disease. About 2% of patients with RCC present with a solitary—usually pulmonary—metastasis. Because survival may occasionally be prolonged, removal of the solitary metastases at the time of nephrectomy is a reasonable course in such patients. Nephrectomy in the face of metastatic disease may also be considered to control severe symptoms, including unrelenting flank pain, intractable hemorrhage, fever, and hypercalcemia secondary to tumor hormone production. Finally, nephrectomy in the face of metastatic disease may be reasonable in patients who are to undergo experimental therapy that requires removal of the primary tumor. Preliminary data suggest that cytoreductive therapy for advanced RCC may improve the response to immunotherapy. This stems from the observation that nearly all those who did have a favorable response to immunotherapy underwent nephrectomy to control local disease initially.

e.   **Immunotherapy.** Because of the very poor prognosis in metastatic disease, interest has been maintained in various immunotherapy protocols. Interferon-α appears to be associated with an objective response rate of 15% to 20%. Interleukin-2 with or without lymphokine-activated killer cells has resulted in 15% to 30% response rates in treated patients. Other therapeutic approaches include gene therapy, tumor vaccines, and monoclonal antibodies (see Chapter 16).

2.   **Partial nephrectomy** is being increasingly considered as standard therapy for selected instances of malignant kidney tumor. Partial nephrectomy is absolutely indicated in cases of solitary kidney, bilateral renal carcinoma, significant renal insufficiency, multiple recurrent tumors (von Hippel–Lindau disease), and established oncocytoma. In addition, it may be considered in cases of familial cancer as well as in cases presenting with small (<5-cm) polar tumors with a normally functioning contralateral kidney.

3.   **Cryoablation and radiofrequency ablation** are being evaluated in patients with multiple and/or bilateral tumors who need or wish to avoid anesthesia and surgery.

a.   **Cryoablation** is a safe procedure that may provide adequate local control in ≥90% of T1 renal cell cancers. Cryoablation was initially used during open surgery or through a laparoscopic approach, but recent reports describe its use as a percutaneous procedure. There are not enough data to evaluate its efficacy in long-term cancer control.

b.   **Radiofrequency ablation** is being used percutaneously to ablate renal tumors under about 4 cm in size. Early results are promising, but longer follow-up will be needed to assess their durability.

II.   **Carcinoma of the renal pelvis and ureter**

A.   **Incidence.** Tumors of the upper urinary tract account for about 5% of urothelial neoplasms. A male-to-female preponderance of 2:1 is noted, with an average age at diagnosis of 65. There is no predilection for side, but tumors occur bilaterally in 2% to 4% of patients.

B.   **Tumor classification**

1.   **Transitional cell carcinoma** accounts for 85% of renal pelvic tumors and 93% of ureteral tumors. The etiology is similar to that of transitional cell carcinoma of the bladder and is thought to involve chemical carcinogens and cigarette smoking. There is a 3:1 male-to-female ratio and a 2:1 Caucasian-to-African American preponderance. More than 20% of patients have multiple, rather than single, lesions at diagnosis. Bladder cancer develops in approximately 50% of patients with ureteral or pelvic cancer. Tumors develop in the contralateral kidney in only 3% of patients with unilateral tumors. About three-quarters of ureteral tumors are in the distal ureter. Two specific groups of patients are at increased risk for the development of renal pelvic tumors.

a.   Persons who for years consume large quantities of **analgesics containing phenacetin or aspirin** have a ninefold greater risk for the development of papillary necrosis and transitional cell carcinoma of the renal pelvis. Tumors in these patients tend to be of a higher histologic grade and stage than are tumors not associated with phenacetin.

   b.   Balkan nephropathy is an environmental tubulo-interstitial renal disease of unknown cause endemic to certain areas of the Balkan Peninsula (the former Yugoslavia, Romania, Bulgaria, and Greece) that lie along the Danube River and its tributaries. Affected patients are at high risk (up to 40%) for the development of renal pelvic cancer. The tumors are frequently bilateral (10% of patients) and of low malignant potential.

   c.   Other risk factors are similar to those described for bladder cancer.

   2.   Squamous cell carcinoma is seen in association with chronic inflammation or irritation (e.g., calculous disease) and accounts for 14% of renal pelvic tumors and 5% of ureteral carcinomas. These tumors tend to invade and metastasize early; the 5-year survival rate approaches zero.

   3.   Adenocarcinoma accounts for fewer than 1% of renal pelvic tumors, occurs predominantly in women, is associated with renal calculus and pyelonephritis, and has a very poor prognosis. Primary adenocarcinoma of the ureter is extremely rare.

C.   Diagnosis. Hematuria is the presenting sign in 80% of patients. Pain with or without obstruction may be seen in 40% of patients. The initial evaluation may be performed by ultrasonography (US), CT, or magnetic resonance imaging (MRI). Intravenous urography (IVU), now rarely performed, displays a radiolucent filling defect that can be confirmed by retrograde pyelography. In patients without obstruction, 85% of tumors are early stage. Voided urinary cytology is not particularly sensitive, but selective cytology and brush biopsy specimens are usually positive for carcinoma. CT or MRI is essential for staging and evaluating regional lymph nodes. Ureteroscopy allows direct visualization and biopsy of suspected lesions. This modality is particularly useful for cases with unexplained filling defects, hematuria, or positive cytology when the diagnosis remains uncertain after conventional diagnostic modalities have been utilized. Angiography is of little use, as the lesions are typically avascular. However, it may demonstrate other causes for renal pelvic filling defects, such as renal artery aneurysms and crossing vessels.

D.   Staging and prognosis. The AJCC staging system is used in renal pelvic and ureteral tumors and correlates with 5-year survival (Table 15.4).

E.   Treatment. Successful treatment depends on the stage and grade of the tumor, irrespective of the surgical procedure employed. In general, low-grade tumors tend to have a good prognosis, whereas high-grade tumors tend to be deeply invasive and have a poor prognosis.

   1.   Nephroureterectomy. Renal pelvic tumors and tumors of the upper two-thirds of the ureter are best treated by radical nephroureterectomy (kidney, adrenal, ureter, and cuff of bladder). When the ureter is left behind, disease may recur in one-third of patients. The overall 5-year survival rate following radical nephroureterectomy is 84%. Laparoscopic nephroureterectomy requires greater operative time compared

Table 15.4. AJCC staging system for ureteral–pelvic tumors and 5-year survival

AJCC Stage	Description	Survival at 5 Years (%)
Primary tumor		
T0	No evidence of primary tumor	
Ta	Neoplasm confined to mucosa	90
TIS	Carcinoma in situ	
T1	Submucosal infiltration only	50–80
T2	Muscular invasion only	17–75
T3	Invasion of periureteral–peripelvic fat or renal parenchyma	
T4	Extension into adjacent organs	5
Lymph nodes		
N1	Single regional lymph node, <2 cm in diameter	
N2	One or more lymph nodes, none >5 cm in diameter	
N3	One or more lymph nodes, >5 cm in diameter	
Metastases		
M1	Distant metastasis	

AJCC, American Joint Committee on Cancer.

with the standard open procedure but has benefits such as decreased patient analgesic requirements, shorter hospitalization, and improved cosmesis. Patients usually are able to resume normal activity more quickly. It appears to be equivalent to the open procedure with regard to cancer control.

2. Distal ureterectomy and reimplantation into the bladder may be used to treat low-grade lesions of the distal one-third of the ureter.

3. Ureteroscopic fulguration/ablation may be used for small lesions <1 cm in size. Neodymium-YAG (yttrium–aluminum–garnet) laser and holmium-YAG laser provide coagulation and ablation of tumors. Ureteroscopic treatment of renal pelvis tumors and ureteral tumors is associated with high recurrence rates. About 40% of renal–pelvic tumors and 25% of ureteral tumors recur after local treatment.

4. Percutaneous therapy allows ablation of tumors in the renal pelvis and upper ureter. Topical therapeutic agents can also be instilled through this route. Percutaneous surgery carries a small theoretical risk of tumor seeding in the nephrostomy tract. Percutaneous ablation may be an acceptable alternative to nephroureterectomy in patients with grade I disease and in patients with grade II disease who are poor surgical risks. Close follow-up surveillance is mandatory.

5. Special situations. In patients with disease in a solitary kidney or synchronous bilateral superficial lesions, a number of alternative approaches are available. These include percutaneous excision and fulguration, partial nephrectomy, bench surgery with autotransplantation, ureteroscopic resection and fulguration, and intrapelvic treatment with bacille Calmette-Guérin (BCG) or chemotherapy. Chemotherapy may be given locally via a nephrostomy tube or ureteral catheter. Intravesical instillation may be used in patients with vesicoureteral reflux.

6. Metastatic disease. The management of metastatic or unresected disease involves platinum-based multiagent chemotherapy, similar to that used in bladder cancer. Postoperative radiotherapy to the ureteral bed is not employed routinely.

F. Follow-up care. There is a 50% to 80% bladder recurrence rate within 18 months. Following surgical removal of tumors of the upper urinary tract, patients should be followed by cystoscopy every 3 months for 3 years, every 6 months for 2 more years, and annually thereafter, provided no recurrences are noted.

III. Carcinoma of the bladder

A. Incidence. Bladder cancer is the second most common genitourinary neoplasm, with >57,000 estimated new cases diagnosed in the United States in 2002. It is estimated that bladder cancer accounts for >12,500 deaths annually. The peak incidence is in persons from 50 to 70 years old, with a male-to-female predominance of almost 3:1.

B. Tumor classification

1. Transitional cell carcinoma accounts for >90% of all cases of bladder cancer.

    a. Papillary transitional cell carcinoma appears as an exophytic frondular lesion. The size and number of lesions vary. This is the most common form of transitional cell carcinoma in the bladder. Most of these tumors are small and noninvasive.

    b. Sessile transitional cell carcinoma appears as a less frondular, more solid lesion with a broad base. These tumors have a greater tendency to be invasive.

    c. Carcinoma in situ is defined by four characteristics: flat, erythematous, multifocal, and high grade. The presence of carcinoma in situ is an indicator of increased biological aggressiveness. Papillary or sessile tumors are more likely to recur or invade when associated with carcinoma in situ.

2. Squamous cell carcinoma accounts for 7% to 8% of cases of bladder cancer and is usually associated with chronic irritation of the urothelium (e.g., schistosomiasis, bladder calculi, foreign bodies).

3. Adenocarcinoma accounts for 1% to 2% of cases and is associated with chronic infection, bladder exstrophy, or urachal remnants in the dome of the bladder. Adenocarcinomas tend to be mucus-secreting tumors.

4. Other types include various types of small cell carcinoma, sarcoma, melanoma, and carcinoid tumors.

C. Etiology

1. Industrial toxins (orthoaminophenols). Continuous contact with aniline dyes, α-naphthylamine, 4-aminobiphenyl, and benzidine used in the rubber, leather, textile, and dye industries may account for up to 25% of instances of bladder cancer.

   2. Cigarette smoking may account for up to 25% to 60% of instances of bladder cancer in developed countries. Smoking leads to deficiency of vitamin B_6 (pyridoxine), which is needed to metabolize orthoaminophenols and endogenous products of tryptophan metabolism. Also, 4-aminobiphenyl may be the carcinogen involved.

   3. Other risk factors include cyclophosphamide, alkylating agents such as thiotepa, and phenacetin-containing analgesics. Radiotherapy of the pelvis is also a risk factor for bladder cancer.

D. Diagnosis

   1. Signs and symptoms. Approximately 80% of patients present with gross, painless hematuria. Approximately 20% of patients with bladder cancer present solely with microscopic hematuria. Ten percent of patients present with symptoms secondary to metastases. Dysuria and irritative symptoms are present in up to 30% of patients—especially those with carcinoma in situ. Secondary urinary infection may be present in about 30% of patients with bladder tumors and should not preclude the search for bladder carcinoma. Upper urinary tract obstruction is rare on initial presentation and is a sign of advanced disease in 50% of cases.

   2. Cystoscopy. Because transitional cell carcinoma is a field-change process, the entire mucosa of the lower tract must be carefully inspected. This includes the vesical, prostatic urethral, and posterior urethral surfaces.

   3. Urinary cytology. Cells for microscopic examination are collected from voided urine or bladder washings. Urinary cytologic study is not sensitive (about 30%) in diagnosing low-grade bladder cancer but is excellent for detecting carcinoma in situ and high-grade lesions (90%). Cytology, when performed by a trained cytologist, has excellent specificity of approximately 90%.

   4. Urinary tumor markers have received increasing attention as a means of diagnosing and following patients with bladder cancer. The most widely used tests are compared in Table 15.5.

Table 15.5. Accuracy of currently available methods of bladder cancer screening

Test Name	Sensitivity (%)	Specificity (%)
Cytology	55	95
BTA stat	70	75
BTA TRAK	65	65
NMP-22	65	80
Urovysion	80	95

Source: Based on data from Glas et al. *J Urol* 2003;169:1975–1982; and Halling et al. *J Urol* 2002;167:2001–2006.

a.   Bladder tumor antigen (BTA) has been shown to be produced by bladder tumor cells and released into the urine. It has been identified as complement factor H-related protein, a protein that may play an important role in protecting cancer cells from the immune system. The original BTA test marketed by Bard was a latex agglutination test that is no longer available in the USA. It has been replaced by two tests with much better sensitivity and specificity: a rapid nonquantitative test (BTA Stat) and a more complex quantitative assay (BTA TRAK). Studies have shown these tests to be more sensitive than cytology, especially for low-grade tumors, but much less specific.

b.   Nuclear matrix proteins (NMPs) form the structural framework of the cell nucleus. Significantly increased concentrations of NMPs have been found in various cancer cells, including bladder cancer. Soluble NMPs can be detected in the urine from bladder cancers using antibodies directed against certain types of NMP (NMP-22).

c.   Immunologic tests. The AuraTech **FDP** (PerImmune) is a rapid immunoassay that detects the urinary fibrin and fibrinogen degradation products associated with bladder cancer. Its 68% sensitivity is higher than that of cytology. The **Immunocyt** test on voided urine employs three monoclonal antibodies specific for two antigens expressed on the surface of transitional cell carcinoma tumor cells. It is designed to be used in conjunction with cytology and improves sensitivity to 86% with a specificity of 79%.

d.   Fluorescence in situ hybridization is used in the Vysis UroVysion Kit that is designed to detect aneuploidy for chromosomes 3, 7, and 17 and deletion of the 9p21 locus in bladder cells found in urine specimens. The sensitivity is about 80%, with a specificity approaching 100%.

e.   Telomerase is an enzyme produced by >30 types of cancer, including >90% of bladder cancers. The test has an overall sensitivity of 70% and specificity of 90%. Sensitivity may be improved in specimens obtained by bladder washings over voided urine. Commercial assays are currently being developed.

5.   Radiologic examination

a.   The IVU demonstrates a filling defect in the bladder only 60% of the time. Small tumors are rarely detected by IVU. Ideally, the IVU should be obtained prior to transurethral resection of any bladder tumor to avoid postoperative changes. In patients with renal insufficiency, diabetes mellitus, or contrast agent allergies, retrograde pyelograms should be performed at the time of cystoscopy or tumor resection.

b.   US is not very useful for the diagnosis or staging of bladder cancer. However, it is very useful in evaluating the renal parenchyma and detecting hydronephrosis. It may also be used to differentiate a soft tissue mass in the bladder from a nonradiopaque stone.

c.   CT with contrast has a sensitivity only slightly higher than IVU in detecting bladder cancer. CT is very useful for clinical staging of patients with more advanced stages of bladder carcinoma. It may demonstrate extravesical extension, nodal involvement, or distant metastases. Thickening of the bladder muscle wall on CT is suggestive, but not diagnostic, of muscle invasion. CT is very sensitive in detecting extravesical disease. In contrast, it is not nearly as sensitive in detecting nodal involvement (false-negative rate of approximately 70%, false-positive rate of approximately 15%). Nodes >2 cm in size will generally be detected by pelvic or abdominal CT.

   d.   MRI is as reliable as CT for staging of invasive or locally advanced disease. It may be useful in patients with contrast agent allergy.

   e.   Metastatic work-up in bladder cancer consists of chest radiograph and bone scan in selected cases. **Chest radiographs** are used as initial screening for pulmonary metastases and for periodic monitoring in treated patients. If the chest film is suspicious for metastatic lesion, a chest CT should be ordered. **Bone scan** is needed only in patients with invasive or locally advanced tumors and skeletal symptoms or elevated serum alkaline phosphatase. Because increased uptake is a nonspecific finding, plain films, CT with bone windows, or MRI should be performed for confirmation. Bone biopsy may be necessary to document metastatic disease.

E.   Stage and grade of tumors
   1.   Staging. The AJCC staging system (Fig. 15.2) has almost entirely replaced the older Jewett classification of urinary bladder cancer (Table 15.6).

   2.   Grading. Bladder tumors are now classified as either low or high grade. This simplified system replaces the previous system of Mostofi in which tumors were designated as grade 1, 2, or 3. Almost all invasive bladder tumors are high grade.

F.   Clinical staging procedures
   1.   Cystoscopy and transurethral resection of bladder tumor (TURBT) are used both to remove as much tumor as possible and to stage the tumor. **Cystoscopy** is used to document the location, size, and appearance of any bladder tumor(s). **TURBT** combined with pathologic examination of the removed tissue allows assessment of the grade and stage of the tumor. **Bimanual examination** should be performed under anesthesia before and after TURBT; it allows assessment of tumor size and any fixation to surrounding pelvic organs or the pelvic side wall. **Mucosal biopsy** should be performed to rule out carcinoma in situ. **Prostatic strip biopsies** should be performed if a high-grade bladder tumor is present (especially near the bladder neck) or if cytology is positive without evident bladder tumor. Prostatic strip biopsies should also be performed to assess the urethra when a neobladder is being considered.

   2.   Radiologic staging includes abdominal and pelvic CT, MRI, chest film, and bone scan, as discussed above. **US** is generally not helpful, but transrectal US may occasionally be used to assess local invasion.

   3.   Other studies include **liver function tests,** especially alkaline phosphatase. Tumor markers such as carcinoembry-

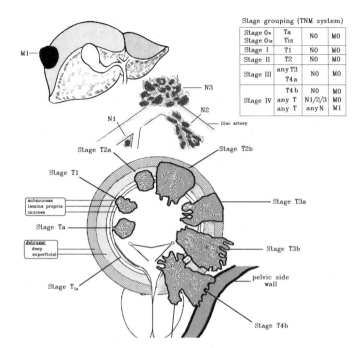

Stage grouping (TNM system)

Stage 0a Stage 0is	Ta Tis	N0	M0
Stage I	T1	N0	M0
Stage II	T2	N0	M0
Stage III	any T3 T4a	N0	M0
Stage IV	T4 b any T any T	N0 N1/2/3 any N	M0 M0 M1

Fig. 15.2.   American Joint Committee on Cancer (AJCC) staging system for bladder carcinoma.

onic antigen may be elevated in 20% of patients with advanced or metastatic transitional cell cancer.

G.   Treatment by stage of disease

1.   Stage 0/I. In 80% of cases, transitional cell carcinoma presents as superficial disease. Of superficial bladder tumors, approximately 60% are Ta, 30% T1, and 10% Tis. Almost all T1 tumors are high grade, and 50% have associated carcinoma in situ. Treatment of superficial disease has as its goal the eradication of as much tumor as possible, prevention or delay of future same-stage recurrences, and prevention or delay of progression to higher-stage disease. **TURBT** is followed by cystoscopic surveillance every 3 months for 2 years, every 6 months for 3 years, and annually thereafter. At any recurrence, the surveillance cycle is repeated from the beginning. A urinary cytologic study should be obtained at each follow-up visit.

a.   Intravesical chemotherapy. Clinical trials have shown no clear advantage with respect to progression, time to appearance of distant metastasis, or duration of survival using various intravesical agents and protocols. However, time to recurrence is often prolonged (Table 15.4).

(1)   Thiotepa was the first intravesical agent to be used for superficial bladder cancer. Its efficacy in reduc-

Table 15.6. AJCC and Jewett staging of bladder cancer

AJCC Stage	Description	Jewett Stage
Primary tumor		
Tx	Primary tumor cannot be assessed	
T0	No evidence of primary tumor	
Ta	Noninvasive papillary carcinoma	0
Tis	Carcinoma in situ	0
T1	Tumor invades subepithelial connective tissue	A
T2a	Tumor invades superficial muscle	B1
T2b	Tumor invades deep muscle	B2
T3a	Tumor invades perivesical tissue—microscopic only	C
T3b	Tumor invades perivesical tissue—macroscopic	C
T4a	Tumor invades prostate, uterus, vagina	C
T4b	Tumor invades pelvic wall, abdominal wall	C
Lymph nodes		
N1	Single regional lymph node, <2 cm in diameter	D1
N2	One or more lymph nodes, none >5 cm in diameter	D1
N3	One or more lymph nodes, >5 cm in diameter	D1
Metastases		
M1	Distant metastasis	D2

AJCC, American Joint Committee on Cancer.

ing recurrence rate is marginal, and it is seldom used today because of the high incidence of myelosuppression and chemical cystitis.

(2) Mitomycin C is an alkylating agent that is minimally absorbed systemically after intravesical instillation and has low toxicity. Instillation of 30 mg of mitomycin C in 50 mL of saline immediately following TURBT may lengthen the time to first recurrence. The standard treatment regimen is 20 mg of mitomycin C in 50 mL of normal saline intravesically, weekly for 6 to 8 weeks. Urinary alkalinization may improve efficacy.

(3) Doxorubicin, epirubicin, and valrubicin are anthracyclines with poor systemic absorption following intravesical instillation. The overall response rate of these agents is about 50%. Doxorubicin is given as 60 mg every 3 weeks for eight treatments. The main role of intravesical anthracycline therapy is to treat patients who have failed BCG treatment and who refuse cystectomy or are poor operative risks.

b. **BCG** has been used as prophylaxis against tumor recurrence (60% response rate), for carcinoma in situ (70% response rate), and for residual carcinoma after TURBT (30% to 60% response rate). In general, the therapy appears to be safe and effective. In contrast to chemotherapeutic agents, BCG not only delays recurrence but also has demonstrated improved progression-free survival. BCG may be used in patients with positive purified protein derivative of tuberculin, as long as no evidence of active tuberculosis infection is documented. BCG is an attenuated strain of *Mycobacterium bovis* that is capable of eliciting a local granulomatous response and occasionally causes disseminated disease. BCG preparations from different manufacturers may vary considerably in therapeutic effectiveness. The mechanism of action of BCG in bladder carcinoma is unknown, but it appears to be immunologically based because interleukin-2 has been found in the urine of patients who have responded to BCG treatment.

(1) **Method of administration of BCG.** There is no standard protocol for BCG administration, and there is no consensus regarding the optimal length of treatment. A recent study confirmed the efficacy of maintenance therapy for carcinoma in situ in which BCG is instilled once a week three times at 3 months, 6 months, and every 6 months to 3 years. This study of maintenance therapy confirmed a reduction in recurrence rate and somewhat improved survival. A description of our current treatment program follows:

(a) Catheterize the patient's bladder with a 16F Foley catheter.

(b) Mix 1 ampule of Tice strain BCG (1×10^8 to 8×10^8 organisms) with 60 mL of saline solution and instill via Foley catheter.

(c) Retain in bladder approximately 2 hours (remove Foley catheter after instillation).

(d) Treat weekly for 6 weeks.

(e) For the second course of treatment, include maintenance therapy (three weekly instillations every 3 months for 1 year).

Wait 2 weeks following TURBT before starting BCG therapy. Perform surveillance cystoscopy and a urinary cytologic study every 3 months during treatment.

(2) **Complications of BCG therapy.** Bladder irritability occurs in 70% of patients for 1 to 2 days. Mild bladder symptoms may be treated with antihistaminic, anticholinergic, antispasmodic, or nonsteroidal anti-inflammatory agents. Toxicities associated with the use of BCG consist of fever (25%) and hematuria (25%). No recent deaths due to BCG treatment have been reported. Systemic disease is called "BCG-osis" and requires antituberculosis therapy. Such patients have prolonged fever, abnormal liver function test results, and pulmonary infiltrates. BCG should not be instilled in patients with an active urinary tract infection.

(3) Follow-up. If recurrent tumor is noted at cysto-scopy, reinstitute BCG therapy weekly for 6 weeks and then proceed with maintenance therapy (three weekly in-stillations every 3 months for 1 year). It has been found that multiple courses of therapy can increase the response rate. If the patient has recurrent or residual disease after two courses of BCG therapy, however, the likelihood of success with additional courses of treatment is minimal. Such patients are at high risk for development of invasive or metastatic cancer and should be considered candidates for intravesical chemotherapy, radiotherapy, or cystec-tomy. Cystectomy should also be considered if the disease involves extensive areas of bladder mucosa or the prosta-tic urethra. The same is true of patients with multiple superficial bladder tumors involving extensive areas of bladder mucosa that cannot be treated by endoscopic means and in whom intracavitary therapy has failed.

c. Management of BCG-refractory disease. About 30% of patients may fail several courses of BCG therapy. **Intravesical interferon-α_{2b}** may produce responses in up to 40% of patients, including those who have failed intra-vesical BCG therapy. After catheterization of the bladder, 100×10^6 U of interferon-α_{2b} is mixed with 30 to 50 mL of normal saline solution and instilled into the bladder. The catheter is withdrawn, and the fluid is retained for about 2 hours. The course is given weekly for 12 weeks and then monthly for 1 year. Mild to moderate flu-like symptoms are the most common adverse response to intravesical inter-feron-α_{2b}. Interferon-α_{2b} may also be combined with BCG for intravesical therapy. Intravesical chemotherapy agents may also be considered for BCG-refractory disease (see above). Under certain circumstances, patients with super-ficial bladder cancer may be candidates for cystoprostatec-tomy (Table 15.7).

d. Prognosis. Superficial transitional cell carcinoma has a documented recurrence rate of 50% to 80%, and most re-currences appear within the first 12 months. Up to 50% of recurrences occur within 3 months, making careful follow-up and patient compliance essential. The prognosis depends on various factors (Table 15.8). Recurrences are most often of the same grade and stage as the original tumor, but up to one-third are of a higher grade. About 5% of stage 0 and up to 25% of stage I cases will develop muscle invasive disease within 5 years.

2. Stage II. More therapeutic options are now available for the patient with clinical organ-confined disease; patient selection has become much more important.

a. TURBT alone may be curative in highly selected pa-tients with low-grade, localized disease invading the super-ficial muscle layers (T2a) and not associated with carcinoma in situ. Recurrence may be expected in almost one-half of pa-tients managed with TURBT alone. Repeat TURBT or cold cup biopsy of the site of the original tumor should be done 3 to 6 weeks after the original resection to determine the pres-ence of residual disease. Close lifelong cystoscopic surveil-

Table 15.7.   Indications for cystectomy in stage 0/1 disease

Failure after two courses of intravesical chemotherapy–
   immunotherapy

Prostatic involvement

Persistent high-grade lesions

Uncontrollable recurrence of Ta disease not amenable to
   transurethral resection

Persistence of tumor in nonfunctioning bladder

lance is necessary if this approach is taken. TURBT alone
may also be appropriate in patients who have undergone
chemotherapy with complete or nearly complete disappearance of tumor.
   b.   External-beam radiotherapy is favored in European centers as curative therapy but is considered second-
line therapy in the United States. Salvage cystectomy may
be necessary in 20% of cases following radiotherapy. The
5-year survival rate (about 30%) is consistently below that
achieved with cystectomy. Nevertheless, external-beam
radiotherapy remains a good option for patients who wish
to avoid surgery or who are poor operative risks.
   c.   Radical cystoprostatectomy. In male patients who
have disease invading the superficial or deep muscle layers
of the bladder, radical cystoprostatectomy with bilateral
pelvic lymph node dissection and ileal loop diversion, conti-

Table 15.8.   Prognostic factors in superficial bladder cancer

Cystoscopic finding		
Tumor size	>5 cm	35% muscle invasion
	<5 cm	10% muscle invasion
Tumor number	Solitary tumors	20–60% recurrence, 5% progression
	Multiple tumors	40–90% recurrence, 15% progression
Pathologic findings		
Stage	Ta	5% progression
	T1, all grades	30% progression
	T1 high grade	50% progression
	Tis	>50% progression (without adjuvant therapy)
Grade	Low	55% recurrence, 5% progression
	High	80% recurrence, 50% progression
Findings at first cystoscopy		
Negative		80% no further recurrence
Positive		10% no further recurrence

nent diversion, or neobladder remains the treatment of choice. If carcinoma in situ or gross tumor involves the prostatic urethra, male patients should undergo simultaneous or delayed **urethrectomy.** In patients with retained urethra, monitoring should include at least annual urethral washings, cytology, and biopsy, if indicated. Positive cytology or biopsy is an indication for urethrectomy. In female patients, anterior exenteration with lymph node dissection and diversion is recommended. Historically, urethrectomy is part of this procedure, but studies have demonstrated that only about 10% of female patients undergoing cystectomy have urethral involvement. Sparing of the urethra is thus a consideration in patients who desire orthotopic bladder replacement. Careful frozen-section examination of the urethral margin should be done at the time of cystectomy to determine the presence of tumor. Female patients with cancer at the bladder neck, diffuse carcinoma in situ, or a positive margin at surgery are not candidates for urethral-sparing orthotopic diversion.

(1) Preoperative radiotherapy. Prospective randomized studies indicate no statistically significant difference in 5-year survival (40% to 70%) between patients receiving **external-beam radiation therapy** (EBRT) in conjunction with cystectomy and patients receiving cystectomy alone. In addition, preoperative radiotherapy has fallen in popularity because of its adverse impact on bowel that may be needed for continent diversion. Those favoring preoperative radiotherapy use one of two approaches: 45 to 50 Gy to the whole pelvis followed by cystectomy 1 to 2 weeks later, or 20 Gy over 5 days followed immediately by cystectomy.

(2) Neoadjuvant chemotherapy is given prior to cystoprostatectomy. The rationale for this approach is that it may downstage the disease by reducing or eliminating the primary tumor or by eliminating micrometastases. The disadvantages of this approach include understaging of the patient's tumor burden and delaying definitive surgical treatment. There is little evidence thus far that neoadjuvant chemotherapy delivers any therapeutic benefit. A variation of this approach is perioperative chemotherapy in which two cycles are given prior to surgery and three cycles afterward.

(3) Adjuvant chemotherapy is given after recovery from cystoprostatectomy is complete. The rationale for this approach is patients with documented metastatic disease may benefit from systemic therapy. The disadvantages include delays induced by prolonged surgical healing or complications and reduced willingness on the part of patients to undergo chemotherapy after major surgery. There is no evidence to suggest that adjuvant chemotherapy in patients with organ-confined disease provides any benefits. For patients with extensive local disease or positive pelvic lymph nodes, cisplatin-based adjuvant therapy may provide a small survival advantage.

d.   Partial cystectomy, sometimes in combination with radiation and chemotherapy, is being increasingly considered as an alternative to radical cystoprostatectomy. The approach has the advantage of preserving bladder and sexual function while avoiding the major surgical risk entailed by radical cystoprostatectomy. Candidates for this approach should have solitary tumor with well-defined margins that is located away from the trigone and bladder neck. There should be no history of prior bladder cancer and no carcinoma in situ documented (except when partial cystectomy is part of a chemotherapy treatment program). Bladder capacity should be generous, and bladder function should be normal. Approximately 10% of patients with bladder cancer fulfill these criteria. The expected recurrence rate is about 50%. Partial cystectomy may be appropriate in patients who have undergone chemotherapy with complete or nearly complete disappearance of tumor.

e.   Bladder-preservation protocols have been proposed as alternatives to radical cystoprostatectomy. A typical protocol involves complete resection of the tumor by TURBT, chemotherapy with methotrexate, cisplatinum, and vinblastine, followed by a course of radiation therapy. Patients not responding are typically referred for radical cystoprostatectomy. Five-year survival of about 50% can be achieved, and 60% to 75% of patients retain use of their bladder. These results are similar to those obtained by TURBT alone in selected patients. Contraindications include hydronephrosis, carcinoma in situ, and tumor burden that cannot be completely resected transurethrally. See Chapter 16 for a complete discussion.

3.   Stage III management is the same as for stage II disease (e.g., radical cystoprostatectomy and urinary diversion or neobladder). However, because a large percentage of these patients are likely to have microscopic disease in their pelvic lymph nodes, some thought should be given to neoadjuvant or adjuvant chemotherapy. If the patient accepts adjuvant chemotherapy, cystectomy and diversion are justified in node-positive disease in an effort to reduce tumor burden. Historically, the most common chemotherapeutic regiments included methotrexate, vinblastine, doxorubicin, and cisplatin (M-VAC) and cisplatin, methotrexate, and vinblastine (CMV). Research has shown that similar efficacy with less morbidity has been achieved with gencytabine and carboplatinum regimens (Chapter 16). Some studies have suggested a longer recurrence-free interval for those given adjuvant therapy, although most studies have shown no effect on disease progression rates and no survival benefit. The median survival for patients receiving M-VAC is about 12 months, with only 3.7% of patients continuously relapse-free at 6 years. With surgery alone or surgery with preoperative external-beam radiation, the 5-year survival rate is 15% to 40% in stage III disease.

4.   Stage IV. Node-positive bladder cancer has a 5-year survival of 15% to 30% following cystectomy. With radiotherapy alone for node-positive disease, the 5-year survival rate is 17%. Involvement of organs outside the pelvis carries a grave prognostic significance, and fewer than 5% of patients survive >5 years. More than 50% of patients with stage IV metastatic bladder cancer die within 1 year. Palliative measures should be undertaken for relief of symptoms. Chemotherapeutic agents as mentioned above may also be administered. See Chapter 16.

IV. Prostate cancer

   A. Incidence and etiology. Prostate cancer is the most common visceral malignancy in male adults and ranks second to lung cancer as a cause of cancer-related deaths in the United States. The American Cancer Society estimates that 189,000 new cases of prostate cancer were diagnosed in 2002 and that approximately 30,200 men will die of the disease. The chance of a man acquiring prostate cancer during his lifetime is about 15%. Prostate cancer mortality appears to be declining since 1995, perhaps owing to aggressive screening for the disease. The cause of prostate cancer is unknown, but several associations have been noted.

   1. Genetic influences. Men with one first-degree male relative with prostate cancer have a 2-fold risk of developing prostate cancer, whereas men with two or three affected first-degree relatives have a 5- to 10-fold risk, respectively. About 10% of prostate cancer cases are believed to be inherited. The incidence of prostate cancer is 50% greater in African American men than in Caucasian men and relatively uncommon in Asians. Men of Scandinavian descent have an increased risk of prostate cancer.

   2. Hormonal factors. Virtually all prostate cancer cells exhibit some degree of androgen dependence. This is supported by the observation that prostate cancer does not occur in eunuchs.

   3. Chemical factors. Workers in the rubber, fertilizer, and textile industries have increased rates of prostate cancer, as do men continuously exposed to cadmium, a known antagonist of zinc. Selenium may have a protective effect.

   4. Diet. A diet high in saturated fat has been associated with increased risk of prostate cancer. On the other hand, antioxidants in the diet such as lycopenes and vitamin E may reduce the risk.

   5. Insulin-like growth factor-1 (IGF-1) has been demonstrated to have both mitogenic effects and antiapoptotic effects on normal prostate epithelial cells. In addition, studies have correlated IGF-1 levels with increased risk of prostate cancer. It is not known why certain individuals have higher circulating levels of this IGF.

   B. Tumor histology and grading. More than 95% of prostatic neoplasms are adenocarcinomas arising from prostatic acinar cells at the periphery of the gland. This contrasts with benign prostatic hyperplasia, which develops from inner periurethral tissues and cells at the transitional zone of the prostate. Squamous cell carcinoma and transitional cell carcinoma of the prostate occur only rarely. Prostate cancer exhibits a wide variety of histologic appearances, even within the same specimen.

   1. Prostatic intraepithelial neoplasia (PIN) consists of benign-appearing prostatic glands lined by cytologically atypical cells. Recently, the grading of PIN has been simplified to include only low-grade and high-grade PIN, based on the prominence of the nucleoli. Low-grade PIN may be ignored. However, high-grade PIN has predictive value in identifying patients at increased risk of having prostate cancer. About 6% of needle biopsy specimens have a finding of high-grade PIN. The risk of cancer on subsequent biopsy in patients with high-grade PIN has been estimated at 20% to 35%. Repeat biopsy within 6 to 18 months should be performed when high-grade PIN is found on needle biopsy.

2.   Adenocarcinoma. The **Gleason system** has replaced all older grading systems such as the Mostofi and the MD Anderson Hospital grading systems. Ignoring cytologic features, Gleason established five grades of glandular morphology. The two most prominent glandular patterns are graded from 1 to 5. The sum of these two grades will range from 2 to 10, with 2 representing the most differentiated and 10 representing the most anaplastic tumors. There is a rough correlation between the Gleason grade and the biological behavior of the tumor, as there is significantly decreased survival associated with grade 4 and 5 tumors.

3.   Sarcomas of the prostate account for <0.5% of all malignant prostatic tumors. Rhabdomyosarcoma, a tumor seen most often in children, is the most frequent type of prostatic sarcoma. Leiomyosarcoma is the most common sarcoma involving the prostate in adults.

4.   Transitional cell carcinoma accounts for 1% to 4% of all prostate carcinomas. Primary transitional cell carcinomas of the prostate present in >50% of cases with stage T3 or T4 tumors and 20% present with distant metastases (bone, lung, and liver). Intraductal transitional cell carcinoma of the prostate appears to involve the prostate via direct extension from the overlying urethra, which is usually involved by carcinoma in situ. Direct invasion from bladder transitional cell carcinoma into the stroma of the prostate may occur.

C.   Diagnosis and staging. Prior to the advent of prostate-specific antigen (PSA) measurement, prostate cancer was usually clinically silent until metastatic disease produced symptoms. Diagnosis depended entirely on routine digital rectal examination (DRE). The digital prostate examination is still very important, but at present, many other studies are important in diagnosis and staging.

1.   PSA is a glycoprotein produced by the prostate and secreted in high concentrations into the seminal fluid cells. Thus, it is specific to the prostate, but not to prostate cancer. Nevertheless, the concentration of PSA in the serum correlates well with pathologic stage and tumor volume. Although controversy continues on the role of PSA in screening asymptomatic men, its utility as a tumor marker in established disease is unquestioned. PSA has a serum half-life of 2 to 3 days. PSA levels are affected by androgen levels, prostate volume, race, and age. PSA levels are somewhat higher in African American men than in Caucasian men without prostate cancer. PSA levels have been interpreted in various ways, including PSA density, PSA velocity, age-specific PSA, and free PSA (Table 15.10).

Although some of these methods may improve detection, they also tend to increase the number of unnecessary biopsies. They appear to be most useful in men with PSA values between 4 and 10, prostates above 45 g in size, and age above 70.

2. DRE was the only screening test for prostate cancer prior to the PSA era. It has long been known that approximately 50% of suspicious lesions on DRE are proven cancerous on prostate biopsy. The positive predictive value of DRE is considerably improved when combined with PSA testing. The main value of DRE is in detecting prostate cancer in men with PSA values below 2.5 ng/mL.

3. Prostate biopsy is most commonly performed today through a transrectal approach under US guidance using a spring-driven biopsy gun (Fig. 15.3).

    a. Indications. Although evidence that prostate cancer screening extends longevity is still inconclusive, we recommend transrectal US-guided prostatic biopsies in men with a life expectancy of >10 years (Table 15.9) who have an abnormal DRE, with or without an elevated PSA level. Abnormalities on DRE include discrete nodules, focal induration, or a diffusely hard prostate. Prostate biopsy is also recommended in men with a normal DRE and an abnormal PSA, although defining PSA abnormality is still controversial. Although a level of >4 ng/mL is considered elevated, other criteria have been proposed in addition to or instead of an absolute cutoff for PSA. These include age-adjusted PSA, PSA velocity, PSA density, and free PSA (Table 15.10).

    b. Patient preparation. Full informed consent should be obtained prior to the procedure, outlining the possible complications of biopsy. Bowel preparation with enema may be necessary in some cases. At our institutions, we routinely use a 3-day course of a quinolone antibiotic such as gaitfloxacin 400 mg PO given the evening before, the morning of, and the morning after biopsy. Patients with valvular heart disease are administered parenteral antibiotics according to the recommendations of the American Heart Association (1 g of ampicillin IM or 1 g of vancomycin IV in those patients allergic to penicillins and 80 mg of gentamicin IM). All anticoagulants and antiplatelet drugs must be stopped for an appropriate period of time. Some **analgesia** is provided by injecting a solution of 1% lidocaine into the rectum. More effective analgesia may be obtained by

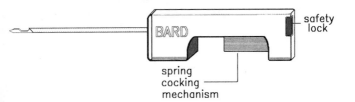

Fig. 15.3. Reusable spring-driven biopsy gun.

Table 15.9. Actuarial table of life expectancies for U.S. men

Age (y)	Life Expectancy (y)	Probability of Death at 1 Year
Birth	73.6	0.0008
30	45.4	0.001
45	31.7	0.004
50	27.4	0.006
55	23.2	0.009
60	19.3	0.01
65	15.7	0.02
70	12.5	0.03
75	9.6	0.05
80	7.1	0.08
85	5.2	0.13
90	3.7	0.19
95	2.7	0.28
100	2.0	0.37

Source: Social Security Administration actuarial tables, 1999.

Table 15.10. PSA parameters suggesting the need for biopsy

Parameters	Age (y) 40–49	50–59	60–69	70–79	
Age adjustment Serum PSA (ng/mL)	0.0–2.5	0.0–3.5	0.0–4.5	0.0–6.5	
Density adjustment Serum PSA/total prostate volume on TRUS >0.15 ng/mL/mL					
Velocity adjustment Serum PSA increase/y	>0.75 ng/mL/y				
Free PSA adjustment	**Serum free PSA (%)** **0–10**	**10–15**	**15–20**	**20–25**	**>25**
Probability of cancer	56	28	20	16	8

PSA, prostate-specific antigen; TRUS, transrectal ultrasonography.
Source: Data from Catalona et al. *JAMA* 1998;279:1542; Carter et al. *JAMA* 1992;267:2215; and Seaman et al. *Urol Clin North Am* 1993;20:653.

injecting 1% lidocaine along the neurovascular bundles of the prostate, beginning at the seminal vesicles and moving outward to the apex. A 25-cm 20-gauge spinal needle is passed through the needle cannula on the transducer, and injection is guided by the transrectal US image.

c. **Transrectal US** is best performed with a 5- to 8 M-Hz hand-held, high-resolution probe with capacity for both transverse and sagittal imaging of the prostate in real time. This probe can be fitted with a cannula that accepts the needle of a spring-loaded biopsy gun, thus allowing multiple cores of tissue to be easily obtained. Insertion of the probe is aided by first performing a DRE. This allows assessment of the adequacy of the rectal space and identifies any relevant prostate abnormalities. With the patient in the left lateral position, the probe is gently introduced with plenty of lubricant. The prostate is imaged first in the transverse plane, then in the sagittal plane. Any hypo- or hyperechoic area are noted.

d. **US findings.** Volume measurement of the prostate is then carried out by measuring its largest transverse diameter, the greatest cephalocaudal length, and its antero-posterior height (Fig. 15.4). Most carcinomas detected by US are hypoechoic regions with irregular borders. However, there are exceptions, and carcinoma may be invisible to US or hyperechoic.

e. **Prostatic biopsy.** US guidance is essential to enable accurate biopsy of suspicious areas as well as systematic sampling of the prostate by biopsy, including areas that appear completely normal. The standard sextant biopsies sample the parasagittal regions of the prostate at the apex, middle, and base of the gland (Fig. 15.5). For glands >50 g by US, 12 cores should be obtained by including the lateral peripheral zone (3 biopsies on each side). The addition of transition-zone biopsies increases detection rates by about

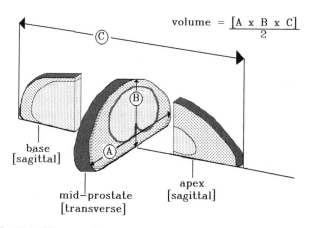

$$\text{volume} = \frac{[A \times B \times C]}{2}$$

base
[sagittal]

mid-prostate
[transverse]

apex
[sagittal]

Fig. 15.4. Ultrasound measurement of prostate volume.

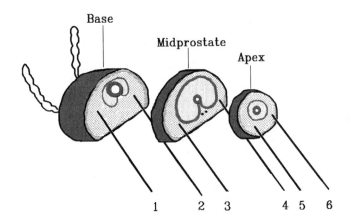

Fig. 15.5.   Standard sextant prostate biopsy.

2% to 4% and is not routinely performed for initial tissue sampling. Biopsy within the transition zone as well as at additional sites in the lateral peripheral zone may be useful in men with PIN undergoing repeat biopsy or men with elevated PSA and negative initial biopsies.

4.   Route of spread. Prostate cancer spreads by lymphatic and hematogenous routes. The primary sites of lymphatic metastases are the external iliac (obturator group), internal iliac, and presacral nodes. In general, the larger and less differentiated the primary tumor, the higher the incidence of lymphatic metastases. Occasionally, the supraclavicular nodes are involved via the thoracic duct. Hematogenous spread to bone, lung, liver, and kidneys occurs late in the disease.

5.   Prostatic acid phosphatase (PAP) was the first biochemical marker for the staging of prostate cancer. About 80% of patients with elevated PAP have metastatic disease. The routine use of PAP for staging has diminished rapidly with the introduction of serum PSA testing. Most patients with elevated PAP have PSA measurements of >20 ng/mL. Thus, PAP no longer provides useful information not available through PSA testing.

6.   Bone scanning is very useful in detecting metastatic disease. Bony metastases occur in about 80% of patients with advanced disease. Of these, about 80% are osteoblastic lesions and 5% osteolytic; the rest are mixed osteoblastic and osteolytic lesions. Phosphate labeled with technetium-99m is rapidly taken up by bone, which is metabolically active. Bone scans are more sensitive than skeletal radiography and are able to detect lesions up to 6 months before they are apparent on x-ray films. However, bone scans are less specific than radiography; increased uptake occurs in arthritis, fractures, Paget's disease, and hyperparathyroidism and after recent trauma. Recent reports have suggested that a bone scan may be omitted if the PSA level is <10 ng/mL in a patient with prostate cancer. We recommend omitting a bone scan in a patient with clinical T2 cancer or lower, a Gleason score of ≤6, and a serum PSA value of <10 ng/mL.

7. CT can assess gross local extension and detect nodal metastases >2 cm. The sensitivity range is from 30% to 75%, and specificity is between 65% and 100%. Staging CT scans are potentially useful only in patients who are being evaluated for EBRT (to create the treatment portals) and in patients who have a serum PSA concentration of >10 ng/mL and a Gleason score of >6.

8. Pelvic lymphadenectomy is generally performed in conjunction with radical retropubic prostatectomy. It is almost always omitted in patients selected for radical perineal prostatectomy, brachytherapy, or EBRT. The external iliac, obturator, and internal iliac lymphatic chains are dissected bilaterally for pathologic examination. Complications include wound infection, lymphocele, and lymphedema of the penis and lower extremities.

9. Partin tables use clinical stage, Gleason sum, and PSA level to predict pathologic findings. The tables have been validated and are quite accurate in predicting organ confinement, extracapsular disease, seminal vesicle involvement, and positive lymph nodes (Appendix II, page 510). The tables should not take the place of clinical judgment, as they predict only pathologic findings, not prognosis.

10. Staging nomenclature. The AJCC staging system (Fig. 15.6) has gradually replaced the Whitmore–Jewett system that was widely used in the past (Table 15.11). In the recent 2002 revision, T2 disease has again been subdivided into three categories as it was in the 1992 version.

D. Treatment will be discussed in terms of clinical organ-confined (stages I and II), locally invasive (stage III and T4, N0, M0), and metastatic (N1, M+ in any combination) disease.

1. Treatment modalities. See Table 15.12. See Chapter 16 for specific information on hormonal and chemotherapeutic agents and Chapter 17 for a discussion of ortho- and brachytherapy.

a. Radical prostatectomy. In organ-confined prostate cancer, radical prostatectomy offers the best chance of long-term disease-free survival (85% at 15 years). Patients with clinical organ-confined disease who have at least a 10-year life expectancy (Table 15.9) and a good operative risk profile are candidates for radical prostatectomy, which may be performed via a retropubic, perineal, or laparoscopic approach. Since the incidence of node-positive disease is >5% in patients with low-grade tumors (Gleason score <6) and/or a PSA level below 10 ng/mL, **pelvic lymphadenectomy** may be omitted in such patients. In this subgroup, radical perineal prostatectomy may also be considered. The prostate is removed en bloc along with the seminal vesicles. The bladder neck is reconstructed and anastomosed to the distal membranous urethra. **Neoadjuvant hormone therapy** has been advocated before radical prostatectomy to induce a lower stage, decrease positive surgical margins, and effect a

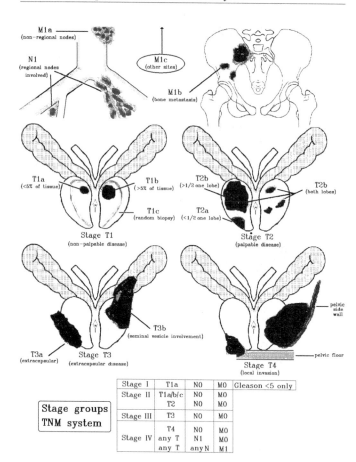

Fig. 15.6.   American Joint Committee on Cancer (AJCC) staging system for prostate cancer.

reduction in long-term cancer recurrence rates. However, pathologic downstaging and a significant difference with respect to PSA progression have not been demonstrated thus far. Permanent incontinence requiring pads or diapers is the most feared complication of radical prostatectomy. Erectile function may be spared by a "nerve-sparing" prostatectomy. However, this approach is not advisable in patients with high pretreatment PSA level or high-grade lesions (Gleason score 8 to 10). The impact of radical prostatectomy on quality of life is summarized in Table 15.13.

b.   EBRT achieves survival rates equivalent to those of radical prostatectomy at 5 and perhaps 10 years following diagnosis (Table 15.14). However, no studies that directly compare EBRT with radical prostatectomy are available.

Table 15.11. AJCC and Whitmore–Jewett staging systems in prostate cancer

AJCC Stage	Description	Whitmore–Jewett Stage
Primary tumor		
Tx	Tumor cannot be assessed	
T0	No evidence of tumor	
T1a	Tumor found incidentally at TURP (<5% of resected tissue)	A1
T1b	Tumor found incidentally at TURP (>5% of resected tissue)	A2
T1c	Nonpalpable tumor identified because of elevated PSA value	B0
T2a	Tumor involves less than half of one lobe	B1
T2b	Tumor involves more than half of one lobe	B1
T2c	Tumor involves both lobes	B2
T3a	Extracapsular extension (unilateral or bilateral)	C1
T3b	Seminal vesicle involvement	C2
T4	Tumor invades adjacent organs or structures	
	Elevated PAP alone	D0
Lymph nodes		
Nx	Regional nodes not assessed	
N0	No regional lymph node metastasis	
N1	Metastasis to regional (pelvic) lymph nodes	D1
Metastases		
M1a	Metastasis to nonregional lymph nodes	D2
M1b	Metastasis to bone	D2
M1c	Metastasis to other sites	D2
	Hormone-refractory metastatic disease	D3

AJCC, American Joint Committee on Cancer; TURP, transurethral resection of prostate; PSA, prostate-specific antigen; PAP, prostatic acid phosphate.

Table 15.12.   Treatment modalities in localized prostate cancer

I. Radical prostatectomy
   a. Retropubic approach
   b. Perineal approach
   c. Laparoscopic approach
II. Radiation therapy
   a. External beam alone
   b. Interstitial radiation
      1. ^{125}I alone with external-beam radiation
      2. ^{103}Pd alone or with external-beam radiation
      3. High-dose ^{192}Ir alone or with external-beam radiation
III. Cryosurgery
IV. Hormone manipulation
   a. Bilateral orchiectomy
   b. Estrogen therapy (diethylstilbestrol)
   c. Progestational agents (megestrol acetate)
   d. Luteinizing hormone-releasing hormone analogs (leuprolide, goserelin)
   e. Antiandrogens (cyproterone acetate, flutamide, bicalutamide, nilutamide)

Furthermore, patients undergoing EBRT are typically older and at a higher stage than those receiving surgery. Prostate cancers with a higher Gleason grade (7) have fared poorly with radiation, and radical surgery has been recommended. The treatment schedule can be tedious—with 6 to 8 weeks usually required for delivery. Radiation therapy offers an alternative treatment in patients who are poor surgical risks or who refuse surgery. Complications of radiation therapy include proctitis (10%), cystitis (5%), and erectile impotence (40% to 50%), especially in patients with preexisting

Table 15.13.   Quality of life after radical prostatectomy

	Baseline (%)	1 Year (%)
Urinary continence		
Total control	80	30
Occasional leak, no pad	10	30
1–2 pads/d	1	20
3 pads/d	<1	5
No control	<1	5
Erectile function		
Adequate erection	75	15
Inadequate erection	15	25
No erection	10	55

Source: Data modified from Stanford et al. *JAMA* 2000;283:354–360.

Table 15.14.   Prostate cancer: disease-specific survival (%) after external-beam radiotherapy

	Group 1	Group 2	Group 3	Group 4
	T1/2 Nx GS = 6	T1/2 Nx GS = 7	T1/2 Nx GS = 8	
		T3 Nx GS = 6	T3 Nx GS = 7	T3 Nx GS = 8
		Tany N+ GS = 6	Tany N+ GS = 7	Tany N+ GS = 8
5 y	96	94	83	64
10 y	86	75	62	34
15 y	73	61	39	27

Tany = any T stage; GS = Gleason score.
Source: Data modified from Roach et al. *Int J Radiat Oncol Biol Phys* 2000; 46:609.

vascular disease. Improved disease-free survival as well as lower complications rates may ensue from the use of three-dimensional conformal radiotherapy.

c.   Brachytherapy has become increasingly popular to treat organ-confined disease. Iodine-125 (half-life 60 days) and palladium-103 (half-life 17 days) give good local control of low-volume disease. Patients with a high probability of organ-confined disease are appropriate candidates for treatment with brachytherapy alone. Such patients include those with stage I or II disease, PSA level of ≤10 ng/mL, and Gleason scores of ≤6. Patients who elect treatment with brachytherapy but do not meet these criteria should be treated with supplemental EBRT. Relative contraindications to brachytherapy include prior transurethral resection of the prostate (TURP) and evidence of outflow obstruction. Prior TURP is associated with irritative symptoms and increased risk of urinary incontinence (up to 50%). Because of postoperative swelling, patients with pretherapy obstruction are at greater risk of postoperative urinary retention. Owing to difficulty in reaching the prostate, patients who weigh over 300 lbs. may not be good candidates for brachytherapy.

(1)   Preoperative preparation should include Fleet enema the evening prior to procedure, perioperative antibiotics (gaitfloxacin 400 mg PO daily or IM/IV if patient cannot take PO), and discontinuance of aspirin, nonsteroidal antiinflammatory drugs, and Coumadin. No cross-matching of blood is necessary.

(2)   Technique. The patient should be in the lithotomy position. A biplanar US probe is placed in the rectum and attached to a stepping unit that moves the probe in 0.5-cm intervals. A perineal template is attached to provide precise placement of the needles into the prostate. US images that match the planning images are obtained. Once the final needle position is established, the seeds are delivered by inserting the needle through the appropriate hole in the template, then through perineal skin and into the prostate under US guidance. At the end of the procedure, flexible cystoscopy may be indicated to retrieve errant seeds in the bladder or urethra.

(3) Postoperative care. The needle puncture sites may be tender or may bleed. Hematuria may be observed in the first 24 hours. Dysuria, frequency, and urgency are very common and should be treated with antimuscarinic agents. Most patients are discharged within 24 hours.

(4) Complications. About one-third of patients have irritative symptoms lasting up to 1 year. About 20% of patients have urge incontinence that gradually improves with time. Diarrhea, blood per rectum, and painful bowel movements are seen initially in one-third of patients. A similar percentage of patients report decreased erectile function. Decreased volume of semen is very common.

(5) Follow-up protocol includes PSA and DRE performed every 3 months for the first 2 years, then every 6 months for 3 years, and then yearly. If any abnormality is noted, biopsy should be considered.

d. Cryotherapy has seen a renewed interest because of improved instrumentation and delivery methods. With use of an approach similar to brachytherapy, multiple cryoprobes are passed into the prostate under US guidance. The mechanism of necrosis in cryotherapy involves intracellular freezing and disruption of intracellular structures. Cell death appears to require temperatures in the range of −20 to −40°C. More than one freezing cycle may be needed for complete tumor ablation. Indications include primary tumor ablation, salvage therapy after other primary therapy (usually EBRT or brachytherapy), and palliative control of local disease. Up to 40% of men may have positive biopsies during the first posttherapy year. Retreatment in such cases may be beneficial. Three-year biochemical recurrence rate following cryotherapy is about 50%. Contraindications include surgical absence of rectum and extensive local disease involving adjacent structures.

(1) Preoperative preparation consists of a Fleet enema the evening prior to the procedure. Order perioperative antibiotics (gaitfloxacin 400 mg PO daily or IM/IV if patient cannot take PO), and discontinue aspirin, nonsteroidal antiinflammatory drugs, and Coumadin. No cross-matching of blood is necessary. Oral antibiotic therapy is continued for 24 hours postoperatively.

(2) Technique. The patient is placed in the lithotomy position, and either general or spinal anesthesia may be used. Cystourethroscopy should be performed at the start of the procedure to assess extent of disease. A suprapubic catheter is placed to permit continuous flow of warm irrigant through the urethra during the procedure. A five-probe technique is standard, placing two probes anteromedially, two posterolaterally, and one posteriorly.

Delivering liquid nitrogen through the probes, two freeze–thaw cycles are generally used. US monitoring is used to follow the freezing process in the prostate.

(3) Postoperative care. The majority of patients can be discharged to home in 1 to 2 days, with a urethral catheter in place for at least 3 weeks.

(4) Complications include injury to the urethra, incontinence (10%), and erectile dysfunction (80%). Urethral fistula is a rare complication. Irritative symptoms may last up to 3 months. Incontinence may occur in up to 10% of cases.

(5) Follow-up protocol is similar to that for brachytherapy. Because of the high local recurrence rate, biopsy should be routinely performed within 12 months of therapy to determine the need for further therapy.

2. **Approach to treatment by clinical stage of disease**
   a. **Prostate cancer screening.** Although the impact of prostate cancer screening and early detection programs is debatable, some recent reports show a 30% drop in the incidence of age-adjusted prostate cancer from 1992 to 1994, a decline in metastatic disease by 60% since it peaked in 1986, and, most importantly, a decline (6%) in prostate cancer mortality between 1991 and 1995 in the United States. However, the mortality from other forms of cancer also declined during this time interval. Thus, it remains unclear whether the decline of prostate cancer mortality can be explained by the increased frequency of PSA-driven therapy during the last decade.

   b. **Stage I** includes T1a disease in which tumor is found incidentally on a TURP specimen, involves ≤5% of tissue resected, and has a Gleason grade of <5. It is critical to ascertain that the patient truly has T1a disease and not T1b disease. This distinction is especially important in patients who are younger than 70 years and might be candidates for curative surgery or radiation therapy. Within 3 months of the initial diagnosis of stage T1a prostate cancer, residual prostate cancer should be ruled out by needle biopsy or repeat transurethral resection. If no residual tumor is found, long-term, age-adjusted survival equal to that of the population without cancer can be expected for those over 70 years old. However, many advocate aggressive therapy for patients under age 55 and recommend radical prostatectomy. In the setting of normal PSA in younger patients with T1a disease, careful discussion between patient and urologist must ensue to ensure that therapy is geared toward the patients' wishes.

   c. **Stage II** includes T1a disease with Gleason grade of ≥5 as well as T1b, T1c, and T2 disease. Either EBRT, interstitial radiation, or radical prostatectomy may be used in treating stage II prostate cancer. Previous TURP has not been an impediment to successful radical surgery. However, patients who have had prior TURP may not be good candidates for interstitial irradiation as there is usually insufficient prostatic tissue remaining after TURP for placement of the radioactive seeds. Since patients aged 75 or older have a life expectancy of <10 years, deferred conservative treatment ("watchful waiting") is a valid option in such cases.

d. Stage III. Between 15% and 30% of newly diagnosed patients have stage T3 prostate cancer. Management options include radical prostatectomy, external-beam radiation with or without interstitial brachytherapy, hormone therapy, and watchful waiting. The choice of therapy must balance the risk of each mode of therapy with the fact that these patients have significant risk of both local and distant failure. **Radical prostatectomy** may be appropriate in a small subgroup of patients with clinical T3 disease who have a serum PSA below 10 ng/mL and a Gleason score of ≤6. Adjuvant hormone or radiation therapy after surgery may improve disease-free interval but not overall survival. Traditionally, stage III disease has been treated with **EBRT** because of the high incidence (35% to 60%) of understaging by clinical methods. Pelvic lymphadenectomy is especially important in this group to determine the best mode of therapy. EBRT may be combined with brachytherapy boost or with hormonal ablation. The use of **neoadjuvant hormonal therapy** with radiation has been shown to reduce local progression and increase metastasis-free survival with a possible survival advantage. Because radiation and hormonally mediated apoptosis appear to be induced by different mechanisms, their interaction may be synergistic. In addition, there is a potential reduction in radiation-associated morbidity. Neoadjuvant hormone therapy is currently considered standard therapy when external-beam therapy is given for locally advanced prostate cancer.

e. Stage IV. Androgen deprivation remains the primary treatment modality in men with metastatic prostate cancer. Hormonal manipulation will achieve a response in up to 90% of patients but does not improve survival.

(1) Immediate versus delayed hormonal therapy remains controversial. The rationale for deferring hormonal management until progression of disease is based on several considerations. Localized prostate cancer is primarily asymptomatic, hormonal therapy is usually efficacious only for up to 3 years, and studies indicate that the 10-year disease-free survival in patients with grades 1 and 2 tumors is >85%, although it is only 34% for grade 3 tumors. Approximately 40% of patients die of other causes because of their age at diagnosis (>70 years). On the other hand, recent data, including those from a large randomized trial, suggest that more patients progressed from M0 to M1 disease (p < 0.001) and that metastatic pain occurred more rapidly in deferred patients. More than twice as many patients required TURP because of local progression. In addition, pathologic fracture, spinal cord compression, ureteral obstruction, and development of extraskeletal metastasis were twice as common in deferred patients. A covariant analytic review of data from the Veterans Administration Cooperative Urological Research Group studies suggests that initiating therapy when patients have minimal metastatic disease may be beneficial. Delayed hormonal therapy may be appropriate for older patients with a life expectancy of ≤10 years and localized prostate cancer (stage T1 or T2) or for patients who value potency over other factors. Early hormonal therapy may be appropriate for younger patients, those with more advanced disease, and patients who do not want the "no treatment" option. In summary, recent data suggest that although survival is unchanged, the quality of life throughout the years one lives may be improved with early hormonal intervention.

(2) Bilateral orchiectomy appears to be the most consistent means of endocrine manipulation. Results are immediate, there is virtually no operative morbidity, and patient compliance is not a problem. Psychological barriers imposed by this surgery have decreased the frequency with which this is performed.

(3) Medical castration may be achieved by a variety of agents. See Chapter 16 for a discussion of their use in prostate cancer. **Combined androgen blockade** is the combination of surgical or medical castration with peripheral antiandrogen blockade in the treatment of advanced prostate cancer. Although not all trials have shown a benefit of combined androgen blockade over conventional therapy, two of the largest controlled trials, the National Cancer Institute Intergroup 0036 Study and the Urological Group of the European Organization on Research and Treatment 30853 Study, demonstrated statistically significant prolonged survival for patients treated by combined androgen blockade compared with those treated by surgical or medical castration alone (particularly for minimal metastatic burden). Combined androgen blockade should be considered in all patients in whom flare-ups must be blocked and in patients who have not responded to monotherapy. **Antiandrogens** may also be considered as monotherapy (see Chapter 16). **Intermittent androgen ablation** is a technique that might improve overall survival by delaying the emergence of androgen-independent clones while improving the overall quality of life. Antiandrogen withdrawal has also been shown to decrease PSA levels. This **antiandrogen withdrawal syndrome** has been demonstrated with nonsteroidal as well as steroidal (e.g., megestrol) antiandrogen agents. A point mutation in androgen-binding receptors that may sensitize tumor cells to the antiandrogen agent is theorized. Aminoglutethimide and ketoconazole can be used to lower serum testosterone quickly in cases involving spinal cord compression secondary to metastases. Regarding **hormone-resistant disease,** there is little effective therapy for patients in whom hormonal manipulation has failed. Palliation may be achieved with focal irradiation to metastatic sites in bone. Strontium-89 has been approved for the management of pain arising from skeletal metastases. Strontium is a radiopharmaceutical that emits a β particle and localizes in bone after intra-venous injection. Approximately 70% to 80% of patients experience pain relief. Chemotherapy has been used in clinical trials and has shown promise in several studies (see Chapter 16).

V.   Testicular and extragonadal germ cell cancer

A.   Incidence. Testis cancer is the most common tumor in boys and men ages 15 to 35 years. Approximately 7,200 new instances of testis cancer were reported in the United States in 1997, with about 350 deaths occurring annually. Testicular tumors make up 1% to 2% of all male malignancies, but 12% of all cancer deaths in patients between the ages of 20 and 35. The incidence is rela-tively higher in people of Scandinavian descent and extremely low in African Americans. A person with testis cancer has a 500-fold greater chance for development of a contralateral tumor than does the general male population; however, simul-taneous bilateral tumors are seen in only 1% to 2% of patients. Patients with a history of cryptorchidism have a 40- to 70-fold in-crease in incidence of testis cancer regardless of whether orchi-dopexy was carried out. Approximately 5% of germ cell cancers arise in extragonadal sites, particularly in the mediastinum and retroperitoneum. About 80% of nonseminomatous testicular tu-mors have abnormalities of chromosome 12p.

B.   Pathology and classification are summarized in Table 15.15.

C.   Diagnosis. Testicular tumors usually present as an asymp-tomatic swelling or mass in the scrotum discovered by the pa-tient. All masses arising from the testis should be considered

Table 15.15.   Classification of testis tumors

I. Germ cell tumors	95%
a. Seminoma	50%
1. Classic (85% of all seminomas)	
2. Anaplastic (5–10% of all seminomas)	
3. Spermatocytic (5–10% of all seminomas)	
b. Embryonal	20%
1. Adult	
2. Juvenile (yolk sac tumor)	
c. Teratocarcinoma (teratoma and embryoma)	10%
d. Teratoma	5%
1. Mature	
2. Immature	
e. Choriocarcinoma	1%
II. Gonadostromal tumors	5%
a. Leydig's (interstitial) cell	
b. Sertoli's cell	
c. Granulosa cell	
III. Secondary (metastatic) tumors	
a. Lymphoma/leukemia	
b. Prostate	
c. Melanoma	
d. Lung	

carcinoma until proven otherwise. Testicular pain is a presenting complaint in only 20% of patients. Systemic symptoms from metastatic disease and hormone production (gynecomastia) are seen in 10% and 5% of cases, respectively. The average delay in diagnosis is 4 to 6 months. Patients with extragonadal tumors often present with pulmonary complaints (mediastinal tumors) or back pain or abdominal mass (retroperitoneal tumors).

  1. **Physical examination** should be performed with the patient standing and facing the examiner. The scrotal examination begins with examination of the uninvolved testis. Both testes should be carefully palpated for size, consistency, and areas of induration. Both spermatic cords and inguinal areas should be examined carefully. A hydrocele, present in 10% of cases, may make examination more difficult. The abdomen should be examined for evidence of nodal disease or visceral involvement. Examination of the chest may reveal pleural effusion or gynecomastia. Finally, the supraclavicular lymph nodes should be palpated.

  2. **Scrotal US** can be very useful in differentiating a testicular mass from epididymitis, hydrocele, spermatocele, testicular torsion, and inguinal hernia. Seminomas appear as circumscribed, homogeneous, hypoechoic lesions, whereas nonseminomatous germ cell tumors (NSGCTs) are typically inhomogeneous lesions with indistinct margins. Microlithiasis is a frequent finding in normal testes and of uncertain significance.

D. **Route of spread.** Testis tumors metastasize in predictable, orderly fashion via the retroperitoneal lymphatics to the perivascular nodes at the level of the renal hilum. Tumors arising in the right testis metastasize primarily to the lymph nodes between the aorta and vena cava below the right renal vein. Tumors on the left side metastasize to the preaortic and paraaortic lymph nodes on the left. Right-sided tumors, unlike left-sided tumors, can cross the midline, making the surgical template for each retroperitoneal procedure different. Iliac and suprahilar nodes are rarely involved without direct extension from the primary nodes. Hematogenous spread to the lungs may be seen with choriocarcinoma or bulky nodal disease.

E. **Staging.** The AJCC staging system (Fig. 15.7) is now widely accepted, but the older Memorial Sloan–Kettering staging system is still frequently preferred because it is more useful clinically (Table 15.16).

  1. **Serum tumor markers** include α-fetoprotein (AFP), the β subunit of hCG (β-hCG), and lactic dehydrogenase (Table 15.17). Almost 85% of mixed germ cell testis tumors will produce an elevation of one or both markers. However, the absence of tumor marker elevation does not rule out primary or metastatic malignancy because as many as 50% of patients with low-volume retroperitoneal disease may have no elevation of tumor markers. The primary role of serum tumor markers is not in staging, but in monitoring disease progression or response to therapy. The level of serum markers may also have prognostic value (see below).

  a. **AFP** is a glycoprotein produced by fetal yolk sac, liver, and the gastrointestinal tract. AFP is not elevated in pure

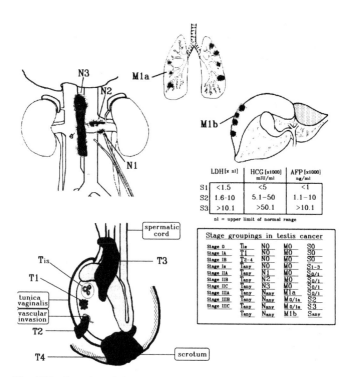

	LDH [x nl]	HCG [x1000] mIU/ml	AFP [x1000] ng/ml
S1	<1.5	<5	<1
S2	1.6-10	5.1-50	1.1-10
S3	>10.1	>50.1	>10.1

nl = upper limit of normal range

Stage groupings in testis cancer				
Stage 0	Tis	N0	M0	S0
Stage IA	T1	N0	M0	S0
Stage IB	T2-4	N0	M0	S0
Stage Is	Tany	N0	M0	S1-3
Stage IIA	Tany	N1	M0	S0/1
Stage IIB	Tany	N2	M0	S0/1
Stage IIC	Tany	N3	M0	S0/1
Stage IIIA	Tany	Nany	M1a	S0/1
Stage IIIB	Tany	Nany	M0/1a	S2
Stage IIIC	Tany	Nany	M0/1a	S3
	Tany	Nany	M1b	Sany

Fig. 15.7.   American Joint Committee on Cancer (AJCC) system for staging of testicular cancer.

seminoma or choriocarcinoma. Because the metabolic half-life of AFP is 5 days, persistence of high levels of AFP 4 weeks after orchiectomy indicates metastatic disease. False-positive results can occur with hepatoma, hepatitis, and bronchogenic, stomach, or pancreatic cancer.

b.   hCG, a glycoprotein produced by syncytiotrophoblastic cells, is composed of an α subunit identical to that of luteinizing hormone and a β subunit unique to hCG. Normal males do not produce significant amounts of β-hCG except from testicular tumors. Serum levels of β-hCG are elevated in 100% of patients with choriocarcinoma (Table 15.17). However, pure seminomas produce only low-grade elevations of β-hCG; marked elevation signifies the presence of associated teratocarcinoma or choriocarcinoma. The half-life of hCG is 24 to 36 hours; persistence of high levels of hCG 7 days after orchiectomy indicates metastatic disease.

c.   Lactic dehydrogenase, particularly isoenzyme 1, is elevated in 30% to 80% of seminomas and 60% of cases with nonseminomatous disease. This test is useful for monitoring treatment when levels of AFP and hCG are normal or have normalized. It may be particularly useful in seminomas that

Table 15.16. AJCC and Memorial Sloan–Kettering staging systems for testis cancer

AJCC Stage	Description	Memorial Sloan–Kettering Stage
Primary tumor		
Tx	Primary tumor cannot be assessed	
T0	No evidence of primary tumor	
TIS	Intratubular tumor (carcinoma in situ)	
T1	Tumor limited to testis, including rete testis	A
T2	Tumor extends beyond tunica albuginea or shows vascular–lymphatic invasion	A
T3	Tumor invades spermatic cord (with or without vascular–lymphatic invasion)	A
T4	Tumor invades scrotum (with or without vascular–lymphatic invasion)	
Lymph nodes		
N1	Regional lymph node mass, <2-cm diameter; multiple nodes <2-cm diameter	B1
N2	Regional lymph node mass <5-cm diameter; multiple nodes <5-cm diameter	B2
N3	One or more regional lymph nodes involved, >5-cm diameter	B3
Metastases		
M1a	Nonregional lymph nodes involved or pulmonary metastases	C
M1b	Other distant metastases	C

AJCC, American Joint Committee on Cancer.

produce no other marker. The lactate dehydrogenase level is included as an indicator of stage in the AJCC staging system (Fig. 15.7).

d. Placental-like alkaline phosphatase is detected in 65% of seminomas. It may be the most sensitive marker for metastatic seminomatous disease and for relapse, but is relatively nonspecific. Elevations may occur in lung, pancreas, stomach, colon, and ovarian tumors.

2. Abdominal CT is the recommended radiologic examination for preoperative staging and metastatic work-up. Although it is not very accurate with low-volume retroperi-

**Table 15.17.   Frequency of elevated
tumor markers in testis cancer**

Histology	Incidence (%)	HCG Elevated (%)	AFP Elevated (%)
Pure seminoma	35	5	0
Embryonal	20	60	70
Teratocarcinoma	10	60	65
Teratoma	5	25	40
Choriocarcinoma	1	100	0

HCG, human chorionic gonadotropin; AFP, α-fetoprotein.

toneal disease, it is excellent for nodal involvement measuring >2 cm. False-positive scans are rare if the cutoff value of 2 cm is used.

3.   Chest CT will identify a small subset of patients with normal findings on chest x-ray films but low-level pulmonary metastases. Currently, chest roentgenography is sufficient to exclude metastatic lung disease if the abdominal CT findings are negative.

4.   Risk stratification is possible based on serum marker level and histologic features. Three different prognostic subgroups have been defined according to the level of serum markers (Fig. 15.7). Patients with serum markers consistent with classification S1 have a good prognosis, those in class S2 have intermediate prognosis, and those in class S3 have poor prognosis. Histologic features with poor prognosis include lymphovascular invasion, percentage embryonal elements, and involvement of the tunica albuginea.

F.   Primary treatment

1.   Testicular tumors. Radical inguinal orchiectomy is indicated in almost all cases with solid testicular mass as the first therapeutic maneuver, even with extensive metastatic disease. Sperm banking should be discussed with the patient interested in preserving future fertility (see Chapter 20). The testicle is approached through an inguinal incision. The spermatic cord is temporarily clamped before the scrotal contents are examined. If the diagnosis of testicular tumor is confirmed, high inguinal orchiectomy is performed, with the spermatic cord ligated and transected at the level of the internal inguinal ring. Transscrotal exploration or needle biopsy of the testis should be avoided for fear of contaminating the lymphatic channels of the scrotal skin.

2.   Extragonadal tumors. For primary extragonadal seminoma, radiotherapy is the primary treatment. For nonseminomatous tumors, primary chemotherapy is given, with surgical excision of residual masses.

3.   Carcinoma in situ may be seen on testis biopsy performed for reasons such as infertility. The malignant potential and appropriate treatment of this finding are still undetermined.

G. Treatment after orchiectomy depends on clinical/pathologic staging and histology. The Memorial Sloan–Kettering staging system is used to guide therapy.

   1. Pure seminoma is exquisitely radiosensitive, and EBRT is the mainstay of treatment after orchiectomy in low-volume disease (see Chapter 17).

   a. Stage A. Prophylactic external-beam radiation to the ipsilateral retroperitoneum (iliac and paraaortic nodes up to the diaphragm) in a dose of 25 to 30 Gy produces cure rates of about 95%. Relapse rate after retroperitoneal radiotherapy is about 4% and usually occurs at sites beyond the irradiated field. These failures are salvageable by chemotherapy or by further radiotherapy to the site of relapse. Although the morbidity of radiation is considered minimal by most urologists, some radiation concerns include infertility, secondary long-term malignancy (stomach, colon), nausea, immunosuppression, and overtreatment in 75% of patients, as the incidence of occult metastasis in clinical stage A seminoma is only 25%. As a result, treatment options after radical orchiectomy other than radiation currently include **surveillance** and adjuvant single-agent chemotherapy using carboplatin. Patients selected for surveillance must be reliable, highly motivated men with small (<3-cm) stage I pure seminoma and negative tumor markers following orchiectomy. The surveillance period is 3 years.

   b. Stages B1 and B2. Treatment is the same as in stage A, with the addition of 10 to 15 Gy to the site of nodal involvement. If the lower aortic or common iliac areas appear involved on CT, the contralateral pelvic nodes are included in the field. Prophylactic supradiaphragmatic radiation is not needed if no radiographic or clinical evidence suggests disease. Prior chest radiation will compromise the patient's capacity to receive full-dose chemotherapy because of marrow suppression and will also increase the risk for pulmonary toxicity (e.g., bleomycin). The 10% to 20% of patients with stage B1 seminoma in whom relapse occurs above the diaphragm respond extremely well to chemotherapy, as seminomas are more chemosensitive than nonseminomas.

   c. Stages B3 and C. Radiation therapy has not been very successful, and combination chemotherapy has now become the primary therapy for high-volume disease. Because of the success of chemotherapy in testis cancer, even with seminoma, the standard of care is to avoid external-beam radiation and proceed with chemotherapy in high-volume disease. During the last 20 years, with new chemotherapeutic agents, the survival of patients with all stages of seminoma has been 95% to 98%. Management of the residual masses in seminomas that are found in 30% to 70% of cases after chemotherapy is controversial. In advanced-stage seminoma following chemotherapy, most resected masses have shown fibrosis and necrosis. Currently, resection is not recommended in cases in which the mass is <3 cm. For larger masses, some centers recommend either radiation, surveillance, or resection and biopsy.

2. NSGCT, unlike seminomas, demonstrate much less radio-sensitivity. Treatment consists of orchiectomy with or without retroperitoneal lymphadenectomy [retroperitoneal lymph node dissection (RPLND)] and with or without combination chemotherapy.

a. **Stage A** (Fig. 15.8) treatment following orchiectomy (for those patients with negative serum markers) is either surveillance or RPLND. The advantages of surveillance are that about 75% of patients will ultimately avoid further surgery. With surveillance, the median time to relapse is 6 months, and detection of disease >2 years after orchiectomy is very rare. The disadvantages are that strict adherence to follow-up is necessary and that if a recurrence is not detected early, increased chemotherapy may be needed.

(1) **RPLND** is presently recommended therapy in North American centers for stage A NSGCTs with features indicative of increased risk such as lymphovascular invasion, extensive embryonal elements, absence of yolk sac, and involvement of testicular tunics or epididymis. Those who are low risk may choose between RPLND and surveillance. Approximately 25% of patients thought to have clinical stage A disease will be understaged and, in fact, have metastatic disease. Cure rates average >90% in pathologic stage A disease after negative RPLND. Of those who relapse, 90% do so within the first 2 years (usually within the chest) and respond well to chemotherapy. Salvage rates of 100% can be achieved. In those with

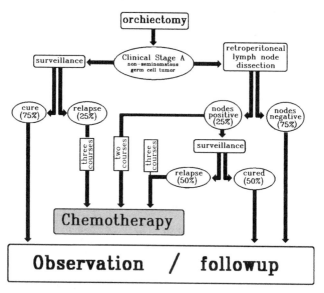

Fig. 15.8. Algorithm for management of clinical stage A nonseminomatous germ cell tumor.

positive RPLND, two cycles of chemotherapy with bleomycin, etoposide, and cisplatin (BEP) can be given immediately after RPLND. Alternatively, surveillance can be performed and three cycles of BEP can be given if relapse occurs.

(2)   **Surveillance.** In patients with low risk for relapse, some centers recommend close surveillance after orchiectomy without RPLND. Approximately 25% of patients with clinical stage A NSGCT will relapse during surveillance. Close follow-up monitoring is mandatory, as 2% to 3% of relapses occur >2 years after orchiectomy.

(3)   **Follow-up.** Patients should be followed monthly during the first year after RPLND and every other month during the second year. Because the incidence of bilateral disease is 12%, the opposite testis must be palpated at each visit. Chest x-ray films and serum markers are checked every 3 months for year 1, every 4 months for year 2, every 6 months for years 3 to 5, and annually thereafter until year 10. CT is performed every 3 months for year 1, every 6 months for year 2, and annually for years 3 to 10.

b.   Stages B1 and B2. RPLND is routinely performed for accurate staging of patients with clinical stages B1 and B2 disease. Patients who are upstaged from clinical stage A to pathologic stage B1/2 are treated in the same manner. Up to 90% of patients can be cured with RPLND alone. Relapsing disease responds well to chemotherapy when discovered early. Nevertheless, the trend is toward giving two cycles of combination chemotherapy following RPLND for pathologic stage B2 and even pathologic stage B1 disease. The relapse rate in pathologic stage B disease without chemotherapy is 50% versus 2% with two cycles of postoperative chemotherapy.

c.   Stages B3 and C. Advanced disease (Fig. 15.9) is best treated with primary chemotherapy. Cisplatin-based regimens achieve an 80% cure rate in stage C disease. RPLND plays a secondary role and is used to confirm the effectiveness of chemotherapy. If CT reveals evidence of persistent nodal disease after chemotherapy, surgical exploration is used to establish the histologic picture. Studies have shown these persistent nodal masses to consist of fibrous tissue in 40% of cases, mature teratoma in 40%, and persistent viable tumor in 20%. With viable malignancy, salvage chemotherapy is necessary (see Chapter 16). Timing of the excision of residual tumor is crucial. Markers must have normalized before surgical excision is undertaken. If not, further chemotherapy is indicated.

VI.   Cancer of the penis is essentially squamous cell cancer of the penile skin. The primary lesion usually occurs on the glans penis or inner surface of the foreskin. Invasion of the corporal bodies and urethra is more common than metastatic disease. Death from penile cancer usually results when local growth leads to sepsis, bleeding, or wasting.

A.   Incidence. Carcinoma of the penis is extremely rare in the United States, accounting for <0.5% of adult male malignancies or 1 to 2 cases for every 100,000. There is a 10- to 20-fold higher

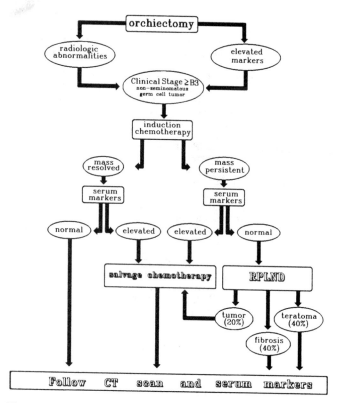

Fig. 15.9. Algorithm for management of stage B3 and higher nonseminomatous germ cell tumor.

incidence in less developed countries, where it may account for up to 10% of cancers in men. Patients tend to present an average of 10 months after the lesion is noted. The average age at presentation is 50 to 70 years.

B.   Etiology. Penile carcinoma is almost never seen in men circumcised at or near birth, leading to speculation that chronic irritation may be a causative factor. Adult circumcision does not confer protection against penile cancer. A viral origin (human papillomavirus type 16) also has been suggested because the incidence of cervical cancer is three- to eightfold higher in women with male partners who have penile cancer. A history of smoking has also been correlated with increased risk of penile cancer.

C.   Classification of penile neoplasms

  1.   Epithelial dysplasias

    a.   Leukoplakia is associated with chronic irritation and often found adjacent to carcinoma.

    b.   Balanitis xerotica obliterans is a severe, chronic inflammatory lesion of the glans (meatus) and foreskin.

2.   Carcinoma in situ consists of malignant changes without invasion through the basement membrane.

   a.   Erythroplasia of Queyrat consists of erythematous velvety plaques on the glans; the condition is often painful and clearly premalignant.

   b.   Bowen's disease is intraepithelial carcinoma of the penile shaft. It is a harbinger of visceral malignancy in 25% of patients.

3.   Squamous cell carcinoma accounts for 98% of cases of penile cancer, with approximately 40% of patients presenting with superficial disease at diagnosis. It is also called epidermoid carcinoma. Verrucous carcinomas (giant condyloma or Buschke–Lowenstein tumor) constitutes approximately 5% of penile cancers. This variant of squamous cell carcinoma spreads locally with a characteristic sharply defined deep margin and has a low metastatic potential. It is usually well controlled with local excision.

4.   Basal cell carcinoma is extremely rare, and fewer than 15 cases have been documented. Treatment is local excision, which is almost always curative.

5.   Melanoma. Fewer than 60 cases have been reported. This presents as a blue–black pigmented papule or ulceration on the glans penis. Surgery is the primary mode of therapy, with radiotherapy of only adjunctive or palliative benefit.

6.   Sarcoma. These may be benign or malignant. Malignant lesions were found on the proximal shaft. The most common malignant lesions are of vascular origin, such as hemangioepithelioma. Local recurrence is characteristic of sarcomas.

7.   Metastatic tumors to the penis are rare, but 75% of them are of genitourinary origin—most commonly bladder and prostate cancers followed by colorectal cancers.

D.   Route of spread is via the regional lymphatics to the superficial and deep inguinal nodes and then to the iliac nodes. Lymphatics from the prepuce drain to the superficial and deep inguinal lymphatics. Lymphatics of the glans, corpora, and urethra drain to the deep inguinal and external iliac nodes. Distant metastases occur in <10% of patients and involve lungs, liver, and bone. Patients with local penile recurrence have a mean survival of 7 years, whereas inguinal nodal recurrence is associated with a mean survival of <2 years.

E.   Diagnosis. Carcinoma of the penis usually begins as a small lesion, most commonly on the glans penis or prepuce. Lesions may be papillary or ulcerative. Most penile carcinomas are not painful, which may account for the long delay in seeking medical attention. It has been reported that up to 50% of patients delay medical treatment for at least 1 year from the time of initial awareness of the lesion. This may be due to patient embarrassment or denial; thus, it is the urologist's responsibility to educate the public and other physicians about the disease. Other symptoms may include penile discharge and dysuria. Approximately 50% of patients have palpable inguinal nodes at the time of presentation, but these are usually inflammatory rather than neoplastic (see below). Diagnosis is established by punch biopsy or excisional biopsy in the operating room. The differential diagnosis includes syphilitic chancre, chancroid, and condylomata acuminata.

F.   Staging. The **Jackson staging system,** based on degree of local invasion and metastases to lymph nodes and other organs, correlates well with 5-year survival. Table 15.18 compares the Jackson and AJCC staging systems. Clinical staging is based on biopsy, urethroscopy, and CT or MRI of the pelvis and abdomen.

G.   Treatment of penile cancer is currently evolving, with the introduction of many penile-sparing modalities. Because most penile carcinomas are initially superficial and located at or near the glans, early diagnosis often makes it possible to avoid radical surgery. Lesions located entirely on the prepuce may be cured by circumcision alone if a 2-cm margin is achievable. Small lesions on the glans may be treated effectively by laser therapy or Mohs technique.

1.   Partial or total penectomy is indicated in most instances of invasive penile carcinoma. Clinical stage T1 tumors require at least partial penectomy to ensure disease-free prox-

Table 15.18.   AJCC and Jackson staging systems in penile cancer

AJCC Stage	Description	Jackson Stage
Primary tumor		
TIS	Carcinoma in situ	
Ta	Noninvasive verrucous carcinoma	I
T1	Invasion of subepithelial connective tissue	I
T2	Invasion of corpus spongiosum or cavernosum	II
T3	Invasion of urethra or prostate	III/IV
T4	Invasion of other adjacent structures	IV
Lymph nodes		
N1	Metastasis in single superficial inguinal lymph node	III
N2	Metastases in multiple or bilateral superficial inguinal lymph nodes	III
N3	Metastases in deep inguinal or pelvic lymph nodes, unilateral or bilateral	III
Metastases		
M1	Distant metastases	IV
Definition of Jackson staging system		
Stage I	Tumor confined to glans or prepuce	
Stage II	Invasion of corpora, no nodal or distant metastases	
Stage III	Tumor confined to penis, regional lymph node metastases present	
Stage IV	Tumor beyond penis, inoperable regional nodes or distant metastases	

AJCC, American Joint Committee on Cancer.

imal margins of 2 cm. Preservation of sexual function may be achieved with 6 cm of remaining corpus cavernosum length. In cases involving the entire shaft or base of the penis, total penectomy and perineal urethrostomy are required.

   a. Inguinal lymphadenectomy. The status of the inguinal lymph nodes and how they are managed are the most important determinants of patient survival in penile cancer.

   (1) Palpable adenopathy is present in about 50% of patients at presentation. Of these patients, only 30% to 60% will have histologic evidence of tumor in lymph nodes. In the remainder, adenopathy is caused by infection or inflammation of the penis. Bilateral inguinal lymphadenectomy is indicated in men who present with palpable inguinal adenopathy that does not resolve after appropriate antibiotic therapy.

   (2) Absent palpable adenopathy. Of the patients without palpable adenopathy at presentation, up to 20% overall will have histologic evidence of nodal disease. This is highly dependent on tumor stage, as only 10% will be positive in T1 tumors, whereas 60% will be positive in T2/3 tumors. Thus, prophylactic bilateral ilioinguinal node dissection should be performed in patients with larger (>5 cm), grade 2 or 3, and more invasive tumors. Delayed lymphadenectomy may be appropriate in selected cases of low-stage, low-volume disease. However, this strategy carries a high risk of recurrence and treatment failure.

   b. Technique of inguinal lymphadenectomy. Bilateral node dissection is associated with a complication rate of 50% and a mortality rate of 1%. Considerable morbidity, including lymphedema, wound necrosis, phlebitis, and pulmonary embolism, may be seen. Changes in technique have limited the complications that were once seen after lymph node dissection; these include sparing the greater saphenous vein and covering the wound with sartorius muscle.

   c. Pelvic lymphadenectomy may be appropriate in healthy, younger patients with pelvic lymph node enlargement on pelvic CT scan. The therapeutic benefit of the operation has not been clearly established.

2. Radiation. External-beam radiation (50 Gy over 5 weeks) has been used as an alternative to partial penectomy. It may be especially useful in younger patients with minimally invasive (T1) lesions to avoid the psychological trauma of penectomy; however, radiation is minimally effective in larger invasive lesions (T2 lesions or higher), and morbidity from radiotherapy in such cases can be quite high. Nearly all patients develop urethritis and edema during radiation therapy; late complications include urethral stricture, fistula formation, meatal stenosis, and discoloration of the penile skin. Another technique to maximize local dose employs **iridium-192** wire brachytherapy. Local control can be achieved in 90% of cases with T1 disease. However, the recurrence rate at 2 years is 63% and 80% by 5 years. Circumcision must be performed before radiation treatment to reduce local morbidity.

3.   Neodymium-YAG laser. Recent trials have demonstrated that with close follow-up, patients with carcinoma in situ and T1 disease of the penis may be effectively treated with the neodymium-YAG laser. This may result in better cosmetic result and the same cure rates. Retreatment with the laser or partial/total penectomy may be necessary in recurrent cases.

4.   Mohs surgery, the meticulous removal of cancerous tissue under microscopic control, is appealing in low-stage penile cancer. Local control may be achieved in >90% of cases. Lesions <1 cm are nearly always successfully treated with Mohs surgery, whereas those >3 cm have a cure rate of only 50%.

5.   Management by stage of disease

   a.   Stage TIS penile cancer (Bowen's disease or erythroplasia of Queyrat) may be successfully treated with topical 5-fluorouracil. Local control rates are good, with excellent cosmetic results. Surgical laser ablation and radiation therapy are also effective modalities for initial treatment.

   b.   Stage Ta disease requires local surgical excision with attention to adequate margins and careful follow-up.

   c.   Stage T1 penile cancer. For the patient with a stage T1 primary tumor and palpable adenopathy, a 4- to 6-week course of antibiotics is prescribed. If the adenopathy resolves, the patient is followed closely. If adenopathy does not resolve, an ilioinguinal lymph node dissection is performed on the affected side, whereas a superficial or modified dissection may be done on the contralateral noninvolved side. In contrast, if the patient develops inguinal adenopathy on one side after a long disease-free interval, a unilateral lymphadenectomy is recommended with observation of the opposite side.

   d.   Stage T2 or T3 penile cancer. For patients with stage T2 or T3 penile cancer and no palpable adenopathy, a bilateral lymph node dissection should be performed for reasons discussed above. Contralateral lymph node dissection is performed because of the 50% chance of contralateral disease developing via lymphatic crossover. Superficial node dissection may be performed on the contralateral side and extended if frozen section indicates any nodal involvement. This reduces the incidence of surgical morbidity.

   e. For **Stage N3** patients, pelvic lymph node biopsy is performed first. Bilateral lymph node dissection is performed only if the result of this pelvic lymph node biopsy is negative. This course is dictated by the fact that cure is rare if pelvic nodal disease is present. Iliac nodes positive for tumor metastases have been found in 15% to 30% of patients with positive inguinal nodes.

   f.   Metastatic disease has been a challenge to urologists. Radiation therapy for node-positive disease has resulted in a <12% cure rate for stages T1, T2, and T3 disease. Most treatment protocols rely on chemotherapeutic agents such as bleomycin, cisplatin, and methotrexate, with methotrexate demonstrating up to a 60% response rate, although this is usually not long-lasting. Combined modalities have in-

cluded postoperative adjuvant chemotherapy and radiation
to positive nodal disease.

H.   Prognosis. For localized disease without metastasis, the
5-year survival rate is 60% to 90%. With inguinal but not iliac
nodal involvement, this drops to 30% to 50%. When iliac nodes
are involved, the 5-year survival rate is 20%. There are no known
5-year survivors among patients with distant metastases.

SUGGESTED READING

Cabanas RM. An approach for treatment of penile carcinomas. *Cancer*
1977;39:456–466.

Carter HB, Epstein JI, Partin AW. Influence of age and prostate-
specific antigen on the chance of curable prostate cancer among
men with nonpalpable disease. *Urology* 1999;53:127–130.

Carter HB, Pearson JD, Metter EJ, et al. Longitudinal evaluation of
prostate-specific antigen levels in men with and without prostate
disease. *JAMA* 1992;267:2215.

Catalona WJ, Partin AW, Slawin KM, et al. Use of the percentage of
free prostate-specific antigen to enhance differentiation of prostate
cancer from benign prostatic disease: a prospective multicenter
clinical trial. *JAMA* 1998;279:1542.

Chen GL, Bagley DH. Ureteroscopic management of upper tract
transitional cell carcinoma in patients with normal contralateral
kidneys. *J Urol* 2000;164:1173–1176.

Chodak GW, Thisted RA, Gerber GS, et al. Results of conservative
management of clinically localized prostate cancer. *N Engl J Med*
1994;330:242–248.

Cookson MS, Herr HW, Zhang ZF, et al. The treated natural history
of high risk superficial bladder cancer: 15-year outcome. *J Urol*
1997;158:62.

Crook J, Grimard L, Tsihlias J, et al. Interstitial brachytherapy for
penile cancer: an alternative to amputation. *J Urol* 2002;167:506.

De La Taille A, Benson MC, Bagiella E, et al. Cryoablation for clinically
localized prostate cancer using an argon-based system: complication
rates and biochemical recurrence. *Br J Urol Int* 2000;85:281.

Donohue JP, Zachary JM, Maynard BR, et al. Distribution of total
metastases in nonseminomatous testis cancer. *J Urol* 1982;128:
315–320.

Epstein JI, Amin MB, Reuter VR, et al. The World Health Organization/
International Society of Urological Pathology consensus classification of urothelial (transitional cell) neoplasms of the urinary bladder. Bladder Consensus Conference Committee. *Am J Surg Pathol*
1998;22:1435.

Fair WR, Cookson MS, Stroumbakis N, et al. The indications, rationale,
and results of neoadjuvant androgens deprivation in the treatment
of prostatic cancer: Memorial Sloan–Kettering Cancer Center results. *Urology* 1997;49(suppl 3A):46–55.

Gettman MT, Blute ML, Spotts B, et al. Pathologic staging of renal
cell carcinoma: significance of tumor classification with the 1997
TNM staging system. *Cancer* 2001;91:354.

Glas AS, Roos D, Deutekom M, et al. Tumor markers in the diagnosis
of primary bladder cancer: a systematic review. *J Urol* 2003;169:
1975–1982.

Greene FL, Page DL, Fleming ID, et al., eds. *American Joint Committee on Cancer (AJCC) cancer staging manual.* 6th ed. New York:
Springer-Verlag, 2002.

Hall MC, Womack S, Sagalowsky AI. Prognostic factors, recurrence, and survival in transitional cell carcinoma of the upper urinary tract: a 30-year experience in 252 patients. *Urology* 1998;52: 594–601.

Halling KC, King W, Sokolova IA, et al. Carcinoma of the penis: analysis of therapy in 100 consecutive cases. *J Urol* 1972;108: 428–430.

Halling KC, King W, Sokolova IA, et al. A comparison of BTA stat, hemoglobin dipstick, telomerase and Vysis UroVysion assays for the detection of urothelial carcinoma in urine. *J Urol* 2002;167: 2001–2006.

Hurley LJ, Libertino JA. Recurrence of nonseminomatous germ cell tumor 9 years postoperatively: is surveillance alone acceptable? *J Urol* 1995;153:1060–1062.

Ianari A, Sternberg CN, Rossetti A, et al. Results of Bard BTA test in monitoring patients with a history of transitional cell cancer of the bladder. *Urology* 1997;49:786–789.

Johansson JE. Watchful waiting for early-stage prostate cancer. *Urology* 1994;43:138–142.

Kirby R. Treatment options for early prostate cancer. *Urology* 1998; 52:948–962.

Koga S, Tsuda S, Nishikido M, et al. The diagnostic value of bone scan in patients with renal cell carcinoma. *J Urol* 2001;166:2126.

Koppie TM, Shinohara K, Grossfeld GD, et al. The efficacy of cryosurgical ablation of prostate cancer: the University of California, San Francisco, experience. *J Urol* 1999;162:427.

Kurth KH. Superficial transitional cell carcinoma: bacillus Calmette-Guérin (BCG) and other intravesical agents. *Curr Opin Urol* 1998; 8:425–429.

Lamm DL, Stogdill VD, Stogdill BJ, et al. Complications of bacillus Calmette-Guérin immunotherapy in 1,278 patients with bladder cancer. *J Urol* 1986;135:272–274.

Lee BR, Jabbour ME, Marshall FF. 13-year survival comparison of percutaneous and open nephroureterectomy approaches for management of transitional cell carcinoma of renal collecting system: equivalent outcomes. *J Endourol* 1999;13:289–294.

Mazeron JJ. Interstitial radiation therapy for carcinoma of the penis using iridium-192 wires: the Henry Mondor experience (1970–1979). *Int J Radiat Oncol Biol Phys* 1984;10:1891–1895.

McCarthy JF, Catalona WJ, Hudson MA. Effect of radiation therapy on detectable serum prostate-specific antigen levels following radical prostatectomy: early versus delayed treatment. *J Urol* 1994; 151:1575–1578.

Mian C, Pycha A, Wiener H, et al. Immunocyt: a new tool for detecting transitional cell cancer of the urinary tract. *J Urol* 1999;161: 1486.

Montie JE, Straffon RA, Stewart BH. Radical cystectomy without radiation therapy for carcinoma of bladder. *J Urol* 1984;131: 477–482.

O'Keefe SC, Marshall FF, Issa MM, et al. Thrombocytosis is associated with a significant increase in the cancer specific death rate after radical nephrectomy. *J Urol* 2002;168:1378.

Pankratz VS, Lieber MM, Blute ML, et al. A comparison of BTA stat, hemoglobin dipstick, telomerase and Vysis UroVysion assays for the detection of urothelial carcinoma in urine. *J Urol* 2002;167: 2001–2006.

Partin AW, Yoo J, Carter HB, et al. The use of prostate-specific antigen, clinical stage and Gleason score to predict pathological stage in men with localized prostate cancer. *J Urol* 1993;150:110–114.

Roach M, Lu J, Pilepich MV, et al. Prostate-specific antigen density (PSAD): role in patient evaluation and management. *Urol Clin North Am* 1993;20:653.

Roach M, Lu J, Pilepich MV, et al. Four prognostic groups predict long-term survival from prostate cancer following radiotherapy alone in Radiation Therapy Oncology Group clinical trials. *Int J Radiat Oncol Biol Phys* 2000;1;47:609–615.

Seaman E, Whang M, Olsson CA, et al. Prostate-specific antigen density (PSAD): role in patient evaluation and management. *Urol Clin North Am* 1993;20:653.

Shalhav AL, Dunn MD, Portis AJ. Laparoscopic nephroureterectomy for upper tract transitional cell cancer: the Washington University experience. *J Urol* 2000;163:1100–1104.

Soloway MS, Briggman JV, Carpinito GA, et al. Use of a new tumor marker, urinary NMP22, in the detection of occult or rapidly recurring transitional cell carcinoma of the urinary tract following surgical treatment. *J Urol* 1996;156:363–367.

Solsona E, Iborra I, Ricos JV, et al. Effectiveness of a single immediate mitomycin C instillation in patients with low risk superficial bladder cancer: short and long-term followup. *J Urol* 1999;161:1120.

Stanford JL, Feng Z, Hamilton AS, et al. Urinary and sexual function after radical prostatectomy for clinically localized prostate cancer. The Prostate Cancer Outcomes Study. *JAMA* 2000;283:354–360.

Storkel S, van den Berg E. Morphological classification of renal cancer. *World J Urol* 1995;13:153–158.

Truong CD, Krishman B, Loa JJ, et al. Renal neoplasm in acquired cystic kidney disease. *Am J Kidney Dis* 1995;26:1–12.

van Bezooijen BP, Horenblas S, Meinhardt W, et al. Laser therapy for carcinoma in situ of the penis. *J Urol* 2001;166:1670.

Wallace DM, Bloom HJC. The management of deeply infiltrating (T3) bladder carcinoma: controlled trial of radical radiotherapy versus preoperative radiotherapy and radical cystectomy. *Br J Urol* 1976; 48:587–594.

Yaycioglu O, Roberts WW, Chan T, et al. Prognostic assessment of nonmetastatic renal cell carcinoma: a clinically based model. *Urology* 2001;58:141.

Zietman AL, Coen JJ, Shipley WU, et al. Radical radiation therapy in the management of prostatic adenocarcinoma: the initial prostate-specific antigen value as a predictor of treatment outcome. *J Urol* 1994;151:640–645.

Zisman A, Pantuck AJ, Dorey F, et al. Improved prognostication of renal cell carcinoma using an integrated staging system. *J Clin Oncol* 2001;19:1649.

16

Medical Management of Genitourinary Malignancy

Ignacio F. San Francisco and Ken Zaner

Malignancies of the genitourinary organs demonstrate widely varying sensitivities to currently available anticancer agents. At one end of the spectrum are germ cell tumors of the testis. As a direct consequence of their high degree of chemosensitivity, such tumors are curable in the vast majority of instances. In contrast, conventional chemotherapy has had essentially no impact on survival in patients with adenocarcinoma of the kidney. Between these two extremes are carcinomas of the bladder and prostate, wherein some success with chemotherapy has been achieved. Impressive rates of response have been achieved with the use of combination chemotherapeutic regimens in bladder cancer. In prostate cancer, however, only modest success with cytotoxic chemotherapy has been achieved, although hormonal management can delay the appearance of metastases.

I. General principles

A. Selective toxicity was first applied successfully in the area of antimicrobial chemotherapy. However, in contrast to the major metabolic differences between microorganisms and normal host cells, the differences between malignant and normal cells are often minimal. As a result, the gap between antitumor effect and intolerable host toxicity ("therapeutic index") is often narrow, limiting the clinical usefulness of many chemotherapeutic agents.

B. Mechanisms of drug activity

1. Cell growth cycle. Both normal and neoplastic cells pass through a qualitatively similar process of cell replication. This cell cycle consists of several phases, which are characterized by specific kinetic or synthetic activities (Fig. 16.1). After the completion of mitosis (M), cells spend a variable period of time synthesizing RNA and proteins (G_1); a phase of DNA synthesis (S) follows, then a second phase of RNA and protein synthesis (G_2). During mitosis, cells divide and two daughter cells are formed. Within any tissue, whether normal or neoplastic, a fraction of cells is not actively replicating; the term G_0 denotes this "resting" phase. Cells in G_0 may be recruited back into the replication cycle via the G_1 phase. Most chemotherapeutic drugs exert their antineoplastic effect by interfering with the synthesis or function of crucial macromolecules. These drugs are often classified according to their activity with respect to the cell cycle. Some agents (cytarabine, methotrexate) are most active against cells in a particular phase and are termed **cycle-specific phase-specific drugs.** Others (cyclophosphamide, doxorubicin) are most active against cycling cells but are not most active during any particular phase of the cycle; they are termed **cycle-specific phase-nonspecific**

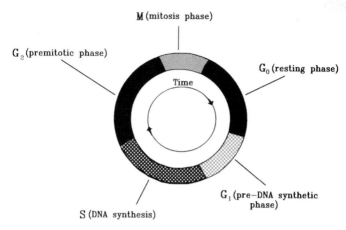

Fig. 16.1.   The cell cycle. M, mitosis; G_1, pre-DNA synthetic phase;
S, DNA synthetic phase; G_2, premitotic phase; G_0, resting phase.

drugs. A third category (carmustine, lomustine) appears to be
active irrespective of whether the cells are replicating; these
are termed **cycle-nonspecific drugs.**

2.   The **log cell kill hypothesis** states that a constant fraction of neoplastic cells will die with any drug treatment,
irrespective of the size of the tumor. For convenience, the
fractional cell kill is often expressed as a logarithm. The ex-
ponential growth of a tumor treated by surgery and then
chemotherapy is depicted in Fig. 16.2. Note that unless
100% of tumor cells are ablated by treatment—an unlikely
result with any currently available chemotherapy regimen—
regrowth is likely. However, multiple treatment cycles delivered at sufficiently frequent intervals can theoretically eradicate all tumor cells completely.

3.   **Drug resistance.** In the preceding example (Fig. 16.2),
complete tumor eradication depended on a number of factors,
including uniform cancer cell sensitivity to the cytotoxic agent
employed. Unfortunately, in the real world, cancer chemotherapy is often unsuccessful—not only because some cancer cells
within a given tumor are not sensitive to a given drug, but also
because initially sensitive cells can acquire resistance to multiple chemotherapeutic agents during the course of treatment.

   a.   Acquired resistance. Generally, if tumor cells are resistant to a particular agent, they will also be resistant to
   other agents in the same class or with a similar mechanism
   of cytotoxic action. Conversely, they will remain sensitive
   to agents with a different mechanism of action.

      (1)   Kinetic resistance is presumed to be a common
      mechanism accounting for the failure of cycle- and phase-
      specific agents to kill neoplastic cells. For example, in
      many human tumors, the bulk of the neoplastic cells are
      in the resting (G_0) phase.

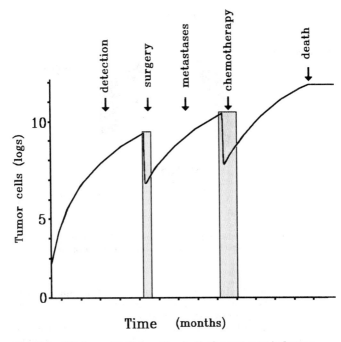

Fig. 16.2.   The log cell kill hypothesis. Each treatment induces a 2 log tumor cell reduction, which, coupled with an intercycle tumor regrowth of 0.5 log, results in a net tumor cell kill of 1.5 log per treatment.

(2)   **Inadequate delivery.** An antineoplastic agent may fail to reach the tumor cells in adequate concentration because of poor perfusion of necrotic tumor, poor absorption from the gastrointestinal tract, or, in the case of tumors of the central nervous system, the blood–brain barrier.

(3)   **Biochemical resistance.** A number of biochemical mechanisms can foil effective drug action, including accelerated drug breakdown, decreased activation, cell-bypass mechanisms, impermeability of cell membranes, and increased repair of cytotoxic lesions. **Multiple-drug resistance** may be conferred by a glycoprotein that enhances drug efflux from cells.

b.   **Natural resistance.** Cancer cells may have an inherent resistance to a drug without previous exposure to the agent, so-called "natural resistance." The theory of natural resistance holds that with increasing tumor size, a steady state is reached in which most cells are no longer rapidly proliferating. Furthermore, the larger the tumor mass, the more likely it is that drug-resistant cells will develop. This theory, although unproven, explains the inverse relationship between tumor size and chemoresponsiveness as well as the superiority of combination chemotherapy over single-drug therapy in many situations.

c. Resistance and apoptosis. Apoptosis is organized cell death in response to various stimuli. Appreciation of apoptosis as a unifying concept in the mechanism of chemotherapy action and resistance has grown recently. Apoptotic cell death is caused by specific biochemical machinery, which is activated by molecular alterations in the cell. A necessary mutation in the cancer transformation process is the loss of some part of the apoptotic machinery. Chemotherapy in many cases can cause sufficient damage to these cells to induce cell death. However, once all of the apoptotic machinery has been lost, the cell becomes resistant to chemotherapy.

C. Toxicity. Cancer chemotherapeutic agents are often associated with frequent and severe adverse effects. Such toxicity may severely limit patient tolerance and the ultimate clinical usefulness of a regimen. It is the responsibility of any physician administering these agents to be familiar with the toxic profile of each drug and to monitor the patient properly so that appropriate action can be taken to limit toxicity. With the exception of nausea and vomiting, the most common toxicities of chemotherapeutic agents derive from their effects on the rapidly growing cells of the bone marrow and epithelium. Adverse effects are discussed in more detail in the section on chemotherapeutic agents.

D. Guidelines for chemotherapy

1. Establish a **pathologic diagnosis.** Antineoplastic drug therapy should never, except in rare circumstances, be instituted without a firm cytologic or histologic diagnosis.

2. Establish the **stage of disease.** In this chapter, tumor–node–metastasis (TNM) staging refers to the most recent American Joint Committee on Cancer system. Proper planning of treatment and follow-up both depend on accurate assessment of tumor stage at the time of diagnosis.

3. Establish the patient's **performance status.** Table 16.1 summarizes the commonly used Karnofsky Performance

Table 16.1. Karnofsky Performance Scale

Rating (%)	Characteristics
100	Normal, no evidence of disease
90	Minor symptoms or signs
80	More pronounced symptoms or signs
70	Cannot work but able to care for self
60	Requires some assistance
50	Requires considerable assistance
40	Requires special care and assistance
30	Severely disabled
20	Hospitalization necessary
10	Death imminent
0	Dead

Scale. In many forms of cancer, the patient's performance status has proved to be one of the most important prognostic factors with respect to tolerance and response to chemotherapy.

4.   Establish **treatment goals.** Realistic goals should be established based on the histologic diagnosis, tumor stage, and patient performance status (Table 16.1). In some diseases, a complete response (CR) is a realistic goal (testis cancer), but in others, palliation or a partial response (PR) is all that can be achieved (bone metastases in prostate cancer).

5.   Consider the **risks and benefits** of chemotherapy.

6.   Establish the appropriate **dose, schedule, and route** of administration.

7.   Establish **response criteria.** It is crucial to define objective response criteria at the initiation of treatment (Table 16.2). The most rigorous response criteria are based on patient survival or reduction in tumor size. When the extent of disease is poorly defined, subjective patient response criteria may be employed (e.g., bone pain in prostate cancer).

8.   Establish a system to monitor **toxicity.** For most agents, this includes determination of white blood cell and platelet counts and performance of liver function tests at regular intervals during and after chemotherapy. For some agents, additional monitors are needed, such as tests of renal function, pulmonary function, and nerve conduction.

E.   **Combination therapy,** in which chemotherapy is combined with surgery and/or radiotherapy, is sometimes indicated. For certain patients who have undergone cancer surgery and manifest known risk factors for relapse or development of metastatic disease, chemotherapy may be indicated even though no evidence of relapse or recurrence is present. This is called **adjuvant therapy.** Examples of known risk factors include a high tumor grade, presence of tumor at resection margins, and intravascular invasion. In contrast, therapy administered before surgery (**neoadjuvant therapy**) is intended to treat undetectable micrometastases and reduce tumor size (**tumor debulking**).

II.   Chemotherapeutic agents

A.   **Alkylating agents** are exemplified by cyclophosphamide and ifosfamide (Fig. 16.3).

Table 16.2.   Clinical criteria for treatment response

Type of Response	Definition
Complete	Complete disappearance of all measurable lesions
Partial	>50% reduction of all measurable lesions No increase in any lesion No new lesions
Stable	<50% reduction of measurable lesions or <25% increase of measurable lesions
Progression	>25% increase of measurable lesions or appearance of new lesions

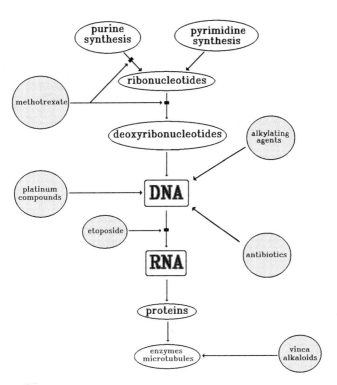

Fig. 16.3. Mechanisms by which chemotherapeutic agents interfere with DNA replication and protein synthesis.

1.   Mechanism of action. As the name implies, this group of agents impairs cell function by substituting alkyl groups for hydrogen atoms on a variety of biologically important molecules. The action of these drugs on DNA interrupts the accurate or complete replication of the DNA molecule and results in mutagenesis or cell death. The alkylating agents are cell cycle specific but not phase specific and thus can kill cells at all points in the growth cycle. In addition, at least some drugs in this class appear also to act on noncycling cells (cycle nonspecific).

2.   Toxicities

   a.   Leukopenia and thrombocytopenia are dose-limiting toxicities that, for most drugs in this class, recover by about 3 weeks. Cyclophosphamide is relatively platelet sparing. The nitrosoureas, in contrast to the other members of this class, cause a nadir in granulocytes and platelets, which occurs at 5 to 6 weeks and may take 8 to 10 weeks to recover.

   b.   Hemorrhagic cystitis can develop in up to 10% of patients during or after cyclophosphamide therapy. Its incidence may be reduced by keeping the patient well hydrated and encouraging frequent emptying of the bladder. Hemorrhagic cystitis from ifosfamide can be particularly severe, and its administration requires concurrent administration with 2-mercaptoethanesulfonic acid (MESNA). See Chapter 1 for the treatment of hemorrhagic cystitis.

c. **Secondary neoplasia.** An increased risk for secondary malignancy is associated with virtually all alkylating agents.

d. **Amenorrhea or azoospermia** is common with all alkylating agents. Azoospermia following chemotherapy lasts for approximately 18 months in most patients but can be permanent.

e. **Pulmonary fibrosis** is uncommon but well described with several alkylating agents, particularly the nitrosoureas and mitomycin C. Periodic pulmonary function testing may be required in patients receiving these agents.

B. **Platinum agents** are exemplified by cisplatin and carboplatin.

1. **Mechanism of action.** These compounds form adducts of the platinum atom to DNA. Several damage-recognition proteins such as high mobility group 1 and 2 (HMG1 and HGM2) recognize cisplatin-damaged structures. Proliferating cells are much more sensitive than those in G_0/G_1, and programmed cell death may be involved.

2. **Toxicities**

a. **Gastrointestinal.** Cisplatin is among the most emetogenic chemotherapy agents currently in use. The advent of 5-hydroxytryptamine-3 (5-HT3) antagonists such as granisetron and odansetron has virtually eliminated the negative impact on the quality of life of patients receiving this drug. Although carboplatin is also emetogenic, it is significantly less so than cisplatin.

b. **Granulocytopenia and thrombocytopenia.** Cisplatin causes only mild granulocytopenia and thrombocytopenia and can therefore be combined with agents that cause greater blood count suppression. In contrast, carboplatin causes dose-limiting suppression of granulocytes and platelets.

c. **Renal tubular damage.** Acute renal tubular necrosis is associated with administration of cisplatin and is often the dose-limiting factor. Renal dysfunction related to platinum develops in approximately 25% of patients. It may be prevented for the most part by vigorous hydration along with mannitol- or furosemide-induced diuresis. On the other hand, carboplatin has much less renal toxicity and does not require large volumes of fluid administration. Carboplatin can be administered to patients with a creatinine clearance of >25 mL/min, whereas cisplatin requires a clearance of >50 mL/min.

d. **Ototoxicity,** manifested as high-frequency hearing loss, is quite common with cisplatin. Periodic hearing tests are recommended.

e. **Peripheral neuropathy** is not uncommon with increasing cumulative doses of cisplatin and can mandate a halt to therapy.

C. Antimetabolites are exemplified by methotrexate, 5-fluo-rouracil (5-FU), and gemcitabine.

1. Mechanism of action. The antimetabolites are a group of low-molecular-weight compounds that structurally resemble normal cell metabolites involved in nucleic acid synthesis. They exert their antineoplastic action by interfering with enzyme systems or by being incorporated into nucleic acids. For example, methotrexate inhibits dihydrofolate reductase, thus interfering with DNA synthesis. Gemcitabine (2′, 2′-difluo-rodeoxycytidine) is a difluorinated analogue of deoxycytidine whose metabolites deplete the intracellular pools of deoxynucleotide triphosphates. The antimetabolites are, for the most part, cycle specific and phase specific, so that the number of cancer cells that can be killed by a single exposure is limited. As a result, increased efficacy requires either more prolonged drug exposure, repeated drug doses, or recruitment of cells into active DNA synthesis. The antimetabolites tend to be the most schedule dependent of all classes of antineoplastic agents.

2. Toxicity. Doses of methotrexate in excess of 80 mg/m^2 require increased hydration, urinary alkalinization, and monitoring of serum levels (Table 16.3). Administration of citrovorum factor (folinic acid) may alleviate the toxicity of methotrexate if given within the first few hours after methotrexate administration. By providing a form of folate, it is hoped that normal cells may be "rescued" without a reduction in the antitumor activity of methotrexate. Additional miscellaneous toxicities include the following:

a. Neurologic toxicity is not uncommon with very high doses of cytarabine and occasionally with 5-FU.

b. Skin hyperpigmentation is occasionally seen with 5-FU.

c. Renal tubular damage. Renal insufficiency requires substantial dose reduction or discontinuance of methotrexate.

d. Gastrointestinal. 5-FU can occasionally cause mild diarrhea. However, the rare patients who are deficient in dihydropyrimidinase can have-life threatening diarrhea, mucositis, granulocytopenia, and thrombocytopenia as a result of 5-FU administration.

D. Topoisomerase-interactive agents include etoposide, topotecan, irinotecan, doxorubicin, daunorubicin, and mitoxantrone.

1. Mechanism of action. Topoisomerase I and II are enzymes that alter the bending characteristics of the DNA molecule, facilitating replication. Topotecan and irinotecan are topoisomerase I inhibitors, whereas the other drugs inhibit predominantly topoisomerase II or both I and II.

2. Toxicities. The predominant toxicity is a dose-dependent granulocytopenia and thrombocytopenia, with a nadir at 10 to 14 days and recovery at 21 to 28 days. Irinotecan can cause severe diarrhea and is usually the dose-limiting toxicity. Doxorubicin and daunorubicin cause cardiotoxicity that increases with increasing cumulative dose. Mitoxantrone less commonly causes cardiotoxicity and is a better choice in elderly patients.

Table 16.3. Toxicity of selected chemotherapeutic agents

Reaction	Alkylating Agents		Antimetabolites		Vinca Alkaloids		Antibiotics	
	CY	CS	MT	FU	VB	VC	DR	BL
Myelosuppression	–	+	+++	++	+++	++	+++	+
Nausea, vomiting	+++	+++	+	++	++	+	++	+
Diarrhea	+	+	++	++	+	–	+	–
Alopecia	++	+	++	+	++	++	+++	++
Nephrotoxicity	–	+++	++	–	–	–	–	–
Neurotoxicity	–	+	–	+	++	+++	+++	–
Cardiac toxicity	–	–	–	–	–	–	+++	–
Pulmonary toxicity	–	–	+	–	–	–	–	+++

CY, cyclophosphamide; CS, cisplatin; MT, methotrexate; FU, 5-fluorouracil; VB, vinblastine; VC, vincristine; DR, doxorubicin; BL, bleomycin.

Nausea and vomiting occur but are less severe than with the platinum compounds.

E. Antimicrotubule agents include the vinca alkaloids (vincristine, vinblastine, and vinorelbine) and the taxanes (paclitaxel and docetaxel).

    1. Mechanism of action. Microtubules are integrally involved in mitosis and are dynamic structures that are in a constant state of polymerization from and depolymerization to the $\alpha\beta$-tubulin heterodimer. The vinca alkaloids bind to the heterodimers and thus block polymerization, whereas the taxanes bind to the polymers and thus block the depolymerization step. The net result is disruption of the microtubule turnover and in turn mitosis. However, there are likely other mechanisms of action also involved.

    2. Toxicities

        a. Myelosuppression. With the exception of vincristine, all of the drugs in this class cause a dose-dependent depression of platelet and granulocyte counts. Surprisingly, paclitaxel has been shown to inhibit the thrombocytopenia caused by carboplatin, and this combination can be given in higher than expected doses.

        b. Neurotoxicity. The vinca alkaloids, particularly vincristine, and the taxanes can produce a dose-related mixed motor–sensory or autonomic neuropathy or both. This toxic effect typically begins with paresthesias of the fingers and toes and often is dose limiting. It can lead to progressive neurologic impairment if treatment is continued.

        c. Anaphylaxis. Severe allergic reactions can be seen with paclitaxel administration, which can be prevented in the majority of patients with premedication with steroids and antihistamines.

        d. Extravasation necrosis. Both vinca alkaloids can produce a severe local tissue necrosis if extravasation occurs during intravenous administration.

        e. Dose-modification factors. Dose reduction or withdrawal may be necessary for all of drugs in the presence of liver dysfunction.

F. Miscellaneous agents such as bleomycin.

    1. Mechanism of action. All the agents in this class are capable of binding with DNA to inhibit its synthesis and that of DNA-dependent RNA. The antibiotics are capable of acting at several phases of the cell cycle and are thus cycle-specific phase-nonspecific agents.

    2. Toxicity

        a. Pulmonary toxicity. Bleomycin can produce a severe, dose-related pulmonary fibrotic process. The cumulative lifetime dose should not exceed 400 U, and pulmonary function should be monitored during treatment. Pulmonary toxicity is characterized by the insidious onset of cough, pleuritic pain, and dyspnea. There is no treatment other than discontinuation of bleomycin, and lung function still may not improve.

        b. Hypersensitivity can be seen idiosyncratically, and patients should be tested with 1 mg of the drug before full dose therapy.

III.   Hormonally active agents

A.   Testosterone, the principal male androgen, is secreted by the testes in response to luteinizing hormone (LH) (Fig. 16.4A). Orchiectomy remains an effective means of reducing serum testosterone levels (Fig. 16.4B). Of the circulating hormone, 98% is bound to sex hormone-binding globulin and albumin and 2% is free. On entry into cells, testosterone is converted by 5α-reductase to its active form, **dihydrotestosterone.** Dihydrotestosterone is then translocated to the cell nucleus. More than 90% of the nuclear dihydrotestosterone is derived from testosterone, the remainder being converted from the weak adrenal androgens androstenedione and dehydroepiandrosterone (Fig. 16.4A). Testosterone provides negative feedback to the hypothalamus and controls the secretion of LH.

B.   LH-releasing hormone (LHRH) agonists include leuprolide and goserelin. Following their administration, LH and testosterone secretion initially increase (the **flare reaction** that occurs in 5% to 10% of patients) and then fall drastically (Fig. 16.4D). Common side effects are impotence, loss of libido, and hot flashes.

C.   Nonsteroidal antiandrogens include flutamide, nilutamide, and bicalutamide. The compounds block the peripheral actions of testosterone, both in the prostate and in the hypothalamus (Fig. 16.4E). Loss of negative feedback to the hypothalamus results in a gradual increase in serum testosterone, which returns to normal after 1 year of treatment. Potency is preserved in 75% of patients. Gynecomastia, diarrhea, and liver dysfunction are common side effects. Nilutamide causes visual disturbances and alcohol intolerance.

D.   Estrogenic compounds such as diethylstilbestrol, conjugated estrogens, and estradiol substitute for the negative feedback effect of testosterone and suppress the secretion of LH. This results in lowering of serum testosterone to castrate levels. Side effects include loss of potency, gynecomastia and breast tenderness, peripheral edema, thrombophlebitis, and pulmonary embolus. Diethylstilbestrol at a daily oral dose of 1 to 3 mg is a cost-effective mode of androgen-withdrawal therapy, but it has been largely replaced by gonadotropin-releasing hormone (GnRH) agonists because of their lower incidence of cardiovascular toxicity and side effects.

E.   Steroidal antiandrogens include cyproterone acetate (not currently available) and megestrol acetate. These compounds produce an estrogen-like effect at the hypothalamus (Fig. 16.4C) as well as a peripheral androgen blockade similar to that of flutamide (Fig. 16.4E). In contrast to estrogenic compounds, steroidal antiandrogens are not associated with significant cardiovascular morbidity. The most frequent side effects are impotence, loss of libido, and breast swelling.

IV.   Biologic and immunologic agents

A.   Bacille Calmette Guérin (BCG) is an attenuated strain of *Mycobacterium bovis* that has been used as an antituberculosis vaccine for many years. It has found major application as intravesical therapy for superficial bladder cancer. BCG appears to have the ability to bind to tumor cells and disrupt epithelium. Following intravesical administration of BCG, increased urine

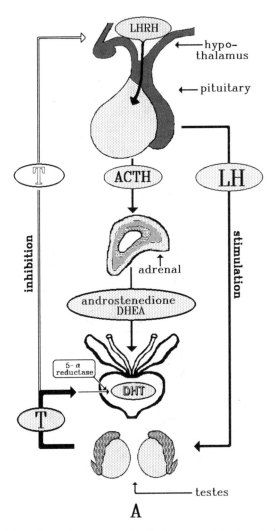

Fig. 16.4. A: Normal hypothalamic–pituitary–gonadal axis. (*continued*)

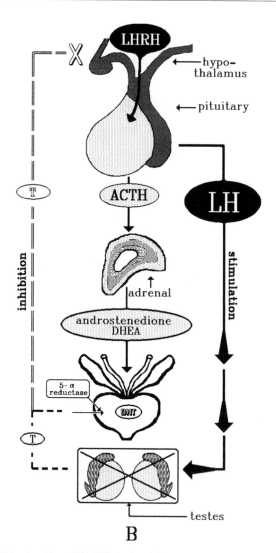

Fig. 16.4.   (*continued*) B: Effect of orchiectomy.

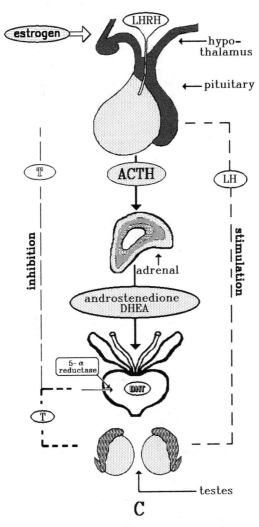

Fig. 16.4. (*continued*) C: Effect of exogenous estrogenic compounds.

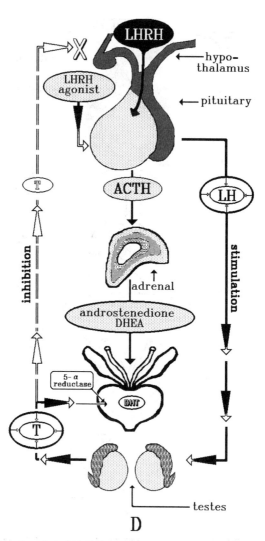

Fig. 16.4. (*continued*) D: Effect of luteinizing hormone-releasing hormone (LHRH) agonists.

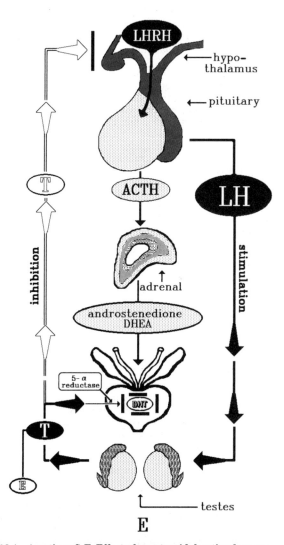

Fig. 16.4. *(continued)* E: Effect of nonsteroidal antiandrogens (flutamide). ACTH, adrenocorticotropic hormone; DHEA, dehydroepiandrosterone; DHT, dihydrotestosterone; T, testosterone.

levels of interleukin-1 (IL-1), Il-2, and tumor necrosis factor have been detected. Major complications are dysuria, urgency, and hematuria. About 5% of patients manifest systemic illness with fever of ≥103°F.

B.   Interferons are a family of molecules subdivided into α, β, γ, and ω subtypes. Interferons appear to augment the effectiveness of cytotoxic T cells and monocytes. Interferon-α2 administered parenterally appears to have some activity in metastatic renal carcinoma. Intravesical administration of interferon-α2 in patients with superficial bladder cancer has produced objective response rates of 40%. The agent has also been used in combination with intravesical BCG. Side effects include fever, malaise, myalgia, headache, anorexia, diarrhea, and mild neutropenia.

C.   ILs are protein products of leukocytes that modulate activity of other leukocytes. IL-2 induces proliferation of T cells and monocytes. IL-2 has been used in metastatic renal cancer, producing a PR in 15% and a CR in 5% of patients.

V.   Renal cell carcinoma

A.   Overview. The medical management of renal cell carcinoma is considered in patients who are not candidates for curative surgery (radical or partial nephrectomy alone) because of metastatic disease or whose disease has recurred after surgery. Renal cell carcinoma extending beyond the limits of surgical resection has proved notoriously refractory to cytotoxic chemotherapy. For this reason, a number of investigations are under way to explore other treatment modes, such as interferon, active specific immunotherapy, and adoptive immunotherapy.

B.   Hormonal therapy in renal cancer. Renal cell carcinoma is not a hormonodependent tumor; nevertheless, progestational agents were originally reported to produce objective response rates of 15% to 20%. Androgens and the antiestrogen tamoxifen also have been noted to have very modest activity in this disease, up to a 2% response rate. Recent studies using more rigid response criteria have failed to substantiate the initial reports, however. These studies have consistently shown that <5% of patients benefit from hormonal therapy. Therefore, these agents are currently not routinely employed.

C.   Chemotherapy. Unfortunately, renal cell carcinoma is considered a chemotherapeutically resistant tumor; therefore, available cytotoxic chemotherapy has had very little impact on this disease. A possible mechanism of resistance is the expression of the multidrug resistance protein (p-glycoprotein/P-170) in the proximal tubule cells where most renal cell carcinomas originate. No single-agent or combination regimen has produced an objective response rate higher than 10%. Vinblastine, 5-FU, and combination chemotherapy regimens are examples of drugs that have been employed with low objective response rates and with increased toxicity, especially in combined regimens.

D.   Immunologic therapy. Currently, immunotherapy is the gold standard in the treatment of metastatic renal cell carcinoma. Renal cancer evokes an immune response, and this treatment may reproduce and enhance this response.

  1.   IL-2. High-dose IL-2 has resulted in 14% response rates in treated patients, with 600,000 to 720,000 IU/kg IV every 8 hours for 5 days for a maximum number of three cycles. The median duration of response is 23 months, although a 4% of mortality rate secondary to toxicity has been described. These doses of IL-2 can produce a severe vascular leak syndrome, which precludes its use in an outpatient or even a community setting. Treatment with lower doses of IL-2 is more appropriate to the community setting. However, the response rates do not appear to be as good as that achieved with high-dose therapy.

2.   Interferon (recombinant leukocyte or human lymphoblastoid interferon) has produced partial regressions in 15% to 20% of treated patients. Median response durations range from 6 to 10 months. The mechanisms of actions are not understood but may include direct tumor-antiproliferative effects and immunostimulatory effects. Intramuscular or subcutaneous doses of 5 to 10×10^6 IU/m^2 have been most often used.

3.   Immunotherapy with previous nephrectomy. In a recent study, patients with metastatic renal cell carcinoma were treated with interferon-α alone (5 mU/m^2) or "debulking nephrectomy" followed by interferon-α. The results showed a significant difference in survival between the two groups, 8.1 versus 12.5 months, respectively. The criteria that should be considered for debulking nephrectomy prior to receiving systemic immunotherapy are the following:

- Greater than 75% tumor debulking possible
- No central nervous system or extensive liver or bone metastases
- Adequate pulmonary and cardiac function
- Eastern Cooperative Oncology Group performance status of 0 or 1
- Biopsy, if performed, showing clear cell-type histology

4.   Other immunologic approaches
a.   Nonmyeloablative allogenic peripheral blood stem cell transplantation. Some studies have shown promising results with response rates up to 50%, but eligibility for this therapy is limited by the need for a human leukocyte antigen–matched sibling donor. This therapy seeks to induce a graft-versus-tumor response.
b.   Future immunotherapy will attempt to introduce more therapeutic specificity. The transfer of cytokine genes to autologous renal carcinoma cells and hybrid cells consisting of tumor and allogeneic dendritic cells may permit new vaccination strategies to induce specific antitumor immunity.

VI.   Urothelial cancer
   A.   Overview. The predominant type of urothelial cancer is transitional cell carcinoma. Chemotherapy has been used for the treatment of urothelial cancer in several clinical settings: (a) superficial bladder cancer amenable to intravesical chemotherapy, (b) low-grade, low-stage urothelial cancer of the upper tract, and (c) advanced local or metastatic cancer from the bladder or upper tract.
   B.   Intravesical therapy. Local and intravesical therapy is appropriate for superficial bladder disease (Tis, Ta, and T1)

Table 16.4.   Intravesical chemotherapeutic agents in bladder cancer

Generic Name	Brand Name	Dose Forms	Dose	
			Initial	Maintenance
Mitomycin C	Mutamycin	5-, 20-, 40-mg vial	20–60 mg weekly × 8	20–60 mg monthly × 12
Thiotepa	Thioplex	15-mg vial	30–60 mg weekly × 6	30–60 mg monthly × 12
Doxorubicin	Adriamycin	10-, 20-, 50-mg vial	60–90 mg q3wk × 8	60–90 mg q6wk × 2, then q12wk × 2

(Table 16.4). This therapy is used to eradicate residual disease, decrease recurrences, and avoid further progression. The most commonly used agent is BCG. Another agent, interferon, directly inhibits the proliferation of bladder tumor cells in vitro and increases bladder tumor cells' surface antigen expression. It decreases the rate of recurrence; in addition, toxicity and local irritation are uncommon. BCG has been compared with interferon for recurrent superficial T1 disease, showing recurrence rates of 39% and 69%, respectively. However, BCG plus interferon has better results in combination, especially in some cases of BCG-resistant transitional cell carcinoma. Other intravesical agents are the chemotherapeutic agents thiotepa (CR 29%, PR 26%), mitomycin C (CR 48%, PR 26%), and doxorubicin (CR 38%, PR 35%). See also Chapter 15.

C. Chemotherapy in locally advanced (stages T2 through T4) disease. Although chemotherapy is not curative for locally advanced disease, it can be of value. Neoadjuvant chemotherapy has the ability to shrink the primary lesion, thus downstaging it, and reduce the incidence of micrometastases, preventing eventual distant metastasis. Although trials have failed to show a consistent survival benefit, it is reasonable to consider multiagent therapy such as methotrexate, vinblastine, doxorubicin, and cisplatin (M-VAC) or taxane-containing regimens in patients with locally advanced disease with acceptable performance status.

D. Chemotherapy in metastatic (stages N2 and M1) disease. At the present time, candidates for systemic chemotherapy include patients who relapse after surgery or radiotherapy and the 10% of patients who present with metastatic disease.

1. Single agents. A number of drugs have demonstrated activity against bladder cancer when used as single agents; for example, cisplatin, the most active agent, has shown a CR of 3% to 9% and a PR of 15% to 35%. Others agents are methotrexate and less active doxorubicin, 5-FU, cyclophosphamide, mitomycin C, and vinblastine. Newer agents with the same activity but less toxicity are paclitaxel, docetaxel, gemcitabine, and ifosfamide. Single agents have shown a limited duration of response; therefore, currently combination chemotherapy regimens are superior and more broadly used for the treatment of advanced transitional cell carcinoma.

2.   Combination regimens. Current results indicate that several combination regimens based on cisplatin are superior to any single agent. The most promising regimens include **M-VAC.** This regimen has yielded an overall response rate of approximately 70%, with a CR in up to 35% of patients. The toxicity of this regimen is severe, however, and experience in managing chemotherapy-induced cytopenias is essential before this or other regimens can be considered. However, newer regimens using taxanes or gemcitabine have shown encouraging results with less toxicity. Currently, the most active regimens are the following:

   a.   M-VAC. Methotrexate 30 mg/m^2 IV days 1, 15, and 22; vinblastine 3 mg/m^2 IV days 2, 15, and 22; doxorubicin (Adriamycin) 30 mg/m^2 IV day 2; cisplatin 70 mg/m^2 IV day 2. Cycles are repeated monthly.

   b.   Gemcitabine 1,000 mg/m^2 days 1, 8, and 15 plus **cisplatin** 75 mg/m^2 day 1 [odds ratio (OR) 50%, CR 20%]. Less toxicity than M-VAC.

   c.   Cisplatin 75 mg/m^2 or 70 mg/m^2 plus **paclitaxel** 175 mg/m^2 or 135 mg/m^2 over 3 hours every 21 days (OR 50% to 70%, CR 15% to 32%).

   d.   Paclitaxel 80 mg/m^2 days 1 and 8; **gemcitabine** 1,000 mg/m^2 days 1 and 8; **cisplatin** 70 mg/m^2 day 1 or **carboplatinum** (OR 78%, CR 28%). Ongoing studies are evaluating some of these regimens in head-to-head comparisons.

3.   Assessment of response. Clear therapeutic goals and parameters of response should be delineated before chemotherapy is instituted. Response to chemotherapy, particularly with combination regimens, appears to occur promptly within 4 to 6 weeks of inception of therapy. Patients who have not demonstrated a response after two cycles should not be subjected to unnecessary morbidity from continued treatment.

4.   Complications. The major toxicities of the agents employed in bladder cancer have been outlined previously. Of particular concern are the nephrotoxicity of cisplatin, cardiotoxicity of doxorubicin, and severe myelosuppression caused by all these agents, with the exception of cisplatin. The use of new agents and combination regimens has improved the secondary toxicity considerably.

VII.   Prostate cancer. Despite increased efforts at screening for prostate cancer, about 10% of patients with prostate cancer present with advanced-stage disease that is not amenable to either surgical or radiation therapy. Although 80% to 85% of the patients with metastatic prostate cancer respond to hormonal manipulation, most of them will progress to a hormone-refractory state within 18 to 24 months. That is why the development of prevention strategies and an effective treatment for hormone-resistant cancer is important.

A.   Chemoprevention in prostate cancer. Based on the very high incidence of this cancer in men, a number of prevention strategies have been tested or considered. The National Cancer Institute is investigating in a randomized double-blind study the role of **finasteride,** an inhibitor of 5α-reductase enzyme, in the prevention of prostate cancer. In this study, patients with normal digital rectal exam and prostate-specific antigen (PSA) level of <3 ng/mL were assigned to finasteride (5 mg/day) or placebo. The preliminary results of this study appear to indicate an advantage to prophylactic finasteride in prostate cancer prevention. Currently, also the National Cancer Institute is studying selenium and vitamin E to confirm their role in the chemoprevention of prostate cancer.

B.   First-line hormonal therapy. The androgen dependency of the human prostate gland has been appreciated for at least 60 years. In many ways, prostate cancer is the male equivalent of breast cancer in women, especially with respect to the role of hormonal manipulation in advanced disease. The neoplastic prostate cell retains a dependency on androgenic hormones for optimal growth, although this dependence is seldom complete. Thus, any agent or procedure that interferes with the production, release, binding, or actions of androgens may potentially inhibit the growth of the prostate cancer cell.

1.   Androgen deprivation continues to be the most frequently used initial treatment for symptomatic metastatic prostate cancer (Table 16.5). Androgen deprivation may be achieved by bilateral orchiectomy or administration of estrogens, nonsteroidal antiandrogens, or synthetic analogues of GnRH. **Bilateral orchiectomy** is currently used only rarely, often in cases of poor compliance with medication schedules. Furthermore, this therapy is permanent and does not lend itself to intermittent hormonal therapy. **LHRH agonists,** such as leuprolide (Lupron) and goserelin (Zoladex), are synthetic analogues of GnRH; both are available in depot forms that allow convenient monthly, three-monthly, or four-monthly injections. LHRH agonists are often administered in conjunction with antiandrogens as a combined androgen blockade for patients with bone metastases. The advantage of this combination is that antiandrogens block the effects of the initial testosterone that surge in the first few days following the LHRH agonist administration. However, there is probably no clear superiority of combined treatment of antiandrogens plus LHRH agonists compared with LHRH agonists alone for the long-term therapy of patients with metastatic prostate cancer. It is not known if the early administration of androgen deprivation therapies results in a survival advantage. Therefore, the times of intervention and deprivation of these two conducts are acceptable.

2. Administration of **estrogens** may be considered when financial barriers preclude the use of LHRH analogues. Estrogens are relatively contraindicated in patients with a history of thromboembolic disease or congestive heart failure. Estrogen is usually administered as diethylstilbestrol at a daily dose of 1 to 3 mg orally. With measurement of serum testosterone levels to monitor effectiveness, the lowest effective

Table 16.5. Antiandrogen therapy

Generic Name (Brand Name)	Dose Forms	How Administered	Dose
LHRH agonists			
Leuprolide acetate (Lupron)	Aqueous solution	SC	1 mg qd
Leuprolide acetate (Lupron)	Depot 7.5-mg lyophilized microspheres	IM	7.5 mg q4wk
Leuprolide acetate (Lupron)	Depot 22.5-mg lyophilized microspheres	IM	22.5 mg q12wk
Leuprolide acetate (Lupron)	Depot 30-mg lyophilized microspheres	IM	30 mg q16wk
Goserelin acetate (Zoladex)	3.6-mg cylindrical implant	SC	3.6 mg q28d
Goserelin acetate (Zoladex)	3-mo cylindrical implant	SC	10.8 mg q12wk
Nonsteroidal antiandrogens			
Flutamide (Eulexin)	125-mg capsules	PO	2 capsules tid
Bicalutamide (Casodex)	50-mg tablets	PO	1 tablet qd
Nilutamide (Nilandron)	50-mg tablets	PO	6 tablets qd × 30 days; 3 tablets qd
Estrogens			
Diethylstilbestrol	1-, 3-, 5-mg tablets	PO	1–3 mg qd
Estradiol (Estrace)	0.5-, 1-, 2-mg tablets	PO	1 mg tid
Esterified estrogens (Estratab)	0.3-, 0.625-, 2.5-mg tablets	PO	1.25 mg tid
Adrenal steroid inhibitors			
Aminoglutethimide (Cytadren)	250-mg tablets	PO	1–2 g qd in q6h doses
Ketoconazole (Nizoral)	200-mg tablets	PO	400 mg tid

LHRH, luteinizing hormone-releasing hormone.

dose should be used. Low-dose radiation (900 to 1,200 cGy in three doses) to the breasts may be administered before diethylstilbestrol is initiated to prevent painful gynecomastia. Hormones can be started 2 to 3 days later. This therapy is often given in conjunction with low doses of warfarin to prevent thromboembolic events. **Antiandrogens** act by binding to androgen receptors in the target cells. Flutamide (250 mg every 8 hours), bicalutamide (50 mg/day), and nilutamide (300 mg/day) are nonsteroidal antiandrogens that are currently used. Of these three agents, bicalutamide is used more frequently because it is taken once daily. This therapy is often associated with fewer side effects than LHRH agonists. **Finasteride** is a 5α-reductase inhibitor that is used as treatment of benign prostatic hyperplasia, and it has shown some effectiveness in combatting hormonosensitive disease when combined with antiandrogen. Finasteride is not routinely used for the treatment of prostate cancer.

C. **Second-line hormonal therapy.** Patients who do not respond initially to hormonal therapy (20%) or who will eventually relapse after an initial response (100%) may respond to alternative hormonal treatment. Therapeutic strategies that have been employed include blockade of adrenal androgen production (aminoglutethimide and **ketoconazole**) and antiandrogens if they have not been used before. If a patient has been on long-term antiandrogens, another option is **antiandrogen withdrawal.** The mechanism by which this maneuver can improve the PSA levels is still unknown, but it is might be explained by a mutation in the androgen receptor. The antifungal imidazoles, typified by **ketoconazole,** have been found to inhibit both adrenal and testicular testosterone production. Ketoconazole (800 mg/day) has produced objective responses in almost 50% of patients with LHRH-refractory prostate cancer. **Glucocorticoids** act by suppressing adrenal steroidogenesis, by inhibition of the pituitary production of adrenocorticotropic hormone (see below).

D. **Cytotoxic chemotherapy**

1. **Factors hindering the use of chemotherapy in prostate cancer.** The role of chemotherapy in prostate cancer remains to be defined. A number of factors, some unique to prostate cancer, hinder attempts at improved definition of this role.

a. **Difficulties in quantifying response.** Most patients with prostate cancer have disease that is not amenable to measurement by standard response criteria.

b. **Poor performance status** is typical of patients with prostate cancer because of their advanced age and debilitation.

c. **Bone marrow reserve is often limited** because of marrow replacement by tumor and previous irradiation. This factor limits patient tolerance of drugs with significant myelosuppressive activities.

2. **Active agents and specific regimens.** A number of active agents have been identified, including estramustine, taxanes, doxorubicin, cyclophosphamide, and cisplatin. In addition, a number of combination chemotherapy regimens

and chemotherapy–hormonal agent combinations have been evaluated. With specific combined regimens such as estramustine plus taxane, a PSA and objective response of >50% can be obtained. Although there is no optimal chemotherapy regimen, combined chemotherapy is likely superior to single agents. Currently, the most effective regimens are **mitoxantrone** (12 to 14 mg/m^2) plus low doses of **corticosteroids** (prednisone 10 mg/day) and **estramustine** (10 mg/kg/day days 1 to 5) plus **docetaxel** (70 mg/m^2 every 3 weeks) with or without corticosteroids (PSA response 68%). Docetaxel (75 mg/m^2 every 3 weeks) can be used as a single agent with a 46% PSA response and a 28% objective response. Further research and trials are needed to find the optimal treatment for patients with hormonorefractory prostate cancer.

VIII. Testicular and extragonadal germ cell cancer

A. Overview. The introduction of highly effective chemotherapeutic regimens for germ cell tumors of the testis has been one of the most important advances in oncology during the last 20 years. The most dramatic impact has been in patients with advanced seminoma and nonseminomatous disease. In these patients, cisplatin-based combination chemotherapy forms the cornerstone of treatment. The initial evaluation and staging of testis cancer are discussed in Chapter 15. For the purposes of this discussion, stage IIA or IIB disease will be termed stage II **nonbulky disease** and stage IIC (metastasis with a lymph node mass of >5 cm in greatest dimension) disease will be called **bulky disease.** The importance of tumor markers in this disease cannot be overemphasized. Germ cell tumors, whether testicular or extragonadal, produce two glycoproteins: the β subunit of human chorionic gonadotropin (β-hCG) and α-fetoprotein (AFP). The relative frequency of elevated markers according to histologic type is given in Table 15.7. In addition to contributing to the initial staging process, serial marker determinations during treatment provide a useful index of response. Their greatest usefulness, however, may be during posttreatment follow-up, when a rising serum marker level may herald a relapse months before any macroscopic evidence of disease is noted.

B. Chemotherapy in early disease

1. Pure seminoma. Because of the exquisite sensitivity of seminomas to radiation therapy (see Chapter 17), chemotherapy plays no role in the initial management of patients with stage I and nonbulky stage II seminomatous disease. Observation after orchiectomy has been suggested because retroperitoneal lymphadenopathy never develops in about 80% of patients. However, the standard of care is still infradiaphragmatic radiation. The small minority of patients who relapse after radiation therapy should nearly all be curable with the use of an appropriate cisplatin-based combination chemotherapy regimen.

2. Nonseminomatous tumors. Patients with early nonseminomatous tumors may undergo retroperitoneal lymph node dissection following inguinal orchiectomy, regardless of the presence of clinical evidence of metastatic disease in the retroperitoneum, and a close clinical follow-up alone following orchiectomy in patients without clinical evidence of metastatic disease (clinical stage A). This policy is based on the high probability of cure with appropriate chemotherapy in the 20% to 30% of such patients who ultimately relapse after orchiectomy alone. A policy of "watchful waiting" in clinical stage A disease places the responsibility for a rigorous surveillance program on both patient and physician. Another alternative for patients with nonseminomatous cancer stage I is two cycles of adjuvant chemotherapy, but this approach is not uniformly accepted. Patients found to have no retroperitoneal disease after undergoing retroperitoneal lymph node dissection (pathologic stage A) can expect cure rates in excess of 90% with no further therapy. In contrast, patients with pathologic stage B disease have a 40% to 50% relapse rate following retroperitoneal lymph node dissection. Postoperative adjuvant chemotherapy has been used in this situation to lower the relapse rate. Results from a large national study of adjuvant chemotherapy for stage B disease suggest that relapses can be eliminated by giving two cycles of platinum-based chemotherapy [bleomycin, etoposide, and cisplatin (BEP)] after retroperitoneal lymph node dissection; however, patients who relapse can virtually all be cured with three cycles of the same regimen given at the time of relapse. Thus, two equally reasonable therapeutic options exist in this situation, and the final choice rests with the patient and physician. In many European centers, retroperitoneal lymph node dissection has been abandoned because of the 50% relapse rate, and primary chemotherapy is used instead.

C. **Chemotherapy in advanced disease**

1. **Initial treatment regimens.** Regardless of histologic type, chemotherapy is the optimal initial therapy in metastatic testis cancer (bulky stage B and stage C) and in primary extragonadal tumors. For patients with stage IIC, three or four cycles of cisplatin-based combination chemotherapy (BEP) are the standard therapies. The best results have been obtained with intensive platinum-based three-drug combinations. This regimen produces CRs in approximately 80% of patients with advanced disease, with an overall cure rate of 70% to 75%. The two most commonly used combinations, which appear to have equal efficacy, are the following:

   a. **BEP.** The following dosages are repeated every 3 weeks for three to four cycles:

      (1) **Bleomycin** 30 U IV days 2, 9, and 16.

      (2) **Etoposide (VP-16)** 100 mg/m^2 IV daily for 5 days.

      (3) **Cisplatin** 20 mg/m^2 IV daily for 5 days.

   b. **Etoposide and cisplatin.** This regimen is a good alternative for patients with compromised pulmonary function who need to avoid the toxicity of bleomycin. The dosages are the same as for BEP, but without bleomycin, and are repeated every 3 weeks for four cycles.

2. **Assessment following induction chemotherapy** involves a careful restaging of the patient by assessing all areas known to have disease previously and repeating tumor marker determinations. Patients in whom markers and all radiographic findings have normalized require close follow-up with no additional treatment.

a. Patients with **pure seminomatous disease** in whom markers normalize but radiographic abnormalities persist also require no further therapy in most cases. In such patients, surgical resection of these areas of suspected residual disease has almost uniformly yielded fibrosis and necrotic tissue without viable tumor.

b. In **nonseminomatous disease** with persistent radiographic abnormalities but normalization of markers, persistent tumor is found in 30% to 40% of patients at surgical exploration, although the remainder will show residual teratoma, a benign component. Thus, whenever it is technically feasible, patients with persistent radiographic abnormalities after induction therapy of nonseminomatous disease should undergo surgical resection. If residual cancer is found, such patients should receive two additional cycles of platinum-based combination therapy with appropriate dose reduction or elimination of bleomycin. Patients with pure nonseminomatous disease who manifest persistently elevated markers after induction chemotherapy should be considered for salvage chemotherapy (see below).

3. Complications of treatment. Platinum-based regimens can produce formidable toxicity. Nausea and vomiting during drug administration can be a severe problem; all patients should receive an antiemetic regimen (dexamethasone plus 5-hydroxytryptamine-3). To minimize potential nephrotoxicity, all patients need to be aggressively hydrated and have their urine output monitored carefully. All these chemotherapy regimens are associated with severe and potentially life-threatening myelosuppression. White cells and platelets must be monitored carefully, and prompt intervention is required at the first sign of infection. Dose reduction and treatment delays need to be avoided, and a dose reduction of etoposide is not recommended unless the day 5 granulocyte count is <1,000, in which case the day 5 etoposide only is held. Miscellaneous toxicity includes mucositis, vinblastine-induced ileus, peripheral neuropathy, alopecia, Raynaud's phenomenon, and bleomycin-induced pulmonary fibrosis.

4. Follow-up after treatment is essential in achieving optimal cure rates in these patients. Most recurrences are within the first year after treatment and nearly all by 2 years. The response rate to subsequent treatment is inversely proportional to the volume of disease, hence the necessity for early detection of recurrent disease. Following achievement of a CR to chemotherapy or surgery, patients should undergo clinical examination, chest roentgenography, and serum marker determination at frequent intervals for the first 2 years of follow-up and at progressively longer intervals thereafter.

5. Chemotherapy for patients with poor-risk disease or after failure of primary chemotherapy involves ifosfamide and cisplatin with etoposide (VP-16) or vinblastine with or without autologous stem cell transplantation. Ifosfamide is an analogue of cyclophosphamide. This regimen, called VIP, results in a CR rate of approximately 33%.

a.   Vinblastine 0.2 mg/kg IV push or etoposide 75 mg/m^2 daily for 5 days.

b.   Ifosfamide 1,200 mg/m^2 IV over 30 minutes days 1 through 5 with MESNA.

c.   Cisplatin 20 mg/m^2 IV over 30 minutes days 1 through 5 with hydration.

6.   Autologous bone marrow transplantation. Patients with progression during platinum-based chemotherapy or failure of prior cisplatin, vinblastine, and bleomycin, etoposide (VP-16), and ifosfamide should be evaluated for autologous bone marrow transplant. In the past, results have been disappointing, with virtually no remissions lasting longer than 1 year. However, more recent studies have shown 15% to 20% long-term disease-free survival when high-dose carboplatin and etoposide are used with autologous bone marrow transplant. Unfortunately, this approach is associated with significant treatment-related toxicity.

IX.   Carcinoma of the penis

Methotrexate, bleomycin, cisplatin, and 5-FU all appear to have some activity against penile cancer. Topical 5-FU has been used with some success in premalignant lesions. Experience with systemic chemotherapy is quite limited in the United States because of the rarity of the disease. Combined therapy with bleomycin and radiotherapy has been reported to be effective. The protocol involves 5,800 cGy of radiation over 38 days combined with 225 mg of bleomycin. More than 90% of patients demonstrated a CR, and 5-year disease-free survival was 70%.

SUGGESTED READING

Adami S. Bisphosphonates in prostate carcinoma. *Cancer* 1997; 80(suppl 8):1674–1679.

Allsbrook WC, Mangold KA, Yang X, et al. The Gleason grading system: an overview. *J Urol Pathol* 1999;10:141–157.

American Joint Committee on Cancer. *AJCC cancer staging handbook.* 5th ed. Philadelphia: Lippincott-Raven, 1998.

Amling CL, Bergstralh EJ, Blute ML, et al. Defining prostate specific antigen progression after radical prostatectomy: what is the most appropriate cut point? *J Urol* 2001;165:1146–1151.

Bolla M, Gonzalez D, Warde P, et al. Improved survival in patients with locally advanced prostate cancer treated with radiotherapy and goserelin. *N Engl J Med* 1997;337:295–300.

Byar DP, Corle DK. Hormone therapy for prostate cancer: results of the Veterans Administration Cooperative Urological Research Group studies. *NCI Monogr* 1988;7:165–170.

Cookson MS, Herr HW, Zhang ZF. The treated natural history of high risk superficial bladder cancer: 15-year outcome. *J Urol* 1997;158: 62–67.

Cox RL, Crawford ED. Estrogens in the treatment of prostate cancer. *J Urol* 1995;154:1991–1998.

Donohue JP, Foster RS. Retroperitoneal lymphadenectomy in staging and treatment: the development of nerve-sparing techniques. *Urol Clin North Am* 1998;25:461–468.

Donohue JP, Roth LM, Zachary JM, et al. Cytoreductive surgery for metastatic testis cancer: tissue analysis of retroperitoneal masses after chemotherapy. *J Urol* 1982;127:1111–1114.

Donohue JP, Thornhill JA, Foster RS, et al. Primary retroperitoneal lymph node dissection in clinical stage A non-seminomatous germ cell testis cancer: review of the Indiana University experience 1965–1989. *Br J Urol* 1993;71:326–335.

Frohlich MW, Small EJ. Stage II nonseminomatous testis cancer: the roles of primary and adjuvant chemotherapy. *Urol Clin North Am* 1998;25:451–459.

Garnick MB. Hormonal therapy in the management of prostate cancer: a historical overview. *Mol Urol* 1999;3:175–182.

Goldenberg SL, Bruchovsky N, Gleave ME, et al. Intermittent androgen suppression in the treatment of prostatic carcinoma: an update. *J Urol* 1997;157:333.

Horenblas S, van Tinteren H, Delemarre JF. Squamous cell carcinoma of the penis. III. Treatment of regional lymph nodes. *J Urol* 1993;149:492–497.

Horwich A, Norman A, Fisher C, et al. Primary chemotherapy for stage II nonseminomatous germ cell tumors of the testis. *J Urol* 1994;151:72–77.

Janetschek G, Hobisch A, Peschel R, et al. Laparoscopic retroperitoneal lymph node dissection for clinical stage I nonseminomatous testicular carcinoma: long-term outcome. *J Urol* 2000;163:1793–1796.

Kattan J, Culine S, Droz JP, et al. Penile cancer chemotherapy: 12 years' experience at Institut Gustave-Roussy. *Urology* 1993;42:559–562.

Krown SE. Interferon treatment of renal cell carcinoma: current status and future prospects. *Cancer* 1987;59:647–652.

Lamm DL, Blumenstein BA, Crissman JD. Maintenance bacillus Calmette-Guerin immunotherapy for recurrent TA, T1, and carcinoma in situ transitional cell carcinoma of the bladder: a randomized Southwest Oncology Group study. *J Urol* 2000;163:1124–1129.

McDougal WS. Carcinoma of the penis: improved survival by early regional lymphadenectomy based on the histological grade and depth of invasion of the primary lesion. *J Urol* 1995;154:364–366.

Messing EM, Manola J, Sarosdy M, et al. Immediate hormonal therapy compared with observation after radical prostatectomy and pelvic lymphadenectomy in men with node-positive prostate cancer. *N Engl J Med* 1999;341:1781–1788.

Moul JW. Prostate specific antigen only progression of prostate cancer. *J Urol* 2000;163:1632–1642.

Osborn JL, Getzenberg RH, Trump DL. Spinal cord compression in prostate cancer. *J Neurooncol* 1995;23:135–147.

Shearer R, Chilvors CED, Bloom HJG, et al. Adjuvant chemotherapy in T3 carcinoma of the bladder. *Br J Urol* 1988;62:558–564.

Thalmann GN, Sermier A, Rentsch C. Urinary interleukin-8 and -18 predict the response of superficial bladder cancer to intravesical therapy with bacillus Calmette-Guerin. *J Urol* 2000;164:2129–2133.

Trigo JM, Tabernero JM, Paz-Ares L, et al. Tumor markers at the time of recurrence in patients with germ cell tumors. *Cancer* 2000;88:162–168.

17

Radiation: External Beam and Brachytherapy

Anthony L. Zietman

Although radiation therapy is used widely in the treatment of genitourinary malignancy, its principles are poorly understood by most practitioners. In some situations, it is the mainstay of treatment (radical radiotherapy). In others, it is used to eradicate microscopically persistent local disease after surgery (adjuvant radiotherapy). In still others, its role is purely palliative. The role of radiation in this setting should not be minimized, as it often contributes to an improved quality of life for the cancer patient. This chapter outlines the basic principles of radiation therapy as they apply to urologic problems.

I. Physics of radiation

A. Types of radiation. Radiation energy consists of high-energy x-rays, γ-rays, or particles (charged or uncharged). These forms of radiation differ mainly in their method of production, degree of penetration into tissue, and biologic effect. Because they are electromagnetic waves that travel at the speed of light, x-rays and γ-rays are sometimes referred to as photons. When high-energy electrons (produced within a linear accelerator) collide with the atomic nuclei of heavy metals such as tungsten, x-rays are emitted. A tungsten target is found in the head of every linear accelerator. In contrast, γ-rays are produced naturally from the decay of isotopes such as iodine-125 (^{125}I) and cobalt-60 (^{60}Co). In other respects, however, γ-rays are identical to x-rays. Particle beams consist of subatomic particles that are either charged (electrons, protons, α-particles) or uncharged (neutrons).

B. Penetrating ability. In general, the greater the energy of the electromagnetic radiation, the greater is its ability to penetrate tissue. High-energy x-rays tend to spare the surface ("skin-sparing effect") and produce their greatest effects in deeper tissues. Modern megavoltage therapy units can produce beams with energy from 2 to 23 million electron volts. Such high-energy beams have eliminated the radiation skin reactions or "burns" characteristic of the lower-energy therapy used a generation ago. In contrast to x-rays, electron particles have very low penetration and are useful for treating surface lesions, while deeper tissues are spared.

C. Measurement of radiation energy. This is based on the amount of ionization (expressed in terms of the quantity of free electrons released) that results when a standardized quantity of air is exposed to radiation. The standard unit of radiation is the **roentgen.** Specifying the amount of radiation in terms of roentgens, however, does not describe the ability of the x-ray beam to penetrate tissue, nor does it describe how much energy is absorbed by the tissue. This is because the penetrating ability of the x-ray beam depends on the energy of the beam and certain characteristics of the irradiated tissue, especially its density. The need to describe the biologic dose of delivered radiation led to the development of other units, such as the rad and, more recently, the gray. The relationship between the roentgen and the gray may be thought of as similar to that between the administered dose of a drug and the absorbed dose.

II. Radiobiology

A. Radiation–tissue interaction. The major effect of radiation in tissues is the ionization of oxygen and water (radiation hydrolysis) to form free radicals (Fig. 17.1). These free radicals are able to react with nuclear and mitochondrial DNA, resulting in breaks in the double strand. Although the cell and the nucleus contain DNA repair molecules, these mechanisms are overwhelmed after a given radiation dose that varies according to radiation type and cell type. Radiation may also affect membrane-bound macromolecules (signaling systems) and initiate

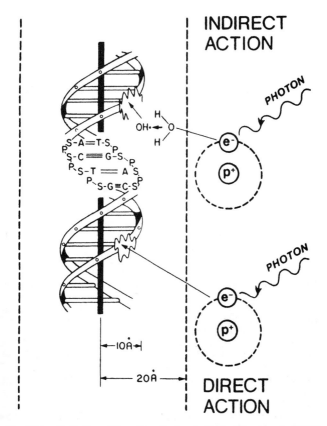

Fig. 17.1. Radiation either directly fractures double-stranded DNA or acts through the production of free radicals.

programmed cell death (apoptosis). The effects of radiation on cellular DNA are instantaneous, but cell death does not usually occur immediately. It is deferred until the cell next attempts to divide. Lethality may not be expressed for several cell growth cycles. When apoptosis is the dominant mechanism, however, a much more rapid form of cell death can occur. This explains the rapid shrinkage of lymphomas treated by radiation.

B.   Factors in the radiation sensitivity of malignant tissues

1.   Intrinsic radiosensitivity. A wide variation in radiation sensitivity exists between tumor types. Generally speaking, lymphomas and seminomas are the most sensitive and melanomas and glioblastomas the least. In between, transitional and squamous cell carcinomas are more sensitive than adenocarcinomas or sarcomas.

2.   Tumor mass. The larger the tumor mass, the greater the number of tumor cells that must be inactivated by radiation. Smaller tumors therefore require lower doses than larger tumors. Some tumors can be so large that the dose of radiation required would be intolerable to the surrounding normal tissue.

3.   Repopulation. Some tumors, when depleted in number of cells, can respond by increasing their proliferative rate to overcome the loss. This may become a limiting factor if the radiation is delivered in too protracted a fashion. Accelerated repopulation may play a role in the rapid recurrence of some transitional cell carcinomas of the bladder after radiation.

4.   Reoxygenation. Hypoxic tissues are less sensitive to radiation, which works in part through the generation of oxygen radicals. Large necrotic tumors may contain a hypoxic core, which limits their curability.

C.   Factors affecting the radiation sensitivity of normal tissues. Normal tissues may be grouped into two types: early and late responding. Early-responding tissues, such as mucous membranes, are quickly depleted because of their rapid turnover time. However, they are easily regenerated after therapy by surviving stem cells and by ingrowth from adjacent untreated mucosa. This explains the rapid development of cystitis and urethritis during radiation treatment for a urologic tumor. These symptoms usually begin to abate within a month after completion of therapy. Late-responding tissues, on the other hand, have slow turnover times and do not express any damage until months or years later. In these tissues, loss of parenchymal cells leads to atrophy, and microvascular obliteration leads to fibrosis. This can result in contraction of the bladder, a chronic rectal ulcer, or erectile impotence. These tissues may be preferentially spared by using multiple small doses of radiation to a high total dose (fractionation). The rationale is that late-responding tissues differ from early-responding tissues and most tumors in that they are capable of repairing small amounts of DNA damage after small doses of radiation.

D.   Delivery of therapeutic radiation

1.   External-beam therapy (teletherapy). This refers to the delivery of radiation from a source some distance from the target. When x-rays are delivered to living tissue, some pass through, and some are absorbed. It is the absorbed dose that interacts with tissues to produce the biologic effects. The unit of absorbed dose was the rad, which is an acronym for "radiation absorbed dose." The rad now has been replaced by the gray (Gy), which equals 100 rads or centigrays (cGy). Patients usually lie on a couch and multiple shaped beams are directed at the tumor. To increase the accuracy of the treatment, patients are usually immobilized with a body cast or mold. Sometimes the target organ itself may be mobile. The prostate gland, for example, may move up to 1 cm in any direction according to rectal or bladder filling. Many centers now track the prostate daily using transabdominal ultrasound (US) and make daily adjustments to ensure that it is the target, rather than a normal tissue, that is being irradiated.

2.   Interstitial therapy (brachytherapy). This is short-distance therapy in which a radioisotope is placed directly within a tumor or body cavity. Different radioisotopes generate radiation with different energies that determine how they can be used. Iodine-125 produces very low-energy radiation. It can thus be left inside a prostate gland indefinitely, and the radiation will not reach any of the surrounding tissues, let alone other people. Other sources such as iridium may be used for prostate implants, but they have a higher energy and would thus represent a radiation hazard if left inside a patient. Brachytherapy is most commonly used to deliver high doses of radiation to an easily accessible organ without delivering much radiation at all to surrounding tissues. The best examples in urologic cancer are prostate and penis.

III.   Clinical radiotherapy

When a patient is referred for radiation therapy, the initial consultation is used to establish the goals and feasibility of such treatment. Curative treatments involve high total doses of radiation to maximize the likelihood of eradicating tumor. Multiple fractions, usually exceeding 30, have to be given to maximize the likelihood of destroying the tumor and minimize normal tissue damage. Adjuvant treatments are also curative, although because only microscopic tumor burdens are faced, lower total doses of radiation can be used. Multiple fractions are again preferred. In palliation, the aim of radiation is to shrink the tumor quickly and end a distressing symptom. Low doses of radiation are sufficient, and they can be given in just a few fractions to minimize inconvenience. Once accepted for therapy, a tumor is carefully localized by clinical examination and all available radiology. This is the process of **simulation,** in which precise **treatment portals** are established. Most modern radiotherapy departments will have a computed tomography (CT) scanner that can be used to generate three-dimensional models of the tumor and surrounding organs. Computers are used to calculate the number and angle of the beams and the doses to be delivered through each beam. **Conformal three-dimensional radiation therapy** is a term used to describe highly accurate multiple-beam radiation that excludes as much normal tissue from treatment as possible. There are some "ultra"-conformal technologies available that, by their accuracy, allow very high doses of radiation to be safely administered. It is assumed that higher doses of radiation translate into higher cure rates. These include intensity-modulated radiation and proton-beam administration techniques.

A. Renal cell carcinoma

1. Primary radiotherapy. Renal cell carcinoma is generally considered radioresistant. Preoperative radiation has been shown to have no impact on survival. Postoperative radiotherapy to the renal bed in doses of 40 to 50 Gy may be given in cases of local extension or nodal metastases. Randomized trials have shown improvements in local control, but there has been no evidence of improved survival. The radiation dose that can be administered to this site is limited by the proximity of the liver and small bowel. Intraoperative radiation and brachytherapy may play a role in the future.

2. Palliative therapy. This is indicated in metastatic renal cell carcinoma for the management of painful bony lesions or spinal cord compression. High doses of 45 to 60 Gy are usually required during a period of 3 to 6 weeks. Treatment needs to be more fractionated than in metastatic hormone-refractory prostate or metastatic bladder cancer because of the remarkable longevity of some patients with renal cell carcinoma.

B. Wilms' tumor. Radiotherapy may be indicated as adjuvant treatment in some cases of Wilms' tumor in childhood. This tumor is very radiation sensitive, and improved survival has resulted from combining radiation with surgical removal of tumor. Radiotherapy in young children has a tendency to slow or even halt vertebral growth. It has been shown that when postoperative chemotherapy is given to children with early-stage disease and favorable histology, adjuvant radiation does not further improve survival. Thus, the current trend is to give radiation only to selected patients, such as those with unfavorable histology, stage III or stage IV disease, positive margins, or gross tumor spillage during surgery. In such cases, 10 Gy is given to the flank. Metastatic sites may also be treated with low-dose radiation in conjunction with systemic chemotherapy.

C. Bladder cancer

1. Primary external-beam therapy. This may be effective in the treatment of invasive bladder cancer and is widely used as a primary modality in some European countries. The 5-year local control is only in the order of 30% to 40%, considerably less than that obtained with cystectomy. For this reason, in the United States, radiation alone is reserved for patients who are poor surgical candidates. The efficacy of radiation, however, may be considerably improved by prior transurethral debulking of the tumor and the synchronous administration of cisplatin, a radiation sensitizer. Much higher rates of local control are possible, and some centers now use this bladder-sparing approach as primary therapy. For cases that are not controlled, the patients undergo prompt salvage cystectomy.

2. Postcystectomy radiation. When a surgically removed tumor is massive and adherent to the pelvic side wall, the risk for local recurrence is extremely high. Postoperative irradiation can be given to a total dose of 45 to 50 Gy, but because the bladder is no longer present to displace the small bowel, small bowel complications (adhesions, stricture) are common. If postoperative irradiation is anticipated, a pelvic sling should be inserted at the time of surgery. Radiation may also be reserved for salvage of local pelvic failure following cystectomy. As it is unsafe to administer the high doses necessary for tumor eradication, cisplatin is usually given concomitantly as a tumor sensitizer.

3. Palliative radiotherapy. In patients with unresectable disease, severe bleeding may develop. Administration of 30 to 50 Gy over 3 to 4 weeks is usually sufficient to stop the hematuria. Bone metastases are treated as for prostate cancer.

D. Prostate cancer

1. Low-risk disease. This is generally defined as T1c to T2a disease with a prostate-specific antigen (PSA) level of ≤10 ng/mL and a Gleason sum of ≤7. These patients are suitable either for external radiation or brachytherapy. Those receiving external beam are given doses of 70 to 76 Gy in divided fractions of 1.8 to 2.0 Gy/day, 5 days a week for a total of 7 to 8 weeks. Brachytherapy is an alternative to external-beam therapy for early-stage disease but is not suitable for men with large-volume or dysfunctional prostates or men who have had a prior transurethral resection of the prostate (TURP). Iodine-125 or palladium-103 seeds are inserted through the perineum under transrectal US guidance (Fig. 17.2). This type of therapy allows a high dose of radiation to be given (145 Gy for iodine or 110 Gy for palladium), but because of the slow decay of the sources, it is given over many months or even years. It is difficult to compare a radiation dose given this way with that delivered by external beam in terms of biologic effect. Medium-term results of brachytherapy are encouraging, and it is the fastest-growing therapy for early-stage prostate cancer. From 60% to 80% of well-selected patients with early-stage, low-risk prostate cancer can expect to be disease-free 10 years later if managed with contemporary forms of radiation therapy.

2. Intermediate-risk prostate cancer. Patients with one or more of the following risk factors are deemed to be at higher risk of bulky primary disease and extracapsular extension: (a) Gleason grade of ≥8, (b) PSA level of >10 ng/mL, and (c) bilaterally palpable disease. Brachytherapy is not usually an option for these tumors unless combined with external radiation to treat extracapsular disease. The standard management is to down-size the tumor with 2 to 4 months of androgen deprivation and, through apoptosis, sensitize it to radiation. Despite the improved progression-free survival rates obtained with combination therapy, cure is less likely because of the high incidence of occult micrometastases. Irradiation of the regional lymph nodes may prevent local progression within the pelvis, but it does not improve survival. Because of potential morbidity, it is now usually omitted.

3. High-risk prostate cancer. Men with multiple high-risk factors have such a high chance for occult systemic disease that androgen deprivation is continued for a full 2 years after the completion of the radiation. Though cure is unlikely, the disease-free survival intervals are greatly extended by such an approach.

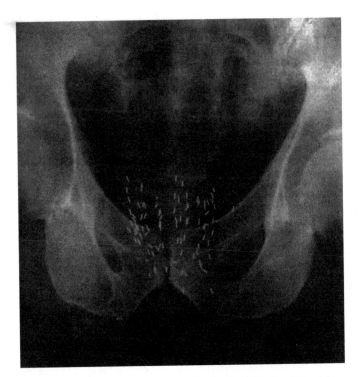

Fig. 17.2.   Radiograph showing the distribution of iodine-125 seeds used in the treatment of localized adenocarcinoma of the prostate.

4.   **Postoperative radiation.** A dose of 60 to 64 Gy over approximately 6 to 7 weeks may be administered to the tumor bed after radical prostatectomy when the likelihood of locally persistent disease is high (e.g., when the surgical margins are positive). The likelihood of lasting local control is very high and is in the order of 80% to 90%. Irradiation of the tumor bed for salvage may be attempted when the PSA rises after radical prostatectomy and a metastatic work-up has proved negative. This is unlikely to be beneficial when the original tumor pathology is of a high grade or seminal vesicle invasion is present. Under these circumstances, the detectable PSA is more likely to represent occult micrometastatic disease than local persistence. Androgen deprivation would be more appropriate.

5.   **Palliation**

a.   **Bone metastases.** These occur frequently in prostate cancer and can be treated with local radiotherapy when androgen ablation has failed. Doses of 8 to 30 Gy given over 1 to 14 days in 1 to 10 treatments are effective at controlling pain 80% of the time. If multiple sites of skeletal pain exist, it might prove more convenient to give a single intravenous dose of the bone-seeking radioisotope strontium-89. When pathologic fracture has occurred, radiation can be given after orthopedic fixation to promote healing.

b. Spinal cord compression. Extradural metastases may lead rapidly to catastrophic paraplegia (Fig. 17.3). This is an indication for urgent treatment with corticosteroids (4 mg of dexamethasone orally every 6 hours) and radiation (generally 30 to 40 Gy).

c. Local tumor progression. This may cause outflow obstruction and bleeding. Although transurethral resection is usually performed for obstruction by prostate cancer, radiotherapy may be considered if operative risk is high, the patient refuses surgery, or previous surgery has failed. Again, doses from 30 to 40 Gy over 2 to 3 weeks may result in a decrease in size of the prostate and abatement of symptoms.

d. Gynecomastia. This is a troublesome complication of estrogen and some antiandrogen therapy such as high-dose bicalutamide (150 mg daily). It can be prevented by breast irradiation (15 Gy in three doses to each breast).

E. Testis cancer. Although chemotherapy is now the major form of treatment for nonseminomatous germ cell tumors and advanced seminoma, radiotherapy is still used regularly in the management of stages A and B seminoma.

1. Stage A disease. Despite orchiectomy, about 25% of patients have occult metastases within the paraaortic lymph nodes. Orchiectomy is therefore followed by administration of 25 Gy over 3 to 4 weeks to these nodal areas. Seminoma is exquisitely radiation sensitive, so low doses that rarely produce any lasting damage to normal tissues within the field are sufficient to eradicate microscopic disease. Radical orchiectomy and adjuvant radiation together in stage A disease result in cure rates of 95% to 98%. The few failures are usually salvaged with chemotherapy.

2. Stage B disease. This is subdivided according to the bulk of the retroperitoneal metastases. In retroperitoneal disease measuring <2 cm in diameter (stage B1), the same radiation treatment is given as in stage A, with the extension of the field into the pelvis to treat the ipsilateral pelvic lymph nodes and the addition of a further 5 to 10 Gy to the mass itself. With this mode of therapy, the 5-year disease-free survival rate is 95%. In patients with 2- to 5-cm diameter disease in the retroperitoneum, radiation still offers an 85% chance of cure and is preferable for men who do not wish to have their fertility compromised by chemotherapy. Those who have bulkier stage B tumors are usually treated by primary chemotherapy, with radiation given to residual masses >3 cm in diameter.

F. Penile and urethral cancer

1. Squamous cell carcinoma of the penis. Although the primary treatment mode in the United States is surgical excision, radiotherapy may be used. Small lesions measuring <3 cm in diameter may be treated with high-dose superficial electron-beam radiation. Cure rates at 3 years approach 90%, and the penis is preserved (Fig. 17.4). Interstitial radiation with iridium is an alternative method of delivering a high dose quickly to a small area. When the lesions exceed 3 cm in size, local control with radiation is less likely and penectomy may

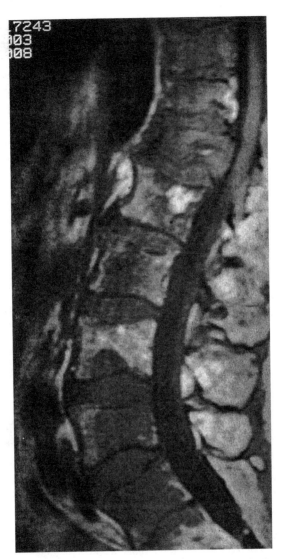

Fig. 17.3. Magnetic resonance image showing spinal cord compression from metastatic prostate cancer. This is an emergency that requires prompt treatment with corticosteroids and radiation.

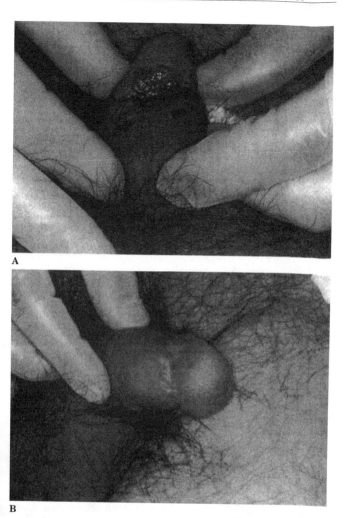

A

B

Fig. 17.4. A small, 1.5-cm penile squamous cell carcinoma before
(A) and 1 year after (B) superficial electron-beam radiation therapy.

be preferred. If the patient declines or is medically unsuitable, then penile irradiation is combined with elective radiation to the inguinal lymph node areas.

2. Urethral cancer. Malignancy in the male anterior urethra can be treated in the same way as penile cancer. Tumors in the posterior urethra are treated in a manner similar to that for prostate cancer, with radiation doses of 60 to 70 Gy to the primary tumor. If the cancers are of the transitional cell type, concomitant cisplatinum can also be given, as for bladder cancer. In female patients, carcinoma of the urethra requires interstitial implantation. This is combined with external-beam radiation to the inguinal and deep pelvic lymph nodes.

IV. Complications of radiotherapy

As previously mentioned, the complications of radiation can be divided into those occurring during or immediately after treatment (early effects) and those occurring months to years later (late effects).

A. Early effects. The early effects of radiation are generally short lived and respond well to symptomatic treatment.

1. Local reactions. These include skin changes and mucositis. High-energy radiotherapy beams, such as those produced by the linear accelerator or cobalt units, tend to spare the skin and produce little erythema. Temporary acute cystitis and proctitis are, however, quite common. Cystitis manifests as urinary frequency and dysuria in the third or fourth week of radiation. It is usually managed by anticholinergic or locally anesthetic medications. If it has an obstructive element, then α blockers may be tried. Proctitis occurs 3 weeks after the start of radiation and usually presents as tenesmus, increased bowel frequency, and occasional rectal bleeding. Diarrhea occurs only when large fields are used to treat pelvic lymph nodes. Proctitis is managed by a low-residue diet, antispasmodic agents, and steroid suppositories. Doses of 25 to 30 Gy will generally affect hematopoiesis within the marrow of the irradiated bones. This can be an issue in patients with bladder cancer or seminoma who have been previously treated by chemotherapy. In these situations, if the white cell count falls below 2,000/mm^3 or the platelet count is <50,000/mm^3, radiation should be stopped until recovery has occurred.

2. Systemic reactions. These can occur after wide-field radiation, such as is given for seminoma. Nausea is common after radiation to the upper abdomen but rarely lasts more than a few days. If it is severe, antiemetics may be prescribed as needed. General fatigability is quite common during external-beam radiation. There are no systemic effects from interstitial brachytherapy.

B. Late effects. Late effects may occur because of parenchymal cell loss leading to tissue atrophy and because of an obliterative endarteritis that may provoke fibrosis. The clinical manifestations depend on the organ irradiated, the state of its vasculature, the radiation dose given, and the radiation fractionation. The degree of early reaction cannot be used to predict the degree of late effects, if any.

1. Kidney. This is a sensitive organ, and radiation nephritis with tubular obliteration has been described in patients who have received 20 to 25 Gy to both kidneys. It manifests as chronic renal failure at least 1 year after radiation. The clinical setting in which it can occur is very uncommon these days, as whole-abdominal irradiation is infrequently used for anything but palliation of lymphoma or ovarian cancer. Unilateral kidney irradiation may lead to hypertension.

2. Ureter. The ureters rarely show any long-term effects from radiotherapy. Stricture is a remote possibility.

3. Bladder. In the days when low-energy equipment was prevalent and daily radiation doses large, radical radiation for bladder cancer was followed by the development of bladder contracture or hemorrhagic cystitis in up to 20% of cases. This problem has now largely been eliminated by the use of small radiation fractions and sophisticated technology. Hyperbaric oxygen has been reported successful in some cases of refractory radiation-induced hemorrhagic cystitis.

4. Prostate and seminal vesicles. Ejaculatory volume is reduced following radiation therapy. Urethral stricture occurs in 1% to 5% of patients undergoing prostate or bladder irradiation. The rate is closer to 15% in patients who have had a prior TURP. Although incontinence rarely occurs after external-beam radiation, it may be seen after prostate brachytherapy in patients who have had a prior TURP.

5. Male and female gonads. These are relatively radiation sensitive. Although the Leydig's cells (and therefore testosterone production) of male adults are quite radioresistant, the spermatogonia are exquisitely sensitive to radiation and are rapidly eliminated by doses of ≥0.8 Gy. The spermatogonia will be replaced in 6 to 24 months, and recovery of the sperm count follows. Permanent azoospermia results only from direct doses of ≥6 Gy. In most major centers, young men treated for seminoma will have their remaining testis shielded with lead to reduce the radiation dose to well below 1 Gy. Sperm banking is not usually recommended unless chemotherapy is to be part of the treatment. Ovaries are more radiation resistant, but permanent sterility can be expected after 12 to 15 Gy of pelvic irradiation.

6. Erectile function. Impotence resulting from radiation may start ≥6 months after therapy. Its incidence may be >50% for those receiving external-beam radiation and approximately 30% to 50% for those receiving prostate implants. It results from the effect of radiation on the proximal corpora to cause a venous leak and the effect on the neurovascular bundles around the prostate. The risk for impotence is higher in older men and those who smoke or have diabetes.

7. Vagina. Vaginal stenosis occurs very infrequently after bladder irradiation. It is more commonly seen after high-dose radiation for cancer of the cervix and uterus. When it occurs and causes sexual dysfunction, it may be treated with lubricants and vaginal dilators.

8. Gastrointestinal tract tissues are sensitive to radiation in doses of ≥50 Gy and can lead to fibrosis, stenosis, and even fistula formation. Most of these effects are minimized by limiting the radiation dose to ≤50 Gy and carefully choosing a radiation-beam arrangement that avoids the small bowel when possible. When treating bladder cancer, radiation oncologists minimize the dose to the small bowel, as this may be required in the future for urinary diversion.

SUGGESTED READING

Bolla M, Collette L. Treatment of prostate cancer with goserelin and radiotherapy. *N Engl J Med* 1997;337:1693–1694.

Kaufman DS, Shipley WU, Griffin PP, et al. Selective preservation by combination treatment of invasive bladder cancer. *N Engl J Med* 1993;329:1377–1382.

Pollack A, Zagars GK, Lewis GS, et al. Preliminary results of a randomized radiotherapy dose-escalation study comparing 70 Gy with 78 Gy for prostate cancer. *J Clin Oncol* 2000;18:3904–3911.

Ragde H, Elgamal AA, Snow PB, et al. Ten-year disease-free survival after transperineal sonography-guided iodine-125 brachytherapy with or without 45-gray external beam irradiation in the treatment of patients with clinically localized, low to high Gleason grade prostate carcinoma. *Cancer* 1998;83:989–1001.

Scardino P, Shipley WU, Vogelzang N, et al., eds. *Textbook of genitourinary oncology.* Baltimore: Williams & Wilkins, 1999.

Shipley WU, Kaufman DS, Thakral HK, et al. Long-term outcome of patients treated for muscle-invasive bladder cancer by tri-modality therapy. *Urology* 2002;60:62–68.

Zelefsky MJ, Fuks Z, Hunt M, et al. High dose radiation delivered by intensity modulated conformal radiotherapy improves the outcome of localized prostate cancer. *J Urol* 2001;166:876–881.

Neurourology

C. Charles Wen and Mike B. Siroky

I. Introduction

The function of the urinary bladder is the storage and expulsion of urine. The pelvic floor is a complex muscle system that acts to support the pelvic organs and promote continence. Neurologic disorders often produce profound dysfunction of the lower urinary tract that may result in urinary retention, urinary incontinence, or both. As a result of dysfunction of the lower urinary tract, the upper urinary tract is often adversely affected, resulting in hydroureteronephrosis, renal failure, urinary stones, or sepsis. Urodynamic testing is discussed in Chapter 7, and urinary incontinence is discussed in Chapter 9.

II. Vesicourethral unit

The urinary bladder is composed primarily of smooth muscle (the **detrusor**). Normal emptying of the bladder is accomplished by contraction of the detrusor muscle accompanied by opening of the bladder neck (**internal sphincter**) and relaxation of the pelvic floor (striated **external sphincter**). Minute-to-minute urinary continence results primarily from closure of the internal urinary sphincter. The external sphincter functions as an auxiliary continence mechanism that is much stronger but much less efficient than the internal sphincter. It is active for short periods of time to prevent leakage of urine during involuntary bladder activity or increased intraabdominal pressure (coughing, straining, or Valsalva maneuver).

    A. Innervation of the vesicourethral unit involves all three divisions of the peripheral nervous system (Fig. 18.1). The detrusor is innervated by the pelvic nerves that arise from sacral segments S2 through S4. These are parasympathetic nerves that secrete acetylcholine as well as other neurotransmitters such as ATP. The hypogastric nerves are sympathetic nerves arising from T10 through T12. They innervate the bladder neck and urethral smooth musculature and secrete norepinephrine. The pudendal nerves are somatic nerves that supply the pelvic floor. Release of acetylcholine at pudendal nerve terminals causes the striated external sphincter to contract.

    B. Central organization of the micturition reflex is hierarchic, with centers located in the cerebrum, posterior hypothalamus, midbrain, pontine reticular formation, and sacral spinal cord (Fig. 18.1). The main function of the pontine center is coordination of the detrusor and its sphincters; suprapontine centers have a net inhibitory effect on the lower centers.

    C. Effects of neurologic lesions vary with their level, extent, and completeness. As a rule, lesions of the cerebrum result in involuntary detrusor contractions that remain coordinated with the sphincters (Fig. 18.2). Lesions of the high spinal cord have the effect of separating the vesicourethral unit from the pontine center, resulting in grossly uncoordinated voiding: **vesicosphincter dyssynergia** (Fig. 18.3). Lesions of the sacral

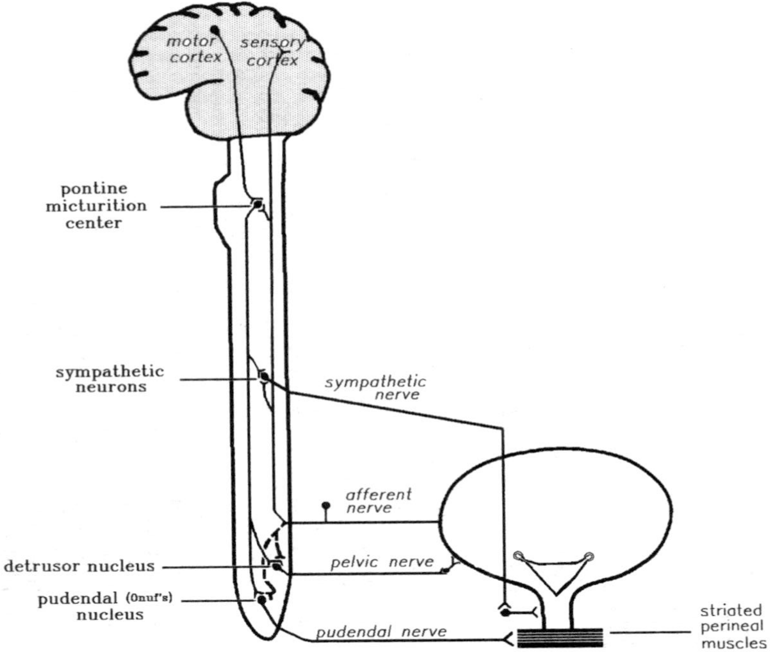

Fig. 18.1.   Neurologic control of micturition involves parasympathetic (pelvic), somatic (pudendal), and sympathetic peripheral nerves. The cerebral cortex inhibits the pontine micturition center, which is responsible for coordinating the bladder and its sphincters during micturition.

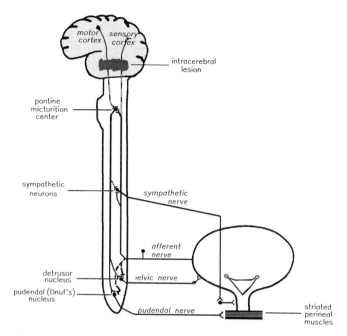

Fig. 18.2. Intracerebral lesions interfere with inhibition of the pontine micturition center.

spinal cord and cauda equina tend to produce a paralyzed detrusor and denervated pelvic floor (Fig. 18.4).

III. Diagnosis

The patient with symptoms of vesicourethral dysfunction requires a careful history and physical examination. Urodynamic testing may or may not be indicated.

A. History. Note any past history of enuresis, urinary infection, calculi, or surgery. In male patients, document the present level of sexual function and note any disturbance of bowel function. The medication history is important. A large number of commonly prescribed drugs may affect voiding function (Table 18.1). The voiding pattern should be elicited in detail, including any frequency (day and night), urgency, incontinence, pain on urination, hesitancy, weak stream, straining to void, dribbling, and incomplete emptying.

B. Physical examination should be focused on the sacral reflexes and sacral sensation. In male patients, perineal sensation is tested by pinprick of the scrotal, penile, and perianal skin. In female patients, the labial and perianal skin should be tested. **Anal tone** is assessed by digital rectal examination. Patients with normal anal tone can voluntarily contract the anal sphincter. Denervation of the perineal floor often manifests as a lax anal sphincter. The **bulbocavernosus reflex** may be tested in several ways. Squeezing the glans penis gently will elicit a

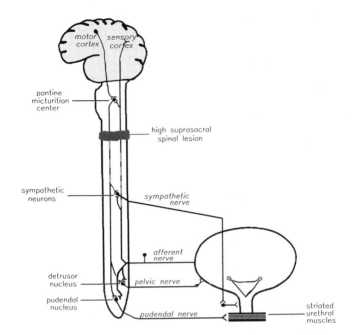

Fig. 18.3.   High suprasacral spinal cord lesions are associated with detrusor hyperreflexia and sphincter dyssynergia.

contraction of the bulbocavernosus muscle, which can be palpated in the perineum. Alternatively, one may elicit the reflex during rectal examination and feel the contraction of the anal sphincter. A variation of this reflex is the "trigonal" reflex, which is elicited by gently tugging on an indwelling Foley catheter and observing the response of the perineal muscles or anal sphincter. The presence of the bulbocavernosus reflex implies that the innervation of the bladder and sphincters is grossly intact. In cases of partial denervation, the reflex may still be present.

IV.   Neurourologic classification
Various systems of classifying urodynamic abnormalities have been proposed. The purpose of these systems is to provide commonly accepted terminology, promote communication, and aid in diagnosis and treatment. The commonly used classification systems are descriptive and do not indicate the cause of the dysfunction (Table 18.2).

V.   Effects of neurologic disease
A.   Spinal cord injury can result from motor vehicle accidents, diving accidents, gunshot wounds, and contact sports. Men are affected much more frequently than women.
   1.   Pathophysiology. Most spinal cord injuries are a combination of contusion, crush, ischemia, and swelling. Thus, some degree of recovery is common; about 50% of spinal cord injuries are ultimately incomplete. Immediately following

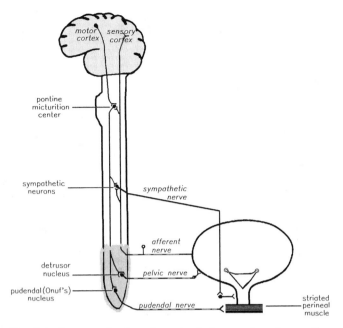

Fig. 18.4. Low sacral and cauda equina lesions produce denervation of the bladder and striated perineal muscles.

Table 18.1. Medications associated with vesicourethral dysfunction

Drug Class	Dysfunction	Examples
Antimuscarinic	Retention	Oxybutynin, tolterodine, antiparkinsonian drugs, phenothiazines
Antispasmodic	Retention	Oxybutynin, dicyclomine, flavoxate
Sympathomimetic	Retention	Pseudoephedrine, ephedrine, phenylephrine, phenylpropanolamine, phentermine, sibutramine
Calcium channel blocking	Retention	Nifedipine, verapamil
Adrenolytic	Incontinence	Prazosin, terazosin, doxazosin, tamsulosin

Table 18.2.   Classification systems used to describe voiding dysfunction

Krane–Siroky	Wein	International Continence Society
Detrusor hyperreflexia	Failure to store	Detrusor
Coordinated sphincters	Because of bladder	Normal
Striated sphincter dyssynergia	Because of outlet	Overactive
Smooth sphincter dyssynergia	Failure to empty	Underactive
Detrusor areflexia	Because of bladder	Urethra
Coordinated sphincters	Because of outlet	Normal
Nonrelaxing striated sphincter		Overative
Nonrelaxing smooth sphincter		Incompetent
Denervated striated sphincter		Sensation
		Normal
		Hypersensitive
		Hyposensitive

suprasacral spinal cord injury, somatic reflexes below the level of injury are often completely abolished (**spinal shock**), including bladder reflexes, resulting in urinary retention. Spinal shock may last for 2 to 12 weeks. The bulbocavernosus reflex is one of the earliest to return. The patient's bladder should be emptied by intermittent catheterization during the period of spinal shock.

2. **Classification of spinal cord injury**

   a.   **Skeletal level of injury** denotes the radiologic determination of the vertebral body with the greatest degree of fracture or injury.

   b.   **Neurologic level of injury** denotes the neurologic determination of the most caudal segment with good motor and sensory function. If dissociation is noted between the motor and sensory levels, both are given. In a **complete** lesion, no function can be elicited below this level. If any nonreflexive movement or sensation exists below the neurologic level of injury, the injury is **incomplete.** Frequently, lack of correlation is found between the neurologic and skeletal level of injury. Because the conus medullaris is located at the L2 and L3 vertebrae, the neurologic level is generally lower than the skeletal level.

   c.   **Grading of motor function** is according to the following scale:

0/5: no movement
1/5: trace of movement

Table 18.3.   Frankel classification of spinal cord injury severity

A	Complete injury, no function below NLI
B	Incomplete injury, some sensation below NLI
C	Incomplete injury, minimal motor function below NLI
D	Incomplete injury, grade 3 movement below NLI
E	Normal motor and sensory function but reflexes remain abnormal

NLI, neurologic level of injury.

2/5: full range of movement with gravity eliminated
3/5: full range of movement against gravity
4/5: full range of movement against resistance
5/5: normal strength and movement

   d.   Frankel grading of completeness of injury is given in Table 18.3. Of all spinal cord injuries, 50% present as Frankel A injury and 30% present as Frankel D. Of patients presenting with Frankel A injuries, >90% are discharged from rehabilitation as Frankel A; 10% improve to Frankel B through D.
3.   High spinal cord injuries (C1 through C8) produce quadriplegia; a significant segment of spinal cord is isolated from higher centers of control (Fig. 18.3).
   a.   Vesicosphincter dyssynergia. When complete, high spinal cord lesions are almost always associated with detrusor hyperreflexia and external sphincter dyssynergia. As mentioned, lesions of the high spinal cord have the effect of separating the vesicourethral unit from the pontine center, resulting in grossly uncoordinated voiding termed **vesicosphincter dyssynergia.** Treatment will be discussed below.
   b.   Autonomic dysreflexia. Autonomic dysreflexia is characterized by significant systolic hypertension, sweating, and paradoxical bradycardia (Fig. 18.5). This syndrome is seen only in patients with spinal cord injury above T6, a viable distal cord, and intact thoracolumbar sympathetic outflow. Of patients with lesions above T6, autonomic dysreflexia may be a significant problem in anywhere from 30% to 85%. Autonomic dysreflexia can be a life-threatening emergency, as systolic blood pressures occasionally exceed 200 mm Hg. The patient complains of severe headache and profuse sweating. Arterial systolic blood pressure is increased by a mean of 40 mm Hg, and diastolic blood pressure is increased by a mean of 25 Hg over baseline. The heart rate is depressed to levels of 60 beats/min or even lower, with the mean decrease being 20 beats/min. Acute episodes of dysreflexia may be associated with bladder distention, fecal impaction, decubitus ulcer, urinary infection, stones, or manipulation of the genitourinary tract. Autonomic dysreflexia may be precipitated during cystometry, cystoscopy, endoscopic surgery, or extracorporeal lithotripsy.

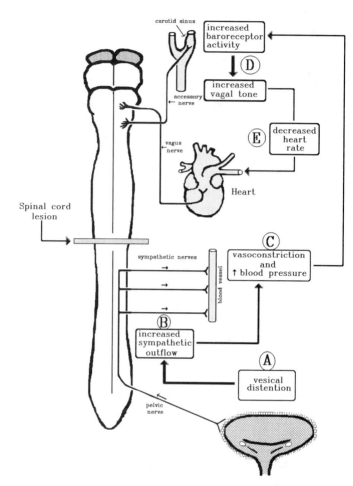

Fig. 18.5. Pathophysiology of autonomic dysreflexia in spinal cord injury.

It can be prevented by spinal anesthesia, but general anesthesia is not effective unless it is quite deep.

4. Low spinal cord injuries (T1 through L5) produce paraplegia. Detrusor hyperreflexia is common; sphincter dyssynergia may coexist depending on completeness of the lesion.

5. Conus (S1 through S5) and cauda equina injury produce bladder areflexia and denervated sphincter in about 75% of patients (Fig. 18.4). The internal sphincter (bladder neck) may be also incompetent in these patients, making them prone to incontinence.

B. The effect of **cerebral lesions,** including those associated with cerebrovascular disease, Parkinson's disease, and brain injury or tumor, on urinary function depends on their location and extent (Fig. 18.2). Cerebral lesions, especially those located in the frontal cortex and internal capsule, tend to produce detrusor hyperreflexia, with coordinated or uninhibited sphincters in the majority of patients (approximately 70%). About 50% of patients who survive stroke have urinary incontinence. Patients with Parkinson's disease may have complex dysfunction caused by a combination of detrusor hyperreflexia, anticholinergic effects of medication, and impaired sphincter control (sphincter bradykinesia). Voiding symptoms are reported in about 25% of unselected parkinsonian patients. About two-thirds of symptomatic patients have detrusor hyperreflexia with coordinated sphincters.

C. Multiple sclerosis produces areas of demyelination in the spinal cord or brain. The site most commonly affected is the cervical spinal cord. Multiple sclerosis is the most important cause of disability in adults between 20 and 45 years old. About 80% of these patients have urologic symptoms. Urinary tract dysfunction tends to correlate with evidence of pyramidal tract dysfunction. Detrusor hyperreflexia is seen in 60% of patients, and about one-third of patients with detrusor hyperreflexia have vesicosphincter dyssynergia. About 20% have detrusor areflexia. The risk for deterioration of the upper tract is less than that in spinal cord–injured patients.

D. Diabetes mellitus is associated with peripheral neuropathy, which may affect the bladder and/or sphincters. About 80% of patients with diabetic bladder dysfunction also have other sequelae of diabetes (retinopathy, neuropathy, vascular disease). The classic urodynamic finding in diabetes is detrusor areflexia, but nearly 50% of patients with diabetes have detrusor hyperreflexia rather than areflexia. This may be caused by concomitant cerebrovascular disease. Patients with detrusor areflexia associated with diabetes also have impaired bladder sensation.

VI. Treatment
The goals of treatment in any type of voiding dysfunction are to (a) reverse the pathologic process whenever possible, (b) alleviate symptoms (especially incontinence) when reversal is not possible, and (c) preserve renal function. It is important to remember that a perfect therapeutic result is rarely obtained in treating voiding dysfunction. A practical treatment plan must take into consideration the underlying disease and its prognosis, the patient's desires, and the family support available to the patient. In most cases, a combination of treatment modes is necessary to achieve satisfactory results.

A. Detrusor overactivity can be a debilitating problem, especially when it causes incontinence. Many options are available in treating the overactive detrusor, which suggests that none is completely effective.

1. Pharmacologic therapy. See Tables 8.4 and 18.3 for a summary of available agents.

a. Antimuscarinic agents continue to be the mainstay of treatment. Side effects common to this group of drugs are dry mouth, blurring of vision, constipation, and drowsiness. Antimuscarinic agents may precipitate acute intraocular hypertension and are contraindicated in patients with angle-closure glaucoma. An ophthalmologic consultation should be obtained for all patients with glaucoma before antimuscarinic medication is prescribed. The prototype agent is oxybutynin hydrochloride in oral doses of 5 mg three times daily. Extended-release formulations of tolterodine and oxybutynin have largely replaced generic oxybutynin as first-line agents because of more favorable side effect profiles. **Intravesical oxybutynin** has been used in some patients who fail oral agents because of side effects. Five milligrams of oxybutynin is dissolved in 50 mg of saline solution and instilled via urethral catheter. The solution is left in the bladder until it is voided or removed by catheterization 4 hours later.

b. **Tricyclic antidepressants** have a combination of anticholinergic and sympathomimetic actions. They may have central effects as well. The prototypic agent is imipramine, used in doses varying from 25 mg at bedtime to 25 mg four times daily. The drug may be used alone or in combination with antimuscarinic agents. Imipramine is contraindicated in patients receiving monoamine oxidase inhibitors.

2. **Biofeedback** may work well in motivated patients and can be used as an adjunct to pharmacologic therapy. In one simple biofeedback technique, the patient keeps a chart to record the timing of voiding and amounts voided. The patient receives rewards or encouragement for increasing the time between voiding, along with antimuscarinic medication. This is often referred to as a Frewen regimen or "bladder drill." More complex methods involve auditory or visual feedback to the patient when bladder contraction occurs to enable the patient to learn techniques to suppress contractile activity.

3. **Electric stimulation** of the vaginal or rectal mucosa can promote urine storage by causing perineal muscle contraction and inhibiting detrusor activity. The stimulation is provided by intravaginal or intrarectal stimulating units.

4. The use of **augmentation cystoplasty** in the treatment of storage failure has recently become widespread. Cystoplasty is most commonly achieved by placing detubularized ileum as a cap on the bladder to increase its capacity. Reported success rates range from 50% to 80%. Following this procedure, many patients will require intermittent self-catheterization.

5. **Supravesical urinary diversion** should be considered in patients with intractable incontinence who demonstrate deterioration of the upper tracts from ureterovesical reflux or obstruction. Continent forms of diversion may be appropriate in some cases.

6. **Botulinum toxin** injected endoscopically into the detrusor has been shown to be an effective treatment for patients who fail or cannot tolerate the side effects of antimuscarinic medications. A total of 300 U of botulinum A toxin can be injected into the detrusor muscle at 20 to 30 sites (approximately

10 U/site), avoiding the trigone. The procedure can be repeated every 6 to 9 months when the effect of the toxin diminishes.

7.   Neuromodulation of sacral nerve roots can be used to treat urge incontinence and urinary retention. Electrodes are surgically implanted in the sacral foramina. Patients are first screened with implantation of a temporary test stimulator. If symptoms are significantly improved, a permanent device can be implanted. Approximately 50% of patients who undergo testing are implanted. Long-term improvements in those implanted have been reported in up to 57% of patients, with up to 50% reoperation rates.

8.   Dorsal rhizotomy can be performed to alleviate bladder spasticity caused by severe detrusor hyperreflexia. Efficacy rates as high as 70% have been reported. Rhizotomy is performed by surgically dividing and denervating the sacral dorsal rootlets to decrease afferent input to motor neurons. These rootlets may also contain sensory and proprioceptive fibers. Implantation of a neurostimulator for the anterior spinal roots allows patients with dorsal rhizotomies to control micturition and possibly erection as well.

B.   Detrusor underactivity

1.   Pharmacologic therapy of the acontractile detrusor is much less successful than therapy of the overactive bladder. Bethanechol chloride has been used for many years for this purpose because its action is somewhat selective for the bladder and gastrointestinal tract and because it can be given by mouth. Bethanechol is capable of increasing the tension in the bladder wall when given in doses of 50 to 100 mg orally four times daily. However, its ability to produce an effective bladder contraction capable of completely emptying the bladder has never been impressive. It may be useful as an adjunct to other methods, such as the Valsalva maneuver, in emptying the bladder. Side effects includes flushing, sweating, headache, diarrhea, gastrointestinal cramps, and bronchospasm.

2.   Intermittent catheterization has been very successful in managing the underactive detrusor. Originally described in patients with spinal cord injury, it may be used to treat a wide variety of voiding dysfunctions. Intermittent catheterization may be combined with antimuscarinic agents to promote dryness. One of the most important factors in promoting patient acceptance of self-catheterization is a positive and supportive attitude on the part of physicians and nurses.

a.   Clean technique. Most patients can be taught to perform intermittent clean self-catheterization. In male patients, the head of the penis is cleansed with povidone–iodine, hexachlorophene, or plain soap, and a 14F straight catheter is inserted into the urethra. In female patients, the urethral meatus is cleansed, and a short 12F female catheter is inserted. Any water-soluble lubricant can be used. The catheters may be cleaned and reused many times. Sterile gloves are not needed. For most patients, the clean technique is the most convenient and cost-effective method of emptying the bladder.

b.   Sterile technique is needed only for patients who are immunocompromised or prone to repeated infection. The only difference from clean technique is that a new, sterile catheter is inserted each time and sterile gloves are used to handle the catheter and prepare the skin.

3.   Valsalva and Crede maneuver is applicable in most paraplegic patients as long as no significant outflow obstruction is present.

C.   External sphincter dyssynergia generally should be treated in male patients to prevent deterioration of the upper tract. Paraplegic patients may be treated with antimuscarinic agents and intermittent self-catheterization. The same regimen may be used in quadriplegic patients if a family member or personal care attendant is available. For quadriplegic patients who cannot perform intermittent self-catheterization, other options may have to be considered.

1.   Pharmacologic therapy is generally not successful. Agents that have been used include baclofen, dantrolene, diazepam, and tizanidine. The use of intrathecal baclofen delivered with a subcutaneous pump has also been reported.

2.   Urethral stents have been implanted to treat external sphincter dyssynergia, but long-term results are not available.

3.   External sphincterotomy is performed by endoscopic resection of the external sphincter. Bladder neck and prostate resection may be required at the same time. Complications of external sphincterotomy include hemorrhage, stricture, and impotence (5% to 10%). About one-third of patients require a second sphincterotomy to correct poor bladder emptying.

4.   Botulinum toxin can be injected into the external urinary sphincter in patients with detrusor sphincter dyssynergia. Under direct vision, 80 to 100 U of botulinum A toxin is injected into the external urethral sphincter at the 3, 6, 9, and 12 o'clock positions. This can also be done for patients with detrusor areflexia who would prefer to void by Valsalva.

D.   Urethral incompetence in patients with neurologic disease is treated in much the same way as in other patients.

1.   Pharmacologic therapy includes pseudoephedrine hydrochloride in oral doses of 30 to 60 mg up to four times daily and phenylpropanolamine hydrochloride in oral doses of 50 mg three times daily. These drugs act to increase muscular tone at the bladder neck and in the urethra. If detrusor instability is present, an antimuscarinic agent may be used concurrently. Sympathomimetic agents should be used with caution in the elderly and in those patients with hypertension, diabetes mellitus, ischemic heart disease, hyperthyroidism, increased intraocular pressure, or bladder outlet obstruction from prostatic hyperplasia. Phenylpropanolamine is contraindicated in patients receiving monoamine oxidase inhibitors.

2.   Sling procedures may be used in selected female patients with type III incontinence resulting from neurologic disease. The sling is composed of autologous rectus fascia, Marlex, Gore-Tex, or Mersilene. In neurologic patients with bladder paralysis, the tension of the sling is adjusted so that urine will be retained, and the patient performs intermittent self-catheterization to empty the bladder. The major complications are operative injury to the urethra or bladder and delayed erosion of the sling into the urethra.

3.   The **artificial urinary sphincter** consists of a periurethral cuff, a pressure-regulating balloon inflated in the prevesical space, and a control valve. In male patients, the cuff can be placed around the urethra (most common) or around the bladder neck and the control valve implanted into the scrotum. In female patients, the cuff is placed around the bladder neck and the control valve is implanted into the labia. Detrusor instability, detrusor hyperreflexia, and diminished bladder compliance are relative contraindications. Approximately one-third of patients require revision of the device at some point. Like all prosthetics, these devices may be complicated by mechanical failure, erosion, displacement, or infection. To reduce the risk for urethral erosion, the device is activated 6 weeks after implantation, when healing has progressed.

4.   **Urethral bulking agents** such as collagen or carbon beads can be implanted via transurethral, periurethral, or antegrade approaches. Bulking agents are injected into the submucosa layer of the proximal urethra. By bulking the submucosal space, coaptation of the urethra is improved and leak point pressures are increased.

E.   Autonomic dysreflexia

The immediate goal of management must be rapid reduction of blood pressure and removal of the precipitating cause, most commonly bladder distention. If very rapid reduction in blood pressure is needed, we prefer a sodium nitroprusside drip at a rate of 25 to 50 µg/min, with a maximum dosage of 200 to 300 µg/min. Alternatively, one can give diazoxide as a bolus of 50 to 150 mg IV every 5 minutes or as an infusion. If less immediate control of hypertension is desired, we use nifedipine given orally or sublingually in a dose of 10 to 30 mg. Severe reflex bradycardia may be managed with intravenous atropine in a dose of 0.4 to 1.6 mg. Long-term prophylaxis of autonomic dysreflexia is accomplished with 1 to 4 mg of prazosin orally twice daily.

SUGGESTED READING

Batista JE, Bauer SB, Shefner JM, et al. Urodynamic findings in children with spinal cord ischemia. *J Urol* 1995;154:1183–1187.

Goldstein I, Siroky MB, Sax DS, et al. Neurourologic abnormalities in multiple sclerosis. *J Urol* 1982;128:541–545.

Hohenfellner M, Pannek J, Bötel U, et al. Sacral bladder denervation for treatment of detrusor hyperreflexia and autonomic dysreflexia. *Urology* 2001;58:28–32.

Kasabian NG, Vlachiotis JD, Lais A, et al. The use of intravesical oxybutinin chloride in patients with detrusor hypertonicity and detrusor hyperreflexia. *J Urol* 1994;151:944–945.

Kershen RT, Atala A. New advances in injectable therapies for the treatment of incontinence and vesicoureteral reflux. *Urol Clin North Am* 1999;26:81–94.

Koldewijn EL, Hommes DR, Lemmens AJG, et al. Relationship between lower urinary tract abnormalities and disease-related parameters in multiple sclerosis. *J Urol* 1995;154:169–173.

Pavlakis AJ, Siroky MB, Goldstein I, et al. Neuro-urologic findings in conus medullaris and cauda equina injury. *Arch Neurol* 1983;40:570–574.

Pavlakis A, Siroky MB, Sax DS, et al. Neurourologic abnormalities in Parkinson's disease. *J Urol* 1983;129:80–83.

Phelan MW, Franks M, Somogyi GT, et al. Botulinum toxin urethral sphincter injection to restore bladder emptying in men and women with voiding dysfunction. *J Urol* 2001;165:1107–1110.

Rudy DC, Awad SA, Downie JW. External sphincter dyssynergia: an abnormal continence reflex. *J Urol* 1988;140:105–110.

Schurch B, Stöhrer M, Kramer G, et al. Botulinum-A toxin for treating detrusor hyperreflexia in spinal cord injured patients: a new alternative to anticholinergic drugs? Preliminary results. *J Urol* 2000; 164:692–697.

Siegel SW, Catanzaro F, Dijkema HE, et al. Long-term results of a multicenter study on sacral nerve stimulation for treatment of urinary urge incontinence, urgency-frequency, and retention. *Urology* 2000;56(suppl 1):87–91.

Siroky MB. Interpretation of urinary flow rates. *Urol Clin North Am* 1990;17:537–541.

Siroky MB. Electromyography of the perineal floor. *Urol Clin North Am* 1996;23:299–302.

Siroky MB, Krane RJ. Neurologic aspects of detrusor hyperreflexia with reference to the guarding reflex. *J Urol* 1982;127:953–957.

Siroky MB, Nehra A, Vlachiotis J, et al. Effect of spinal cord ischemia on vesico-urethral function. *J Urol* 1992;148:1211–1214.

Staskin DS, Vardi Y, Siroky MB. Post-prostatectomy continence in the parkinsonian patient: the significance of poor voluntary sphincter control. *J Urol* 1988;140:117–118.

Pediatric Urology

Elise De and Stuart B. Bauer

In addition to a detailed understanding of embryology and physiology, pediatric urology requires sensitivity toward the special emotional needs of sick children and their parents. With recent advances in surgery, intensive care technology, and chemotherapy, children are surviving conditions that were previously devastating and often fatal. Continuing advances in the field of reconstructive surgery offer the potential for highly successful management of these challenging diseases.

I. Wilms' tumor (nephroblastoma)

A. Incidence. Wilms' tumor accounts for approximately 10% of childhood cancers. Annual incidence in the United States is 450 to 500 cases. The tumor simulates the development of a normal kidney with blastemal, epithelial, and stromal components. Unilateral tumors present at a median age of 37 months in boys and 43 months in girls; bilateral tumors are usually diagnosed earlier. Wilms' tumor can be sporadic or, in 1% to 2% of cases, familial. The familial form is an autosomal dominant trait with incomplete penetrance; the *FWT1* gene on chromosome 17q and the *FWT2* gene on chromosome 19q have been linked to two groups of families. A number of syndromes are associated with Wilms' tumor (Table 19.1). Overall, about 5% of patients with Wilms' tumors have associated genitourinary anomalies (hypospadias, cryptorchidism, renal fusion, and other anomalies).

B. Histology is one of the most important predictors of clinical outcome. A **favorable histology** is one without anaplastic features as defined by nuclear diameter, chromatin content, and mitotic figures. Anaplasia can be focal or diffuse and is present in 5% of tumors. Clear cell sarcoma and rhabdoid tumors are also considered **unfavorable histology.** Overall, unfavorable histology is seen in about 12% of patients with Wilms' tumor.

C. Diagnosis. The most common presentation is a large, firm, unilateral abdominal mass (80%). Less common are abdominal pain (30%) and nausea and vomiting (20%). About 12% of patients have distant metastases at presentation.

Approximately 50% of patients have hypertension, and half present with hematuria. Anemia may be present, and results of liver function tests may be abnormal in the presence of metastatic disease. A complete exam for associated anomalies or venous obstruction is essential. Radiographically, the diagnosis and essential staging are made by ultrasound (US) and confirmed by computed tomography (CT). Chest radiography is essential as well. Wilms' tumor must be differentiated from hydronephrosis, polycystic kidney, and neuroblastoma.

D. Staging is summarized in Table 19.2. It is essential to stage accurately preoperatively in order to follow protocol adjuvant therapies.

Table 19.1. Syndromes that incorporate Wilms' tumor

Syndrome	Features	Risk of Wilms' (%)	Genetics
Denys–Drash	Male pseudo-hermaph-roditism	90	*WT1* gene
	Renal mesangial sclerosis		of 11p13 mutated
WAGR	Aniridia GU anomalies Mental retardation	42	*WT1* gene of 11p13 deleted
Beckwith–Wiedemann	Hemihypertrophy, organomegaly Omphalocele Adrenal tumors Hepatic tumors	5–20	linked to 11p15

WAGR, W̲ilms' tumor, A̲niridia, G̲U̲ abnormalities, R̲etardation; GU, genitourinary.

E.   Treatment of Wilms' tumor involves a multimodal approach that includes surgical removal, chemotherapy, and radiotherapy. Survival approaching 100% can be achieved in earlier-stage disease.

1.   Surgical removal via the transperitoneal approach is the mainstay of treatment for unilateral tumors and provides important staging information. Complete resection without spillage is of the utmost importance to avoid relapse and/or the need for irradiation. Radical nephrectomy without formal lymph node dissection is performed if palpable nodes are not detected. Surgical complications occur in 11% of cases, most

Table 19.2.   Summary of staging of Wilms' tumor (according to National Wilms' Tumor Study Group)

Stage	Description
I	Tumor confined to kidney, completely excised without spillage or capsular rupture
II	Tumor beyond kidney but completely excised or spillage confined to flank
III	Residual nonhematogenous disease present but confined to abdomen
IV	Hematogenous metastases (e.g., brain) or nonabdominal lymph node metastases
V	Bilateral disease: Stage each according to above criteria

From Neville and Ritchey, *Urol Clin North Am* 2000; 27:435–442.

commonly hemorrhage and small bowel obstruction. Bilateral biopsy should be performed in patients with bilateral tumors; resection should be attempted only after preoperative chemotherapy and reevaluation for partial resection versus further chemotherapy.

2. Chemotherapy is indicated in all stages of Wilms' tumor regardless of histologic type (vincristine and actinomycin D in the lower stages, adding doxorubicin, cyclophosphamide, etoposide, and/or carboplatin, in some cases dropping actinomycin D in the higher stages).

3. Radiotherapy. In patients with favorable histology, radiotherapy is reserved for stage III or higher advanced disease. With unfavorable histology, radiotherapy is also given in stage II disease.

II. Neuroblastoma is the most common intraabdominal malignancy of infancy. A poorly differentiated neoplasm of the adrenal gland, it is a neoplasm derived from neural crest cells that typically occurs in infants and young children. See Chapter 23 for a complete discussion.

III. Vesicoureteral reflux is caused by primary or secondary incompetence of the ureterovesical valve mechanism. During bladder contraction, urine passes in a retrograde direction into the ureter. The degree of reflux is graded according to the classification system of the International Reflux Study (Table 19.3). Grading is based on the appearance of contrast agent in the collecting system during voiding cystourethrography (VCUG).

A. Incidence. Studies of asymptomatic children have estimated an incidence of 17%, whereas vesicoureteral reflux is present in 70% of infants with urinary tract infection. More importantly, between 30% and 50% of children with reflux will have renal scarring. Reflux is the second most common cause of prenatal hydronephrosis and accounts for 37% of cases. Adults with urinary tract infection (UTI) have a 5% incidence of reflux.

B. Etiology

1. Primary reflux is caused by lateral displacement of the ureteral orifice during embryogenesis and a shorter intramural tunnel for the ureter, resulting in a poor muscular backing. A weaker valve mechanism is therefore available to close the orifice during bladder contractions.

Table 19.3. International classification of vesicoureteral reflux

Grade of Reflux	Degree of Reflux
1	Ureter only
2	Ureter and pelvis, no dilatation
3	Mild dilatation of ureter, pelvis, and calyces; minimal forniceal blunting
4	Moderate ureteral tortuosity, pelvic and calyceal dilatation
5	Gross dilatation, tortuosity of ureter, papillae obliterated

2.   Ureteral duplication is commonly associated with reflux into the lower pole ureter, again owing to its abnormally short intramural tunnel (see below).

3.   Ureteral ectopia without ureterocele may be associated with reflux.

4.   Abnormalities of the bladder wall such as diverticula, radiation cystitis, and cyclophosphamide (Cytoxan) cystitis may predispose to vesicoureteral reflux. UTI may be associated with transient reflux, due to the inflamed bladder wall.

5.   Elevated intravesical pressure from any cause may lead to reflux. Common causes are posterior urethral valves, detrusor hyperreflexia, and prostatic enlargement in adults.

6.   Prune-belly syndrome is a congenital condition characterized by deficient anterior abdominal musculature, bilateral cryptorchidism, bilateral megaureter, and often bilateral vesicoureteral reflux.

7.   Iatrogenic reflux may result from any surgical procedure that disrupts the trigonal muscle, such as prostatectomy. Resection of the ureteral orifice can also produce reflux.

8.   Dysfunctional voiding or elimination syndromes can lead to reflux. Voiding patterns should always be elicited in the medical history.

C.   Diagnosis. Vesicoureteral reflux rarely causes symptoms. Most instances of reflux present as recurrent UTI or pyelonephritis. In more advanced stages, the patient may present with uremia or hypertension. The intravenous urography (IVU) findings are usually normal in lower grades of reflux. The VCUG is the definitive examination and must include a voiding phase; in some cases, reflux may be seen only during the elevated intravesical pressures associated with micturition. In addition, in visualizing the urethra, the voiding phase of the VCUG may allow the diagnosis of outflow obstruction to be made (e.g., posterior urethral valves).

D.   Treatment

1.   Medical management is indicated in cases of low-grade vesicoureteral reflux without outlet obstruction or another abnormality. Good patient compliance is necessary. Long-term antibiotic suppression with a regimen of amoxicillin (neonate), trimethoprim/sulfamethoxazole, nitrofurantoin, or other antibiotic agent at one-fourth to one-half the usual dose daily is commonly used. Depending on the grade of reflux as determined by VCUG, the age of the patient at diagnosis, and unilateral versus bilateral disease, a considerable number of instances of vesicoureteral reflux will resolve spontaneously without surgical correction (Table 19.4). If the patient remains asymptomatic, urine cultures are obtained periodically (e.g., every 3 months) during treatment. US and radionuclide cystogram should be obtained at yearly intervals. If acute ("breakthrough") infection occurs, a full course of appropriate antibiotics is given and a prophylactic regimen is then instituted. Some clinicians perform a dimercaptosuccinic acid scan to look for renal scarring at this juncture. Surgery is often recommended after breakthrough UTI.

2.   Surgical therapy is indicated in patients with high-grade primary reflux (grades 4 and 5), those with low-pressure

Table 19.4. Resolution of vesicoureteral reflux with antibiotic prophylaxis

Grade of Reflux	Resolution (%)
1	90
2	60
3	50
4	30
5	0

reflux and significant hydroureter, and patients in whom medical management has failed. Although failure can be defined in various ways, most agree that persistence of reflux after 3 to 4 years of antibiotic prophylaxis, multiple "breakthrough" infections, new or increased renal scarring, deterioration of renal function, and noncompliance with medication are indications for surgical therapy. In patients with minimal hydroureter, creation of a ureteroneocystostomy with the Leadbetter–Politano, Cohen, Glenn Anderson, or extravesical techniques has a 98% cure rate. Approximately 1% of patients have obstruction of the ureterovesical junction after ureteral reimplantation that requires reoperation. In patients with massive ureteral dilatation, tapering of the distal ureter may be necessary during reimplantation. Rarely, temporary supravesical diversion is necessary in patients who are severely uremic.

IV. **Obstruction of the upper urinary tract**

   A. **Ureteropelvic junction obstruction**

      1. **Incidence.** The ureteropelvic junction is the most common site of urinary tract obstruction in children and the most common cause of prenatal hydronephrosis (48%). The vast majority of instances are congenital in origin. With routine prenatal US, the majority of cases of ureteropelvic junction obstruction are detected before birth. Children who escape diagnosis in infancy can present later with either urinary infection or episodic abdominal pain. There is a predilection for the left side (67%), and boys are affected twice as often as girls.

      2. **Associated findings** include contralateral obstruction of the ureteropelvic junction (10%), contralateral renal agenesis (5%), and vesicoureteral reflux (10%).

      3. **Pathophysiology**

         a. The exact etiology has not been determined, but an **intrinsic muscular defect** is likely the most common cause, either an interruption of the circular fibers or an abnormality of the collagen matrix. Impaired peristalsis through the ureteropelvic junction results.

         b. **Aberrant blood vessels** that cross the ureteropelvic junction anteriorly and supply the lower renal pole account for approximately one-third of cases.

         c. **Less common causes** include valvular mucosal folds, persistent fetal convolutions, stenosis or stricture, and upper ureteral polyps.

    d.   Secondary obstruction of the ureteropelvic junction may occur with high-grade vesicoureteral reflux, which leads to the development of a tortuous ureter and kinking at the point of fixation. Periureteral fibrosis and external compression are possible but usually in an older population.

  4.   Diagnosis

    a.   Symptoms and signs. Obstruction of the ureteropelvic junction occurs in varying degrees. The majority of children now present for evaluation in infancy with a history of antenatal hydronephrosis. Approximately 30% of older children present with UTI. Others may present with a palpable flank mass, intermittent pain, vomiting, or failure to thrive. The pain may be confused with pain arising from the gastrointestinal tract. Fluid intake can exacerbate the pain by transiently increasing the intrarenal pressure proximal to the point of obstruction. The patient may present with gross or microscopic hematuria (25%) with or without a history of antecedent trauma. In cases of bilateral obstruction of the ureteropelvic junction, a child may present with uremia.

    b.   Radiologic examination. Increasingly, hydronephrosis is diagnosed antenatally by maternal US. Subsequent imaging can determine whether the etiology is ureteropelvic junction obstruction. US will show pelvic and calyceal dilatation with a ureter of normal caliber. Traditionally, the IVU demonstrates a delayed nephrogram and delayed excretion of contrast agent in high-grade obstruction. However, obstruction of the ureteropelvic junction can be mild or intermittent and may become evident only during periods of diuresis. Thus, many provocative tests have been devised, such as the nuclear diuretic renogram (the diuretic IVU has been largely replaced). The nuclear agent merceptoacetyltriglycine, a radiopharmaceutical cleared primarily by tubular secretion and somewhat by glomerular filtration, provides differential function, data on washout from individual kidneys, and with Lasix assessment of fluid challenge. For equivocal cases, the Whitaker test can be performed, although it is used only rarely in children.

    c.   Antegrade perfusion of the kidney (Whitaker test). Following percutaneous nephrostomy, the nephrostomy catheter is perfused at a rate of 10 mL/min while the perfusion pressure is measured. The intravesical pressure, monitored simultaneously with an intravesical catheter, is subtracted from the intrapelvic pressure. In the presence of obstruction of the upper urinary tract, a higher perfusion pressure is required to achieve a given perfusion rate. A differential intrapelvic pressure of >20 cm H_2O is considered diagnostic of obstruction. Although false-positive and false-negative results can occur, the overall accuracy of the test is approximately 90%. Its major disadvantage is the requirement for percutaneous nephrostomy.

  5.   Treatment

    a.   Conservative management is indicated in patients with minimal objective evidence of obstruction, normal renal function, no symptoms, and no history of infection.

    b. Surgical pyeloplasty is indicated for children if symptoms that can be attributed to the obstruction are present or if differential function on nuclear scan falls below 35%. If the lower ureter is not well visualized, cystoscopy and retrograde pyelography should be performed in conjunction with pyeloplasty. The **Anderson–Hynes dismembered pyeloplasty,** the most commonly employed procedure to correct this anomaly, involves excision of the ureteropelvic junction segment, reanastomosis of the ureter to the pelvis, and repositioning of any associated or aberrant vessels posterior to the anastomosis. Other techniques include flap-type and incisional–intubated repairs, for example, a long spiral flap to provide extra ureteral length. Open techniques render an 85% to 100% success rate. Endoscopic techniques using incisure have been employed successfully in older children, and laparoscopic techniques (including robotic assistance) have been used in younger children.

    c. Nephrectomy should be considered in patients with complete or nearly complete absence of renal function (<5% to 10%).

B. Duplication of the kidney, renal pelvis, and ureter. A system of standardized terminology is presented in Table 19.5.

    1. Incidence. Duplication of the upper urinary tract is one of the most common congenital malformations, approximately 1 in 125 (0.8%) of the population. The female-to-male ratio is probably about 3:2, and unilateral duplication is six times more frequent than bilateral.

    2. Associated malformations. Duplication of the ureter itself is usually of no clinical significance, but associated prob-

Table 19.5.   Definition of terms in upper urinary tract duplication

Term	Definition
Duplex kidney	Kidney with two pelvicalyceal systems
Bifid pelvis	Duplex kidney with single ureter
Bifid ureter	Duplex kidney with two ureters that join outside bladder; older term is "incomplete duplication of ureter"
Double ureter	Duplex kidney with two ureters that do not join; older term is "complete duplication of ureter"
Ectopic ureter	Ureter that drains to abnormal site
Lateral ectopia	Ureteral orifice lateral to normal position
Caudal ectopia	Ureteral orifice at or distal to bladder neck
Intravesical ureterocele	Ureterocele located entirely within bladder
Ectopic ureterocele	Ureterocele located at or distal to bladder neck

lems such as reflux or obstruction may require treatment. Because of the development of the mesonephric duct, the ureteral orifice draining the upper pole segment will be located in the bladder in a position caudal and medial to the orifice draining the lower pole segment (Meyer–Weigert rule).

a.   Vesicoureteral reflux is the most common problem associated with complete duplication of the ureter. Reflux, which occurs in 30% of cases, is much more likely to occur into the lower pole ureter because it inserts laterally into the bladder and has a shortened intramural segment. Rarely, when the ureter inserts into or below the bladder neck at the level of the sphincter, reflux occurs into the upper pole ureter alone. Reflux into both ureters may occur when the orifices are in close proximity.

b.   Ureteral ectopia. Any ureter that does not insert onto the trigone may be considered ectopic. Thus, lateral displacement is, strictly speaking, a form of ectopia; in practice, however, the term is reserved for insertion onto or distal to the bladder neck. Ureteral ectopia has a female-to-male predominance of 3:1, and about 10% of instances are bilateral.

(1)   Location. If the ectopic ureter is located in the proximal female urethra, the result is usually obstruction, reflux, or both. These patients often present with recurrent UTIs. If the location of the ureter is distal to the external sphincter, the patient invariably presents with continuous incontinence despite a normal voiding pattern. An ectopic ureter also may insert into the vestibule, vagina, or uterus, again leading to continuous incontinence. An ectopic ureter in male patients inserts most commonly into the prostatic urethra, although it may insert into the ejaculatory duct, seminal vesicle, or vas deferens/epididymis (Table 19.6). These patients can present with UTIs or epididymitis but not incontinence, because the ectopic ureter in males never inserts below (distal to) the external sphincter.

(2)   Association with duplication. In female patients, an ectopic ureter is part of a duplication anomaly in >80% of cases and almost always affects the upper pole ureter. The converse is not true; only about 3% of completely duplicated ureters are ectopic. In males, the ectopic ureter is part of a single rather than a duplicated system.

c.   Ureterocele is a term describing a cystic dilatation of the terminal or intramural portion of the ureter; it usually is associated with the upper pole ureter in a completely du-

Table 19.6.   Location of orifice in ureteral ectopia

Male Patients (%)		Female Patients (%)	
Urethra	50	Urethra	35
Seminal vesicle	30	Vestibule	35
Ejaculatory duct	15	Vagina	25
Vas deferens	5	Uterus	5

plicated system (80%), although single-system ureterocele is possible. Ureterocele occurs in females four times more often than in males. Approximately 10% of ureteroceles are bilateral. The ureteral orifice may be located entirely within the bladder (intravesical ureterocele), at the bladder neck, or within the urethra (ectopic ureterocele). In girls, an ectopic ureterocele can prolapse into the urethra, and as such it is one of the most common causes of infravesical obstruction in girls. Antibiotic prophylaxis should be prescribed to any patient with ureterocele because of the risk of obstruction and pyuria.

d. **Ureteropelvic junction obstruction** of the lower pole is possible and should not be overlooked.

3. **Diagnosis.** US may demonstrate the presence of a dilated, dysplastic upper pole segment in duplication. If both segments of a duplicated kidney are functioning, the IVU usually demonstrates this (Table 19.7). Not infrequently, however, the renal upper pole segment may have little or no function and thus will not be visualized on IVU. The presence of a duplication with nonfunction of the upper pole segment is suggested on IVU by (a) downward displacement of the lower pole calyces by the upper pole ("drooping lily" sign), (b) discrepancy between the size of the kidney and the small number of calyces seen, and (c) change in the renal axis, with the upper pole displaced laterally away from the vertebral bodies. This displacement results in an increased distance between the kidney and vertebral bodies on the affected side in comparison with the contralateral side. Radionuclide studies may demonstrate a degree of function in an upper pole segment not visualized by IVU. When ureterocele is present, bladder films on IVU may demonstrate a characteristic filling defect referred to as a "cobra head" deformity. US findings include a dilated ureter, and the ureterocele appears as a thin-walled cystic structure protruding into the lumen of the bladder. A VCUG should be performed in every patient with duplication to rule out vesicoureteral reflux into the ipsilateral lower pole or contralateral ureters; ureterocele can often be seen within the bladder early in the filling phase. Cystoscopy is needed to assess the location of the ureteral orifices and the extent and boundary of any existing ureterocele, but this may be performed at the time of planned corrective surgery. Retrograde contrast studies may be useful in some cases of ectopic ureter.

Table 19.7. Radiologic findings in duplication with ureterocele

Radiologic Finding	Upper Pole (%)	Lower Pole (%)
IVU: nonfunction	90	5
IVU: delayed function	10	75
VCUG: reflux	15	45

IVU, intravenous urogram; VCUG, voiding cystourethrogram.

4. Treatment of ureteral duplication depends on the presence of reflux or obstruction and on the degree of impairment of renal function in the upper and/or lower pole moieties of the kidney.

a. When **reflux** is present in one or both ureters of a duplicated system and neither ureterocele nor ectopia can be demonstrated, reflux is treated in the same manner as a single-system refluxing ureter. In the absence of hydroureter, prophylactic antibiotics (to help prevent pyelonephritis) and annual radiologic follow-up will demonstrate spontaneous resolution in about 50% of patients. In patients placed on such a regimen, breakthrough infections, progressive renal scarring, and noncompliance with treatment are indications for surgical correction of the reflux. In patients with hydroureter or very high-grade reflux (grade V), surgical correction should be the initial mode of therapy. In approximately 10% of patients, reflux may cause severe damage to the lower pole renal unit, sometimes making heminephrectomy necessary.

b. Ectopic ureter. In patients who have an ectopic ureter, with or without an associated ureterocele, treatment depends on the function of the ectopic upper pole segment. If upper pole function is poor or absent, upper pole heminephrectomy and ureterectomy are indicated. If upper pole renal function is good, a ureteropyelostomy from upper to lower pole may be undertaken. Alternatively, if reflux into the lower pole ureter is present, excision of the ureterocele and reimplantation of the common sheath should be performed.

C. Megaureter denotes a dilated ureter and may occur as a result of various conditions. Primary megaureter consists of an adynamic 3- to 4-cm segment of ureter next to the ureterovesical junction. Secondary megaureter implies a problem either extrinsic to or distal within the urinary tract (e.g., abnormal bladder function and/or obstruction of the bladder outlet) that secondarily affects the ureterovesical junction. Megaureter can be further categorized based on etiology of the dilatation: (a) refluxing, (b) obstructed, (c) both refluxing and obstructed, and (d) neither refluxing nor obstructed.

1. Pathophysiology

a. Primary obstructive megaureter is thought to be caused by defective peristalsis in the intramural ureter. A catheter usually can be passed easily in a retrograde manner through the aperistaltic segment, which cannot be done in cases of true ureteral stenosis or extrinsic compression of the ureter. The lesion is bilateral in 25% of instances, affects the left ureter three times as often as the right, and affects boys three times as commonly as girls. The contralateral kidney is absent or dysplastic in 10% of instances. Children with primary obstructive megaureter may be asymptomatic (e.g., most cases of antenatal diagnosis) or may present with recurrent urinary tract infection, hematuria (gross or microscopic), or flank pain.

b. Secondary obstructive megaureter is often bilateral and results from obstruction of the bladder outlet secondary to posterior urethral valves, neurogenic bladder dysfunction with bladder pressures of >40 cm H_2O (especially myelodysplasia), or functional voiding disorders. In such patients, hypertrophy of the bladder wall can lead to secondary obstruction of the ureterovesical junction.

c. Vesicoureteral reflux is a very common cause of ureteral dilatation. It may result from primary dysfunction of the ureterovesical junction or secondary incompetence of the ureterovesical junction caused by obstruction of bladder outflow, neurogenic dysfunction, or functional voiding disorders.

d. Other causes of megaureter in the absence of obstruction or reflux include residual dilatation from obstruction or reflux in the past, high rates of urine flow (diabetes insipidus, polydipsia from any cause), and bacterial infection.

2. Diagnosis. Megaureter is most commonly detected by US, especially prenatal US. A ureter of >7 mm in diameter is diagnostic, with 5 to 7 mm equivocal. There is a relatively greater dilatation of the distal ureter than of the proximal ureter or renal pelvis. In mild cases, only the distal third of the ureter is dilated, and the remainder of the upper urinary tract remains normal. A VCUG should be performed in all cases to rule out reflux and to detect obstruction of bladder outflow. Diuretic radionuclide renogram provides information regarding renal function and obstruction. In some cases, endoscopy may need to be performed to assess the bladder trigone and permit retrograde studies of the ureter.

3. Treatment depends on the severity and etiology.

a. Primary megaureter without reflux or obstruction. Because megaureter repair in infancy has a higher complication rate, expectant management is preferred where possible. Antibiotic prophylaxis, frequent imaging with US (every 3 months), urinalysis, and observation for symptoms allow some cases to resolve spontaneously. If renal function worsens, UTI becomes an issue, or a severe case fails to improve, surgery is indicated.

b. Megaureter with reflux. When reflux is present, the indications for surgery are similar to those discussed in the vesicoureteral reflux section. Intraoperatively, megaureter requires excision of the distal ureter, excisional or tapering infolding, and reimplantation of the ureter.

c. Obstruction or neurogenic bladder. When obstruction of bladder outflow is the cause, treatment of the primary lesion may lead to subsequent resolution of the ureteral dilatation. Thus, a period of time should elapse after the initial surgery before deciding on the secondary megaureter repair.

d. Severe cases. Ureterostomy and vesicostomy are options when renal function or infectious complications necessitate.

V. Obstruction of the lower urinary tract

A. Posterior urethral valves are the most common cause of obstruction of bladder outflow in male neonates and infants. They represent 10% of cases of prenatally diagnosed hydronephrosis overall; conversely, two-thirds of cases of posterior urethral valves are diagnosed antenatally. These valves represent mucosal folds at the distal prostatic urethra that cause varying degrees of obstruction. Type I valves extend distally from the verumontanum and insert anteriorly near the margin of the membranous urethra. They are thought to arise owing to the mesonephric ducts inserting abnormally into the cloaca. Type II valves are no longer thought to be obstructing valves but rather hypertrophy in response to another obstructing lesion; they extend proximally from the verumontanum to the bladder neck. A type III valve is a circular diaphragm distal to the verumontanum at the level of the membranous urethra. It is thought to represent incomplete dissolution of the urogenital membrane.

1. **Associated findings. Oligohydramnios** occurs because of low intrauterine production of urine and may be associated with **pulmonary hypoplasia** (50% mortality). High-pressure reflux during the prenatal period may lead to **renal dysplasia. Postnatal vesicoureteral reflux** is present in one-third to one-half of patients and portends a worse prognosis; one-third of these cases resolve spontaneously after valve ablation. **Bladder dysfunction** is common and, depending on the urodynamic findings, may require anticholinergic medications, clean intermittent catheterization, and/or bladder augmentation.

2. **Diagnosis.** Currently, diagnosis is most commonly made by screening antenatal US. Previously, neonatal physical exam demonstrating a palpable hypertrophied bladder and/or dilated ureters and pelves could be appreciated. Poor urinary stream may or may not be present. In some newborns and infants, only nonspecific symptoms such as failure to thrive, uremia, hypertension, or anemia indicate that there is a problem. In severe cases, electrolyte abnormalities may lead to seizures or cardiac arrhythmias. Older children may present with incontinence, vague abdominal complaints, UTI, distended bladder, thin urinary stream, or hematuria. Urinary extravasation (usually at the calyceal fornix) may result in urinary ascites at any age.

3. **Imaging.** US is usually the first diagnostic tool, demonstrating bilateral hydroureteronephrosis and a large, thick-walled bladder in severe cases. IVU can demonstrate the same. The VCUG is the most diagnostic examination and will show a heavily trabeculated bladder, prominence of the bladder neck, dilatation of the posterior urethra, and focal narrowing of the stream at the site of the valves. Vesicoureteral reflux should be sought. Intraoperatively, endoscopy will visualize the valves if flow from the bladder is induced by suprapubic pressure.

4. **Treatment** of urethral valves ranges from temporizing catheterization to endoscopic fulguration to surgical urinary diversion.

   a. In a **nonuremic child,** it is agreed that fulguration should be the primary treatment. Even the smallest urethra can usually be navigated given today's technology. Antegrade pressure can be achieved by the Crede maneuver and fulguration using a cautery wire or electrode performed in retrograde fashion to ensure that the sphincter is not injured. In the rare infant in whom the urethra is too small, either suprapubic ablation via a transvesical approach or temporary diversion by cutaneous vesicostomy can be performed. When the child is older, valve ablation and closure of the vesicostomy are performed.

b.   Azotemia, acidosis, or sepsis. In children with metabolic abnormalities, temporary bladder drainage should be established by urethral catheter or suprapubic tube. After resolution of the azotemia, sepsis, and/or electrolyte abnormalities, transurethral fulguration of the valves can be performed. In the most severe instances of hydronephrosis, azotemia may not resolve completely after catheterization because of obstruction at the ureteropelvic and/or ureterovesical junction, poor ureteral peristalsis, permanent renal dysfunction, or occasionally catheter-induced bladder irritability. There is controversy in the literature as to whether valve ablation, vesicostomy, or supravesical diversion provides the best chance of recovering renal function. Approximately one-third of patients with severe enough disease to require diversion of the upper urinary tract progress to renal failure by puberty. Overall, the prognosis for posterior urethral valves has improved dramatically since the original studies in the 1970s noted mortality rates of 50% by adolescence. Currently, neonatal deaths are seen in only 2% to 3% of cases, and long-term data are not yet complete.

c.   Vesicoureteral reflux. Valve ablation results in spontaneous resolution of vesicoureteral reflux in approximately one-third of patients. One-third of patients have complications due to their reflux and require surgical correction. The remainder do well with antibiotic prophylaxis, and decisions regarding reimplantation depend on overall progress.

d.   Prenatal intervention. Vesicoamniotic shunts and antegrade ablation of valves have been performed in utero in severe cases, with obvious risks. Data demonstrating improved prevention of renal dysfunction and other complications such as pulmonary hypoplasia versus perinatal management have not been published to date.

B.   Anterior urethral valves are congenital urethral diverticula that, when filled, balloon into and obstruct the urethral lumen. The presentation is similar to that of posterior urethral valves except for the VCUG findings. Management is similar except the surgical options include both endoscopic and open urethral repair.

VI.   Maldescent of the testis

Cryptorchidism refers to congenital failure of descent of the testis into the scrotum. Classification of its eventual location varies. The testis is either palpable or nonpalpable on physical examination. More accurately, at the time of surgery, the testis can be confirmed as absent, intraabdominal, intracanalicular, extracanalicular, or ectopic (e.g., perineal). The most common location is at the external inguinal ring. The etiology of cryptorchidism is multifactorial and results from a number of hormonal and mechanical factors (e.g., the gubernaculum); the exact relationship of events has yet to be described.

A. Incidence. The testes normally descend into the scrotum at 7 months of gestation. The incidence of cryptorchidism decreases with age and gestational weight; it is 30% in premature infants, 3% in newborns, 1.0% at 3 months, and 0.75% to 1.0% at 1 year of age. Seventy percent descend spontaneously by age 3 months.

B. Associated findings. A patent processus vaginalis is present in 90% of patients, and inguinal hernia is present in 25%. Unilateral cryptorchidism in an otherwise normal child is generally an isolated finding; however, bilateral cryptorchidism, especially when associated with any degree of hypospadias, may be a sign of an intersex state such as adrenogenital syndrome or one of the androgen-insensitivity syndromes. Bilateral cryptorchidism is also found in "prune-belly" syndrome, exstrophy of the bladder, pituitary disorders, testicular feminization, and dozens of other syndromes.

C. Diagnosis. In infants and newborns, absence of one or both testes is usually noted on routine physical examination. In true cryptorchidism, the scrotum on the affected side may be underdeveloped. A retractile testis is a normally descended testis that is pulled into the pubic area by the cremaster muscle. In such cases, the scrotum is normal and the testis can be manipulated gently back into the scrotum. Retractile testes do not require surgery and resolve spontaneously at puberty; they should be followed until then.

    1. Imaging. In instances of bilateral cryptorchidism or nonpalpable unilateral cryptorchidism, US, CT, or magnetic resonance imaging may demonstrate the presence and location of the testis or testes. However, imaging is only 44% accurate, and surgical exploration is indicated in any case. Therefore, there is little reason to request radiologic evaluation.

    2. The **human chorionic gonadotropin (hCG) stimulation test** can be used to distinguish bilateral cryptorchidism from bilateral anorchia. If follicle-stimulating hormone (FSH) is elevated, bilateral anorchia likely exists and the hCG stimulation test is not necessary. After the baseline serum testosterone has been measured, the child is given 1,000 to 1,500 U of hCG IM daily for 4 days. On the fifth day, the serum testosterone level will be many times its baseline value if normally responsive testes are present. In addition to a diminished or absent response to exogenous hCG, patients with bilateral anorchia will demonstrate elevated levels of luteinizing hormone (LH) and FSH initially. Regardless of the results of these tests, surgical exploration will have to be performed.

    3. Diagnostic laparoscopy may be very helpful in the evaluation and treatment of cryptorchidism, as described below.

D. Treatment

    1. Hormonal therapy with hCG or LH-releasing hormone has been reported to cause descent of the cryptorchid testis in about 20% of patients, although success depends heavily on the location of the testis before treatment.

    2. Surgical exploration is currently the treatment of choice in most patients and should be carried out prior to

1 year of age. The surgical approach depends on preoperative examination. Palpable testes should be explored inguinally. Dissection of the spermatic cord usually provides enough length to reach the scrotum. If not, the Prentiss maneuver can allow more length by routing the testis medial to the inferior epigastrics. With the advent of laparoscopy, non-palpable testes are explored through diagnostic laparoscopy. Blind-ending vessels denote anorchia, and no further therapy is indicated. Inguinal vessels necessitate inguinal exploration. If the cryptorchid testis appears rudimentary, orchiectomy is indicated: Ten percent of these contain viable germ tissue. If a viable testis is found during laparoscopy, the vessels can be ligated as the first stage of the Fowler–Stephens two-stage repair. The second stage can be completed as an open or laparoscopic technique in 6 months after collateralization via the vasal and cremasteric circulation. In any technique, the testis is secured in a dartos pouch in the scrotum.

E. **Complications and sequelae**

   1. **Testicular neoplasia.** The prevalence of cryptorchidism in patients with germ cell tumors is 10%. One in 2,550 men with cryptorchidism will develop a germ cell tumor compared with 1 in 100,000 of the general male population, a 40-fold difference. Intraabdominal testes seem to account for a disproportionate number of malignancies in cryptorchid testes. The data are not complete on whether orchiopexy influences the risk for testicular cancer, but it does facilitate the exam over time. Of patients with unilateral cryptorchidism in whom neoplasia develops, about 15% will have a tumor in the contralateral, normally descended testis. In a newly diagnosed postpubertal male patient under the age of 35 years, the cryptorchid testis should be removed; in patients older than 35, the risk for development of testis cancer is less than the risk associated with anesthesia.

   2. **Infertility.** In studies measuring paternity (as opposed to spermiograms), 75% to 87% of men with unilateral cryptorchidism and 33% to 53% of those with a history of bilateral cryptorchidism were able to father children. Histologic evidence of Leydig cell hypoplasia is observed as early as 1 month of life. Abnormalities of the vas and epididymis are present in 30% to 90% of patients. Testicular biopsy can still demonstrate spermatogenesis for assisted reproductive technologies.

   3. **Torsion of the testicle** may occur rarely in the cryptorchid testis.

VII. **Torsion of the testis.** Testicular torsion results in twisting of the spermatic cord and occlusion of the venous or arterial supply to the testis. Thus, testicular torsion is a true vascular emergency. If not treated emergently (within 4 to 6 hours after onset of pain), complete infarction of the testis results, followed by atrophy of the testis. Although testicular torsion can occur at any age, the age incidence is bimodal, with the condition most common during adolescence (ages 10 to 20 years) and less common in the neonatal period. Fifty percent of cases of torsion occur during sleep. Testicular torsion is broadly classified into two types.

A. **Extravaginal.** This form is seen in neonates. The entire testis and tunica twist in a vertical axis on the spermatic cord as a consequence of incomplete fixation of the gubernaculum to the scrotal wall, which allows free rotation within the scrotum.

B.   Intravaginal. This more common form of torsion is found in adolescents and adults. A congenital high investment of the tunica on the cord, which produces the "bell-clapper" deformity, allows the testis to rotate on the cord (Fig. 19.1). Because this anomaly is bilateral, there is a significant risk for a contralateral metachronous torsion. Spasm of the cremaster muscle causes the right testis to rotate clockwise and the left counterclockwise as observed from the foot of the bed.

1.   Clinical features. The classic presentation of sudden and severe testicular pain, nausea, vomiting, and a high testis with local tenderness is diagnostic. Not infrequently, one can elicit a past history of similar attacks, which presumably represent intermittent episodes of torsion. Physical examination reveals exquisite testicular tenderness. The testis lies transversely and more cephalad than normally. If one can palpate the epididymis in an anterior location at this stage, the diagnosis of torsion is strongly supported.

2.   Differential diagnosis. The most frequent misdiagnosis is that of epididymoorchitis (Table 19.8), which is generally less acute and usually accompanied by a urinary infection or prostatitis. Although the maneuver is not always reliable, elevation of the testicle increases pain in torsion and decreases pain in epididymoorchitis (Prehn's sign). Although rare, torsion of the appendix testis—a remnant of the müllerian duct—presents in a similar fashion. The tenderness, however, is well localized to the upper pole of the testis, and a characteristic blue dot sign on the skin of the scrotum may be appreciated (Fig. 19.2).

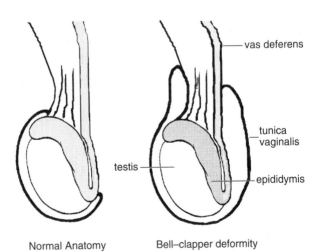

Fig. 19.1. Normal testicular anatomy compared with the "bell-clapper" deformity, characterized by high insertion of the tunica vaginalis on the cord.

Table 19.8. Differentiating spermatic cord torsion from acute epididymoorchitis

	Torsion	Inflammation
Mode of onset	Abrupt	Few hours to days
Affected testis	Higher than opposite	No change in position
Epididymis	Usually nonpalpable	Palpable and tender
Urethral discharge	Absent	May be present
Cremasteric reflex	May be absent	Usually present
Response to elevation	No change in pain	Pain relieved
Fever	Usually absent	May be present

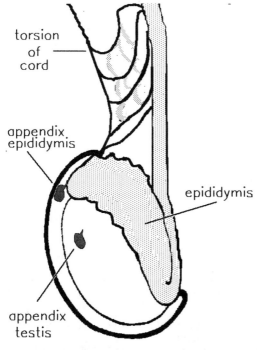

Fig. 19.2. Common causes of acute scrotum in childhood include torsion of the spermatic cord, appendix testis and epididymis as well as epididymitis.

3. Diagnosis. It is almost axiomatic to consider an acutely painful swollen testis in an adolescent as torsion until it is proven otherwise at surgery. Color Doppler and color duplex Doppler sonography to assess arterial flow and radionuclide scanning with [^{99m}Tc]pertechnetate have been used with an accuracy of 90%. Both methods are based on the premise that arterial flow to the testis is decreased in torsion and increased in epididymitis. Unfortunately, no method is totally reliable, and testicular imaging is only an adjunct to a good history and physical examination.

4. Treatment depends on the interval from onset of pain to presentation in the emergency department. Within 4 hours of onset, manual detorsion of the testicular cord under local anesthesia should be attempted. (Remember that the testes twist toward the midline as seen from the feet.) If manual detorsion is successful, elective bilateral orchidopexy is indicated within the next few days. If detorsion is not successful, immediate surgical exploration is indicated. If the presentation is between 4 and 24 hours after onset of pain, immediate surgical exploration, detorsion, and bilateral orchidopexy should be performed. If >24 hours has passed since onset of pain, surgical exploration is indicated, but preservation of testicular function is doubtful. A nonviable testis should be removed and a testicular prosthesis placed. This is to prevent infectious complications and the potential of autoimmune injury to the contralateral testicle.

VIII. Exstrophy of the bladder

Exstrophy of the bladder is a congenital defect characterized by ventral herniation of the bladder through the anterior abdominal wall. It is part of the exstrophy–epispadias complex, all of which are thought to be due to premature rupture of the cloacal membrane. The rectus muscles and pubic symphysis are widely separated owing to a deficient mesenchymal layer, and the posterior wall of the bladder fills the defect. Incidence is 3.3 per 100,000 live births in the general population and 1 in 70 offspring of affected individuals. There is a 2.3:1 male predominance. In male patients, complete epispadias (a condition in which the urethra opens onto the dorsal aspect of the penis) may be present, and the clitoris is bifid in female patients.

A. Associated findings. Bladder exstrophy is associated with abnormalities of the abdominal wall, pelvis, external genitalia, testicular descent, and rectum (incontinence and rectal prolapse). Epispadias and a shortened penis are observed in the male and bifid clitoris in the female. Vesicoureteral reflux is present in 100% of cases after closure of the bladder. Inguinal hernias (82% of boys and 11% of girls) should be repaired at the time of initial surgery.

B. Treatment is initiated in the neonatal period. Diagnosis by prenatal US provides the opportunity to deliver near a medical center specializing in treatment of exstrophy. In the delivery room, the umbilical cord should be tied off at its base with 2-0 silk and the bladder covered with saline and saran wrap to prevent denudation. Staged reconstructions over the years have been modified to the current: closure of the bladder, at least posterior urethra, and abdominal wall with osteotomies at birth and bladder neck reconstruction and ureteral reimplantation at age 4 to

5 years. The epispadias repair can be done at 6 to 12 months if not performed as a single-stage newborn repair. The corpora are mobilized for penile lengthening, and the urethral plate is tubularized to the end of the glans. Continence success rates from staged early reconstruction are 67% to 90% and approach 80% in terms of continence and preservation of renal function. There are no comprehensive data on single-stage repairs, although early success has been reported.

IX. Hypospadias

Hypospadias is a congenital defect of the penis resulting in a proximal (ventral) urethral meatus, ventral curvature (chordee), and ventral deficiency of the foreskin. Hypospadias is classified by the location of the meatus as (a) glanular, (b) coronal, (c) penile, (d) penoscrotal, or (e) perineal (Fig. 19.3).

A. Inheritance. Hypospadias has a multifactorial mode of inheritance that is not sex-linked. The incidence of hypospadias in subsequent offspring varies between 0% and 25%, depending on the severity of the hypospadias in the index child and presence of hypospadias in other family members.

B. Associated findings. Undescended testis is found in 10% of all patients with hypospadias, but this incidence increases to 30% in patients with a penoscrotal or perineal opening. An inter-

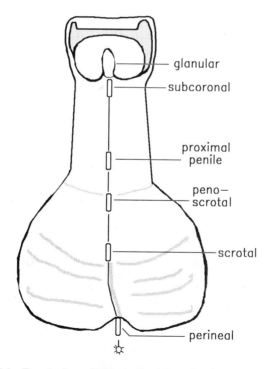

glanular

subcoronal

proximal penile

peno—scrotal

scrotal

perineal

Fig. 19.3. Terminology of hypospadias is based on location of the meatus after repair of any ventral chordee.

sex state is found in approximately one-third of patients with hypospadias and undescended testicles. Such patients should be carefully evaluated. Karyotyping should be performed to be certain that these persons are not females with virilized genitalia.

C.   Treatment involves the surgical repair of chordee when present and urethral reconstruction by one of many techniques. The most common in use today is the tubularized incised urethral plate or Snodgrass repair. Other procedures include a meatus-based flap, an island pedicle flap, or a free skin graft from the dorsal foreskin. Patients with hypospadias should not be circumcised because the foreskin often is required for surgical reconstruction. Depending on the type of repair, approximately 10% to 20% of patients develop urethrocutaneous fistula requiring secondary closure. Overall results are excellent.

X.   Disorders of sexual differentiation

A.   Disorders of chromosomal sex occur when the number or structure of the X or Y chromosome is abnormal.

1.   Klinefelter's syndrome (seminiferous tubule dysgenesis) is the most common major abnormality of sexual differentiation, with an incidence of approximately 1 in 1,000 males. Patients often present after the time of expected puberty and are diagnosed incidentally. Patients characteristically have small, firm testes, impaired sexual maturation, azoospermia, gynecomastia, and elevated levels of urinary gonadotropins. Hyalinization of the seminiferous tubules is a typical histologic finding. The common karyotype is either a 47XXY pattern (classic form) or 46XY/47XXY (mosaic form, milder phenotype), due to nondisjunction during meiosis. Plasma levels of LH and FSH are high, the latter being a consequence of damage to the seminiferous tubules. Mean plasma levels of estradiol are also elevated, leading to insufficient masculinization and enhanced feminization. Most patients benefit from injections of testosterone cypionate or testosterone enanthate. Surgery is the only available means to correct the gynecomastia. Surveillance for breast carcinoma (eightfold greater risk) should be instructed. Paternity can sometimes be achieved with intracytoplasmic sperm injection (ICSI).

2.   XX male syndrome is a rare disorder in which a 46XX karyotype is present. Eighty percent of patients have the Y-linked testis-determining factor (SRY), presumably from translocation of a fragment of the Y chromosome to the X chromosome. This occurs in about 1 in 20,000 to 24,000 male births. Affected persons lack female internal genitalia and have a male psychosexual identification. Ten percent have hypospadias. Clinical features in those with the *SRY* gene resemble those in Klinefelter's syndrome, including small testes, gynecomastia, azoospermia, and hyalinization of the seminiferous tubules; genitalia are otherwise usually normal. Plasma gonadotropin and estradiol levels are elevated and mean testosterone levels are low. Management is similar to that of Klinefelter's syndrome. All are infertile.

3.   Turner's syndrome (gonadal dysgenesis) is characterized by sexual infantilism, short stature, shield chest, webbed neck, neonatal lymphedema, primary amenorrhea, and bilateral streak gonads in phenotypic females. Multiple congenital anomalies are noted; 10% to 20% have cardiac anomalies, most commonly coarctation of the aorta, and 30% to 60% have renal anomalies. The incidence is 1 in 2,500 live births. The karyotype varies: 45X in 50%, mosaicism in 30% to 40%, and isochrome X in 12% to 20%. The mosaic patients who contain Y-chromosomal material have a 30% chance of developing gonadoblastoma, and therefore gonadectomy is indicated at diagnosis. Mosaicism with a normal chromosomal complement (46XX/45XO) lessens the severity of the gonadal abnormality, and the likelihood of menses and breast development is greater in such cases. Plasma gonadotropins are elevated from the neonatal period to 4 years of age, normalize until age 10, and then rise to abnormally high levels thereafter. Management involves administration of recombinant human growth hormone with the anabolic steroid oxandrolone during childhood in an effort to increase the final adult height. Estrogen replacement therapy should be given at the time of expected puberty to patients without spontaneous feminization. Gonadectomy is indicated in mosaics when *SRY* material is present in the karyotype because of the possible development of gonadoblastoma. Maternity can be achieved in some patients.

4. Mixed gonadal dysgenesis is a disorder in which phenotypic males or females have a testis on one side (usually intraabdominal) and a streak gonad on the other. Müllerian structures accompany the streak gonad and wolffian structures the testis. Most have 45X/46XY mosaicism, thought to be due to difficulties with mitotic anaphase. After congenital adrenal hyperplasia, it is the most common cause of ambiguous genitalia reported in neonates. The phenotype ranges from Turner's syndrome (see above) to ambiguous genitalia to phenotypic male. Two-thirds are raised as girls. Gonadal tumors develop in 15% to 20% of patients. In phenotypic females, prophylactic gonadectomy should be performed. In phenotypic males, all streak gonads should be removed and testes may be preserved with close observation if they can be brought to a scrotal location. Wilms' tumor is also associated with mixed gonadal dysgenesis (e.g., in Denys–Drash syndrome), and screening is indicated.

5. Dysgenetic male pseudohermaphroditism. The karyotype is 45X/46XY or 46XY, and patients have bilateral dysgenetic testes. Ambiguous genitalia and müllerian structures are dependent on relative testicular function.

6. True hermaphroditism is a condition in which both a functional ovary and testis or an ovotestis (60% of gonads) is present. Seventy percent of cases have a 46XX karyotype, 10% have a 46XY karyotype, and the remainder are chimeric (e.g., 46XX/47XXY). Three-fourths are sufficiently masculinized to be raised as boys. Most of these patients have hypospadias, and half have incomplete labioscrotal fusion. Most phenotypic females have an enlarged clitoris, a urogenital sinus, and a hypoplastic uterus. The internal genitalia tend to follow the ipsilateral gonad. At puberty, a variable degree of feminization or masculinization occurs. Breast development occurs in three-fourths, and half menstruate. Hormonal

replacement is initiated as needed. Sex assignment depends
largely on external and internal anatomic findings in the
newborn, and external genitalia should be modified accordingly. Fertility is possible in females but has not been reported in males. Gonadal tumors occur in 10% of patients
with 46XY karyotype and 4% with 46XX. Therefore, once gender assignment has been established, unnecessary gonadal
and internal genital structures are removed.

B. Disorders of gonadal sex are characterized by an abnormal differentiation of the gonads without a chromosomal
abnormality.

   1. Pure gonadal dysgenesis is a syndrome in which phenotypic females have a 46XX karyotype, streak gonads with
   otherwise normal internal and external genitalia, sexual infantilism, and no somatic anomalies. Growth is normal. It
   has been observed to be an autosomal recessive trait within
   families. Estrogen deficiency is variable, and feminization occurs in 40%. Management with estrogen replacement therapy is started at puberty and is maintained throughout life.

   2. Complete gonadal dysgenesis occurs in 46XY females
   with streak gonads but otherwise normal internal and external genitalia. Sexual infantilism persists, and amenorrhea is
   noted. Risk of gonadal tumors is 30%. Gonadectomy and hormone replacement at puberty are indicated.

   3. Absent testis syndrome occurs in 46XY males with absent testes in whom endocrine function of the testis was variable during embryogenesis and fetal development. The clinical
   features range from absent or incomplete virilization of the
   external genitalia to bilateral anorchia in otherwise normal-
   appearing males. The degree of virilization depends on the
   timing of testicular failure during gestation—that is, whether
   it occurred before or after the development of the seminiferous
   tubules and the onset of Leydig's cell function. Müllerian inhibiting substance production prior to testicular failure leads
   to regression of müllerian structures. Management depends
   on the clinical features. Depending on the patient's phenotype,
   either estrogen or androgen replacement therapy is given to
   allow appropriate secondary sexual development.

C. Disorders of phenotypic sex

   1. Female pseudohermaphroditism is a disorder of the
   46XX female in which the ovaries and müllerian derivatives
   are normal, but the feminization of the external genitalia is
   abnormal. Virilization of the female fetus is secondary to excess androgens from either the maternal circulation or the
   fetal adrenal gland.

      a. Congenital adrenal hyperplasia is the most com-
      mon cause of ambiguous genitalia in the newborn. It is also
      the most common cause of female pseudohermaphrodit-
      ism. In males, the phenotype is precocious puberty, not am-
      biguous genitalia.

         (1) Pathophysiology. The etiology of congenital ad-
         renal hyperplasia is a deficiency in one of the five follow-
         ing enzymes of adrenal steroid production: 21-hydroxylase
         (95% of cases), 11β-hydroxylase (5% of cases), 3β-hydroxy-
         steroid dehydrogenase, 17-hydroxylase, and cholesterol

side-chain cleavage enzyme (rare). The end result is low cortisol and up-regulation of adrenocorticotropin. In the first three defects listed, resultant androgen production is too high and often aldosterone too low.

(2) Diagnosis. Congenital adrenal hyperplasia can be mild or severe. In the severe form, decreased mineralocorticoid production can lead to life-threatening salt wasting and dehydration. This usually happens in the first weeks of life. Failure to recognize this problem can result in severe hypotension and ultimately to circulatory collapse. Adrenal crisis is a urologic neonatal emergency. In addition to a complete history and physical examination (including a family history of sudden infant death), measurement of serum electrolytes, chromosomal analysis, and determination of enzymatic defect should be performed. 21-Hydroxylase deficiency results in elevated plasma 17-hydroxyprogesterone by radioimmunoassay, 11β-hydroxylase deficiency leads to elevated plasma 11-deoxycortisol and 11-deoxycorticosterone, and 3β-hydroxysteroid dehydrogenase deficiency leads to elevated 17-hydroxypregnenolone and dehydroepiandrosterone. Prior 24-hour urine collections are now only necessary for evaluating response to therapy. Abdominal and pelvic US are necessary to confirm müllerian structures.

(3) Management of congenital adrenal hyperplasia should focus on the issues of salt-wasting crisis, degree of virilization, and psychosocial concerns surrounding the sexual assignment of the child. Replacement therapy with cortisone and mineralocorticoids is essential to prevent salt wasting. In addition, a properly treated child can maintain fertility if gender remains chromosomal. Surgical intervention involves reconstruction of the genitalia (clitoral reduction and creation of a vaginal introitus and labial skin folds), which can be performed either during early infancy or later in childhood.

b. Exogenous androgens and progestogens represent another cause of female pseudohermaphroditism. In the past, progestational agents with androgenic side effects were administered during pregnancy to prevent abortion, resulting in virilization of the female fetus. Female pseudohermaphroditism may also occur when the mother has a virilizing ovarian or adrenal tumor.

2. Male pseudohermaphroditism results from inadequate virilization of the 46XY male embryo.

a. Abnormalities in androgen synthesis lead to incomplete virilization of the fetus. The phenotypes range from penoscrotal hypospadias to phenotypic female. There are five known defects of testosterone synthesis within the adrenal gland, each involving a crucial enzymatic step in the conversion of cholesterol to testosterone. They exhibit autosomal recessive inheritance. The enzymes cholesterol side-chain cleavage enzyme, 3β-hydroxysteroid dehydrogenase, and 17α-hydroxylase are common to the synthesis of other adrenal hormones in addition to androgens, and their deficiency leads to congenital adrenal hyperplasia and male pseudohermaphroditism. Glucocorticoids are deficient in all three; mineralocorticoids are elevated in 17α-hydroxylase deficiency and deficient in the first two. On the other hand, 17,20-lyase and 17β-hydroxysteroid oxidoreductase deficiency are involved only in androgen synthesis. A deficiency in either leads solely to male pseudohermaphroditism. In the latter, a phenotypic female can become virilized at puberty owing to gonadotropin-increasing androgen concentrations. Müllerian structures are absent in all five defects because of intact müllerian inhibiting substance.

b.   Abnormalities of androgen action may cause impaired male development as a result of resistance to androgen action in target cells.

(1)   Deficiency of 5α-reductase is an autosomal recessive disorder associated with failure of dihydrotestosterone formation from testosterone, resulting in normal male wolffian duct derivatives but defective masculinization of the external genitalia. Phenotype ranges from severe **perineoscrotal hypospadias** to marked ambiguity with a blind vaginal pouch opening into the urogenital sinus. At puberty, variable degrees of masculinization occur with increased levels of testosterone sometimes changing a female phenotype to male.

(2)   Androgen receptor disorders. The most common of these disorders is **complete testicular feminization,** due to loss of the androgen receptor on Xq11 and 12. Since androgen lacks effect but the müllerian inhibiting substance effect is unchanged in utero, neither müllerian nor wolffian structures are present. The gonads can be abdominal or labial and have the histologic appearance of undescended testes. The clitoris is normal or small, and the vagina is short with a blind ending, but the external genitalia are unambiguously female. As a newborn, testosterone, dihydroxytestosterone, and gonadotropin levels are normal. With puberty, estradiol increases secondary to increased gonadotropin; therefore, breast development, general habitus, and distribution of body fat are female in character. Because of increased tumor formation in the undescended testis (2% to 5%), gonadectomy is recommended after puberty and feminization. **Partial androgen resistance** is known as **Reifenstein's syndrome;** the phenotype can vary from a normal-appearing infertile man to marked ambiguity.

c.   Leydig cell aplasia/LH receptor abnormalities lead to an XY male with phenotype ranging from female (short vagina, absent müllerian structures) to male phenotype with sexual infantilism.

SUGGESTED READING

Atala A, Keating M. Vesicoureteral reflux and megaureter. In: Walsh PC, Retik AB, Vaughan ED, et al., eds. *Campbell's urology.* 8th ed. Philadelphia: Saunders, 2002:2053–2116.

Carr MC. Anomalies and surgery of the ureteropelvic junction in children. In: Walsh PC, Retik AB, Vaughan ED, et al., eds. *Campbell's urology.* 8th ed. Philadelphia: Saunders, 2002:1995–2006.

Diamond DA. Sexual differentiation: normal and abnormal. In: Walsh PC, Retik AB, Vaughan ED, et al., eds. *Campbell's urology.* 8th ed. Philadelphia: Saunders, 2002:2395–2427.

Dome JS, Coppes MJ. Recent advances in Wilms tumor genetics. *Curr Opin Pediatr* 2002;14:5–11.

Gearhart JP. Exstrophy, epispadias, and other bladder anomalies. In: Walsh PC, Retik AB, Vaughan ED, et al. *Campbell's urology.* 8th ed. Philadelphia: Saunders, 2002:2136–2196.

Glassberg KI, Braren V, Duckett JW, et al. Suggested terminology for duplex systems, ectopic ureters and ureteroceles. *J Urol* 1981;132: 1153–1154.

Gonzales ET. Posterior urethral valves and other urethral anomalies. In: Walsh PC, Retik AB, Vaughan ED, et al., eds. *Campbell's urology.* 8th ed. Philadelphia: Saunders, 2002:2207–2230.

Koff SA, Wagner TT, Jayanthi VR. The relationship among dysfunctional elimination syndromes, primary vesicoureteral reflux and urinary tract infections in children. *J Urol* 1998;160:1019.

Mandell J, Colodny AH, Lebowitz R, et al. Ureteroceles in infants and children. *J Urol* 1980;123:921–926.

Neville HL, Ritchey ML. Wilms' tumor: overview of National Wilms' Tumor Study Group results. *Urol Clin North Am* 2000;27:435–442.

Retik AB, Borer JG. Hypospadias. In: Walsh PC, Retik AB, Vaughan ED, et al., eds. *Campbell's urology.* 8th ed. Philadelphia: Saunders, 2002:2284–2333.

Ritchey ML. Primary nephrectomy for Wilms' tumor: approach of the National Wilms' Tumor Study Group. *Urology* 1996;47:787–791.

Schlussel RN, Retik AB. Ectopic ureter, ureterocele, and other anomalies of the ureter. In: Walsh PC, Retik AB, Vaughan ED, et al., eds. *Campbell's urology.* 8th ed. Philadelphia: Saunders, 2002: 2007–2052.

Schneck FX, Bellinger MF. Abnormalities of the testes and scrotum and their surgical management. In: Walsh PC, Retik AB, Vaughan ED, et al., eds. *Campbell's urology.* 8th ed. Philadelphia: Saunders, 2002:2353–2394.

Weiss RM, Biancani P. Characteristics of normal and refluxing ureterovesical junctions. *J Urol* 1983;129:858–861.

Witherow R, Whitaker RH. The predictive accuracy of antegrade pressure flow studies in equivocal upper tract obstruction. *Br J Urol* 1981;53:496–499.

Male Reproductive Dysfunction

Ronald E. Anglade and Robert D. Oates

I. Definitions

Infertility is defined as the inability to achieve a pregnancy resulting in live birth after 1 year of unprotected intercourse (**primary infertility**). Couples who have been fertile in the past, but have fewer than the desired number of children, have **secondary infertility.** Fifteen percent of couples in the United States cannot achieve an unassisted pregnancy. A male factor can be identified in nearly 60% of these couples (20% male factor only and 40% joint subfertility).

  A. **Indications for infertility work-up.** Couples should have a joint infertility evaluation at 1 year, unless the following factors are present: (a) in males: bilateral cryptorchidism, testicular torsion, previous unexplained infertility, prior chemotherapy; (b) in females: advanced maternal age (over 35 years), irregular or absent menses, previous unexplained infertility, history of pelvic inflammatory disease.

  B. **Goals** of the evaluation of an infertile male should be the identification of (a) reversible conditions, (b) irreversible conditions that may be managed by assisted reproductive technologies (ART), (c) irreversible conditions (including genetic and chromosomal abnormalities) that could adversely affect any offspring, and (d) medical conditions relevant to infertility.

II. Normal hypothalamic–pituitary–gonadal axis

Abnormalities of the hypothalamic–pituitary–gonadal axis (Fig. 20.1) account for approximately 1% to 5% of diagnoses in a male infertility clinic. They are commonly referred to as pretesticular causes.

  A. The **hypothalamus** is the site of production of gonadotropin-releasing hormone (GnRH), which reaches the anterior pituitary via the portal venous system. GnRH is produced in the basal medial hypothalamus and the arcuate nucleus. The pulsatile release of GnRH depends on multiple stimuli including catecholamines, dopamine, and serotonin. The hypothalamus begins generating GnRH pulses at around the time of puberty. GnRH levels are highest at night and in the spring. Endorphins, estrogen, and androgen can inhibit GnRH release.

  B. The **anterior pituitary** secretes two important hormones (gonadotropins) that control testicular function: luteinizing hormone (LH) and follicle-stimulating hormone (FSH). Pituitary function and gonadotropin release depend on the pulsatile stimulation of GnRH at nearly 60-minute intervals. LH and FSH are glycoproteins with α and β subunits that are linked by noncovalent bonds. The biologic properties of each hormone are determined by its hormone-specific β subunit. Conversely, the α subunits are identical in LH and FSH as well as in other human glycoprotein hormones. **LH** is released into the systemic circulation in a pulsatile fashion after GnRH binds the cell surface

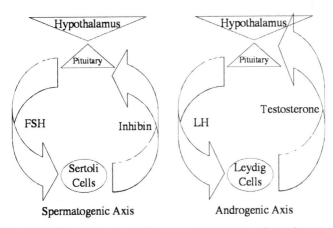

Fig. 20.1. Hypothalamic–pituitary–gonadal axis. Gonadotropin-releasing hormone (GnRH) secreted by the hypothalamus induces release of follicle-stimulating hormone (FSH) and luteinizing hormone (LH) from the anterior pituitary. FSH acts on Sertoli cells to stimulate spermatogenesis, whereas LH induces testosterone production from the Leydig cells.

receptor. LH is the major stimulus to testosterone production by Leydig cells, while testosterone exerts a negative feedback on pituitary LH release. **FSH** acts on Sertoli cells and is responsible for the initiation and maintenance of spermatogenesis. It also causes increased production of müllerian-inhibiting factor, aromatase, and inhibin. The latter is a polypeptide secreted by Sertoli cells that has a negative inhibitory effect on pituitary FSH release.

C.   The **testis** is responsible for sperm production as well as testosterone synthesis and secretion.

1.   Germ cells are found along the basement membrane within the seminiferous tubules. They constitute approximately 70% to 80% of the mass of the testis. Spermatogenesis proceeds by the production of increasingly mature and differentiated germ cells (Fig. 20.2). Fully formed spermatozoa are finally extruded into the lumen of the seminiferous tubule. Mature spermatozoa are produced in about 71 days. FSH and high intratesticular concentrations of testosterone are required for germinal epithelium maturation.

2.   Leydig cells are located in the interstitium between the seminiferous tubules and produce testosterone in response to pituitary LH stimulation. The mean adult serum level of testosterone is 600 ng/dL (range 250 to 1,000 ng/dL). Approximately 7.0 mg of testosterone is produced daily in a normal adult male. Most of the plasma testosterone (60%) is bound to sex hormone-binding globulin, and some (38%) is bound to serum albumin. The remaining 2% (free testosterone) is the physiologically active portion. A small amount of estradiol is also produced by the Leydig cells.

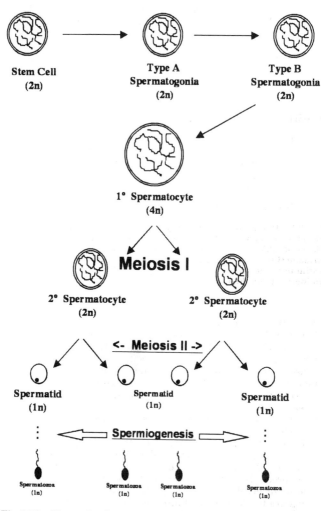

Fig. 20.2.   The cycle of spermatogenesis proceeds from the diploid spermatogonia through two meiotic reduction divisions to the motile, haploid spermatozoan.

3. Sertoli cells are contained within the seminiferous tubules and lie slightly offset from the inside surface of the basement membrane. FSH action in the testis appears to be targeted toward Sertoli cells, which act as an intermediary between the germinal epithelium and pituitary gland. Tight junctions between adjacent Sertoli cells create an effective blood–testis barrier. The polypeptide inhibin, which suppresses FSH release, is secreted by Sertoli cells.

III.   Normal testicular and ductal anatomy

  A. The **human testes** are paired oval structures weighing approximately 15 to 20 g in the adult male, with a longitudinal length of 4.5 to 5.1 cm. The testis is covered by the tunica albuginea, a dense and fibrous capsule. Fibrous septa divide the testis into many lobules and segregate the seminiferous tubules. These long, V-shaped tubules terminate in the rete testis toward the posterior and central superior segments of the testis. They are composed of supporting cells (Sertoli cells and peritubular cells) as well as the germinal elements that differentiate to form mature spermatozoa. The epithelium of the rete testis is flat and cuboidal. Efferent ductules emerge from the rete in the superior testis and coalesce in the caput epididymis to form a single epididymal tubule. Blood supply to the testis is via the internal spermatic artery as well as the cremasteric and vasal arteries. Venous return is via the veins of the pampiniform plexus, these eventually joining to form a single gonadal vein that empties into the renal vein on the left side and into the inferior vena cava on the right. The veins of the pampiniform plexus are intimately associated with the testicular (internal spermatic) artery.

  B. The **epididymis** is divided into three segments: the head (caput), body (corpus), and tail (cauda). Spermatozoa exit the testis via six to eight tiny tubules, collectively called the efferent ducts. These tubules quickly merge into a single tubule in the caput epididymis. Pseudostratified columnar epithelium lines the epididymal tubule in this region. Sperm in the caput epididymis have limited fertilization ability and are relatively immotile. As they travel through the epididymis, their motility and capacity to penetrate through the egg membrane increase progressively. Blood supply is via the deferential artery and branches of the testicular vessels.

  C. The **vas deferens** is a thick-walled structure that is embryologically derived from the mesonephric duct. From the cauda epididymis to the ejaculatory duct, where it joins the ipsilateral seminal vesicle, each vas deferens is 25 to 45 cm long. The terminal, dilated segment of each vas deferens where it joins the ejaculatory duct is called the **ampulla** of the vas. The outer adventitial layer contains a rich neurovascular network. The lumen of the vas deferens is the continuation of the convoluted epididymal ductule in the tail of the epididymis and is lined with pseudostratified columnar epithelium. Roughly one-third of the sperm in the ejaculate comes from the tail of the epididymis and the remainder from the ampulla.

  D. The **seminal vesicles** are lobulated structures, approximately 5 to 10 cm long and 2 to 5 cm wide, found lateral to the vasal ampullae on each side. *The seminal vesicles do not store sperm* but rather produce a fluid rich in fructose and coagulation

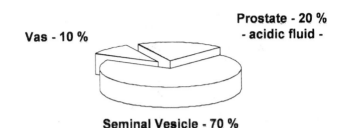

Fig. 20.3. Components of the seminal fluid. The majority of the fluid contained in each ejaculate is produced by the seminal vesicles and is alkaline. A lesser amount is contributed by the prostate, and a small amount arrives from the testis via the vas deferens.

factors. Seminal vesicle fluid accounts for approximately 70% of the ejaculate volume, prostatic secretions contribute 20%, and vasal fluid containing sperm accounts for only 10% (Fig. 20.3). The luminal epithelium is of the pseudostratified columnar type.

E. The **ejaculatory duct** is the confluence of the seminal vesicle duct and the ampulla of the vas. It courses through the prostate to terminate at the verumontanum.

F. The **prostate** is a glandular structure situated between the bladder neck and external sphincter. Fibromuscular stroma surrounds the glands of the prostate. Prostatic ducts empty into the urethra through multiple openings in the verumontanum.

IV. Neurophysiology of ejaculation

Ejaculation consists of three distinct phases:

A. Emission is the initial deposition of the seminal fluid components from the vasa, vasal ampullae, prostate, and seminal vesicles into the posterior urethra. It is mediated by efferent sympathetic fibers emanating from T10 through L2.

B. Bladder neck closure via coaptation of the circular smooth muscle fibers of the bladder neck occurs throughout the entire ejaculatory event to prevent reflux of seminal fluid into the bladder.

C. Antegrade propulsion of seminal fluid is mediated by somatic efferents arising from S2 through S4 and results in forceful expulsion of seminal components through the urethra. This is the result of rhythmic contractions of the bulbocavernosus, ischiocavernosus, and pelvic floor muscles. Pelvic splanchnic nerves relay afferent sensory stimuli from the prostate, vas deferens, and seminal vesicles to the cord, whereas the sensory division of the pudendal nerve is responsible for the transmission of information coming from the genital skin afferents. The ejaculatory reflex center, located between T12 and L2, is thought to integrate higher cerebral neural inputs, the sensory fiber afferents from the genital region, and the sympathetic and somatic efferent motor outflow to coordinate the various components of the ejaculatory reflex.

V. Spermatogenesis is the series of events occurring in the seminiferous tubule that leads to the production of mature spermatozoa from spermatogonia (Fig. 20.2). Forward motility is acquired during transport through the epididymis. The three major phases of spermatogenesis are as follows:

A. Spermatocytogenesis. Spermatogonia type A mitotically divide into the slightly more differentiated type B spermatogonia, which then replicate their DNA to produce primary spermatocytes (4N).

B. Meiosis I and II. Primary spermatocytes undergo the first meiotic reduction division and halve their DNA content, the daughter cells being known as secondary spermatocytes (2N). The second meiotic reduction division then occurs with the resultant haploid cells termed spermatids (N).

C. Spermiogenesis. Spermatids are morphologically transformed into spermatozoa during spermiogenesis (nuclear elongation and flattening, acrosome formation, and shedding of residual cytoplasm).

VI. Clinical evaluation of the infertile couple

In treating infertile couples, the physician is dealing with young, healthy persons who are nevertheless faced with a profound organic dysfunction: the inability to procreate. It is best to take a direct, factual, yet sensitive approach to the psychological implications of infertility. In most instances, successful treatment of infertility requires that the urologist work closely with a gynecologist and occasionally an endocrinologist. The proper treatment of infertile couples often involves counseling and psychological support in addition to surgical or medical therapy.

A. History. Information regarding the duration of the relationship and attempts to conceive is essential in establishing that infertility exists. It is imperative to determine whether either partner has ever been pregnant or caused pregnancy in other relationships. One should take a survey of the sexual development of the male partner during childhood and puberty, including the timing and nature of pubertal changes as well as any history of undescended testicles, hypospadias, gynecomastia, mumps, herniorrhaphy, or scrotal surgery. A history of **cryptorchidism** is particularly important because the incidence of bilateral abnormalities is high even in unilateral cryptorchidism. The development and maintenance of libido, potency, and ejaculatory function should be noted. **Retrograde or absent ejaculation** is most often caused by diabetic autonomic neuropathy, sympatholytic drugs, or retroperitoneal surgery. A history of urethritis or epididymitis may suggest genital tract obstruction as the cause of infertility. Some **prescription medications** and **spermatotoxins** may adversely affect spermatogenesis or sperm motility (Table 20.1). Self-administered agents may also be detrimental to spermatogenesis, especially marijuana (reversible depression of spermatogenesis, likely secondary to alterations in the hypothalamic–pituitary–gonadal axis) and alcohol (probably a direct effect at the testicular level). Cigarette smoking has adverse effects on sperm count, motility, and morphology. The spermatogenic function of the testis is extremely sensitive to radiation and may be completely destroyed by as little as 80 cGy.

B. Physical examination in infertile male patients may provide a specific diagnosis or suggest the focus for the ensuing

Table 20.1.   Partial list of spermatotoxins

Dilantin	Valproic acid
Alcohol	Anabolic steroids
Cannabis	Cimetidine
Colchicine	Spironolactone
Nicotine	Nitrofurantoin
Sulfasalazine	Calcium channel blockers

work-up. The examination is best performed with the patient standing in a warm room.

1.   Testes. The size and consistency of the testes should be assessed, as spermatogenesis is often reduced or absent in small testes with an abnormal consistency. The normal testis is about 4.5 cm long and 2.5 cm wide, with a volume of >20 mL. Because the seminiferous tubules account for approximately two-thirds of the mass of the testis, patients with diminished spermatogenesis have a decreased testicular volume. Even in markedly atrophic testes, the Leydig cells may be preserved and testosterone production may be relatively normal.

2.   Spermatic cord/penis. Any asymmetry of the spermatic cords should be noted. The vas deferens and epididymis should be palpated for areas of tenderness or induration, which may be indicative of obstruction. The presence of both vasa must be clearly documented. **Bilateral absence of the vasa** is rare but may occur in up to 2% of infertile male patients. Both spermatic cords should be palpated for the presence of varicoceles (see below). Abnormalities of the urethral meatus or any penile anatomic features that could interfere with normal intercourse and delivery of ejaculate to the vagina should be evaluated.

3.   Digital rectal examination is generally unnecessary in the male infertility evaluation. It should, however, be performed in older men per American Urological Association guidelines.

C.   Laboratory evaluation

1.   Semen analysis is the single most important component of the laboratory evaluation of the infertile male patient. The semen should be collected after 48 to 72 hours of abstinence from ejaculation. The specimen should be kept at room temperature and delivered to the laboratory within 1 hour. At least two separate samples should be collected within a period of 4 to 6 weeks. Minimum adequate parameters of semen analysis found in fertile men are summarized in Table 20.2, and definitions of the various terms used to describe deficient semen parameters are listed in Table 20.3.

a.   Seminal fluid comprises the combined secretions of the prostate, seminal vesicles, and bulbourethral glands. Seminal volume normally varies from 1 to 5 mL, of which the prostate contributes 20% and the seminal vesicles 70%. If the seminal vesicles are absent, atrophic, or nonfunctional or if bilateral obstruction of the ejaculatory ducts is present, the volume of the semen will be low (<1 mL) and the pH will

Table 20.2. Semen analysis: standards of adequacy

Ejaculate volume	>2.0 mL
Sperm density	>20 million sperm/mL
Percent motility	>60%
Forward progression	>2 (scale 1–4)
Morphology	>30% normal forms

Adapted from World Health Organization, 1992.

be acidic (<7.0) as the semen will consist mostly of prostatic fluid. The initial portion of the ejaculate contains most of the spermatozoa. Following ejaculation, **coagulation** occurs secondary to seminal vesicle factors. Within 5 to 20 minutes, **liquefaction** of the coagulum by proteolytic enzymes in the secretions of Cowper's glands, the prostate, or both results in the formation of a semiviscous fluid. In some instances, delayed liquefaction (>1 hour) is observed; its significance is unknown.

b. The **fructose assay** is a technique to measure the amount of fructose in the semen semiquantitatively. Fructose is secreted by the seminal vesicles, and an absence of fructose in the azoospermic patient indicates either bilateral seminal vesicle aplasia or bilateral ejaculatory duct obstruction. However, if the seminal fluid volume is normal and the pH alkaline in an azoospermic patient, seminal vesicle fluid must be present and therefore fructose will be present. Under these circumstances, there is no need to perform the test. Conversely, if the semen volume is low (<1 mL) and the pH is acidic (<7.0) in an azoospermic patient, then the seminal vesicles are not contributing to the ejaculate and the evaluation of fructose will not be helpful. Therefore, by using the parameters of semen volume and pH, contribution or lack of contribution to the ejaculate from the seminal vesicles can be determined and a fructose assay will not be helpful.

c. **Sperm density** varies over a wide range in fertile and infertile men and is poorly correlated with the conception rate. Thus, it is difficult to define a "normal" sperm density.

Table 20.3. Semen analysis nomenclature

Normozoospermia	Sperm density >20 million/mL
Oligozoospermia	Sperm density <20 million/mL
Azoospermia	Sperm density = 0
Asthenozoospermia	Motility <50%
Teratozoospermia	Morphology <30% normal forms
Oligoasthenoteratozoospermia	Density, motility, morphology less than minimal standards of adequacy
Aspermia	Absence of ejaculate

Although 20 million spermatozoa per milliliter is commonly accepted as the lower limit of normal, as many as 10% of fertile men have a sperm density of <20 million per milliliter. Only azoospermia is absolutely associated with sterility.

d.   Sperm motility, morphology, and function are perhaps more important than sperm density, although poor motility and low density usually coexist. Normal motility is defined as at least 60% of the sperm moving in a straight line at good speed. The forward progression score is a characterization of the direction and speed of the motile sperm fraction and is as important a parameter as the overall percentage of motile sperm. Asthenospermia (poor motility) may be secondary to improper collection methods, intrinsic factors, varicoceles, etc. The spermatozoa must rapidly penetrate the cervical mucus and gain access to the cervical canal because the acidic vaginal secretions are able to immobilize spermatozoa within 1 to 2 hours. In contrast, spermatozoa may remain motile within the crypts of the uterine cervix for a period of 2 to 8 days, forming a sperm reservoir from which sperm may be constantly transported to the fallopian tubes. Fertilization of the ovum also requires that the spermatozoa undergo a final process of maturation in the female genital tract, called **capacitation.** Because of the complexity of this process, it is not surprising that estimates of sperm motility as commonly performed are a very crude index of fertilizing capacity. Sperm of normal morphology have smooth and oval heads with an acrosome that is well defined and comprises 40% to 70% of the total surface area of the sperm head. There should be no defects in the tail, midsection, and neck, nor any cytoplasmic droplets larger than half the size of the sperm head.

2.   Analysis of sperm function is accomplished by looking at how sperm actually "work" in a biologic system. In vitro and in vivo assays of sperm–mucus interaction define how the sperm penetrate and move in cervical mucus, which may be quite different from the motility they exhibit in a semen analysis. Fertilizing ability is the most critical attribute of sperm, and a sense of potential capability can be gained with the zona-free and human zona pellucida assays.

a.   In vitro mucus penetration tests, commercially available in kit form, are designed to assess the ability of sperm to cross cervical mucus. The patient's sperm are mixed with either human or bovine cervical mucus in a capillary tube to determine how far they can travel within a standardized period of time.

b.   In vivo penetration testing, called the postcoital or Sims—Huhner test, is performed at the time of ovulation, when the partner's cervical mucus is most receptive to sperm penetration. The cervical mucus is examined under the microscope for motile spermatozoa within several hours of intercourse. The presence of 10 to 20 actively motile sperm per high-power field is considered normal. It is important to realize that an abnormal test result may indicate a deficiency of sperm motility as well as abnormalities of cervical mucus. Infections, presence of antisperm antibodies, and poor timing of the test may contribute to abnormal test results.

c.   In vitro fertilization testing has become possible with the development of the **sperm penetration assay,** which measures the percentage of zona-free hamster eggs (eggs stripped of their zona pellucida) penetrated by the patient's sperm and the number of sperm that have gained entry into each oocyte. Although each laboratory has its own normal values, the sperm penetration assay can be quite predictive of the ability of a subject's sperm to fertilize oocytes, in both natural and in vitro environments. The hemizona assay measures the ability of the patient's spermatozoa to bind to receptors on the human zona pellucida. This test is currently under further investigation and refinement and is not widely available.

d.   The **antisperm antibody assay** is used to detect antibodies directed against sperm surface antigens in the semen. Antisperm antibodies detected in the serum are thought to be less significant clinically. Testicular trauma, previous genital infections, or genital tract obstruction may predispose to elevated antisperm antibody levels. The immunobead test is one of the most precise antisperm antibody tests currently in use; it can detect immunoglobulin A or immunoglobulin G binding to sperm and is considered clinically relevant if >20% to 50% of sperm demonstrate binding to the polyacrylamide beads.

e.   **Sperm DNA integrity assays** have been developed to measure the structural integrity of DNA within the sperm. The assumption is that sperm DNA of infertile men is more susceptible to strand breaks and will be unable to fertilize oocytes appropriately. The preliminary data suggest that individuals with high levels of DNA strand breaks still have difficulty with conception even using ART. Examples of these tests are the sperm chromatin structure assay, terminal deoxyribosyltransferase-mediated fluorescein-dUTP nick end labeling (TUNEL) reaction, and the single cell gel electrophoresis (COMET) assay. Currently, these tests are not recommended for routine clinical use.

3.   Hormonal assays

a.   **FSH, LH, and testosterone** are measured to detect abnormalities in the hypothalamic–pituitary–testicular axis. Such abnormalities account for a small percentage of patients with infertility. Interpretation of these tests is complicated by the wide range of normal values and by the considerable overlap between normal and abnormal. In men with mild oligospermia or motility deficiencies, hormonal abnormalities are rarely striking and often require provocative tests before they become manifest. No significant difference in levels of testosterone or estradiol exists between normal and oligospermic men. FSH may be elevated in both azoospermia and oligospermia. In general, only the severely oligospermic or azoospermic patient benefits from hormonal assessment.

b.   **Elevation of prolactin** secondary to a pituitary microadenoma may result in suppression of FSH and LH output

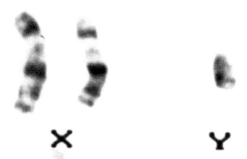

Fig. 20.4.   Sex chromosomal constitution of a male with pure 47XXY Klinefelter's syndrome.

and is usually suspected when symptoms and signs of testosterone deficiency are noted.

D. Genetic assessment. Men with nonobstructive azoospermia or severe oligospermia may have an underlying genetic defect. A karyotype may reveal aberrations in chromosome number (e.g., Klinefelter's syndrome, 47XXY; mosaic Klinefelter's syndrome, 46XY/47XXY) (Fig. 20.4) or chromosome structure (e.g., abnormal Y chromosomes, translocations). Chromosomal abnormalities are found in approximately 10% of azoospermic men, 5% of severely oligospermic men, and 1% of normospermic men.

1. Y-Chromosomal microdeletion assay. The long arm of the Y chromosome has two stretches of DNA that contain genes involved in sperm production (Fig. 20.5). The first is termed AZFa and the second contains AZFb and AZFc. Approximately 13% of men with nonobstructive azoospermia and cytologically normal Y chromosomes have a microdeletion involving one or more of these regions. Approximately 50% of men with isolated AZFc deletions and no sperm in their ejaculate will have sperm retrieved from the testis tissue that can be used in conjunction with in vitro fertilization to effect fertilization, embryo development, and pregnancy. Men with long deletions (AZFb and c) or AZFa deletions have not been found to have intratesticular sperm.

2. Syndromes of vasal aplasia, such as congenital bilateral absence of the vas deferens (CBAVD), are predominantly a consequence of mutations in both alleles of the cystic fibrosis transmembrane conductance regulator genes (*CFTR*). If the combination of the two abnormalities is "severe," clinical cystic fibrosis will be present. However, if the phenotypic manifestation of the two anomalies is "less severe," the patient may present clinically with one of the vasal aplasia syndromes but no recognizable pulmonary or pancreatic pathology. In this case, both partners should undergo *CFTR* gene testing. If the patient's partner is found to have a *CFTR*-allele mutation (she would be a "carrier"), the couple should be counseled regarding the possibility of having an offspring with clinical cystic fibrosis or, if male, CBAVD.

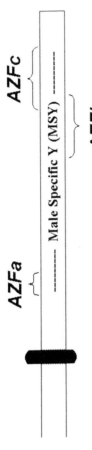

Fig. 20.5. The "male-specific" portion of the long arm of the Y chromosome. The AZFa region contains at least two genes necessary for optimal sperm production. In a small number of azoospermic men, the AZFa region is deleted. The AZFb and AZFc regions are actually one long stretch of DNA with various points where deletion may happen. There are numerous gene families that may be necessary for maximal spermatogenesis.

E. Radiologic evaluation

1. **Transrectal ultrasound** (TRUS) is now the initial diagnostic modality for documenting ejaculatory duct obstruction and seminal vesicle/vasal absence or aplasia. Ejaculatory duct obstruction should be suspected in azoospermic or severely oligoasthenospermic patients with a low semen volume. A previous history of recurrent prostatitis, perineal pain, hematospermia, epididymal pain, or pain with ejaculation is often present. It is important to note that the diagnosis is not excluded if the volume is low normal. TRUS will demonstrate dilated seminal vesicles and ejaculatory ducts and occasionally a midline prostatic cyst in cases of ejaculatory duct obstruction. If the diameter of the seminal vesicle is >1.5 cm in the anteroposterior diameter, obstruction is likely to be present. TRUS also helps define the depth of resection that may be necessary as treatment of ejaculatory duct obstruction as it provides a picture of the interior of the prostate. In cases of CBAVD, TRUS is clearly able to demonstrate the anatomic deficiencies of the vasal ampullae and seminal vesicles. Because the intrarenal collecting system, ureters, seminal vesicles, vasa, and distal two-thirds of the epididymis share a common embryologic precursor, renal US should be obtained in patients with syndromes of vasal aplasia to rule out renal anomalies.

2. **Vasography,** now infrequently performed, permits radiologic visualization of the entire vas deferens from the most proximal straight portion to the ejaculatory duct and is indicated only in patients with vasal obstruction in the inguinal or pelvic area. It is not required in the patient with spermatogenic dysfunction at the time of testis biopsy or in the patient with ejaculatory duct obstruction that was clearly imaged by TRUS. Retrograde contrast injection toward the epididymis should never be performed.

3. **Scrotal US** is not helpful in the routine evaluation of male infertility.

VII. Male reproductive abnormalities

A. **Low-volume azoospermia.** When no sperm are found in the ejaculate of the patient with a semen volume of <1 mL, either ejaculatory duct obstruction or one of the syndromes of vasal aplasia will usually be the cause.

1. **Ejaculatory duct obstruction** may have either an acquired or a congenital cause. Congenital midline prostatic cysts may be of müllerian origin and can outwardly compress the terminal portions of the ejaculatory ducts as they course through the prostate. These are easily seen with TRUS. Prior prostatic inflammation may result in scarring and occlusion of the ejaculatory ducts. In this circumstance, no intraprostatic dilation of the ducts will be seen, although there will be vasal ampullary and seminal vesicle dilation. Complete ejaculatory duct occlusion is manifested by low-volume azoospermia, but partial ejaculatory duct obstruction may present as low semen volume, severe oligoasthenospermia out of proportion to what might be expected from the testis size, and consistency combined with hormonal data.

2. CBAVD and congenital unilateral absence of the vas deferens (CUAVD) are clinically mild forms of a phenotypic spectrum that includes cystic fibrosis. The presence of abnormalities (e.g., mutations, deletions of base pairs) in both the maternal and the paternal copies of the cystic fibrosis transmembrane conductance regulator (*CFTR*) gene leads to defective protein action. As a result, pulmonary and pancreatic ductal secretions are thick and tenacious. In addition, nearly all male patients with cystic fibrosis have bilateral vasal aplasia and are infertile. CBAVD and CUAVD are limited, "mild" clinical expressions of *CFTR* dysfunction in which no pulmonary or pancreatic pathology is evident, but vasal absence is still present. Prior to commencing infertility treatment, cystic fibrosis mutation analysis is critical in both partners to define their risk, as a couple, of transmitting maternal and paternal *CFTR* gene anomalies. TRUS is able to demonstrate seminal vesicle anatomic abnormalities including aplasia, hypoplasia, or cystic dysplasia. The vasal ampullae are typically absent.

B. Normal-volume azoospermia. When the semen volume is normal, ejaculatory duct obstruction and CBAVD are not likely etiologies. Either an obstruction exists to sperm flow between the testis and vasal ampullae (implying normal spermatogenesis), or the ductal system is patent but spermatogenesis is markedly deficient.

1. Vasal or epididymal occlusion may be congenital or acquired. The seminal fluid volume will be of normal quantity because so little of it is contributed by the vasal and epididymal component. Congenital epididymal obstruction is typically located at the vasal–epididymal junction. Acquired causes are numerous, the most common being vasectomy. Inflammation of the vas and epididymis may lead to scarring and point occlusions, most commonly in the epididymis. Tuberculous vasitis and epididymitis may completely obliterate large luminal sections, making reconstruction impossible. Young's syndrome is characterized by bronchiectasis and gradual epididymal obstruction by inspissated epididymal secretions. The testis size and consistency are normal, as spermatogenesis is unaffected. Serum FSH, LH, and testosterone are all within an adequate range, reflecting an uncompromised spermatogenic and androgenic axis. The epididymis may be firm and full, which can be appreciated only with careful and thorough physical examination.

2. Spermatogenic failure that is sufficiently severe will lead to azoospermia. As explained above, the semen volume is relatively unaffected. Clinical clues to this diagnosis include small testes, reflective of a lack of spermatogenic cell mass. The consistency may be soft or firm, depending on the level of interstitial fibrosis that exists. In most instances, Leydig cells are unaffected and testosterone production remains normal. If serum FSH is elevated, the problem is within the seminiferous tubules, and the pituitary is responding appropriately with a compensatory increase in its output of FSH (hypergonadotropic hypogonadism). If the FSH is undetectable, then a hypothalamic or pituitary anomaly is present in which testicular stimulation is absent (hypogonadotropic hypogonadism).

C. Hypergonadotropic hypogonadism is the end result of multiple conditions that limit spermatogenesis.

1. Klinefelter's syndrome occurs in 1 in 500 live births. Men with Klinefelter's syndrome may present not uncommonly with an initial complaint of infertility. The karyotype reveals an extra X chromosome (47XXY). Testes are small and firm. Gynecomastia may be present. Hormonal evaluation reveals elevated LH and FSH, whereas testosterone may be low.

2. XX male syndrome is seen in 1 in 10,000 males and results from translocation of the sex-determining gene from the Y chromosome to either an autosome or one of the X chromosomes. Occasionally, an abnormality in one of the other genes is involved in the testis-determination cascade. These patients are phenotypically male with absent spermatogenesis. They are missing the "spermatogenesis" genes located on the long arm of Y that are required for optimal spermatogenesis.

3. Y-chromosome microdeletions are found in approximately 10% to 15% of azoospermic men and in approximately 6% of severely oligospermic men. AZFc microdeletions are the most common. Microdeletions involving the AZFa and AZFb deletions are rare, as are point mutations involving spermatogenesis genes. Other genes are actively being searched for and will likely help explain the remainder of the azoospermic population, for whose condition there is presently no recognizable etiology.

4. Toxic/inflammatory injury includes bilateral mumps (adult onset), viral orchitis, radiation, or chemotherapy. Such injury may temporarily or even permanently suppress spermatogenesis. A proper history will elicit these causes.

D. Hypogonadotropic hypogonadism results from either pituitary and/or hypothalamic disorders. Serum testosterone and gonadotropin levels are typically very low, often undetectable. Panhypopituitarism may result from pituitary tumors and the treatment regimens employed.

1. Kallmann syndrome (congenital hypogonadotropic hypogonadism associated with anosmia) is an X-linked disorder with phenotypic manifestations that include anosmia, infertility, deficient virilization (gynecomastia, cryptorchidism), bimanual dyskinesis (upper body mirror movements), among many others. The causative gene is *KAL1* located on the short arm of the X chromosome (Xp22.3 region). This gene encodes a protein anosmin that plays a key role in the migration of GnRH neurons and olfactory nerves to the hypothalamus during fetal development. Treatment usually consists of human chorionic gonadotropin (hCG; induces virilization via Leydig cell secretion of testosterone) followed by recombinant human FSH (induces spermatogenesis).

2. Prader–Willi syndrome is also a form of hypogonadotropic hypogonadism but also includes obesity, mental retardation, cryptorchidism, and diabetes mellitus as clinical features. Genetically, deletion of a region on chromosome 15 or uniparental disomy for chromosome 15 is most often found.

3.   Anabolic and androgenic steroid abuse suppresses pituitary LH release, leading to decreased intratesticular testosterone production. The end result is severe oligospermia or azoospermia. Although the effects are thought to be reversible, long-term pituitary suppression has been reported. Extremely low, even undetectable FSH and LH levels in a well-virilized patient with normal to high testosterone levels are the keys to this diagnosis.

E.   Oligoasthenospermia (low sperm density and poor sperm motility) is merely a description of the semen analysis and is not sufficient for etiologic diagnosis. **Varicocele** is the most common surgically correctable cause of oligospermia. A varicocele occurs when the veins of the pampiniform plexus become dilated and tortuous in the spermatic cord. It occurs unilaterally (almost always on the left) in 80% of patients and bilaterally in 18%. The diagnosis is best made after the patient has been standing upright in a warm room for several minutes. Varicoceles have been reported in about 15% of the fertile male population. Although varicocele may be found more frequently in infertile male patients (40%), the pathophysiology of infertility in association with varicocele is unclear. Testicular arterial blood flow and temperature elevation with decreased Leydig cell function have been demonstrated and may affect the contralateral testis as well. Partial ejaculatory duct obstruction and various toxins are two of the other possible causes of oligospermia in the infertile male patient. Finally, the etiology of oligoasthenospermia is often not apparent from the history and/or physical examination. In this regard, its cause is "idiopathic," but it is more than likely that genetic and environmental mechanisms will soon be found to explain the most severe cases. Immunologic infertility may be suspected in the presence of considerable sperm clumping or agglutination, poor or absent motility with relatively normal sperm density, an abnormal postcoital test result, an unexpectedly poor result in the hamster egg penetration test, or a history predisposing to the development of antisperm antibodies (e.g., vasectomy). The patient's semen should be tested for antibodies against sperm by the techniques described above.

VIII.   Therapy of male reproductive dysfunction

A.   Low-semen-volume azoospermia (<1.0 mL)

1.   Ejaculatory duct obstruction is clearly defined by TRUS. Transurethral resection is carried out if TRUS has defined a midline cystic structure or intraprostatic dilation of the ejaculatory ducts. Excision of the roof of the cyst at the level of the verumontanum allows decompression of the cyst and relief of ductal obstruction. This may also be done with the use of urologic lasers. If there is no midline cyst, incision into the surface of the ejaculatory duct itself on the floor of the prostate is carried out. If the ejaculatory ducts are not dilated and are fibrotic, transurethral resection will not be helpful. Direct ductal sperm aspiration will be the treatment of choice (see below).

2.   Vasal aplasia coexists with absence or aplasia of the seminal vesicles as a consequence of improper mesonephric duct development. No reconstruction is possible in these cases. As spermatogenesis is adequate and at least the caput epididymis is always present, it is possible to achieve pregnancy through a combination of microsurgical sperm aspiration (MESA) and intracytoplasmic sperm injection (ICSI). ICSI involves microinjection of a single sperm into an oocyte. Sperm that are surgically harvested from the epididymis have little capacity to fertilize but can readily participate in all the post-fertilization events required for embryo development. When ICSI is used for fertilization of oocytes with sperm obtained by MESA, the results are superior to those obtained with conventional in vitro fertilization techniques (which require the sperm to fertilize the oocyte), and ICSI is now the preferred treatment for these patients. Sperm can be retrieved on the day of oocyte harvesting or can be obtained at a time remote from ICSI and cryopreserved. This type of specimen can be subdivided into many cryovials, each serving as the sperm source for a future ICSI cycle. With this approach, MESA needs to be carried out only once. Percutaneous epididymal sperm aspiration is an alternative approach but is limited in terms of amount of sperm recovery and ability to cryopreserve several specimens.

B. Normal-semen-volume azoospermia

   1. Primary spermatogenic failure is not a surgically correctable lesion. FSH levels are typically elevated. Although testicular biopsy has traditionally been advocated, a thorough physical examination and review of relevant laboratory values will usually be enough for diagnosis. Testicular sperm extraction is a form of excisional therapeutic biopsy of the testis. Sperm are obtained with microscopic assistance from the excised specimen, and ICSI is performed with those individual spermatozoa. Approximately 50% of azoospermic men will have some sperm within their testis tissue that can be used in conjunction with ICSI. Both frozen-thawed and fresh tissue can be employed. The obvious worry is that if the etiology of the patient's azoospermia is genetic (e.g., microdeletion of the AZFc region on the Y chromosome), transmission to his offspring may occur. There is no absolute correlation between the results of a testis biopsy histologic pattern and whether sperm will be found in the retrieved tissue. In some studies, approximately one-third of patients initially diagnosed with Sertoli cell-only histology had intratesticular sperm at the time of testicular sperm extraction. This new therapy has dramatically changed the approach to the nonobstructive azoospermic patient, as no diagnostic biopsy is therefore necessary. Fertilization and pregnancy rates with testicular sperm extraction have been lower than those obtained with ejaculated or epididymal sperm in most studies, but biologic paternity can be realized in a population that had very little chance until recently.

   2. Secondary spermatogenic failure occurs as the result of pituitary or hypothalamic dysfunction, which may be of congenital or acquired causes, as mentioned above. Medical therapy in these instances depends primarily on manipulation or replacement of the gonadotropins FSH and LH. To induce virilization, hCG can be administered. This will stimulate Leydig cell production of testosterone. If fertility is also a goal of therapy, pure FSH or a combination of FSH and LH also needs to be administered to induce spermatogenesis. Once a steady state has been reached (often after 12 months of continuous therapy), hCG may be all that is required to maintain ongoing spermatogenesis.

3. Epididymal and vasal obstruction may be amenable to reconstructive microsurgery. A combination of history, physical examination, and laboratory results often points to an obstructive pathology, and there is no need for a testis biopsy before definitive reconstruction. At this initial surgery, the level of obstruction is determined. Obviously, if the patient had a prior vasectomy, that will be the likely site of blockage. Microsurgical expertise is required to optimize the patient's chances for a successful outcome.

a. Vasectomy reversal is carried out in those men who wish to restore their fertility potential. Postoperative patency rates are excellent but do depend on the number of years since the vasectomy. However, there is no precipitous drop-off after 10 years, an untrue "fact" that has been propagated by both urologists and gynecologists for years (Fig. 20.6). The longer the duration, the more likely it is that a secondary site of obstruction has developed in the epididymis. Although some surgeons will always perform an anastomosis of one end of the vas to the other (**vasovasostomy**), others will move back to the epididymis if no sperm are found in the testicular end of the vas and create a vasal–epididymal tubule connection (**vasoepididymostomy**). This is performed at a location where the epididymal tubule contains sperm, thus ensuring that the anastomosis is proximal to any secondary obstructive site and that the epididymal tubule is patent from the testis to

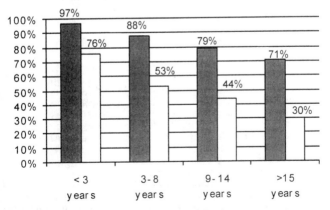

Fig. 20.6. Patency and pregnancy rates following vasovasostomy. Gray columns indicate patency rates; white columns indicate pregnancy rates. (Adapted from Belker et al. Results of 1,469 microsurgical vasectomy reversals by the Vasovasostomy Study Group. *J Urol* 1991;145:505–511.)

that point. Pregnancy rates do not equal patency rates, as female factors and poor sperm activity may limit the chances of conception.

b.   Microsurgical reconstruction of congenital or post-inflammatory occlusions almost always involves vasoepididymostomy. Patency and pregnancy rates depend on the microsurgical experience of the surgeon and the level at which the anastomosis occurs. There appears to be little difference between the cauda and corpus of the epididymis in regard to these rates, but there is a definite decrease in both when the anastomosis is to the caput region.

c.   MESA is carried out when reconstruction is not possible. MESA should also be considered at the time of reconstruction, so that if the attempt does not lead to sperm in the ejaculate, at least a cryopreserved specimen can be used as the sperm source for ICSI. Obviously, before vasal or epididymal sperm are extracted and frozen, the couple must have decided that they would indeed carry out an ICSI cycle with any cryopreserved sperm if that were their only option.

C.   Ejaculatory dysfunction. Anejaculation is a common result of spinal cord injury, and some impairment of fertility will be present in almost all of those so injured. In addition to the difficulties with ejaculation, testicular spermatogenic function may also be compromised. Possible etiologies for this suppression are numerous and include chronic infection of the urinary tract, debilitating associated illnesses (e.g., decubitus ulcers, respiratory infections), disruption of the normal thermoregulatory mechanisms, infrequency of ejaculation, and hormonal derangements. This is an important aspect of the total evaluation of these patients, because once a semen specimen has been obtained (see below), the need for advanced reproductive therapies such as in vitro fertilization may arise. The therapy of these couples therefore includes two main considerations: (a) How do we best obtain the semen specimen? (b) Once we have it, how do we most efficiently use it to help the couple achieve pregnancy (Table 20.4)?

1.   Spinal cord injuries above T10. If the spinal cord injury is above the T10 level, the lower cord may be alive and reflexive, the sympathetic innervation of the vasal ampullae, seminal vesicles, bladder neck, and prostate should be intact, the putative integration center at T12 and L1 should be functional, the sensory afferents reaching the cord at S2 through S4 and the efferents exiting the cord at this same level to innervate the periurethral musculature should all be uninjured, and the tracts leading to and from the integration center should be complete. Therefore, because the entire ejaculatory reflex arc is in place, all that is missing are the influences from the cortical regions and other higher centers.

a.   Penile vibratory stimulation (PVS) is the first line of therapy for the anejaculate spinal cord–injured patient. It is performed by placing a vibrator on the frenular surface of the glans penis and delivering a sensory stimulus to the ejaculatory integration center. This will activate the center, and if a certain threshold is exceeded, a normal ejaculatory reflex will be initiated and lead to antegrade ejaculation.

Table 20.4. Pregnancy rates and adjunctive reproductive techniques employed in couples in which the male partner has spinal cord injury

Technique	Total No. of Cycles	No. of Successful Couples/ Total No.	% Pregnancy Rate/Cycle
Self-insemination	—	5/8	—
Intrauterine insemination			
Natural cycle	11	0/6	0
Clomiphene citrate	6	1/4	17
Human menopausal gonadotropin	19	4/8	21
Gamete intrafallopian transfer	9	5/6	56
In vitro fertilization	5	2/7	29

Adapted from Nehra et al. *J Urol* 1996;155:554–559.

The vibrator does not need to be fancy or expensive as a simple massage unit will suffice. The key element is the tip that is used. Ideally, it must be conical in shape so that the vibratory stimulus is focused on a small surface point and not diffuse, as occurs with the round-headed units. Of men with cervical cord injuries, approximately 60% to 75% will ejaculate with PVS, and approximately 50% of patients with injuries at the thoracic level will do so (Fig. 20.7). Obviously, the lower cord segment must be active and able to generate reflex responses. If the lower extremities are flaccid and the bladder atonic, PVS is unlikely to be effective, as these signs demonstrate a lack of activity in the lower cord and it is unlikely that any sensory stimulus from the sacral area will actually reach the integration center. Why all patients with active lower cords do not respond to PVS is unknown.

b. Technique. In general, once the vibrator is placed, an erection occurs immediately. An increase in penile tumescence and rigidity heralds impending ejaculation. Immediately following emission, the periurethral musculature contracts and semen is rhythmically discharged. If PVS is effective in inducing antegrade ejaculation, the couple can easily be taught how to perform it. In this way, a semen specimen is obtained by the patient at home. This substantially eases the financial burden without increasing inconvenience. In the periovulatory period, PVS is carried out and the collected seminal fluid is inseminated onto the cervical area. In this way, the couple may be able to achieve conception naturally without the need for medical intervention. If the semen specimen is poor or if the couple is unsuccessful after 6 to 12 months of home insemination, more advanced strategies can be employed, such as intrauterine insemination, in vitro fertilization, or ICSI.

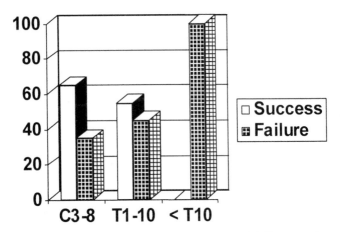

Fig. 20.7. Penile vibratory stimulation: success and failure rates in spinal cord injury patients.

    c. Autonomic dysreflexia may occur in patients with lesions above neurologic level T6 when ejaculating because the sympathetic nervous system is being activated. Either giving sublingual calcium channel blockers 10 minutes before PVS is begun or simply stopping the stimulation and raising the patient's head is usually all that is needed to abort the dysreflexia. It is important, however, always to have the first trial in the clinician's office to be prepared for any potential severe dysreflexic side effects.

2. Spinal cord injury below T10. If the damage to the spinal cord has occurred to segments below neurologic level T10, it is unlikely that a full ejaculatory reflex loop is still intact. There is interruption of the pathway from the integration center to the sympathetic nuclei (a lesion just above the integration center but below the sympathetic outflow tract at T10 through L2) or somewhere below the integration center, which impairs the transmission of sensory impulses from the afferents or motor impulses through the efferents. In this case, PVS will not be effective in eliciting an antegrade ejaculation. Two options are available in this situation: rectal probe electroejaculation and direct sperm harvesting.

    a. Rectal probe electroejaculation should be thought of as the next most appropriate maneuver, as it involves no incisions, can be performed repeatedly in an office setting if the patient has no sensation in the rectal area, and provides a semen specimen that can possibly be used for less complicated adjunctive reproductive techniques such as intrauterine insemination. Direct retrieval of sperm from the ductal system is an invasive operative intervention that provides smaller numbers of sperm. In general, it is used only in conjunction with in vitro fertilization or ICSI.

b. Technique. In rectal probe electroejaculation, contraction of the vasal ampullae and seminal vesicles is electrically induced with a probe so that "ejaculation" occurs. Typically, semen simply drips from the urethral meatus. Most often, the bladder neck also tightens to prevent retrograde flow of semen. If seminal fluid does travel in a retrograde direction, it can be recovered after completion of the stimulations.

In all cases, the bladder is emptied before the initiation of electric stimulation, and 20 to 30 mL of an appropriate buffer is left indwelling. This optimizes the environment in which the sperm will be should they move in a retrograde direction. Once the semen is collected, the various sperm parameters (count, motility, forward progression) determine what reproductive technique will be used to try to achieve pregnancy.

c. Results. Overall, approximately 10% of spinal cord–injured patients will have extremely poor semen parameters. With the availability of ICSI, however, these men may also be able to achieve biologic paternity. With the combination of intrauterine insemination and in vitro fertilization, approximately 50% of couples will achieve pregnancy (Table 20.4). It is important to understand that concomitant female factors do exist in a fair number of couples that may prevent conception.

3. Retroperitoneal lymph node dissection may cause an ejaculation in a small percentage of men. In a male patient who has had a unilateral orchiectomy, the baseline level of sperm production in the remaining testis may be significantly impaired. Approximately 25% of men in this situation will have an exceedingly poor production potential in that gonad, and adjuvant therapy such as chemotherapy may be additionally detrimental. This factor must always be kept in mind during determination of how best to achieve pregnancy once semen has been retrieved. Nerve-sparing retroperitoneal lymph node dissection often leaves the sympathetic chain intact, and no deficit in ejaculatory ability is noticed. However, if the retroperitoneal lymph mode dissection was performed before the development of modifications that maintain the integrity of the sympathetic nerves or if the nerves had to be sacrificed, a failure of emission may occur. Most patients will sense a fairly normal orgasmic experience, but there will be no antegrade flow of semen. In contrast to what occurs in the spinal cord–injured patient, the afferent sensory impulses and the augmentative cortical stimuli will activate the ejaculatory integration center. The normal temporal sequence of events is preserved, and the patient "feels" the "build-up" and "release" sensations associated with ejaculation and the rhythmic contractions of the periurethral musculature. PVS is obviously ineffective in these men, as the entire problem is the interruption of the efferent motor outflow via the sympathetic nerves to the seminal structures; it is not failure of initiation or control of the ejaculatory reflex, as it is in the spinal cord–injured male patient. Rectal probe electroejaculation is the treatment of choice for these men, as semen specimens can be easily obtained. Because rectal sensation is completely intact, a general or spinal anesthetic is required. As in the spinal cord–injured patient, the determination of which adjunctive reproductive technique will be used to achieve conception is based in part on the semen parameters. If they are particularly poor, in vitro fertilization or ICSI may be the most efficient option. However, if the sperm count and motility are excellent, several cycles of intrauterine insemination may be carried out. It is important to consider that each cycle of sperm retrieval involves anesthesia for the patient, and each specimen obtained should therefore be cryopreserved at the very least. A good overall approach is to cryopreserve the first trial specimen recovered and make plans based on the results. If the counts are low, one of the thawed vials will suffice as the sperm source for ICSI. If the specimen is adequate, one of the vials may be used for intrauterine insemination. In addition, this subdivided specimen can be considered as a backup if a fresh sample is to be collected on the day of ovulation (intrauterine insemination) or oocyte harvesting (in vitro fertilization or ICSI).

4. Retrograde ejaculation may be have neurologic or anatomic causes (Table 20.5). It occurs when the bladder neck does not coapt tightly during emission, so that the path of least resistance is into the bladder instead of the urethral meatus. It is a common misconception that retrograde ejaculation is present in spinal cord–injured patients and patients who have undergone retroperitoneal lymph node dissection. Occasionally this is true, but most often an ejaculation and failure of emission are the predominant outcomes of these two situations. The etiologies of retrograde ejaculation can be divided into two main groups: neurologic and anatomic. The history of the patient will be most revealing. If the patient has never noticed an antegrade ejaculate, it is likely that the reason is idiopathic or "occurred" before puberty. Many patients, such as those with diabetes mellitus, may describe a

Table 20.5. Etiologies of retrograde ejaculation

Neurologic
  Spinal cord injury
  Retroperitoneal lymph node dissection
  Diabetes mellitus
  Transverse myelitis
  Multiple sclerosis
  Pharmacologic (α-sympatholytic medications)
  Idiopathic

Anatomic
  Prior bladder neck surgery
  Transurethral resection of prostate
  Transurethral resection of bladder neck

gradual onset of failure of antegrade ejaculation, whereas others can pinpoint an exact temporal onset, such as following an extensive retroperitoneal lymph node dissection. It is important to ask whether the patient has noticed whitish fluid admixed with urine during the first void subsequent to intercourse. In addition, it is interesting to note whether there have been times when the patient actually has had an antegrade flow of semen and in what particular situations that might occur. It has been reported that ejaculation with a full bladder may lead to antegrade semen flow, perhaps through a different reflex mechanism that leads to closure of the internal sphincter.

   a.   Diagnosis of retrograde ejaculation. The simplest way to diagnose retrograde ejaculation is through examination of the postejaculate urine specimen. The steps the patient and clinician should follow are listed below. It is critical to have the patient empty his bladder before ejaculation so that the volume of the postejaculate mixture of urine and semen is small, which makes analysis and processing far easier. There is no reason to catheterize the patient after ejaculation if his voiding pattern is normal, as he will be able to discharge whatever is in the bladder himself—usually 10 to 15 minutes after ejaculation. The final volume of this second urination is typically 30 to 40 mL.

   (1)   Patient instructions. (a) Void to completion; (b) ejaculate and capture any antegrade material; (c) void to completion immediately afterward; (d) label the specimen "postejaculate urine."

   (2)   Clinician instructions. (a) Grossly examine the specimen, note the presence of seminal fluid, and measure and record pH; (b) centrifuge specimen for 5 minutes; (c) reconstitute the pellet to 1 mL; (d) calculate the concentration (millions/mL) and motility parameters. In this fashion, an accurate estimation of the number of sperm released into the posterior urethra (the sperm count) can be made. If there is a relatively large number of sperm in the postejaculate urine with no antegrade ejaculate produced, then the diagnosis of retrograde ejaculation is secure. If the specimen is azoospermic, it may indicate either failure of emission (no seminal fluid will be noticed in the postejaculate urine specimen) or a combination of retrograde ejaculation and testicular failure or obstruction of the proximal ductal system (seminal fluid present indicating emission but no sperm seen in the postejaculate urine). This is not an uncommon occurrence in a patient after retroperitoneal lymph node dissection who may also have a spermatogenic failure in the remaining gonad.

   b.   Treatment of retrograde ejaculation. Treatment objectives depend in part on the etiology. If the cause is anatomic, the bladder neck is fixed in an open position, and closure with medical therapy will not be successful. In this case, the mixture of urine and semen must be optimized for use with intrauterine insemination. This is best done by adjusting the pH, both before and during processing. The patient should be instructed to ingest bicarbonate (four 650-mg tablets) 1 hour before anticipated ejaculation. This will usually alkalinize the urine component of the mixture. The ideal pH is between 7.5 and 8.5. The patient should also ingest 2 full glasses of water at that time so that the urine portion is dilute. The specimen should be immediately processed with standard sperm medium and prepared for intrauterine insemination as per the laboratory protocol. Only in the rare circumstance of inadequate motility (most affected by a suboptimal milieu) is catheterization with instillation of 30 mL of sperm medium into the bladder necessary before ejaculation. If intrauterine insemination is unsuccessful, then more aggressive therapies should be considered. If the etiology is neuropathic, an attempt at pharmacologically inducing bladder neck coaptation is worthwhile. This involves stimulation of the circular fibers with α-sympathomimetic agents such as 60 mg of pseudo-ephedrine every 6 hours beginning 24 to 48 hours before expected ejaculation. This technique is successful in approximately 30% of cases of retrograde ejaculation following retroperitoneal lymph node dissection. Occasionally, the patient will mention that he noticed antegrade semen flow while on "cold medications" that probably contain agents such as pseudoephedrine. If antegrade semen flow is restored, medication is begun 1 day before ovulation, and intercourse is often all that is required to achieve pregnancy. If medical therapy fails to reverse the direction of seminal flow, processing of the postejaculate urine sample for use with adjunctive techniques is carried out as described above. In addition, pseudoephedrine given prior to intercourse has been helpful in improving antegrade flow in mild cases of retrograde ejaculation.

D. Oligoasthenoteratospermia

1. Elimination of spermatotoxins. The first step in the treatment of oligoasthenoteratospermia is identification and possible elimination of spermatotoxins. Semen analysis should be repeated 2 to 3 months after discontinuation of any identified toxic agents.

2. Medical therapy. Clomiphene citrate, hCG, tamoxifen citrate, oral kallikrein, pentoxifylline, and folinic acid have been used for the medical treatment of oligoasthenoteratospermia. Double-blind, placebo-controlled studies have been few. Those that have been performed do not indicate efficacy. Recently, carnitine supplementation has been proposed as a possible treatment for motility disorders. At this point, placebo studies have not shown an improvement in fertility rates.

3. Surgical therapy

a. Varicocelectomy. A varicocele is found in approximately 15% of fertile men and 40% of infertile men. Surgical correction (varicocelectomy) results in improvement in semen analysis in 40% to 70% of patients. Pregnancy occurs in approximately 40% of couples within 1 year of treatment. Open surgical techniques in which subinguinal, inguinal, or retroperitoneal incisions are employed show roughly similar rates of success. It is important to preserve the testicular artery and lymphatics. Laparoscopy confers no benefit in comparison with the subinguinal approach. Angiographic techniques have been described for selective catheterization of the internal spermatic veins and for treatment of occlusion by injection of sclerosing agents or use of intravenous balloons or stainless-steel coils. The pregnancy rate with these techniques appears to be comparable with that for surgical ligation of the varicocele, although contrast reactions and venous injury may occur.

b. Partial obstruction of the ductal system may occur at the level of the ejaculatory ducts or epididymis. Surgical correction via transurethral resection of the ejaculatory duct or microsurgical reconstruction may lead to a normalization of semen parameters. The clues to the diagnosis of partial ejaculatory duct obstruction are reduced semen volume and seminal deficiency out of proportion to what would be expected from the history, physical examination, and hormonal evaluation. TRUS is ideal to confirm a suspected diagnosis.

4. ART

a. Intrauterine insemination is often the first therapeutic step after all maneuvers to manage each partner have not led to pregnancy. At the time of ovulation, a semen specimen is processed to remove the seminal fluid and concentrate the sperm fraction, which is then placed into the uterine cavity via a transcervical catheter. This delivers sperm to the upper reproductive tract, closer to the fallopian tubes, where fertilization occurs. It is performed in an office setting without the need for anesthesia. The female partner may be regulated with oral medications to time ovulation more precisely. Parenteral medications may also be added to stimulate multiple follicular development and increase the chances of conception by increasing the number of oocytes released. Appropriately selected couples will have success in 15% to 20% of cases.

b. In vitro fertilization involves the incubation of harvested oocytes with processed spermatozoa in in vitro culture. Fertilized oocytes (embryos) are then either transferred to the uterine cavity with a transcervical catheter or cryopreserved if of adequate quality. The success of in vitro fertilization depends on both oocyte and sperm quality. Fertilization rates are generally in the range of 60% to 70%, with term delivery achieved in 30% of couples. In vitro fertilization is recommended if sperm quality is adequate and the couple has failed a protocol of intrauterine insemination. If the sperm have been shown to lack fertilizing ability or if they are expected to lack such capacity (sperm harvested from the epididymis) or if there are too few sperm in the ejaculate to initiate in vitro fertilization, then ICSI is employed.

c. In ICSI, delicate micromanipulation equipment is used to place an individual spermatozoan into the cytoplasm of a harvested oocyte. This procedure bypasses all mechanical fertilization barriers. It is particularly useful

in situations of severe oligospermia and when the spermatozoa are functionally deficient. Embryos develop in 60% to
80% of manipulated oocytes, with a "take-home-baby" rate
of approximately 30% per cycle.

SUGGESTED READING

American Urological Association. Male infertility best practices policy of the American Urological Association: optimal evaluation of
the infertile patient and management of obstructive azoospermia.
AUA update series lesson 38, vol XXI.

Belker AM, Thomas AJ, Fuchs EF, et al. Results of 1,469 microsurgical vasectomy reversals by the Vasovasostomy Study Group. *J Urol*
1991;145:505–511.

Damani M, Master V, Meng MV, et al. Post-chemotherapy azoospermia: fatherhood with sperm from testis tissue using intracytoplasmic sperm injection. *J Clin Oncol* 2002;2:930–936.

McCallum TJ, Milunsky JM, Munarriz R, et al. Unilateral renal agenesis (URA) associated with congenital bilateral absence of the vas
deferens (CBAVD): phenotypic findings and genetic considerations.
Hum Reprod 2001;16:282–287.

Mulhall J, Oates RD. Vasovasostomy and vasoepididymostomy. In:
Krane RJ, Siroky MB, Fitzpatrick J, eds. *Operative urology.* London:
Churchill Livingstone, 2000:383–392.

Nehra A, Werner MA, Bastuba M, et al. Vibratory stimulation and
rectal probe electroejaculation as therapy for patients with spinal
cord injury: semen parameters and pregnancy rates. *J Urol* 1996;
155:554–559.

Oates RD. Male infertility. In: Noble J, ed. *Primary care in general
medicine.* 3rd ed. St. Louis: Mosby Year Book, 2000.

Oates RD. Cystic fibrosis and congenital bilateral absence of the vas
deferens: update on genetic etiology, phenotypic findings, and
therapeutic alternatives. *Contemp OB/GYN* 2000;45:77–86.

Oates RD. Genetic considerations in the treatment of male infertility.
In: Thornton K, ed. *Infertility and reproductive medicine clinics of
North America.* New York: Elsevier Science, 2002.

Oates RD, Brown L, Silber SJ, et al. Clinical characterization of 42
oligospermic or azoospermic men with microdeletion of the AZFc
region of the Y chromosome, and of 18 children conceived via intracytoplasmic sperm injection. *Hum Reprod* 2002;17:2813–2824.

Oates RD, Lobel SM, Harris DH, et al. Efficacy of intracytoplasmic
sperm injection using intentionally cryopreserved epididymal
spermatozoa. *Hum Reprod* 1996;11:133–138.

Sadeghi-Nejad H, Oates RD. Treatment of male infertility. In: Collins
RL, Siefer DB, eds. *Office infertility: principles and practice.* New
York: Springer-Verlag, 2001.

Silber SJ, Nagy Z, Liu J, et al. The use of epididymal and testicular
spermatozoa for intracytoplasmic sperm injection: the genetic implications for male infertility. *Hum Reprod* 1995;10:2031–2043.

Wang Z, Milunsky J, Yamin M, et al. Analysis of 100 cystic fibrosis mutations in 92 patients with congenital bilateral absence of the vas
deferens by mass spectroscopy. *Hum Reprod* 2002;17:2066–2072.

World Health Organization. *WHO laboratory manual for the examination of human semen and sperm-cervical mucus interaction.* 3rd ed.
Cambridge: Cambridge University Press, 1992.

Priapism

Meir Daller, Ricardo M. Munnariz, and Irwin Goldstein

I. Definition and classification

Priapism is a pathologic condition of penile erection that persists beyond or is unrelated to sexual stimulation. The term "priapism" is derived from the Greek word *Priapus,* one of the fertility gods who was often depicted as having a giant phallus. Priapism is a significant medical condition that requires evaluation and may require emergency management. The incidence of priapism in the general population is low (about 1 in 100,000 persons/year). **Ischemic** (venoocclusive) **priapism** is the most common form of priapism. It is characterized by pain and the absence of venous outflow. Because of the prolonged increased intracavernosal pressure, there is also absence of cavernous arterial inflow. Ischemic priapism beyond 4 hours is a compartment syndrome requiring emergent medical intervention. Potential consequences are irreversible corporal fibrosis and permanent erectile dysfunction. **Arterial (nonischemic) priapism** is a less common form of priapism caused by unregulated cavernous inflow. The erection is usually painless and not fully rigid. Nonischemic priapism requires evaluation but is not generally a medical emergency.

II. Etiology of ischemic priapism

A. Pharmacologic agents are responsible for up to 80% of cases (Table 21.1).

1. Intracavernosal injection of vasoactive drugs for the management of erectile dysfunction is the most common cause of drug-induced priapism. The risk of priapism after intracavernosal injection of vasoactive agents such as papaverine and prostaglandin E_1 or a combination of those agents is higher in men with psychogenic, neurogenic, or pure cavernosal arterial insufficiency.

2. Antihypertensive drugs (phenoxybenzamine, labetalol, prazosin) are thought to induce priapism through their α-adrenergic blocking activity, preventing or delaying physiologic detumescence, or by direct relaxation of the smooth muscle of the corpus cavernosum.

3. Anticoagulants such as heparin are hypothesized to induce priapism through a relatively hypercoagulable state that occurs after therapy is discontinued. Patients on hemodialysis are susceptible to priapism due to recurrent heparinization. Warfarin has also been associated with priapism.

4. Although **tricyclic antidepressants** have rarely been associated with priapism, **trazodone,** a widely used antidepressant and hypnotic, is commonly associated with prolonged erections and priapism. The most likely mechanism is α-adrenergic blockade, which interferes with the normal detumescence mechanism. **Antipsychotic drugs** such as phenothiazines have also been associated with ischemic priapism, most likely due to dopamine D_1-receptor blockade

407

Table 21.1.   Etiology of ischemic priapism

Drugs
  Intracavernosal agents
    Papaverine, prostaglandin E_1, phenoxybenzamine
  CNS–active drugs
    Trazadone, benzodiazepines, phenothiazines, risperidone
  Antihypertensive agents
    Prazosin, phenoxybenzamine, labetalol, Ca^{2+} channel blockers,
      β blockers, hydralazine
  Anticoagulants
    Heparin, warfarin
  Hormonal agents
    Testosterone, gonadotropin-releasing hormone, tamoxifen
  Illicit drugs
    Cocaine and marijuana

Parenteral nutrition

Miscellaneous
  Carbon monoxide, black widow spider venom, alcohol

Hematologic disorders
  Hyperviscosity states
    Polycythemia
  Hemoglobinopathies
    Sickle cell anemia, thalassemia
  Immunologic disorders
    Lupus, protein C deficiency

Metabolic disorders
  Gout, diabetes, nephrotic syndrome, renal failure, amyloidosis,
    Fabry's disease

Neurologic disorders
  Spinal cord lesions, autonomic neuropathy, spinal stenosis

Malignancies
  Leukemia, prostate cancer, urethral cancer, metastatic renal
    cancer, multiple myeloma

Idiopathic

and to a lesser degree by their antihistamine, antiserotonergic, anticholinergic, and α-adrenergic blocking properties.
5.   **Illicit drugs** such as **cocaine,** by either intranasal or topical administration, have become a common cause of ischemic priapism. The pathophysiologic mechanism is complex and multifactorial. On the one hand, cocaine is a potent norepinephrine reuptake inhibitor, which may deplete neuronal norepinephrine stores and prevent detumescence. On the other, it is a potent serotonin reuptake inhibitor, which may cause central nervous system stimulation and peripheral vasodilation. **Marijuana** has also been associated with priapism.
6.   In the past, when **parenteral hyperalimentation** contained high-fat emulsions, ischemic priapism was frequently

reported. Several pathophysiologic mechanisms such as hypercoagulability, fat embolism, capillary thrombosis, and decreased capillary blood flow have been hypothesized to cause the development of parenteral hyperalimentation-induced ischemic priapism.

7. The administration of **androgens and antiestrogens** (tamoxifen) has been associated with ischemic priapism.

8. Toxins (**black widow spider venom**) may cause priapism. Following the bite of the black widow spider, local symptoms (swelling, erythema) develop rapidly. Systemic symptoms may take up to 6 hours to develop and include muscle cramps, particularly of the abdomen and back, muscle pain, numbness and tingling of the palms of the hands and bottoms of the feet, drooling, and sweating. Priapism is due to uninhibited release of neurotransmitters in the cavernosal tissue.

B. **Hematologic disorders,** especially hemoglobinopathies, are the most common cause of priapism in the pediatric population. The incidence of sickle cell disease in African Americans is estimated to be 8%, and the majority of patients with sickle cell disease will experience an episode of priapism by the age of 20. The vast majority of sickle cell priapisms occur during nocturnal erections. Patients may have short-term episodes tasting from 5 minutes to 3 hours that resolve spontaneously (**stuttering priapism**). It is possible that the combination of abnormal erythrocytes, low oxygen tension, and decreased corporal pH during prolonged nocturnal erections may induce the formation of irreversible sickle cell erythrocytes that prevent venous outflow and normal penile detumescence. Other hyperviscosity states such as **leukemia** and **polycythemia** have also been associated with priapism. The pathophysiology is probably similar to that in sickle cell anemia.

C. **Metabolic disorders** such as amyloidosis and Fabry's disease are infrequent causes of priapism. The most likely pathophysiologic mechanism is due to cavernosal outflow obstruction.

D. **Neurologic disorders.** Spinal cord injury, spinal stenosis, and autonomic neuropathy are rare causes of priapism; in these cases, the priapism generally resolves spontaneously or requires minimal intervention.

E. **Idiopathic.** The etiology of ischemic priapism is unknown in approximately 30% to 50% of cases. A comprehensive evaluation should be done in every case of priapism to rule out any underlying cause such as hematologic abnormalities.

III. **Pathophysiology of ischemic priapism** involves an imbalance of the vasoconstrictive and vasorelaxing mechanisms, leading to a closed penile compartment syndrome biochemically characterized by hypoxia, hypercapnia, and acidosis. Prolonged corporal smooth muscle exposure to these conditions results in muscle refractory to constricting agents and irreversible damage to erectile tissue with subsequent corporal fibrosis. Acidosis attenuates trabecular smooth muscle contractility to α-adrenergic agonists. Furthermore, hypoxemia activates a cascade of endothelial cell reactions characterized by increased neutrophil adhesion, decreased mitochondrial respiratory chain activity, and an increase in intracellular calcium.

Table 21.2.   Etiology of arterial (high-flow) priapism

Blunt perineal trauma
Penetrating perineal trauma
Cavernosal artery laceration
Idiopathic: unrecognized trauma

Re-establishing corporal blood flow during the management of ischemic priapism is associated with reperfusion of ischemic tissues that may generate harmful reactive oxygen species.

IV.   Arterial (nonischemic) priapism results from unregulated cavernous arterial flow due to acute perineal trauma. This leads to the formation of an arterial–lacunar fistula. Turbulent arterial flow into the fistula causes unregulated release of endothelial nitric oxide, a potent vasodilator and anticoagulant that prevents penile detumescence and clotting of the arterial–lacunar fistula. Arterial priapism is characterized by a permanent painless partial erection, almost always with normal penile axial rigidity during sexual activity. If arterial priapism is associated with persistent inadequate penile erection during intercourse, one must suspect that the traumatic event, which resulted in a lacerated cavernosal artery, was also severe enough to cause endothelial injury, leading to arterial obstructive pathology. Alternatively, the traumatic event may cause corporal tissue injury that results in corporal venoocclusive dysfunction. In such cases, vascular testing (duplex Doppler ultrasound and dynamic infusion cavernosometry and cavernosography) is indicated to differentiate cavernosal artery insufficiency from venous leak and to determine if vascular reconstruction is appropriate to reestablish potency (Table 21.2).

V.   Diagnosis

   A.   Ischemic priapism. The diagnosis of priapism is usually made by history and physical examination (painful erection that does not involve the glans). General diagnostic tests recommended include complete blood count, platelets, differential, reticulocyte count, hemoglobin electrophoresis, urine analysis, and urine screening for metabolites of cocaine or for psychoactive drugs. Prostate-specific antigen is also recommended to rule out the possibility of invasive prostate cancer into the cavernosal bodies. Assessment of corporal blood flow status *must* be carried out *in all patients* by either corporal aspirate (color, consistency, corporal blood gas) or penile duplex Doppler ultrasound and repeated after treatment has been performed to continuously assess the status of cavernosal arterial blood inflow.

   B.   Arterial priapism. The diagnosis of high-flow priapism is usually made by history (perineal trauma is almost always reported by patients) and by physical examination (partial, *nonpainful* erection). Duplex Doppler ultrasound is a noninvasive modality that allows easy visualization and localization of the arterial–lacunar fistula.

VI.   Management

   A.   Ischemic priapism. Prior to manipulating the priapistic penis, penile anesthesia (dorsal nerve, subcutaneous local penile shaft block, or circumferential penile block) and/or systemic analgesia should be considered to minimize patient discomfort and to maximize the efficacy of any invasive therapy. Important aspects in the management of sickle cell disease–associated priapism are oxygenation, hydration, alkalinization, and exchange transfusions to increase the hematocrit value to >30%. Nasal O_2 should be administered to patients with sickle cell disease to keep saturation above 92%.

 1. **α-Agonist injection** alone may be successful, especially in cases of intracavernosal drug–induced priapism. Phenylephrine is the drug of choice because of its relatively pure α-agonist profile (1 mL or 1 mg of phenylephrine is drawn up and mixed with 9 mL of normal saline for injection). Inject 0.3 to 0.5 mL of this mixture, using a 27- or 29-gauge needle, directly into the corpus cavernosum. Allow 10 to 15 minutes between repeat injections. Maximum dose is 1.5 mg.

 2. **Technique of corporal irrigation.** After appropriate local anesthesia, a 16- to 18-gauge needle is inserted perpendicularly into the lateral corpus cavernosum and 20 to 30 mL of blood is withdrawn through a three-way stopcock. Once bright red blood is obtained, aspiration can be stopped. Simple aspiration may be successful in cases of priapism lasting <24 hours.

 3. **α-Agonist irrigation** using dilute solutions may be combined with corporal aspiration. A dilute solution of phenylephrine is made by adding 10 mg (1 ampule) to 500 mL of normal saline. If phenylephrine is not available, epinephrine may be substituted (1 mg in 1,000 mL of normal saline). A syringe containing 20 to 30 mL of α-agonist solution is attached to the three-way stopcock and used to irrigate the corpora. If needed, additional blood is aspirated until detumescence is achieved. After withdrawal of the needle, firm pressure should be applied for 5 minutes to prevent hematoma formation. The penis is then wrapped snugly with an elastic bandage.

 4. **Follow-up.** Successful treatment outcome should be assessed by physical examination of the penis. In cases of partial resolution, interval assessment of corporal blood flow status by corporal aspirate or penile duplex Doppler ultrasound is mandatory. If the episode of priapism has been successfully resolved, the patient may be discharged home with detailed instructions, follow-up, and oral analgesics. In the case of partial resolution or ischemic edema, persistent partial erection, or persistent pain, inpatient observation is recommended. Adrenergic agonists may be administered (intracavernosal and/or oral) on an interval basis to induce complete detumescence.

 5. **Surgical shunting.** If, after repeated first-line interventions over several hours, no resolution of the ischemic priapism can be achieved, surgical shunts such as the Winter procedure are indicated (Fig. 21.1). In the vast majority of cases, distal shunts are effective. Proximal shunts are not more efficacious than distal shunts and in addition have a higher complication rate.

 6. **Prognosis.** The most important predictor of maintenance of premorbid erectile function is the **duration of the priapism.** Hence, rapid intervention is a necessity. Men with

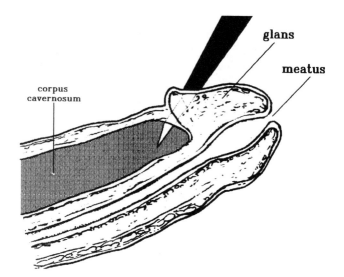

Fig. 21.1. Winter procedure to produce a cavernosoglanular fistula for ischemic priapism.

<24 hours of priapism have a 92% probability of returning to premorbid erectile function in contrast to 22% if the priapistic episode extends for >7 days.

B.   Arterial priapism. This form of priapism is not a compartment syndrome and thus is ***not a medical emergency.*** Patients may be treated electively with selective internal pudendal arteriography and superselective embolization. Autologous clot injection will temporarily occlude the lacerated artery, allowing the injured vessel to heal. The use of metal coils is associated with permanent and irreversible occlusion of the cavernosal arteries, leading to erectile dysfunction.

VII.   Clitoral priapism is a rare condition characterized by prolonged erection of the clitoris causing engorgement, swelling, and pain in the clitoris and immediate adjacent area. The most common etiology is the use of antipsychotic agents, especially trazodone hydrochloride. Withdrawal of the medication is usually successful as treatment.

SUGGESTED READING

Adeyoju AB, Olujohungbe AB, Morris J, et al. Priapism in sickle-cell disease: incidence, risk factors, and complications—an international multicentre study. *Br J Urol Int* 2002;90:898–902.

Eland IA, Van Der Lei J, Stricker BHC, et al. Incidence of priapism in the general population. *Urology* 2001;57:970–972.

Fiorelli RL, Manfrey SJ, Belkoff LH, et al. Priapism associated with intranasal cocaine abuse. *J Urol* 1990;143:581.

Fowler JEJ, Koshy M, Strub M, et al. Priapism associated with the sickle cell hemoglobinopathies: prevalence, natural history, and sequelae. *J Urol* 1991;145:65–68.

Hakim LS, Kulaksizoglu H, Mulligan R, et al. Evolving concepts in the diagnosis and treatment of arterial high flow priapism. *J Urol* 1996;155:541–548.

Hamre MR, Harmon EP, Kirkpatrick DV, et al. Priapism as a complication of sickle cell disease. *J Urol* 1991;145:1.

Junemann KP, Alken P. Pharmacotherapy of erectile dysfunction: a review. *Int J Impotence Res* 1989;1:71.

Kulmala RV, Letonen TA, Tammela TL. Preservation of potency after treatment for priapism. *Scand J Urol Nephrol* 1996;30:313–316.

Winter CC, McDowell G. Experience with 105 patients with priapism: update review of all aspects. *J Urol* 1988;140:980.

Witt MA, Goldstein I, Saenz de Tejada I, et al. Traumatic laceration of the intracavernosal arteries: the pathophysiology of non-ischemic, high flow, arterial priapism. *J Urol* 1990;143:129.

Zelissen PMJ, Stricker BHCh. Severe priapism as a complication of testosterone substitution therapy. *Am J Med* 1988;85:273.

Sexually Transmitted Diseases

Khalid Badwan and Mike B. Siroky

I. Introduction

The urologist may encounter **sexually transmitted diseases** (STDs) or genital dermatologic diseases in male patients and is responsible for their diagnosis and treatment. In the United States, about 15 million new cases of STDs occur annually (Table 22.1). Patients with STDs usually present with complaints of urethral discharge ("drip"), dysuria, or genital skin lesions. Worldwide, approximately 25 different infectious diseases are spread primarily by sexual contact. In the United States, the majority of new infections in males are due to human papilloma virus (HPV), *Chlamydia, Trichomonas,* and genital herpes simplex virus (HSV), in that order. Up to 60% of patient contacts may be asymptomatic despite being infected. Without treatment, they may become potentially infective carriers. Cultures should be obtained from sexual partners, and they should be treated as needed. Infection with multiple organisms is common (e.g., gonorrhea and nongonococcal urethritis). The U.S. Public Health Service recommends voluntary testing of all patients with STDs for human immunodeficiency virus (HIV).

II. HPV is the cause of genital warts, also called condylomata acuminata.

A. Virology. HPV types 6 or 11 cause the vast majority of visible genital warts. However, HPV types 16, 18, 31, 33, and 35 are found occasionally in visible genital warts and have been associated with erythroplasia of Queyrat, Bowen's disease, and squamous carcinoma of the penis. Patients with obvious genital warts may be infected simultaneously with multiple HPV types.

B. Epidemiology. HPV infection is now the most common STD in the United States, especially among young patients. As many as 50% of sexually active adults test positive for genital HPV infection, the vast majority being unrecognized and asymptomatic.

C. Diagnosis. The incubation period is long, typically 1 to 2 months. Diagnosis is based on the characteristic appearance of the lesion. Application of dilute acetic acid solution (3% to 5%) to suspicious areas may be performed to identify subclinical disease. HPV-infected areas turn white. On the glans and inner prepuce, the lesions are typically exophytic. On skin surfaces, they tend to be small and papular. In circumcised men, the penile shaft is the most common site, whereas in uncircumcised men, the glans penis and inner aspect of the foreskin are the most frequent sites. Approximately 5% of patients with genital warts will have intraurethral warts. Large condylomata with propensity for local invasion are called Buschke–Lowenstein tumors. Biopsy may be indicated with atypical or large lesions.

D. Treatment choice is determined by wart area, wart count, anatomic site, morphology, cost, and patient preference. Podophyllin (25% in benzoin) is carefully applied weekly to each le-

Table 22.1.   Estimated new cases annually of sexually transmitted diseases in the United States

Human papilloma virus	5,500,000
T. vaginalis	5,000,000
C. trachomatis	3,000,000
Genital herpes	1,000,000
Gonorrhea	650,000
Syphilis	70,000

From Centers for Disease Control, 2000.

sion and washed off after 4 hours. Podofilox 0.5% solution or gel is available for self-application bid for 3 days followed by 4 days without therapy. This cycle may be repeated up to four times. Imiquimod 5% cream is applied three times a week at bedtime and washed off 6 to 10 hours later. Treatment may extend for up to 16 weeks. Trichloroacetic acid in 80% to 90% solution may be applied carefully only to warts and allowed to dry. This treatment can be repeated weekly, if necessary. Other treatment options include cryotherapy and surgical removal, both of which may be beneficial for patients who have a large number of warts or extensive involvement. Intraurethral warts may be treated with 5-fluorouracil cream (intraurethral once a week for 3 weeks) or endoscopic cauterization. For lesions limited to the foreskin, circumcision may be considered.

E.   Prevention. It is likely that condoms do not provide reliable protection against HPV. Because the virus may reside in clinically uninvolved skin, successful removal of visible warts does not reduce the patient's risk of transmitting the virus to sex partners. Nevertheless, sex partners should be evaluated for warts and other STDs and treated appropriately.

III.   *Chlamydia trachomatis* is the most common bacterial cause of STD in men. The most common clinical manifestation of chlamydial infection is urethritis. From 5% to 10% of the young male population may have asymptomatic infection.

A.   Nongonococcal urethritis (NGU). Urethritis in men has traditionally been classified as gonococcal and nongonococcal. *C. trachomatis* has been established as the most frequent cause of NGU, accounting for about 30% of cases. This leaves a group of cases now designated as **nonchlamydial, nongonococcal urethritis** (NCNGU), in which the etiology is unclear. Organisms that may cause NCNGU are *Mycoplasma genitalium, T. vaginalis, Ureaplasma urealyticum,* and herpes simplex. Gonorrhea and chlamydial infection often coexist.

1.   Clinical features. The presentation is usually a thin, mucoid urethral discharge associated with dysuria and meatal pruritus. The incubation period in NGU (5 to 10 days) is longer than in gonococcal infection (2 to 7 days). Reiter's syndrome (arthritis, uveitis, urethritis) may also be present.

2.   Diagnosis is made by urine-based diagnostic tests based on detecting chlamydial DNA by polymerase chain reaction (PCR). These tests are highly specific for chlamydia and can detect nonviable as well as living bacterial DNA. Previous methods of chlamydial culture have been replaced by these newer tests. The patient should be instructed to abstain from voiding for 2 hours. The first void is collected in a sterile container and sent to the laboratory for chlamydial PCR testing. Gonorrheal PCR testing can be done simultaneously. To detect *T. vaginalis,* a wet smear can be prepared by mixing a drop of urethral exudate with 1 mL of normal saline solution.

3.   Treatment of NGU due to *Chlamydia* or *Ureaplasma* infection is 1 g of oral azithromycin or 100 mg of oral doxycycline twice daily for 7 days. Alternative treatments include ofloxacin or erythromycin. All sex partners should be evaluated and treated.

B.   Epididymitis in sexually active men under the age of 35 is due to *C. trachomatis* in about 50% of cases and *Neisseria gonorrhoeae* in the remaining 50%. Urethritis frequently accompanies sexually transmitted epididymitis. **Treatment** with empirically chosen antibiotics is indicated before culture results are available. The Centers for Disease Control recommends the combination of ceftriaxone (250 mg IM as a single dose) plus doxycycline (100 mg PO bid for 10 days) for the treatment of acute epididymitis this is most likely sexually transmitted.

IV.   *T. vaginalis* is a flagellated protozoan that causes vaginal infection in women who are often asymptomatic carriers. In males, *T. vaginalis* may cause asymptomatic infection or symptomatic urethritis, prostatitis, or epididymoorchitis. Incubation period averages 1 week but can range from 4 to 28 days. *T. vaginalis* infection may account for 15% of cases of NCNGU urethritis.

A.   Diagnosis. Male patients may complain of dysuria, testicular pain, or lower abdominal pain. There may be mucopurulent penile discharge in 25% to 50% of cases or signs of prostatitis or epididymitis. As there is a high rate of coinfection with *N. gonorrhoeae* and other STDs, always test for syphilis, *N. gonorrhoeae, C. trachomatis,* HIV, hepatitis B, and hepatitis C in patients with suspected *T. vaginalis* infection. Trichomonads appear as ovoid-shaped parasites with flagellae on saline wet mount of urethral discharge. The saline wet mount is positive in only 60% of cases, and recent voiding may make the test less sensitive because trichomonads may be washed away. Anaerobic cultures will be positive within 48 hours in 95% of cases.

B.   Treatment is 2 g of metronidazole orally as a single dose or 250 mg PO tid for a week. Erythromycin base 500 mg PO qid for 7 days may be used for persistent or recurrent urethritis.

V.   HSV may cause painful vesicles on the genital skin. The vast majority of cases are caused by HSV type 2 (Table 22.2).

A.   Clinical features. The incubation period varies from 1 to 30 days, but 3 to 5 days is typical. Almost all have painful ulcerative lesions on the prepuce, glans, or shaft of the penis; 80% have tender lymphadenopathy, 60% fever, 45% dysuria, and 25% urethritis. The clinical course is less severe for recurrences. Sacral autonomic neuropathy may result in acute urinary retention. Proctitis may occur in men having anal sex.

Table 22.2. Clinical features of sexually transmitted genital skin ulcers

Disease	Incubation	No./Size	Induration	Pain	Adenopathy
Syphilis	10–90 d	Single/variable	Yes	No	Yes
Chancroid	2–5 d	Multiple/variable	No	Yes	Yes
LGV	3–30 d	Single/small	No	No	Yes
GI	Up to 3 mo	Single/large	No	No	No
HSV	3–5 d	Multiple/small	No	Yes	Yes

LGV, lymphogranuloma venereum; GI, granuloma inguinale; HSV, herpes simplex virus.

B.   Diagnosis is made clinically by noting vesicles on an ery-thematous base. These do not follow a dermatomal distribution. Viral culture and PCR are both sensitive methods of viral de-tection. To culture, a vesicle should be ruptured with a sterile needle and the base rubbed with the swab. Smears can be pre-pared for Tsank staining by scraping lesions and staining with Giemsa or Wright stain. These may demonstrate multinucle-ated giant cells, which indicate infection with HSV or varicella-zoster virus.

C.   Treatment. Famciclovir has replaced acyclovir. Although its mechanism of action is similar, famciclovir has more favor-able pharmacokinetics that enable less frequent dosing. Its bioavailability is approximately 75% (versus 10% to 20% for acyclovir), and prolonged intracellular levels are achieved. Dosing for acute HSV infection is 250 mg orally three times daily for 5 days (equivalent to 200 mg of acyclovir five times daily for 7 to 10 days). Therapy shortens the duration of pain and reduces viral shedding and duration of systemic symp-toms. However, it does *not* eliminate latent virus, nor does it affect the risk of recurrence. Recurrent HSV infection can be treated with 125 mg of famciclovir orally twice daily for 5 days. Suppressive dosing is 125 to 250 mg orally twice daily. Sup-pressive therapy is indicated in patients with more than six recurrences per year.

VI.   Gonorrhea is caused by *N. gonorrhoeae,* an intracellular gram-negative diplococcus. The incubation period is 3 to 7 days after sexual contact, and symptoms develop within 14 days in 90% of cases. Asymptomatic disease may occur in either sex but is much more common in women than in men. Up to 35% of men will have concomitant chlamydial infection. Among homosexual men, the pharynx is affected in 40% and the rectum in 25%. Ure-thritis is the presenting complaint in >95% of infected men. Acute complications include epididymitis, orchitis, and prostatitis. Ure-thral stricture is a late complication.

A.   Diagnosis is by urethral smear and culture on special media. Specimen should be collected using calcium alginate ure-thral swabs. The presence of **intracellular** gram-negative diplo-cocci on smear is diagnostic. Pharyngeal cultures are obtained if history suggests infection. If only extracellular organisms are seen, one must depend on results of culture for a definitive diag-nosis, although in some cases, a clinical decision to treat may be made. *Neisseria* grows best at 35° to 37°C in a 3% to 5% carbon dioxide environment on Thayer–Martin medium to prevent over-growth by other organisms. Direct immunofluorescence is a rapid assay and has a sensitivity of 84% and specificity of 100% in men. DNA probes have a sensitivity of 90% to 98% and a speci-ficity of 82% to 98%. Ligase chain reaction has a sensitivity of approximately 100% and a specificity of 99%. Direct gram stain diagnosis remains the preferred method of diagnosis today.

B.   Treatment. Uncomplicated infection may be treated with 125 mg of intramuscular ceftriaxone, 400 mg of oral cefixime, 500 mg of oral ciprofloxacin, or 400 mg of ofloxacin. Approxi-mately 25% of men with gonorrheal infection have concomitant infection with *C. trachomatis.* Thus, a regimen for *Chlamydia* infection as outlined in Table 22.3 should also be prescribed. If a patient has severe allergies, 2 g of intramuscular spectinomycin may be used. All sex partners should be evaluated and treated. Patients under age 18 should not receive quinolones. Cases of gonorrhea resistant to quinolones have been reported sporadically, although they remain extremely rare in the United States.

VII. Genital molluscum contagiosum appears as raised papules with a central depression on the scrotum or shaft of the penis. The lesions are caused by a poxvirus that has an incubation period of 2 to 7 weeks. Diagnosis is by clinical appearance. Treatment consists of opening each lesion with a pointed applicator dipped in liquid phenol or use of cautery, cryotherapy, or lasers. This condition is highly associated with HIV infection.

VIII. Syphilis is caused by the spirochete *Treponema pallidum*. The disease presents initially as a primary genital ulcer, called a chancre, appearing most commonly on the glans penis. The ulcer is typically nontender and has well-defined borders. Syphilis is considerably more common among African Americans and in the southeastern regions of the United States.

A. Pathology

1. Primary stage. *T. pallidum* may enter through open skin or through intact mucous membrane. After multiplying at the site of inoculation, spirochetes enter the regional lymph nodes and the bloodstream. After an incubation period ranging from 10 to 90 days, the chancre of primary syphilis appears at the site of inoculation and is accompanied by regional lymphadenopathy. Chancre may appear on the genitalia or any site of inoculation. The untreated chancre typically is present for 1 to 6 weeks.

2. Secondary stage. Approximately 6 weeks after the primary chancre heals, a diffuse maculopapular rash develops, involving the palms and soles of the feet. Generalized lymphadenopathy and systemic symptoms of fever, malaise, and joint pains are also common. This phase will typically last 1 to 2 months. During both the primary and the secondary stages of syphilis, the patient is infectious to others.

3. Latent-phase syphilis is characterized by lack of symptoms and signs, with the presence of a positive serologic test for syphilis. Patients are not infectious during this phase, which may last up to 20 years.

4. Tertiary-stage syphilis is characterized by destructive lesions of the aorta, central nervous system, bones, and skin.

B. Diagnosis. Syphilis may present in a multitude of ways and has been called the "Great Imitator." The diagnosis is made by scraping the base of the ulcer and examining the serous material with a dark-field microscope for motile spirochetes (*T. pallidum*).

1. Antibody tests. Results of nonspecific serologic tests [e.g., VDRL (Venereal Disease Research Laboratory); RPR (Rapid Plasma Reagin)] do not become positive until 1 to 3 weeks after the appearance of the ulcer and return to normal in almost all patients treated for primary syphilis.

2. Specific treponemal tests include the fluorescent treponemal antibody absorbed (FTA-ABS) and microhemagglutination assay for antibody to *T. pallidum* (MHA-TP).

Table 22.3.   Antibiotic therapy of sexually transmitted disease in male patients

STD	Likely Organisms	Therapy	
		Recommended	Alternative
Gonorrhea	N. gonorrhoeae	Ceftriaxone 125 mg IM or cefixime 400 mg PO or ciprofloxacin 500 mg PO or ofloxacin 400 mg PO	Spectinomycin 2 g IM
Nongonococcal urethritis	C. trachomatis	Azithromycin 1 g PO or doxycycline 100 mg PO bid × 7 d	Erythromycin 500 mg PO qid × 7 d or ofloxacin 300 mg PO q12h × 7 d
	T. vaginalis	Metronidazole 2 g PO or metronidazole 250 mg PO tid × 7 d	Erythromycin 500 mg PO qid × 7 d
Syphilis	T. pallidum	Benzathine penicillin G 2.4 mg IM	Doxycycline 100 mg PO bid × 14 d Ceftriaxone 1 g IM qid × 4 doses

Disease	Organism	Treatment	Alternative
Chancroid	*H. ducreyi*	Ceftriaxone 250 mg IM *or* azithromycin 1 g PO *or* erythromycin 500 mg PO qid × 7 d	Ciprofloxacin 500 mg PO bid × 3 d
Granuloma inguinale	*C. granulomatis*	Doxycycline 100 mg PO bid × 7–28 d	TMP/SMX DS 1 tab PO bid × 14 d
LGV	*C. trachomatis*	Doxycycline 100 mg PO bid × 21 d	Erythromycin 500 mg PO qid × 21 d Azithromycin 1 g PO Sulfasoxazole 500 mg PO qid × 21 d
Genital warts	HPV types 6 and 11	Podophyllin 25% in benzoin	Cryotherapy Imiquomid 0.5% 3/wk Trichloroacetic acid Surgical removal
Genital herpes	HSV type 2	Famciclovir 125 mg PO tid × 5 d	Acyclovir 200 mg PO 5 times daily × 7–10 d

TMP/SMX, trimethoprim/sulfamethoxazole; DS, double strength; LGV, lymphogranuloma venereum; HPV, human papilloma virus; HSV, herpes simplex virus.

Treponemal tests are more sensitive and more specific than nontreponemal tests for the diagnosis of syphilis. Results of the FTA-ABS (fluorescent *Treponema* antibody absorption) test become positive earlier and usually remain positive for life. In contrast to the VDRL, the FTA-ABS very rarely gives a false-positive result. Therefore, the FTA-ABS and MHA-TP should be used to confirm a positive nontreponemal test or when there is a clinical suspicion for syphilis in a patient with a negative nontreponemal test. Since treponemal tests remain positive even after successful treatment, they are not good markers for disease activity or recurrence.

C. Treatment for primary syphilis is 2.4 ×10^6 U of benzathine penicillin G given intramuscularly. If the patient is penicillin-allergic, give 100 mg of doxycycline orally twice daily for 2 weeks or 1 g of ceftriaxone intramuscularly every other day up to four doses. Tetracycline or erythromycin may also be used as alternative agents.

IX. Chancroid, caused by *Haemophilus ducreyi,* resembles the lesion of primary syphilis. The ulcer may be painful with or without adenopathy. An estimated 10% of patients with chancroid have coexisting syphilis or HSV infection.

A. Diagnosis. An irregular, painful ulcer develops on the penis 2 to 5 days after exposure. In contrast to syphilis, multiple lesions are common. Tender inguinal lymphadenopathy develops usually unilaterally within 1 to 2 weeks in about half of untreated patients. The diagnosis is confirmed by gram stain of material from the base of the ulcer, which may reveal gram-negative coccobacilli in chains or clusters.

B. Treatment options include azithromycin (1 g PO in a single dose), ceftriaxone (250 mg IM in a single dose), erythromycin, or ciprofloxacin. Painful fluctuant buboes may be decompressed by needle aspiration.

X. Granuloma inguinale (donovanosis) is a chronic infection of genital and perigenital skin caused by

T. vaginalis
Candida albicans
C. trachomatis
N. gonorrhoeae
HSV

It has an unusually long incubation period (up to 3 months). The genital ulcer is nontender and indurated. Subcutaneous inguinal granulomas develop. Diagnosis is confirmed by demonstrating the organism within monocytes (Donovan bodies) in tissue obtained from the ulcer base. Primary treatment is doxycycline (100 mg orally for 3 weeks); alternative options include trimethoprim/sulfamethoxazole, ciprofloxacin, and erythromycin. Sex partners need to be examined and treated.

XI. Lymphogranuloma venereum (LGV) is rare in the United States but endemic to areas of the Caribbean, Central America, Southeast Asia, and Africa. The causative organism is *C. trachomatis,* serotypes L1, L2, and L3. The organism does not penetrate intact skin and must be acquired by contact with an active lesion. The disease is characterized by a small, transient genital lesion appearing 3 to 30 days after sexual contact and very tender inguinal lymphadenopathy evident 2 to 6 weeks after contact. The primary lesion is similar to that of herpes but nontender. It may be difficult to differentiate from syphilis. The second phase, characterized in male patients by unilateral lymphadenopathy (buboes), may include constitutional symptoms such as fever, chills, myalgias, and malaise. A third phase consisting of proctocolitis may appear many years later. In homosexual men, proctitis may be a presenting symptom.

A. **Diagnosis** is best made by culture of infected tissue obtained by needle aspiration. However, culture of *C. trachomatis* is difficult; an isolate is obtained only 30% of the time. Serology (complement fixation) is not specific for this infection, as other chlamydial infections may cause elevated antibody titers. However, a complement fixation titer of >1:64 along with the typical clinical findings is considered diagnostic of LGV.

B. **Treatment** is doxycycline 100 mg PO bid for 21 days. Surgical drainage of infected buboes may also be necessary. Alternative antibiotics include erythromycin (500 mg PO qid for 21 days), azithromycin, and sulfisoxazole. Ulcers are healed at 7 days in 50% of cases, at 14 days in 80%, and at 28 days in 100%. The relapse rate is 3% to 5%.

XII. **Acquired immunodeficiency disease syndrome** (AIDS) is due to infection by HIV. In the United States, 41,000 new cases of AIDS are diagnosed per year, 50% in patients younger than 25 years. AIDS predisposes to opportunistic infections of the genitourinary tract. The infectious, inflammatory, and malignant conditions associated with AIDS are prone to progression and development of secondary complications (abscess formation, recurrence, systemic infection).

A. **Infections and inflammatory conditions**

1. **Kidney.** AIDS-related kidney infections include cytomegalovirus, *Aspergillus,* and *Toxoplasma.* Generally, patients at risk have advanced AIDS with impaired immune systems. **AIDS-related nephropathy** is an ill-defined condition characterized by azotemia, proteinuria, and focal segmental glomerulosclerosis on renal biopsy. This entity must be considered in patients who are seropositive for HIV and have significant proteinuria. The disease is more prevalent among young black males. Treatment consists of antiretroviral agents.

2. **Prostate.** In some studies, nearly 10% of men hospitalized for AIDS-related infections are diagnosed with bacterial prostatitis. Clinical features include fever, obstructive urinary symptoms, and low back pain. Treatment requires prolonged course of antibiotics (i.e., fluoroquinolones) to overcome poor tissue penetration in the prostate. Prostatic abscesses are known to occur in HIV patients and require urgent open or transrectal drainage to avert frank sepsis.

3. **Testes and epididymis.** Testicular atrophy is a common finding and is multifactorial (endocrine disturbance, recurrent fevers, drug toxicity). Epididymoorchitis is common and often complicated by progression to chronic infection and abscess formation.

4. **Genitourinary malignancies.** AIDS is known to predispose to a number of malignancies. Traditionally, central nervous system tumors and Kaposi's sarcoma are closely associated with AIDS. The blunted immune surveillance system also predisposes to urologic malignancies such as squamous cell carcinoma (penis), melanoma, and testicular cancers.

5.   Voiding dysfunction is related to peripheral and central neuropathy seen in AIDS patients. Urinary retention is seen in as many as 50% of patients with advanced AIDS. Less common is detrusor hyperreflexia (25%). Clean intermittent catheterization with or without antimuscarinic agents is the preferred treatment.

6.   Stones. AIDS patients treated with indinavir, a protease inhibitor, are prone to urolithiasis. Indinavir stones are radiolucent and undetectable by computed tomography.

XIII.   Candidiasis involving the **glans or foreskin** is most often seen in uncircumcised men with poor hygiene. Additional risk factors include diabetes mellitus and immunosuppression. Candidal balanitis is often associated with vaginal candidiasis in the female partner. Clinical features include bright red patches or papules on the foreskin and glans. **Diagnosis** is made by culture or scraping some of the lesion for a potassium hydroxide prep to look for yeast cells. **Treatment** is miconazole nitrate or clotrimazole creams (apply bid to affected area for 2 to 3 weeks, then reevaluate result). Oral therapy with fluconazole (150 mg PO once) is also effective but more costly.

XIV.   Pediculosis pubis is due to *Phthirus pubis,* the pubic louse. Most common presentation is pruritus or the presence of lice or nits (eggs) on the pubic hair. Diagnosis is made by gross or microscopic identification of the lice or nits. Recommended treatment is permethrin 1% creme rinse or lindane 1% shampoo applied to the affected area. Some patients may require retreatment after 1 week.

XV.   Scabies is due to *Sarcoptes scabiei,* the scabies mite. Sexual transmission is common in adults. The predominant symptom is intense pruritus. Typical findings consist of excoriated maculopapular lesions on the genitalia. Scrapings from a lesion may reveal the mite or eggs on microscopic examination. Treatment consists of permethrin 5% cream applied to all areas of the body from the neck down and washed off after 8 to 14 hours. Alternatives include topical lindane 1% lotion or sulfur 6% ointment. Bedding and clothing should be decontaminated or removed from body contact for at least 72 hours.

SUGGESTED READING

Burstein GR, Zenilman JM. Nongonococcal urethritis—a new paradigm. *Clin Infect Dis* 1999;28(suppl 1):S66.

Cates W. Estimates of the incidence and prevalence of sexually transmitted diseases in the United States. *Sex Transmit Dis* 1999; 26(suppl):S2–S7.

Centers for Disease Control. *Tracking the hidden epidemics. Trends in the STD epidemics in the United States.* Atlanta: Centers for Disease Control, 2000.

Krieger JN, Jenny C, Verdon M, et al. Clinical manifestations of trichomoniasis in men. *Ann Intern Med* 1993;118:844–849.

Krieger JN, Verdon M, Siegel N, et al. Risk assessment and laboratory diagnosis of trichomoniasis in men. *J Infect Dis* 1992;166: 1362–1366.

Kwan DJ, Lowe FC. Genitourinary manifestations of the acquired immunodeficiency syndrome. *Urology* 1995;45:13–27.

McNagny SE, Parker RM, Zenilman JM, et al. Urinary leukocyte esterase test: a screening method for the detection of asymptomatic chlamydial and gonococcal infections in men. *J Infect Dis* 1992; 165:573.

Rosen T, Brown TJ. Genital ulcers: evaluation and treatment. *Dermatol Clin* 1998;16:673–685.

Sobel JD, Nagappan V, Nyirjesy P. Metronidazole-resistant vaginal trichomoniasis—an emerging problem. *N Engl J Med* 1999;341: 292–293.

Stamm WE. *Chlamydia trachomatis* infections: progress and problems. *J Infect Dis* 1999;179(suppl 2):S380.

Stamm WE, Hicks CB, Martin DH, et al. Azithromycin for empirical treatment of the nongonococcal urethritis syndrome in men: a randomized double-blind study. *JAMA* 1995;274:545.

Totten PA, Schwartz MA, Sjostrom KE, et al. Association of *Mycoplasma genitalium* with non-gonococcal urethritis in heterosexual men. *J Infect Dis* 2001;183:269–276.

Surgical Disorders of the Adrenal Gland

Meir Daller and Mike B. Siroky

The adrenal glands are small, yellowish, triangular endocrine glands located at the superior and medial aspect of each kidney. In the past, adrenal disease usually became manifest because of systemic symptoms and signs resulting from a change in gland function. The availability of computed tomography (CT) has made detection of asymptomatic adrenal masses more common. This chapter describes a systematic approach to the evaluation, diagnosis, and treatment of the adrenal mass. A classification of primary adrenal lesions is given in Table 23.1, and a list of common sources of metastatic lesions in the adrenal gland is given in Table 23.2.

I. Surgical anatomy and embryology

The adrenal gland—triangular on the right, crescent shaped on the left—caps the superomedial pole of each kidney (Fig. 23.1). The cortex is the visible part of the adrenal gland and is distinguished from perirenal fat by its dark yellow color, finely granular surface, and firm consistency. The medulla is dark red in color and friable. Each adrenal gland weighs approximately 6 g, and its average dimensions in adults are approximately $5.0 \times 3.0 \times 0.6$ cm.

A. Blood supply. The adrenal glands receive their arterial blood from three sources: (a) the inferior phrenic artery, (b) the abdominal aorta, and (c) the renal artery. The arrangement of the adrenal veins is much simpler than that of the arteries and is important surgically. On the left side, vascular control of the adrenal vein is easy because the adrenal vein is long (3 cm), empties into the left inferior phrenic vein, and takes an oblique course downward to enter the left renal vein. On the right side, vascular control of the adrenal vein is more difficult as it is much shorter on this side (0.6 cm) before emptying directly into the posterior part of the inferior vena cava. This presents the risk for injury to the vena cava with disastrous hemorrhage.

B. Embryology. The suprarenal glands embryologically comprise two distinct parts: the cortex and the medulla. The cortex is derived from mesoderm and is a groove in the coelom between the base of the mesentery medially and the mesonephros and undifferentiated gonad laterally. This close proximity explains why ectopic cortical tissue has been described below the kidneys and associated with the testes or ovaries. The medulla is derived from the ectoderm and is developed from migrating cells of the neural crest. This migration of nervous cells forms the ganglia of the sympathetic trunk and of the sympathetic plexuses. It also forms the paraganglia, which secrete catecholamines (i.e., the chromaffin tissue).

II. Radiology of the adrenal

A. Plain abdominal radiography has a limited role in the evaluation of adrenal neoplasms. However, such films can detect

Table 23.1. Differential diagnosis of primary adrenal masses

Neoplastic
  Adrenocortical hyperplasia
  Adenoma
  Carcinoma
  Pheochromocytoma
  Neuroblastoma
  Ganglioneuroma
  Medullary carcinoma

Nonneoplastic
  Adrenal cyst and pseudocyst
  Adrenal abscess
  Adrenal hematoma
  Amyloidosis
  Myelolipoma and other hamartomas
  Wolman disease (familial xanthomatosis)

adrenal calcifications in adults with tuberculosis or histoplasmosis or an old hematoma. In addition, they can detect calcifications in children following neonatal adrenal hemorrhage or in association with neuroblastoma.

B. Ultrasound. Ultrasound examination of the abdomen is economical and safe and can be useful for serial evaluation of adrenal growth. It can differentiate between a cyst and a solid adrenal mass. It can evaluate vascular involvement or liver metastases. Although the adrenal glands can be identified in most patients with ultrasound, this technique is somewhat limited because it does not give the explicit anatomic definition seen on a CT scan or magnetic resonance imaging (MRI).

C. CT. For patients with known or suspected adrenal lesions, CT has become the imaging procedure of choice. It can precisely identify the size, location, appearance, presence of local or vascular invasion, lymph node involvement, and presence of distant metastases in the majority of patients. An attenuation of ≤10 HU is fairly diagnostic of adrenal cortical adenoma (96% specificity). Intravenous contrast agent may be useful in defining enhance-

**Table 23.2. Most common primary
sites for adrenal metastases**

1. Lung
2. Female breast
3. Melanoma
4. Renal cell carcinoma
5. Extraadrenal lymphoma
6. Leukemias
7. Pancreatic carcinoma
8. Colonic carcinoma
9. Ovarian carcinoma

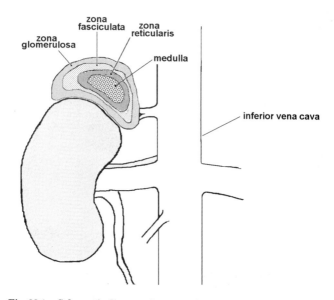

Fig. 23.1. Schematic diagram drawn to depict the anatomic relations of the adrenal gland and demonstrate the three zones of the cortex surrounding the medulla. Not drawn to scale.

ment of an adrenal lesion. Washout is a measurement of the percentage decrease between the initial enhancement (80 seconds) and the delayed enhancement (10 minutes). A large decrease is a high-percentage washout, and a small decrease is a low-percentage washout. Washout of >50% seems to be specific for benign adrenal adenoma, whereas a washout of <50% is fairly specific for metastasis. The physiology of washout is not well understood.

D. MRI. MRI can demonstrate anatomic information, extension into adjacent structures, and the relationship between adrenal tumors and major vessels. It can also offer substantial information to help discriminate between benign and malignant adrenal lesions. MRI is particularly useful in patients with suspected pheochromocytomas and is the imaging procedure of choice when a patient has biochemical data suggesting catecholamine excess. Nonfunctioning adrenal adenomas appear on T2-weighted images similar to normal adrenal tissue, whereas pheochromocytomas exhibit high signal intensity on the enhanced T2-weighted imaging. MR angiography using gadolinium may be useful to delineate the anatomic relationships between adrenal tumors and vascular structures.

E. Radioisotope scanning/positron emission tomography. Radioisotope imaging relies on function rather than anatomy. Analogues of substrates required for adrenal hormone synthesis can be radiolabeled and used to localize functional adrenal adenomas and pheochromocytomas. Available radiopharmaceuticals include [^{131}I]6-iodomethylnorcholesterol,

[^{131}I]19-iodocholesterol, and [^{75}Se]selenomethylnorcholesterol. Hypersecreting tumors such as cortisol, aldosterone, and androgen-secreting adenomas demonstrate radiocholesterol uptake, whereas primary and secondary adrenal malignancies appear as "cold" areas. Adrenal medullary scintigraphy requires radioiodinated meta-iodobenzylguanidine (MIBG) guanethidine analogues such as [^{131}I]MIBG and [^{123}I]MIBG, which are specifically concentrated in the sympathomedullary system. [^{131}I]MIBG scintigraphy localizes pheochromocytoma as focal increased adrenal uptake with 86% sensitivity and 99% specificity. [^{123}I]MIGB has higher sensitivity for pheochromocytoma with 100% sensitivity and 85% specificity. Masses of <1.5 to 2 cm. in diameter and tumors with extensive necrosis and/or hemorrhage may be undetected. Iodocholesterol-labeled analogues may be particularly useful in patients who have extraadrenal pheochromocytomas. Positron emission tomography tracers are currently being evaluated but not yet widely used.

F. Vascular studies such as angiography of the adrenal glands have been supplanted by noninvasive imaging techniques. Venous sampling may be rarely useful to localize the site of hormonal secretion.

G. Fine-needle aspiration biopsy of adrenal masses should be reserved for cases that require tissue confirmation of suspected metastases (sensitivity 80% to 100%).

III. Incidentally discovered adrenal mass

An adrenal mass noted on CT is considered an "incidentaloma" when there is no history or physical finding suggesting an adrenal functional disorder or mass. Such adrenal masses are noted in approximately 1% to 5% of all abdominal CT studies in adults. Among cancer patients, three-fourths of incidentalomas represent metastases, whereas in noncancer patients, more than two-thirds are benign lesions. The approach to adrenal incidentalomas is focused on distinguishing benign and nonhypersecreting from malignant or hormone-secreting adrenal masses that require further therapy (Fig. 23.2). A large number of these are benign cortical adenomas (about 50%), adrenal cysts/pseudocysts (15%), and nodular hyperplasia (12%). Approximately 5% are pheochromocytomas that require surgical removal (Table 23.3). Among patients with no endocrine complaints, clinically inapparent adrenal masses are most often nonfunctioning tumors (approximately 70%). About 10% of patients with incidentaloma have subclinical hypercortisolism.

A. Associated syndromes. Multiple endocrine neoplasia type 1 (MEN-1) is an autosomal dominant familial cancer syndrome characterized by tumors of the parathyroid, endocrine pancreas, and anterior pituitary gland. Incidentally detected lesions of the adrenal cortex, for example, adenoma, carcinoma, or nodular bilateral hyperplasia, have been reported in 30% to 40% of MEN-1 cases. Multiple endocrine neoplasia type 2 consists of medullary thyroid carcinoma, parathyroid hyperplasia, and pheochromocytomas. Pheochromocytoma has also been associated with von Hippel–Lindau disease.

B. Hormonal evaluation. For almost all patients, an overnight (1-mg) dexamethasone suppression test and determination of fractionated urinary and/or plasma metanephrines should

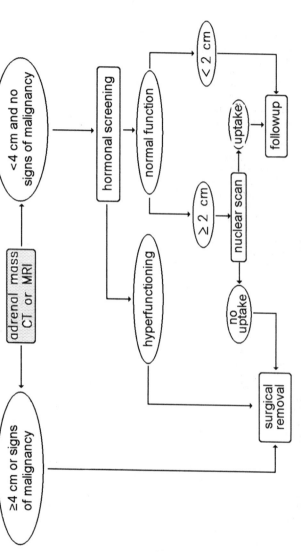

Fig. 23.2.   Algorithm for evaluating an adrenal incidentaloma.

Table 23.3.   Relative frequency of adrenal "incidentalomas"

Cortical adenoma	50%
Cyst/pseudocyst	15%
Nodular hyperplasia	12%
Myelolipoma	10%
Metastases	10%
Pheochromocytoma	5%
Adrenal carcinoma	2%

be performed to rule out hypercortisolism and functioning
pheochromocytoma. Patients with imaging characteristics indicating a myelolipoma or an adrenal cyst may not need hormone
evaluation. In patients with hypertension, serum potassium and
a plasma aldosterone concentration/plasma renin activity ratio
should be performed to rule out primary aldosteronism.

C. Follow-up is carried out to detect interval changes in mass
size or the development of hormone overproduction. Although
the vast majority of adrenal lesions remain stable, from 5% to
25% may enlarge during follow-up. Hormone overproduction
(usually hypercortisolism) may develop in up to 20% of patients
during follow-up but is unlikely in a patient with a lesion <3 cm.
The onset of catecholamine overproduction or hyperaldosteronism during long-term follow-up is very rare. A reasonable protocol is to obtain a repeat CT scan at 6 to 12 months after the
incidentaloma is first detected. Repeat hormone evaluation at
1 year should consist of an overnight 1-mg dexamethasone suppression test and urine catecholamines/metabolites. If there is
no change on follow-up, there are no data to support continued
radiologic evaluation. If some increase in size is detected, either
intervention or further follow-up is indicated. Whether further
hormone monitoring is indicated in stable patients is unclear at
present.

IV. Specific benign lesions

A. Adrenal adenoma, the most common benign adrenal
mass, is found in 2% to 10% of all autopsies. Many are hormonally active, resulting in primary hyperaldosteronism (Conn's
syndrome) or hypercortisolism (Cushing's syndrome).

1. Diagnosis. Size is an important determinant in distinguishing adenoma from carcinoma. The vast majority of
adrenal adenomas are <6 cm in diameter, although rarely
they can be up to 10 cm in diameter. In contrast, >90% of
adrenal carcinomas are >6 cm in diameter. Since MRI may
underestimate size, lesions **>5 cm** should be explored. Histologically, there are two types of adrenal adenomas: those that
contain a high percentage of intracytoplasmic lipid (70%) and
those that do not (30%). Thus, the presence of intracytoplasmic lipid is fairly specific for adrenal cortical adenomas and
can be used to distinguish the lesion from others such as
metastasis, hemorrhage, and other primary adrenal neoplasms. Clear cell carcinoma of the kidney also contains an
abundance of intracytoplasmic lipid and can confuse the
issue when these metastasize to the adrenal gland.

2.   Conn's syndrome, clinically characterized by hypertension and hypokalemia, is due to hypersecretion of aldosterone. Adrenal adenomas causing hypersecretion of aldosterone (aldosteronomas) may be single, multiple, or bilateral. The increased aldosterone production causes sodium retention, potassium loss, extracellular volume expansion, and suppression of plasma renin activity. Most of the symptoms of Conn's syndrome are caused by hypokalemia (muscle weakness, polydipsia, polyuria). Hyperaldosteronism is found in 50% of hypertensive patients with significant hypokalemia. In 80% of patients with Conn's syndrome, a unilateral adrenal adenoma is found that is amenable to adrenalectomy. Although primary aldosteronism accounts for <2% of all cases of hypertension, the disease is important because these hypertensive patients are amenable to surgical cure.

3.   Cushing's syndrome is due to endogenous overproduction of cortisol. Pituitary causes of Cushing's disease are five times more common than adrenal causes. Both pituitary and adrenal causes are far more likely to occur in women than in men. Adrenal adenomas typically secrete only mildly excessive amounts of glucocorticoids. If there is evidence of virilization or mineralocorticoid excess, adrenal carcinoma should be suspected. The most common manifestations of Cushing's syndrome are obesity, hypertension, muscle weakness, emotional lability, and glucose intolerance.

4.   Treatment. All hormonally active adrenal adenomas should be removed surgically. Nonfunctioning adenomas, especially those measuring <3 cm in diameter, may be followed by serial CT at 3, 6, and 18 months. Additionally, biopsy specimens can be taken from adenomas 3 to 6 cm in size by CT or ultrasound. If any increase in size is noted on follow-up, repeat biochemical assessment and adrenalectomy are indicated. Either open or laparoscopic adrenalectomy is an acceptable procedure for the resection of an adrenal adenoma. The laparoscopic approach, when performed by surgeons experienced in the technique, may have advantages such as decreased postoperative pain, reduced ileus, decreased length of hospital stay, and the potential for earlier return to work.

B.   Adrenal cysts are often unilateral and more frequent in females. The most common cause (45%) is an endothelial cyst composed of dilated lymph channels. Calcification may be found in up to 15% of these cysts and does not imply malignancy. The fluid in these cysts may be clear or milky. Hemorrhage into a cyst is easily identified by MRI. **Pseudocysts,** which represent about 40% of adrenal cysts, are probably a result of adrenal hemorrhage into normal adrenal or an adrenal tumor. CT is characterized by a smooth, round, low-density mass, usually with thin walls. MRI appearance may range from that of a simple cyst to a more complex picture consistent with soft tissue, septation, and hemorrhage. Complicated cysts may require aspiration or surgical resection to exclude malignancy.

C.   Myelolipomas are benign neoplasms of the adrenal cortex composed of mature adipose cells and hemopoietic tissue in varying proportions. Most are hormonally inactive. In most cases, the fatty component is virtually diagnostic on CT imaging. On MRI, the fatty component appears hyperintense on T1-weighted and intermediate in signal on T2-weighted images. Since the risk of hemorrhage and malignancy is low, asymptomatic adrenal myelolipomas can be treated conservatively.

D.   Adrenal hemorrhage may be spontaneous, traumatic, or related to anticoagulation. CT findings may indicate a unilateral or bilateral mass, initially hyperdense, which shows gradual resorption during follow-up. MRI of adrenal hemorrhage also reflects evolution from acute to chronic stages as the hemoglobin in the lesion breaks down. On ultrasound, adrenal hemorrhage appears as an anechoic mass that may displace or compress the upper pole of the kidney.

E.   Hamartomas include multiple mixed connective tissue tumors such as myelolipomas, adenolipomas, and lipomas. These benign, nonfunctioning tumors account for <5% of all adrenal masses. Often, they can be diagnosed on the basis of a high fat content on CT or MRI.

F.   Ganglioneuromas are derived from medullary neural crest cells. They are extremely rare nonfunctioning tumors that represent the mature form of neuroblastoma. Ganglioneuromas are diagnosed in the same manner as any adrenal mass. Surgical adrenalectomy is the preferred treatment because the diagnosis cannot be made preoperatively with certainty and because rare instances of degeneration into neuroblastoma have been reported.

V.   Primary malignant lesions

A.   Adrenal carcinoma is a highly malignant tumor, fortunately quite rare (1 case per 1.7 million), accounting for only 0.2% of all cancer deaths. Five-year survival rates of approximately 35% are expected. Adrenal carcinoma metastasizes most commonly to the lung, liver, and regional lymph nodes. Staging of adrenal carcinoma is given in Table 23.4.

Adrenal cancer occurs at all ages from early infancy to the eighth decade of life. A bimodal age distribution has been reported, with the first peak occurring before the age of 5 years and the second in the fourth to fifth decade. The sexual incidence of nonfunctioning adrenal carcinoma is approximately equal, but female patients are far more likely to have a func-

Table 23.4.   Staging of adrenal carcinoma

T1	Tumor ≤5 cm without local invasion
T2	Tumor >5 cm without local invasion
T3	Tumor any size with local extension but no invasion
T4	Tumor any size with invasion of adjacent organs
N0	No lymph node involvement
N1	Lymph node involvement
M0	No distant metastases
M1	Distant metastases present

Stage I: T1, N0, M0
Stage II: T2, N0, M0
Stage III: T1 or T2, N1, M0
Stage IV: Any T, any N, M1 or T3, N1 or T4

Table 23.5.   Endocrine manifestations of adrenal carcinoma

Cushing syndrome (30%)
Virilization and precocious puberty (22%)
Feminization (10%)
Primary hyperaldosteronism (2.5%)
Combined hormone excess (35%)
Polycythemia (<1%)
Hypercalcemia (<1%)
Hypoglycemia (<1%)
Adrenal insufficiency

tional carcinoma. Thus, females tend to be diagnosed somewhat earlier because of virilization, whereas males are older and have a somewhat worse prognosis. There is no predilection for one side of the body over the other. About 70% of adrenal carcinomas are hormonally active by clinical evidence, and patients tend to present most commonly with a combination of virilization and Cushing's syndrome (Table 23.5). Nonfunctioning adrenal carcinoma typically presents with fever, weight loss, abdominal pain, back pain, abdominal fullness, or symptoms related to metastases. In children, adrenal carcinoma is the most common cause of Cushing's syndrome, whereas in adults, adrenal hyperplasia is much more common. However, hormonally active adrenal carcinoma still accounts for 30% of instances of Cushing's syndrome in adults. More than 90% of tumors are >6 cm in size when first discovered.

   1. **Biochemical studies** are important in the initial diagnosis and in providing postoperative tumor markers (Table 23.6). It is important to remember that even in patients without clinical endocrinopathy, elevated levels of steroids such as pregnenolone may be demonstrated in many cases of adrenal carcinoma. The hallmark of this tumor is markedly elevated levels of urinary 17-ketosteroids. Plasma cortisol and urinary free cortisol may also be elevated, whereas plasma levels of adrenocorticotropin are depressed. Even high doses of dexamethasone do not suppress the urinary steroid levels. It is

Table 23.6.   Adrenal cortex: normal biochemical values

Test	Male Patients	Female Patients
Urine (24 h)		
17-Hydroxysteroid	3–15 mg	2–12 mg
17-Ketosteroid	0.9–6.1 mg	0–3.1 mg
Free cortisol	10–50 µg	10–50 µg
Plasma		
Cortisol 8 A.M.	4–22 µg/dL	4–22 µg/dL
Cortisol 5 P.M.	3–17 µg/dL	3–17 µg/dL

Values may vary according to method and laboratory.

advisable to rule out pheochromocytoma in all patients with adrenal mass to avoid a hypertensive crisis on induction of anesthesia.

2.   Radiologic diagnosis is based primarily on CT and MRI with T2-weighted images. Cross-sectional imaging may show downward displacement and axis change in the ipsilateral kidney, but demonstration of this finding usually requires a mass larger than 2 to 3 cm in diameter.

3.   Radionuclide studies based on radiocholesterol labeled with ^{131}I have been used to diagnose adrenal masses. In general, the degree of uptake correlates with the secretory activity of the gland. Radiocholesterol scanning cannot reliably differentiate carcinoma from adenoma, however, because either may have increased uptake or low uptake.

4.   Fine-needle aspiration is most useful in the evaluation of cystic masses, but even in this case, it is of questionable value. A clear aspirate may be indicative of a benign cyst, whereas bloody fluid may indicate either a benign or a malignant lesion. Even when the aspirate is bloody, however, the lesion is much more likely to be benign than malignant. Unless there is evidence of biochemical abnormality, a small adrenal cyst can be followed in the same manner as small adrenal adenomas. Cytologic examination of adrenal cyst fluid is difficult because there is little published experience.

5.   Percutaneous biopsy guided by CT or ultrasound has been reported to be useful in the differential diagnosis of solid adrenal masses. Tissue can be obtained in >95% of biopsies, and it is possible to differentiate between benign and malignant disease in >85% of these samples. The technique is useful and may obviate the need for surgery. Rare complications include pancreatitis.

6.   Treatment of all primary adrenal carcinomas is surgical. Currently, laparoscopic surgery is not recommended for known adrenal carcinoma or large adrenal masses. This is because adrenocortical carcinoma may require radical en bloc resection with or without local lymphadenectomy in close proximity to the great vessels. If complete resection of an adrenocortical carcinoma cannot be achieved, as much as possible of the tumor should be removed. Solitary recurrences or metastases should also be removed surgically, if possible. Long-term disease-free status has been produced by complete resection of adrenocortical carcinoma, whereas long-term remissions have followed surgical resection of hepatic, pulmonary, or cerebral metastases. If the carcinoma is functioning, perioperative administration of glucocorticoids is essential because the contralateral adrenal is likely to be suppressed (Table 23.7). Complete recovery of contralateral adrenal function generally requires many months, during which time steroid support must be continued. Steroid replacement is not necessary in cases of nonfunctioning adrenal carcinomas. Chemotherapy with the steroid synthesis-blocking agent mitotane (ortho-para-DDD [dichlorodiphenyl dichloroethane]) in doses of 2 to 6 g daily is available in patients with metastatic disease, but the response rate is poor. Cisplatin, etoposide, and ketoconazole have been found to induce regression in some patients. Transarterial em-

**Table 23.7.   Perioperative steroid
replacement for adrenalectomy**

Cortisone acetate 100 mg IM
  1. Evening before surgery
  2. Morning of surgery
  3. In recovery room

Cortisone acetate 75 mg IM q8h
  1. First postoperative day
  2. Second postoperative day

Cortisone acetate 75 mg IM q12h
  1. Third postoperative day
  2. Fourth postoperative day

Cortisone acetate 25 mg PO bid with fludrocortisone 0.1 mg PO

Continue for at least 1 mo postoperatively

bolization may also help induce partial remission. Radiotherapy is of little use except for palliation of bony metastases.

7.   Prognosis of adrenal carcinoma is generally poor, with a mean survival of approximately 18 months. Generally, children with adrenocortical carcinoma have a better prognosis than adults. Highly aggressive tumors can progress rapidly within a few months. With aggressive surgical therapy, the mean survival increases to 48 months, and survival as long as 10 years has been described for some patients undergoing vigilant monitoring and aggressive surgery for local recurrences or distant metastases. Cures have been achieved for patients operated on at the early stages of adrenal cancer while the tumor was still encapsulated.

B.   Pheochromocytoma is a rare tumor derived from neural crest tissue. There are approximately 400 new instances yearly in the United States. Pheochromocytoma is found in 0.1% to 0.4% of hypertensive patients. Although approximately 90% are adrenal in origin, the tumors can arise wherever chromaffin cells are located, such as the paraaortic sympathetic ganglia and the organs of Zuckerkandl at the aortic bifurcation. Pheochromocytoma is often loosely described as following the **"rule of 10s,"** which states that 10% are malignant (and metastasize), 10% are multiple, 10% are bilateral, and 10% are extraadrenal; of the ectopic pheochromocytomas, 10% are above the diaphragm. Many cases of bilateral pheochromocytoma are part of MEN-2 (Sipple's syndrome), which includes medullary carcinoma of the thyroid and parathyroid hyperplasia. Pheochromocytoma is found in 50% of patients with Sipple's syndrome. An increased incidence of pheochromocytoma is also associated with neurofibromatosis and von Hippel–Lindau disease. Malignant tumors tend to be large and metastasize to bones, lung, liver, and spleen.

1.   Diagnosis is based on the clinical picture of hypertension (episodic or sustained), severe headaches, palpitations, and sweating found in >90% of cases. Paradoxically, orthostatic hypotension is frequently found as a result of diminished plasma volume. An acute hypertensive crisis may be precipi-

Table 23.8.   Adrenal medulla: normal biochemical values

Test	Normal Range
Urine (24 h)	
Vanillylmandelic acid	2–10 mg
Epinephrine	0–15 µg
Norepinephrine	11–86 µg
Metanephrine	<1.3 mg
Plasma (30 min supine)	
Epinephrine	>50 pg/mL
Norepinephrine	40–410 pg/mL

Values may vary according to method and laboratory.

tated by almost any stimulus to the sympathetic nervous system, especially induction of anesthesia or administration of contrast medium or monoamine oxidase inhibitors, which block the metabolism of catecholamines. A rare phenomenon is "micturition syncope," which is precipitated by voiding in a patient with pheochromocytoma of the bladder wall.

2.   Biochemical abnormalities include elevated levels of catecholamines and their metabolites in the plasma and urine (Table 23.8). Because >50% of secreted catecholamines appear in the urine as metanephrine, normetanephrine, or vanillylmandelic acid (VMA), these substances may be measured to estimate catecholamine production.

a.   Measurement of urine and plasma catecholamines is carried out by specific methods such as chromatography or radioimmunoassay. Before collecting urine, obtain specific instructions on diet and drug restrictions from your laboratory.

b.   Although provocative tests are rarely used, the **glucagon test** may be helpful in those patients whose hypertension is paroxysmal. After administration of 1 mg of glucagon SC, both blood pressure and catecholamine levels will rise markedly within 2 minutes.

c.   The **clonidine test** involves administration of 0.3 mg of clonidine; this will produce a drop in norepinephrine and epinephrine levels below 500 pg/mL in patients with neurogenic hypertension but not in those with pheochromocytoma.

d.   In general, a high ratio of VMA to catecholamines in the urine indicates a large tumor, whereas a low ratio indicates a small tumor.

e.   Elevation of only epinephrine—not norepinephrine—in the serum indicates a tumor arising in the adrenal medulla. This is because only medullary tissue can methylate norepinephrine into epinephrine.

3.   Radiologic diagnosis plays an important role in localizing these tumors. MRI is very useful in identifying pheochromocytomas, as they appear like a "bright light" on T2 images. MRI is especially useful in identifying extraadrenal tumors. Coronal and sagittal views can be reconstructed to give excellent detail of the surrounding structures and vascular involvement.

4.   Radionuclide studies include the scanning agent MIBG, which is concentrated in storage granules of adrenergic cells. It may be used to detect pheochromocytoma in the adrenal as well as in extraadrenal sites.

5.   Treatment of pheochromocytoma is surgical excision; the operative approach depends on the location and number of tumors.

  a.   Perioperative management is extremely important in preventing intraoperative malignant hypertension or postoperative hypotension. Preoperative oral **phenoxybenzamine** is titrated (initial dose of 20 to 40 mg/day increased by 10 mg daily) until blood pressure is nearly normalized. As opposed to prazosin, phenoxybenzamine binds irreversibly to α-adrenergic receptors and thus provides stable blood pressure control even in the face of a severe catecholamine surge. In addition, all patients should be well hydrated preoperatively. If tachycardia or arrhythmias are present preoperatively, a β-adrenergic blocking agent such as propranolol may be given orally. If hypertension is a problem intraoperatively despite α-adrenergic blockade, it may be controlled rapidly with sodium nitroprusside. Hypotension is a feared complication in the immediate postoperative period; however, it should not be a problem in patients well prepared and maintained with intravenous fluids. Finally, blood sugar should be monitored; with removal of the catecholamine stimulus to gluconeogenesis, fatal hypoglycemia may occur.

  b.   The surgical approach is dictated by the known or suspected location of the tumors. If a tumor has been localized to the adrenal, a thoracoabdominal incision permits exposure of the adrenal and systematic exploration of the abdominal cavity. If an ectopic tumor or bilateral tumors are suspected, a transverse epigastric "chevron" incision is recommended. With either incision, palpation of the obvious tumor mass is kept to a minimum, but careful palpation for other tumors is mandatory. The operative mortality for intraabdominal pheochromocytoma is 1% to 4%. If pheochromocytoma of the bladder wall is present, segmental resection with pelvic lymph node sampling is usually sufficient therapy. Recently, laparoscopic adrenalectomy has been performed to remove incidentally found adenomas and small, single pheochromocytomas. This procedure can be carried out in either transperitoneal or retroperitoneal fashion. Laparoscopic adrenal surgery for pheochromocytoma is a difficult and demanding task that must be performed by an experienced surgeon.

  c.   Prognosis in benign pheochromocytoma is very favorable, although local recurrence is possible. Thus, urinary VMA and metanephrine should be measured every 6 months for 3 to 5 years postoperatively. Malignant pheochromocytoma has a 5-year survival of 33% to 44%. Survival after demonstration of metastases is <3 years in the vast majority of patients. Prognosis appears worse with

extraadrenal than with adrenal tumors. There is no effective chemotherapy, and radiation therapy is only palliative.
C.   Neuroblastoma is a highly malignant tumor of childhood derived from neural crest cells. Approximately 75% are found in the abdominal cavity, most commonly (50%) in the adrenal gland. The remainder may occur in ectopic locations: the cervical sympathetic chain (4%), thorax (15%), or pelvis (4%). Neuroblastoma accounts for 6% to 8% of all childhood malignancies. Approximately 50% of neuroblastomas are found in children younger than 2 years. Seventy percent of patients have metastatic disease at the time of presentation.

    1.   Diagnosis. There are no specific symptoms in neuroblastoma. Approximately 70% of patients present with an abdominal mass, 50% have abdominal or bone pain, 28% have weight loss or failure to thrive, and malaise or weakness is present in 18%. Physical findings may include hepatomegaly or a fixed abdominal mass that often extends across the midline.

        a.   Biochemical and laboratory studies. Although hypertension is rare, neuroblastoma often produces excess amounts of catecholamines. In >80% of patients, the level of VMA or homovanillic acid in the urine is elevated and may be used as a tumor marker. Anemia is very common in disseminated disease. Bone marrow aspirate will reveal tumor cells in up to 70% of cases.

        b.   Radiologic studies. In up to 50% of patients with intraabdominal tumor, neuroblastoma is characteristically calcified in a central, finely stippled pattern. Calcification in neuroblastoma is five times as common as in Wilms' tumor and may be used to differentiate between the two tumors. Typically, neuroblastoma causes a downward and outward displacement of the kidney on intravenous urography. CT is helpful in delineating the mass and documenting extension, especially involvement of the vena cava. Chest roentgenography, skeletal films, and bone scan should be performed to complete the metastatic survey. MIBG has been used to identify primary and metastatic lesions. Staging is as follows (Evans):

Stage I: Tumor is organ-confined
Stage II: Regional spread but not across midline
Stage III: Tumor extending across midline
Stage IV: Distant metastases
Stage IV-S: Small primary and distant metastases to liver, skin, or bone marrow but negative findings on bone films

    2.   Treatment involves a combination of surgical removal, radiation therapy, and chemotherapy. In stage I, stage II, and some stage III tumors, complete surgical removal is usually possible. The abdominal tumor is explored through a transverse incision. Tumor that cannot be removed totally should be treated by subtotal resection and clipping of the margins for postoperative radiotherapy. Although neuroblastoma is radiosensitive, radiation therapy is mainly a palliative maneuver. In instances of very large tumors thought to be unresectable, preoperative radiation should be given to reduce tumor size and permit a "second-look" operation. In unresectable stage III tumors, radiation in doses of 2,500 to 3,000 rads is commonly given. Radiation is also given to palliate painful bone metastases. With residual (stage III) or disseminated disease (except stage IV-S), chemotherapy is indicated with cyclophosphamide, vincristine, and dacarbazine. Infants with stage IV-S disease generally have an excellent prognosis following surgical removal of the primary tumor only. Bone marrow transplantation is still being tested as a part of various chemotherapeutic protocols. Labeled MIBG may also prove helpful with targeted radiation therapy.

3. Prognosis. Patients who present at 1 year of age or younger have a much better prognosis (80% cure rate) than do older children (20% cure rate). In addition, one-third of infants present with metastatic disease compared with two-thirds of older children. The tumor metastasizes to liver most commonly in infants and to bone most commonly in older children. Maturation of neuroblastoma to a more benign tumor (ganglioneuroma) may occur spontaneously in 5% to 10% of patients and implies an excellent prognosis.

VI. Metastatic lesions

Metastases to the adrenal gland from distant sites are found in approximately 12% to 25% of autopsies. As expected, these metastases are more often bilateral and multiple than localized. Common sites of origin are listed in Table 23.2. The adrenals may be involved in systemic diseases such as Hodgkin's disease, lymphosarcoma, and leukemia.

SUGGESTED READING

Alexander F. Neuroblastoma. *Urol Clin North Am* 2000;27:383–392.

Avisse C. Surgical anatomy and embryology of the adrenal glands. *Surg Clin North Am* 2000;80:403–415.

Barzon L. Adrenocortical carcinoma: experience in 45 patients. *Oncology* 1997;54:490–496.

Barzon L, Boscaro M. Diagnosis and management of adrenal incidentalomas. *J Urol* 2000;163:398–407.

Barzon L, Pasquali C, Grigoletto C, et al. Multiple endocrine neoplasia type 1 and adrenal lesions. *J Urol* 2001;166:24–27.

Berruti A. Mitotane associated with etoposide, doxorubicin, and cisplatin in the treatment of advanced adrenocortical carcinoma. Italian Group for the Study of Adrenal Cancer. *Cancer* 1998;83:2194–2200.

Boscaro M, Barzon L, Fallo F, et al. Cushing's syndrome. *Lancet* 2001;357:783–791.

Brandi ML. Guidelines for diagnosis and therapy of MEN type 1 and type 2. *J Clin Endocrinol Metab* 2001;86:5658–5671.

Grumbach MM, Biller BM, Braunstein GD, et al. Management of the clinically inapparent adrenal mass ("incidentaloma"). *Ann Intern Med* 2003;138:424–429.

Janetschek G. Laparoscopic surgery for pheochromocytoma. *Urol Clin North Am* 2001;28:97–105.

Stratakis CA. Adrenal cancer. *Endocrinol Metab Clin North Am* 2000;29:15–25.

Udelsman R. Radiology of the adrenal. *Endocrinol Metab Clin North Am* 2000;29:27–42.

Young WF Jr. Management approaches to adrenal incidentalomas: a view from Rochester, Minnesota. *Endocrinol Metab Clin North Am* 2000;29:159–185.

Fluid and Electrolyte Disorders

Peter A. Zeman and Mike B. Siroky

I. Physiology

A. Total body water constitutes about 50% of body weight in adult women and 60% in adult men. The total body water is divided into **extracellular fluid** (ECF) (about one-third) and **intracellular fluid** (ICF) (about two-thirds).

B. ECF comprises interstitial fluid (about three-fourths) and plasma (about one-fourth). The major cation in the ECF is sodium; the major anions are chloride, bicarbonate, and plasma proteins.

C. ICF constitutes most of the body water. The major cations are potassium and magnesium; the major anions are phosphates and proteins.

D. Physiologic mechanisms maintain proper plasma osmolality and serum sodium concentration by regulating body water. These mechanisms may be divided into extrarenal and intrarenal types. Extrarenal mechanisms are thirst, pituitary secretion of antidiuretic hormone (ADH), and adrenal secretion of mineralocorticoids. Intrarenal mechanisms are the water permeability of the collecting duct (affected by ADH), sodium and chloride resorption in the distal tubule (affected by mineralocorticoids), and the volume delivered to the distal tubule.

E. Volume depletion or **hypovolemia** is caused by loss of sodium and water in varying proportions (Table 24.1). Such volume contraction may be accompanied by normal serum sodium levels, hyponatremia (serum sodium <135 mEq/L), or hypernatremia (serum sodium >150 mEq/L) (Table 24.2). If sodium and water are lost in approximately isotonic proportions (e.g., ileostomy), the serum sodium concentration remains normal and the ICF volume is little affected. If the loss is hypotonic (e.g., nasogastric suction, diarrhea, severe glycosuria), hypernatremia will result. However, the clinical signs of hypovolemia will be attenuated by movement of water from the intracellular space to the ECF. Hypertonic loss does not occur naturally. However, if naturally occurring isotonic or hypotonic losses are replaced with water only, the effects of hypertonic loss are reproduced (i.e., hyponatremia with hypovolemia).

F. Volume excess refers to expansion of the ECF from retention of varying proportions of sodium and water (Table 24.3). If this expansion of ECF is clinically evident, edema or ascites may be noted. The cause may be renal failure, cardiac failure, or liver disease.

II. Sodium and volume disorders

A. Volume depletion is most commonly caused by gastrointestinal losses, administration of diuretics, primary and secondary renal disease, adrenal disease, and sequestration of fluids—"third-space loss." Depending on the severity of the volume depletion, the manifestations include poor skin turgor,

Table 24.1.   Causes of volume depletion

I. Gastrointestinal
  A. Emesis or nasogastric drainage
  B. Diarrhea
  C. Bowel fistulas
     1. Ileostomy
     2. Colostomy
II. Renal
  A. Salt-wasting nephropathy
     1. Medullary cystic disease
     2. Polycystic disease
     3. Interstitial nephritis
     4. Analgesic nephropathy
     5. Partial urinary obstruction
  B. Renal tubular acidosis, proximal type
  C. Osmotic diuresis
     1. Glucose (diabetes mellitus)
     2. Loop diuretics
     3. Osmotic diuretics (urea, mannitol)
     4. Radiographic contrast media
  D. Water diuresis
     1. Central diabetes insipidus
     2. Nephrogenic diabetes insipidus
  E. Postobstructive diuresis
III. Adrenal insufficiency
IV. Sequestration
  A. Large surgical wound
  B. Ileus
  C. Burns
  D. Peritonitis

Table 24.2.   Causes of hypovolemic states classified by serum sodium levels

Hyponatremia	Normal Serum Sodium	Hypernatremia
Nasogastric suction	Ileostomy	Nasogastric suction
Diarrhea	Biliary fistula	Sweating
Renal disease	Pancreatic fistula	Diarrhea

Table 24.3.   Causes of volume excess

  I. Acute and chronic renal failure
 II. Congestive heart failure
III. Liver cirrhosis
 IV. Water intoxication
     A. Psychogenic polydipsia
     B. Transurethral resection syndrome
  V. Inappropriate secretion of ADH (Schwartz–Bartter syndrome)
     A. Carcinoma of lung, duodenum, pancreas
     B. Pulmonary disease
        1. Viral or bacterial pneumonia
        2. Tuberculosis
        3. Aspergillosis
     C. CNS disorders
        1. Encephalitis and meningitis
        2. Stroke
        3. Brain tumors
        4. Brain abscess
        5. Subdural hematoma
        6. Guillain–Barré syndrome
        7. Head trauma
     D. Anesthesia
     E. Generalized trauma

ADH, antidiuretic hormone.

postural hypotension, and dry mucous membranes (5% depletion); weakness, apathy, sunken eyes, and hypotension (10%
depletion); or shock and coma (15% depletion). The serum
sodium is often normal, but the blood urea nitrogen is elevated
out of proportion to the creatinine. The hematocrit and serum
albumin concentration are also elevated. If renal and adrenal
functions are normal, the urinary sodium concentration is very
low (serum sodium <15 mEq/L), the urine is highly concentrated (osmolality >600 mOsm/L and specific gravity >1.020),
and its volume is decreased. Under these circumstances, the
cause is most likely gastrointestinal—vomiting or diarrhea.
Substantial ECF volume may be sequestered in the peritoneal
cavity with peritonitis or pancreatitis and in the bowel lumen
with ileus. If the urinary sodium is >20 mEq/L, one should suspect underlying salt-wasting renal disease, Addison's disease,
diabetes insipidus, or previous administration of diuretics.
Administration of diuretics is the most common cause and is
accompanied by hypokalemia in most instances. Salt-wasting
renal disease is usually accompanied by a serum creatinine
level in excess of 3 mg/dL. Addison's disease is characterized by
hyperkalemia.
   1. Postobstructive diuresis refers to excessive and prolonged polyuria following relief of urinary obstruction. The
phenomenon is caused by a combination of physiologic diuresis (urea osmotic diuresis), pathologic diuresis (impairment of
renal salt and water reabsorption), and iatrogenic diuresis

(glucose osmotic diuresis and water diuresis resulting from intravenous therapy). The impairment of renal salt and water reabsorption is caused by short-term unresponsiveness to ADH and mineralocorticoid. Another factor may be elevated levels of atrial natriuretic peptide, which produces natriuresis and diuresis.

a. Diagnosis. True postobstructive diuresis is rare and occurs only following relief of bilateral urinary obstruction or relief of obstruction of a solitary kidney. The typical patient at risk is one with moderate to severe azotemia caused by chronic outflow obstruction. In addition to azotemia, laboratory values may indicate hyperkalemia and metabolic acidosis. Urinalysis will reveal low specific gravity (1.002 to 1.10), low osmolality (<400 mOsm/L), and low urine sodium (<40 mmol/L). The mean duration of diuresis is 2.2 days, but in 72% of instances, the duration is ≤2 days. The median urine volume excreted is approximately 8 L.

b. Management is facilitated by identifying as early as possible patients who are at greatest risk for development of a high-volume prolonged diuresis leading to sodium, potassium, and volume depletion. It is useful to follow therapy by daily determination of supine and upright blood pressure, body weight, and serum and urine electrolyte levels.

(1) Low-risk patients have no peripheral edema, congestive heart failure, or mental confusion. Azotemia is mild (serum creatinine <2.0 mg/dL). They can be allowed free oral intake of fluids. Intravenous fluid replacement is necessary only if one or more of the following are present: orthostatic hypotension, tachycardia, mental confusion, hyponatremia, or urine output >200 mL/h. Intravenous fluids consist of 50% normal saline solution or 5% dextrose in 50% normal saline solution plus 20 mEq of potassium chloride. The hourly rate should be half the amount of the previous hourly urine output.

(2) Moderate-risk patients are characterized by the presence of one or more of the following: mild peripheral edema, congestive heart failure, and azotemia (serum creatinine <4.0 mg/dL). Therapy is essentially the same as for low-risk patients except that intravenous fluid replacement should be started early in treatment.

(3) High-risk patients have one or more of the following: a serum creatinine level above 4.0 mg/dL, mental obtundation, congestive heart failure, and noticeable peripheral edema. Intravenous fluid therapy as mentioned above should be instituted after obstruction is relieved. If the patient is hyponatremic, urine output is replaced milliliter for milliliter with normal saline solution. Appropriate amounts of potassium, calcium, and bicarbonate may be added. As the serum creatinine falls below 4.0 mg/dL and as the body weight falls, the rate of diuresis should fall as well.

B. Volume excess in urologic patients is caused most commonly by concomitant medical disorders such as congestive heart failure, acute and chronic renal failure, and liver cirrhosis. A syndrome of inappropriate ADH secretion has been de-

Table 24.4. Symptoms and signs of post-TURP syndrome

Cardiovascular	Neurologic
Early	
Bradycardia	Restlessness
Hypertension	Confusion
Dyspnea	Visual disturbances
Cyanosis	Twitching
Angina	Seizures
Late	
Hypotension/shock	Obtundation/coma

TURP, transurethral resection of prostate.

scribed in various conditions. The inappropriate secretion of ADH causes impaired renal excretion of water and mild ECF expansion, usually without edema, leading to a secondary natriuresis from the kidney. The postoperative and posttraumatic patient may have mild increases in ADH secretion. Overzealous fluid therapy in these patients will result in mild fluid overload and hyponatremia.

The **posttransurethral resection syndrome** (Table 24.4), specific to urology patients, occurs in 2% to 10% of patients undergoing transurethral resection of the prostate (TURP) and is characterized by cardiovascular and neurologic manifestations. The incidence depends in a general way on gland size and resection time (Table 24.5). It is caused by absorption of excessive amounts of irrigating fluid from the prostatic fossa during transurethral prostatectomy. The solute in these isotonic irrigating fluids is most commonly sorbitol or glycine. Once these solutes are metabolized, the effect is equivalent to the administration of solute-free water—hence the term "water intoxication." Because the ECF is expanded and hyponatremia results, the neurologic manifestations are attributable to edema of the brain cells; however, some investigators place more emphasis on the role of the hyponatremia itself. In addition, glycine (but

Table 24.5. Variables affecting the incidence of post-TURP syndrome

Variable	Incidence (%)
Gland size	
<45 g	0.8
>45 g	1.5
Resection time	
<90 min	0.7
>90 min	2.0

TURP, transurethral resection of prostate.

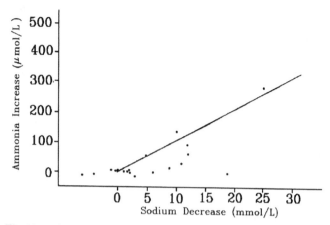

Fig. 24.1.   Correlation between increase in blood ammonia level and decrease in serum sodium observed in patients undergoing transurethral resection of the prostate with 1.5% glycine irrigation. (Adapted from Shepard et al. The role of ammonia toxicity in the post transurethral prostatectomy syndrome. *Br J Urol* 1987;60:349.)

not sorbitol or mannitol) may be metabolized to ammonia, and hyperammonemia has been documented in about one-third of patients receiving glycine irrigation during TURP (Fig. 24.1). Glycine should avoided as an irrigating fluid. The use of high-frequency vaporation electrodes has also been shown to reduce the incidence of transurethral syndrome.

Treatment should be individualized according to the severity and type of symptoms as well as the presence of preexisting medical conditions.

1.   Predominantly neurologic symptoms. In most patients with mild neurologic manifestations and serum sodium concentrations above 110 mEq/L, induction of diuresis with intravenous furosemide (20 to 40 mg) is usually sufficient to correct the imbalance. Furosemide may be ineffective because of low serum sodium levels, and in such cases, 1 to 2 g of mannitol/kg IV may be given. In patients who are comatose or manifest seizures, more rapid correction of the hyponatremia by administration of 3% normal saline solution (1 L/12 h) is indicated, in addition to administration of anticonvulsants and general metabolic support. Administration of hypertonic saline solution is not necessary in patients without severe neurologic manifestations and, in fact, is contraindicated in patients with signs of cardiovascular overload. There is no specific remedy for hyperammonemia caused by glycine metabolism. The patient usually recovers within 12 to 24 hours with general supportive care.

2.   Predominantly cardiovascular symptoms. These patients should be aggressively managed as if they had pulmonary edema. Early monitoring with a Swan–Ganz catheter is recommended. Endotracheal intubation should be considered if the patient becomes severely dyspneic or hypoxemic. If the capillary wedge pressure is elevated, diuretic therapy should be instituted to reduce volume excess. In severe cases, shock may ensue and should be treated with infusion of colloids and adrenergic drugs.

III.   Metabolic acid–base disorders

A.   **Metabolic acidosis** is a systemic disorder resulting from accumulation of fixed acid with decreased plasma bicarbonate concentration. Acid may accumulate because of its ingestion, increased endogenous production, or impaired excretion. Metabolic acidosis is classified according to the presence of either "elevated anion gap" or "normal anion gap." The anion gap is defined as the difference between the serum sodium concentration and the sum of the serum chloride and bicarbonate. The presence of an increased anion gap (>14 mEq/L) implies the addition of acid to the system, such as occurs in renal failure, ketoacidosis, lactic acidosis, and poisoning with salicylates, methanol, or ethylene glycol. A normal anion gap (12 mEq/L) implies the loss of bicarbonate with retention of chloride, which occurs in renal tubular acidosis, urinary diversion, pancreatic fistula, and diarrhea.

1.   **Renal failure** results in metabolic acidosis with increased anion gap. This is because (a) with reduction in glomerular filtration, there is inability to excrete sulfates and phosphates; and (b) with reduced tubular mass, there is inability to form sufficient urinary ammonium and thus excrete acid.

2.   **Renal tubular acidosis** is characterized by a renal tubular defect leading to inability to acidify the urine. This condition results in a hyperchloremic (normal anion gap) acidosis. In contrast to patients with renal failure, patients with renal tubular acidosis have little or no reduction in glomerular filtration. Daily alkali therapy usually corrects the metabolic derangement. Two types of renal tubular acidosis are recognized:

   a.   **Distal (type I, classic)** renal tubular acidosis is characterized by inability of the distal tubule to excrete hydrogen ion. Hypokalemia is a frequently associated finding.

   b.   **Proximal (type II, bicarbonate-wasting)** renal tubular acidosis is characterized by inability of the proximal tubule to absorb adequate amounts of filtered bicarbonate.

3.   **Urinary diversion** is performed to divert urine from the bladder to the skin or to fashion a bladder substitute with various intestinal segments including stomach, jejunum, ileum, transverse colon, and sigmoid colon (Table 24.6). A variety of unique metabolic derangements may be seen in patients who have bowel segments interposed in the urinary tract. Except for stomach (see below), most are associated with various degrees of metabolic acidosis.

   a.   **Jejunum** is characterized by an enormous capacity for allowing solutes and water to move passively across the mucosa. Hypertonic urine in the jejunal lumen leads to loss of sodium, chloride, and water.

   b.   **Ileum** has a much lower absorptive capacity than jejunum, and the absorptive process is much slower. It has been shown that the ileum actively absorbs ammonium

Table 24.6. Electrolyte changes following urinary diversion

Bowel Segment	pH	Na	Cl	K	Incidence (%)	Treatment
Stomach	–	0	–	–	5	H₂-Blocker omeprazole
Jejunum	–	–	–	–	25–40	Saline infusion
Ileum	–	0	–	0;–	75	Alkalinization, chlorpromazine, nicotinic acid
Colon	–	0	–	–	75	Alkalinization, chlorpromazine, nicotinic acid

+, increased; –, decreased; 0, no change.

and chloride from the urine. Potassium and urea are also absorbed passively by the ileum.

    c. Colon has absorptive processes similar to those in the ileum, except that there is less propensity to absorb potassium.

4. **Acid–base disturbances** following urinary diversion vary in character and degree depending on the particular segment of bowel, the contact time between the urine and bowel mucosa, and the presence of impaired renal function.

    a. Jejunal conduit is sometimes performed in patients who require a high urinary diversion and in patients who have received radiation to the ileum. In 25% to 40% of patients with jejunal conduits, a syndrome characterized by nausea, vomiting, anorexia, and muscle weakness develops in the early postoperative period. Laboratory tests reveal a hyponatremic, hypochloremic, hyperkalemic acidosis with azotemia. The pathogenesis involves significant losses of sodium and chloride from the jejunum into the urine in the lumen (Fig. 24.2). The salt loss triggers increased aldosterone production in an attempt to conserve sodium. Aldosterone acts on the distal renal tubule to promote resorption of sodium and hydrogen ions with excretion of potassium. This process, however, results in a concentrated, potassium-rich, sodium-poor urine. On entering the jejunal conduit, the potassium is absorbed and even more sodium is lost. Urea is also absorbed passively from the conduit, which, when combined with the contracted ECF and diminished glomerular filtration rate, results in azotemia. The syndrome is more likely to occur as the length of the jejunal conduit increases. The treatment is oral replacement with sodium chloride tablets as well as correction of acidosis with bicarbonate (300 to 600 mg of sodium bicarbonate PO three times daily). Acutely hypovolemic patients require intravenous therapy with normal saline solution and bicarbonate.

    b. Ileal conduit has a low incidence of clinically significant metabolic complications and is preferred for patients

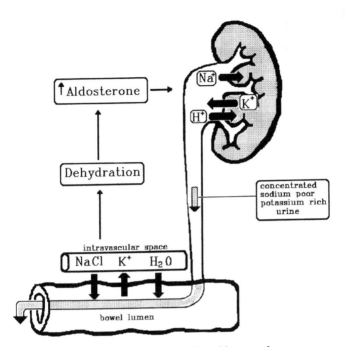

Fig. 24.2. The pathophysiology of the jejunal loop syndrome.

with renal insufficiency. Although mild metabolic acidosis is present in most patients with ileal conduit, clinical symptoms develop in only 5% to 10% of patients. Serum electrolyte determinations reveal increased chloride, decreased bicarbonate, and normal or low potassium levels. Hyperchloremic acidosis in a patient with ileal conduit implies the presence of some degree of intrinsic renal failure, obstruction of the conduit, or excessive conduit length. If there is conduit dysfunction, catheter drainage of the conduit may be sufficient. Most patients with laboratory evidence of acidosis should be treated even if asymptomatic to prevent mobilization of bone calcium. Most patients respond well to oral administration of 15 to 30 mL of potassium and sodium citrate (Polycitra) in water four times daily. Agents specifically meant to block chloride absorption may also be used: 25 to 50 mg of chlorpromazine twice daily or 400 mg of nicotinic acid twice daily.

c. Colon conduits may be constructed from transverse colon or sigmoid colon. In terms of metabolic complications, colon conduits offer no advantages over ileal conduits and are more likely to lead to hypokalemia than ileal segments. Treatment is the same as for ileal segments except that oral potassium supplementation may be required.

d. Ureterosigmoidostomy is a form of continent urinary diversion that was widely used to substitute for the bladder before the advent of the ileal conduit, but it is rarely used today. In this operation, the ureters are anastomosed in a nonrefluxing manner to the sigmoid colon, which acts as a reservoir for both urine and feces. Nearly 80% of patients with ureterosigmoidostomy exhibit some degree of hyperchloremic acidosis. Potassium loss may occur because of chronic diarrhea. Metabolic acidosis is seen most often, in its severest form in patients with some degree of renal insufficiency. Thus, renal insufficiency is a relative contraindication to this form of urinary diversion. Treatment is similar to that described above for ileal conduits, with the aim being to maintain the serum bicarbonate level at nearly normal levels. In acutely ill patients, rectal tube drainage is rapidly effective in restoring acid–base balance; it should be combined with administration of intravenous fluids containing additional potassium (20 to 40 mEq of potassium chloride/L) and bicarbonate (1 to 2 ampules of sodium bicarbonate).

   e.   Continent urinary diversions are increasingly being used as a bladder substitute. Despite the long contact time between urine and bowel mucosa, there has been a rather low reported incidence of hyperchloremic acidosis in these patients. The treatment is the same as for patients with ileal segments described above.

B.   Metabolic alkalosis may occur as a result of several different mechanisms:

   1.   Loss of chloride in excess of sodium accompanied by contraction of ECF occurs because of protracted vomiting, nasogastric suction, and the use of potent diuretics. This contraction alkalosis is the most common cause of metabolic alkalosis. Because the patient is depleted of chloride, the renal tubule increases its absorption of filtered bicarbonate, producing metabolic alkalosis. The urinary chloride concentration is usually very low (<10 mEq/L). Treatment is aimed at correcting the salt and water deficit with intravenous salt solutions and correcting the accompanying hypokalemia.

   2.   Excess renal absorption of bicarbonate without ECF contraction occurs when the renal tubule is stimulated to resorb sodium by aldosterone or cortical mineralocorticoids. Filtered bicarbonate is resorbed with the sodium, and chloride is lost in the urine (urinary chloride >20 mEq/L). This mechanism is seen in hyperaldosteronism, Cushing's syndrome, and Bartter's syndrome. Metabolic alkalosis may also result from ingestion of alkali and severe potassium depletion. The underlying disorder is treated, and potassium deficits are corrected. Spironolactone may block the effects of aldosterone and other mineralocorticoids on the renal tubule.

   3.   Gastrocystoplasty. Stomach actively secretes hydrogen and chloride ions into the lumen, resulting in acidic urine and release of bicarbonate into the bloodstream. This excess bicarbonate is excreted in the urine and partially neutralizes the acid secreted by the stomach segment. The acid secretion is, however, mainly stimulated by gastric distention after ingestion of a meal. Thus, the patient has episodes of metabolic alkalosis. Treatment consists of 300 mg of cimetidine four times daily or 20 mg of omeprazole daily, which is a potent inhibitor of gastric acid secretion.

IV. Potassium

A. Potassium balance is primarily determined by the kidneys, which serve as the major organs of potassium excretion. Total body potassium is partitioned such that 64% is in the ICF and 24% is in the ECF, including plasma; thus, changes in the serum potassium concentration only roughly indicate the status of total body potassium. The serum potassium level may change because of (a) alteration in total body potassium stores or (b) alteration in the transcellular partition of potassium. Total body potassium is decreased with excessive gastrointestinal or renal losses. The kidneys are unable to eliminate potassium completely from the urine even in the face of severe potassium depletion, as they can sodium. The total body potassium is increased with acute renal failure. The transcellular distribution of potassium in the body is affected by the following:

1. Serum pH. In systemic acidosis from any cause, hydrogen ions enter cells in exchange for potassium, causing hyperkalemia. Despite the fact that potassium depletion may exist in a patient with metabolic acidosis, the serum potassium level may be normal or even increased. Systemic alkalosis has the opposite effect.

2. Insulin and glucose cause movement of potassium into cells and may cause hypokalemia.

B. Hypokalemia is defined as a serum potassium level of <3.5 mEq/L and may develop secondarily to inadequate oral intake (rarely), gastrointestinal losses (gastric, intestinal, colonic, or biliary), or urinary losses (renal tubular acidosis, osmotic diuresis, hyperaldosteronism, hyperadrenalism). Patients who undergo ureterosigmoidostomy are prone to the development of hypokalemia in association with the classic hyperchloremic acidosis because of colonic loss of potassium from passive diffusion and chronic diarrhea. Hypokalemia is also a potential problem in patients with postobstructive diuresis.

1. Manifestations may be neuromuscular (weakness, paresthesias, depression of deep tendon reflexes, paralysis), cardiac [electrocardiographic (ECG) abnormalities, increased sensitivity to digitalis], and nonspecific (nausea, irritability, nephropathy). ECG findings include flattened T waves, presence of U waves, and depressed ST segments.

2. Treatment consists of replacement of the potassium deficit by the oral route whenever feasible. This may be accomplished with 10% potassium chloride liquid supplement in doses of 40 to 60 mEq daily. Intravenous therapy is reserved for patients unable to tolerate oral feedings or those with severe hypokalemia. In general, not more than 100 mEq IV should be given daily to avoid overcorrecting the problem and producing hyperkalemia. Concomitant alkalosis should be corrected with bicarbonate.

C. Hyperkalemia, defined as a serum potassium level in excess of 5.0 mEq/L, may result from acute renal failure, adrenal insufficiency, or major trauma, especially crush injuries. As mentioned previously, systemic acidosis causes transcellular redistribution of potassium and elevates the serum potassium level. Hemolysis of red cells in the blood sample is a common artifactual reason for hyperkalemia.

1. **Manifestations** are potentially more life threatening than those of hypokalemia. Cardiac manifestations become common at potassium levels above 6.5 mEq/L. Clinically, these include bradycardia, hypotension, and arrhythmias. ECG findings are peaked T waves, depressed ST segments, prolonged PR intervals, and widened QRS complexes. Neuromuscular manifestations also can occur, resembling those described under hypokalemia. If hyperkalemia is suspected by clinical or ECG evidence, treatment should be initiated while laboratory confirmation is awaited.

2. **Treatment** of hyperkalemia involves measures that move potassium into cells, antagonize the toxic effects of potassium, or promote excretion of potassium from the body.

a. **Glucose and insulin** given intravenously cause a rapid shift of potassium into the intracellular compartment. One ampule of 50% dextrose (25 g of dextrose) with 10 U of regular insulin should be infused intravenously over 5 minutes. Potassium levels should begin to fall within 30 to 60 minutes.

b. **Sodium bicarbonate** causes systemic alkalosis, which promotes movement of potassium intracellularly. One ampule of 7.5% sodium bicarbonate (44.6 mEq of bicarbonate) may be given intravenously over 5 minutes. A second ampule can be given after 15 to 30 minutes if ECG changes persist or do not improve. Alternatively, 90 mEq of sodium bicarbonate may be added to 1 L of intravenous fluid containing 5% or 10% dextrose and given over a 3-hour period.

c. **Calcium gluconate** antagonizes the toxic effects of hyperkalemia on the myocardium and neuromuscular tissues. Five to 10 mL of 10% calcium gluconate should be given intravenously over 2 minutes with constant ECG monitoring. If ECG abnormalities do not improve within 5 minutes, a second dose may be given. Although calcium acts rapidly, its effect is short-lived, and other means of reducing extracellular potassium should also be used. Calcium may induce arrhythmias in patients receiving digitalis and should be given only with careful rhythm monitoring and when defibrillating equipment is available.

d. **Ion-exchange resins,** such as Kayexalate, work by exchanging potassium for sodium. It is important to remember that approximately 1.5 mEq of sodium is added to the body for each 1.0 mEq of potassium removed; thus, patients are at risk for cardiovascular overload. The recommended oral dosage is 20 to 50 g of Kayexalate dissolved in 200 mL of 20% sorbitol solution given every 4 hours. If more rapid action is desired or if oral intake is not feasible, Kayexalate may be given as a rectal enema (50 g of Kayexalate powder dissolved in 200 mL of 20% dextrose solution).

e. **Hemodialysis** is effective in the treatment of hyperkalemia but is usually reserved for situations in which it is necessary for other reasons, such as acute uremia (see Chapter 25).

V. Calcium

A. Calcium balance depends on the interaction of intestinal absorption, bone storage, and renal tubular excretion. This balance is maintained by the combined actions of vitamin D and parathyroid hormone (PTH). More than 98% of total body calcium is stored in bone, and approximately 45% of total serum calcium is bound to protein (primarily albumin). The remainder constitutes the ionized fraction, which is physiologically active and controls PTH secretion.

  1. PTH acts to elevate the serum calcium level by mobilizing calcium from bone, increasing renal tubular resorption of filtered calcium, and increasing intestinal absorption of calcium. In addition, PTH promotes renal tubular excretion of phosphate.

  2. Vitamin D promotes intestinal absorption of calcium and phosphorus and also mobilizes skeletal calcium into the serum; however, vitamin D is inactive until it is metabolized to its active form (1α,25-dihydroxycholecalciferol) in the kidney. The rate of this metabolic conversion is controlled by PTH. By this mechanism, the parathyroid gland controls the intestinal absorption and bone storage of calcium.

B. Hypercalcemia is a potentially life-threatening complication of neoplastic disease (or cancer chemotherapy). It has been estimated that 10% to 20% of patients with malignancy have hypercalcemia. Although most commonly associated with breast and lung tumors, lymphomas, and leukemias, almost any malignancy can produce hypercalcemia. In most solid tumors, hypercalcemia is the result of bone metastases, but osteolysis from tumor production of prostaglandins has been reported rarely. Finally, ectopic production of PTH, termed **pseudohyperparathyroidism,** in solid tumors accounts for approximately 2% of instances of hypercalcemia and is most commonly caused by squamous cell carcinomas of the lung (33%), renal carcinoma (33%), and gynecologic tumors. The differential diagnosis of hypercalcemia should include primary hyperparathyroidism, immobilization, vitamin D intoxication, use of thiazide diuretics, and sarcoidosis. Patients with hypercalcemia may present with changes in mental status (psychosis, obtundation, coma), gastrointestinal function (nausea, vomiting, constipation, abdominal pain), or urinary function (polyuria, nocturia). ECG changes include a shortened QT interval and occasionally arrhythmias. **Treatment** of acute hypercalcemia may involve various strategies. The presence of stupor or coma, renal failure, or cardiac arrhythmia in association with a serum calcium level of >15 mg/dL is termed hypercalcemic crisis and requires urgent treatment as follows:

  1. Saline diuresis is induced by rapid intravenous infusion of normal saline solution or lactated Ringer's solution at a rate of 250 to 500 mL/h. Presentation of a large sodium load to the renal tubule enhances calcium excretion in the urine. Clearly, careful monitoring of the central venous pressure is required, especially in patients with cardiac disease, and the central venous pressure should not be permitted to rise above 10 cm H_2O. Furosemide should be given simultaneously in doses of 20 to 40 mg IV every 2 hours to enhance calcium excretion further and maintain the water diuresis.

2.   Glucocorticoids may be used when less rapid reduction of serum calcium is desirable (e.g., in chronic hypercalcemia associated with malignancy). Sixty milligrams of oral prednisone per day will reduce the serum calcium over several days. Glucocorticoids affect serum calcium by decreasing the rate of bone metabolism, decreasing intestinal absorption of calcium, and promoting its renal excretion.

3. In instances of severe hypercalcemia (serum level >15 mg/dL) that are refractory to standard treatment, mithramycin has been effective. Because of potential side effects such as thrombocytopenia, renal failure, and hepatic failure, mithramycin should not be used as a first-line agent in the treatment of hypercalcemia. The drug is given by slow intravenous infusion (15 to 25 μg/kg) during 4 to 6 hours. A hypocalcemic effect is seen within 12 hours and lasts 3 to 7 days. Rapid reduction of serum calcium can be achieved by **hemodialysis**, which is the treatment of choice in patients with oliguric renal failure. Perhaps the most rapid reduction of serum calcium follows intravenous administration of 15 to 50 mg of **sodium ethylenediaminetetraacetic acid (Na-EDTA)** per kilogram over 4 hours, but this agent can cause nephrotoxicity.

C.   Hypocalcemia may be secondary to vitamin D deficiency, bowel malabsorption, magnesium deficiency, hypoparathyroidism, pseudohypoparathyroidism, and acute pancreatitis. Apparent hypocalcemia can result from hypoalbuminemia because, as discussed previously, approximately 45% of the serum calcium is bound to albumin. In hypoalbuminemia, the ionized calcium level is unaffected, and the patient will not manifest signs of hypocalcemia. Because most hospital laboratories report total serum calcium rather than ionized calcium, one must estimate the ionized calcium level by assessing the serum albumin and serum calcium levels together. A useful rule of thumb is that each fall of 1 g/dL in serum albumin accounts for a decrease of 0.8 mg/dL in serum calcium.

1.   Renal failure commonly leads to hypocalcemia. As discussed, the kidneys convert vitamin D to its active form, and this function is impaired in renal failure. Another factor in renal failure is hyperphosphatemia, which promotes precipitation of calcium in bone and other tissues. Hypocalcemia from enhanced bone deposition of calcium may occur rarely in patients with osteoblastic bone metastases from carcinoma of the prostate, breast, or lung.

2.   Paresthesias, especially in the circumoral area, may be an early symptom of hypocalcemia. Tetany (increased neuromuscular irritability) is the classic sign of hypocalcemia. Latent tetany may be elicited by tapping over the facial nerve to produce twitching (Chvostek's sign) or by inflating a blood pressure cuff above systolic pressure for 3 minutes to produce carpal spasm (Trousseau's sign). Other manifestations include psychosis, development of cataracts, and prolongation of the QT interval on the ECG.

3. **Treatment** of hypocalcemia depends on the acuteness of onset and the likelihood of laryngeal spasm or convulsions or both. The onset of tetany caused by **acute hypocalcemia** requires emergent treatment with 20 mL (2 ampules) of 10% calcium gluconate IV over 15 minutes. It is important to remember that alkalosis decreases the ionized calcium concentration and can potentiate the effects of hypocalcemia. Also, magnesium depletion interferes with PTH responsiveness and thus can cause hypocalcemia. If the serum magnesium is <0.8 mEq/L, severe magnesium depletion is present and should be corrected with 1 to 2 g of 10% magnesium sulfate IV over 15 minutes. Following acute therapy, calcium can be provided intravenously (600 mg of calcium gluconate/L of 5% dextrose in water) or orally (2 to 4 g of elemental calcium/day).

VI. **Magnesium**
After potassium, magnesium is the second most important intracellular cation and is an activator of many metabolic enzymes. Magnesium is absorbed in the ileum and excreted by the kidney.

A. **Hypomagnesemia** may occur because of dietary deficiency, malabsorption, or renal losses. The most common clinical condition producing magnesium deficiency in the United States is chronic alcoholism, with its associated malnutrition, malabsorption, and alcohol-induced magnesuria. Renal magnesium wasting in urologic patients may occur in renal tubular acidosis, the diuretic phase of acute tubular necrosis, drug-induced nephrotoxicity (aminoglycosides, *cis*-platinum), and therapy with loop diuretics. Clinically, the symptoms of hypomagnesemia resemble those of hypocalcemia and include seizures, personality changes, and cardiac tachyarrhythmias. As discussed previously, hypomagnesemia may be the cause of hypocalcemia. **Treatment** involves administration of 2 to 3 g of magnesium sulfate IV over 1 to 2 minutes followed by 1 g IM every 4 to 6 hours, depending on the patient's magnesium level and clinical status.

B. **Hypermagnesemia** occurs most commonly in patients with renal failure who receive magnesium-containing antacids or laxatives such as milk of magnesia, Mylanta, and Maalox.

1. **Hemiacidrin and stone disease.** Urologic patients are at particular risk from the use of hemiacidrin (Renacidin) to accomplish chemolysis of urinary (struvite) stones (see Chapter 14). Hemiacidrin is a mixture of magnesium hydroxycarbonate, magnesium acid citrate, and calcium carbonate. The magnesium in hemiacidrin replaces the calcium in urinary stones, thus producing a more soluble salt. However, infusion of hemiacidrin into the infected upper tract at high pressure may lead to magnesium toxicity. This is also a problem in patients with ileal segment diversion because magnesium is absorbed through the ileal mucosa. Magnesium toxicity is manifested as hypotension, nausea, and vomiting, usually at serum levels of between 3 and 5 mEq/L. At serum levels of 7 mEq/L, drowsiness and depression of deep tendon reflexes ensue. At serum levels above 12 mEq/L, respiratory arrest and coma are likely. During stone chemolysis with hemiacidrin, daily determinations of magnesium and phosphate are indicated.

2. Treatment of hypermagnesemia in patients undergoing hemiacidrin infusion consists of immediate cessation of infusion. The patient should receive 10% calcium gluconate (10-mL ampule) IV over 5 minutes, and diuresis should be induced by intravenous administration of saline solution with 20 to 40 mg of furosemide. If symptoms of hypermagnesemia persist, hemodialysis is indicated.

SUGGESTED READING

Bogaert GA, Mevorach RA, Kim J, et al. The physiology of gastrocystoplasty: once a stomach, always a stomach. *J Urol* 1995;153: 1977–1980.

Fontaine E, Barthelemy Y, Houlgatte A, et al. Twenty-year experience with jejunal conduits. *Urology* 1997;50:207–213.

Grundy PL, Budd DWG, England R. A randomized controlled trial evaluating use of sterile water as an irrigant fluid during transurethral electrovaporization of the prostate. *Br J Urol* 1997; 80: 894–897.

Hahn RG. Irrigating fluids in endoscopic surgery. *Br J Urol* 1997;79: 669–680.

McDougal WS. Metabolic complications of urinary intestinal diversion. *J Urol* 1992;147:1199–1208.

Shepard RL, Kraus SE, Babayan RK, et al. The role of ammonia toxicity in the post transurethral prostatectomy syndrome. *Br J Urol* 1987;60:349–351.

Stampfer DS, McDougal WS, McGovern FJ. The use of bowel in urology: metabolic and nutritional complications. *Urol Clin North Am* 1997;24:715–722.

Vaughn ED Jr, Gillenwater JY. Diagnosis, characterization, and management of post-obstructive diuresis. *J Urol* 1973;109:286–292.

Renal Failure, Dialysis, and Renal Transplantation

Ricardo M. Munnariz, Andrew Kramer, and Gennaro Carpinito

The urologist is frequently required to manage patients with acute or chronic renal failure (CRF). Most commonly, the urologist is asked to evaluate a patient who has acute oliguria, increased serum creatinine, or both, and the role of the urologist is to rule out a correctable obstruction. Less often, urologic surgery is required in a patient known to have chronic renal insufficiency. In both circumstances, an understanding of acute and CRF is essential to proper patient management.

I. Renal function tests

A. Glomerular filtration rate (GFR). This is one of the best indicators of renal function and reflects the total filtration of all functioning nephrons. The normal value for GFR is about 120 mL/min in men and 95 mL/min in women. GFR tends to diminish with aging (or the comorbidities associated with aging) at a rate of about 0.75 mL/min/year.

1. **Creatinine clearance.** Although the best estimate of GFR is obtained by measuring inulin clearance, the creatinine clearance provides an approximate measure that is accurate enough for clinical use. Because creatinine is also secreted by the kidney, the creatinine clearance overestimates GFR by as much as 20%, especially in the diseased kidney. Creatinine clearance tends to fall with aging, as skeletal muscle mass is reduced. Over relatively short periods of time, the plasma creatinine is inversely proportional to the creatinine clearance; thus, a rise in plasma creatinine from 0.8 to 1.6 mg/dL may indicate a fall of 50% in the GFR (Fig. 25.1). The creatinine clearance is measured by collecting urine over a predetermined time period (2 hours, 6 hours, 24 hours) and measuring the creatinine content of the urine ($Creat_{urine}$), urine volume per minute (Vol_{urine}), and plasma creatinine ($Creat_{plasma}$). The creatinine clearance (C_{cr}; mL/min) is obtained from the following formula: $C_{cr} = [Creat_{urine}\ (mg/dL) \times Vol_{urine}\ (mL/min)]/Creat_{plasma}$ (mg/dL). To obtain the correct value for creatinine clearance, attention must be paid to the units in the preceding equation. If the laboratory does not report urine or serum creatinine in milligrams per deciliter, the figure must be converted to these units. *The total urine volume must be converted to milliliters per minute by dividing the volume (milliliters) by the collection period (e.g., 1,440 minutes for 24-hour collection).*

2. **Estimating GFR.** Several formulas may be used to estimate the GFR without collecting 24-hour urine samples. These formulas can be used in only patients with stable renal function. The **Cockroft–Gault equation** allows the creatinine clearance to be estimated from the plasma creatinine level

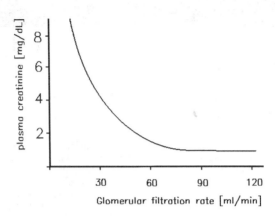

Fig. 25.1.   Idealized relationship between plasma creatinine level and glomerular filtration rate.

in patients with stable plasma creatinine: C_{cr} (mL/min) = [(140 − age) × body wt (kg)]/[Creat$_{plasma}$ (mg/dL) × 72]. This formula corrects for the decline in creatinine production with age and the increased creatinine production with increasing body weight. Because of diminished creatinine production in women, the value obtained must be multiplied by 0.85 in women.

3.   Blood urea nitrogen (BUN) is much less useful than the plasma creatinine in estimating GFR because (a) the rate of urea production is not constant and (b) approximately 40% to 50% of the filtered urea is passively reabsorbed in the proximal tubule. Thus, in the face of hypovolemia associated with enhanced proximal sodium and water reabsorption, the BUN will rise out of proportion to any change in GFR.

B.   Tests of tubular function

1.   Proximal tubule reabsorption results in conservation of electrolytes, glucose, and amino acids. To determine proximal tubular function, compare urine and blood levels of a compound (X) that is reabsorbed in the proximal tubule to calculate percentage tubular reabsorption ($T_{reabsorption}$): $T_{reabsorption} = [(1 − U_X/P_X)/(U_{cr}/P_{cr})] \times 100$, where U_X is the concentration of compound X in urine, P_X is the concentration of compound X in plasma, U_{cr} is the concentration of creatinine in urine, and P_{cr} is the concentration of creatinine in plasma. This formula can be used for amino acids, electrolytes, calcium, and phosphorus.

2.   Distal tubular function is best evaluated by testing the concentrating and diluting ability of the kidney. Under conditions of water deprivation, the normal kidney can concentrate the urine to 1,200 mOsm or a specific gravity of 1.030. A first-voided specimen after an overnight fast is adequate to test concentrating ability. A specific gravity of ≥1.023 indicates intact concentrating ability. Concentrating ability tends to decline with age after 45 years.

II. Acute renal failure
A. Definition. Acute renal failure is a sudden renal deterioration over a period of hours to days, resulting in the failure to maintain fluid and electrolyte homeostasis and excrete nitrogenous waste products. Acute renal failure can also be defined operationally as an increase in serum creatinine of >0.5 mg/dL, an increase of >50% over the baseline value, or a decrease in creatinine clearance of 50%.

B. Oliguria is defined as a urine output of ≤400 mL/24 h; it typically occurs in acute renal failure but is not an invariable finding. **Anuria** (total cessation of urine output) is rare. It is important to remember that oliguria is a relative state that depends on the patient's fluid intake and renal concentrating ability. In the face of poor concentrating ability, even a rate of 1,000 mL/24 h may not be sufficient to remove body wastes. Urine volumes of ≥500 mL/24 h are noted in about 25% of patients with acute renal failure.

C. Symptomatic uremia may manifest in patients with acute renal failure with various physical signs and symptoms. Owing to fluid overload, hypertension and peripheral edema may result. Gastrointestinal symptoms such as nausea, vomiting, and upper gastrointestinal bleeds are common in the patient with an acute exacerbation in renal function. Neurologic signs include mental status changes, encephalopathy, coma, and seizures. Hematologic manifestations may include bleeding and anemia. Electrolyte disturbances are frequent as well, including hyponatremia, hyperkalemia, hypermagnesemia, hypocalcemia, and hyperuricemia. Last, pruritus is very common in the acute renal failure patient, especially in the arms and legs.

D. Classification. The most useful classification system recognizes acute renal failure caused by prerenal, renal, and postrenal factors (Table 25.1).

1. Prerenal azotemia results from hypoperfusion of the kidneys and may be caused by a wide variety of conditions (Table 25.1). A fall in systemic blood pressure or plasma volume from any cause leads to the release of norepinephrine and angiotensin in an attempt to maintain the perfusion of vital organs such as the heart and brain. Renal vasoconstriction leads in turn to a decreased GFR and azotemia. Thus, it is important to realize that renal ischemia may be present even in the face of normal systemic blood pressure. A rise in BUN and plasma creatinine may be the only manifestation of renal hypoperfusion. BUN may be elevated out of proportion to creatinine. The renal tubules respond to a lowered GFR by increasing the absorption of sodium and water. Renal hypoperfusion may also be present in cardiac failure and cirrhosis with ascites. In advanced hepatic cirrhosis, a progressive decline in renal function, termed hepatorenal syndrome, may occur.

2. Renal azotemia. Acute tubular necrosis (ATN) is the most common cause of azotemia due to parenchymal dysfunction. The pathophysiology of ATN is poorly understood, but it is known that necrosis of renal tubules with plugging of their lumina by necrotic debris plays a major role. Renal ischemia is a common cause for ATN, discovered initially in surgical patients in whom the aorta or renal artery was clamped

Table 25.1.   Causes of acute renal failure

I. Prerenal azotemia
  A. Volume depletion
    1. Hemorrhage
    2. Gastrointestinal losses (vomiting, diarrhea, fistulas)
    3. Renal losses (nephritis, glycosuria, diuretics)
    4. "Third space" losses (pancreatitis, peritonitis, intestinal obstruction)
    5. Burns
  B. Circulatory disorders
    1. Congestive heart failure
    2. Hypotension/shock
    3. Cirrhosis with ascites
    4. Sepsis
  C. Local renal ischemia
    1. Bilateral renal artery occlusion
    2. Prostaglandin inhibitors
    3. Bilateral renal vein thrombosis
    4. Cyclosporin and tacrolimus (vasoconstriction of small renal vessels)

II. Renal azotemia
  A. Acute tubular necrosis
  B. Urate nephropathy
  C. Vasculitis
  D. Hemolytic uremic syndrome
  E. Acute interstitial nephritis
  F. Acute glomerulonephritis

III. Postrenal azotemia
  A. Urate nephropathy
  B. Bilateral staghorn calculi
  C. Bilateral ureteral obstruction
  D. Bladder outlet obstruction

for periods of time. Certain medications have been implicated as causes of ATN, including nonsteroidal antiinflammatory drugs (NSAIDs), angiotensin-converting enzyme inhibitors, cyclosporin, and aminoglycosides (Table 25.2). Acute interstitial nephritis (AIN) is less common than ATN. This classically presents with fever, eosinophilia, and rash. Certain medications implicated in causing AIN are penicillins, cephalosporins, sulfa derivatives, furosemide, thiazides, captopril, valproic acid, dilantin, NSAIDs, and cimetidine. ATN is generally considered to have three phases:

    a. The **oliguric phase** usually begins within 24 hours after an acute renal insult such as ischemia or administration of nephrotoxic agents. The onset of ATN is much more insidious with aminoglycoside toxicity; typically, a rise in plasma creatinine becomes apparent only after ≥7 days of drug administration. Patients who continue to produce reasonable amounts of urine despite a progressive rise in plasma creatinine and BUN are said to have nonoliguric ATN. The maintenance of normal urine output in some pa-

Table 25.2.   Drugs associated with acute renal failure

Aminoglycosides
Anesthetics
Iodinated contrast media
Nonsteroidal antiinflammatory agents

tients with ATN may be caused by a less marked fall in GFR or an increased degree of tubular dysfunction leading to diminished concentrating ability. The first appears more likely; patients with nonoliguric ATN have been shown to have a better prognosis overall than patients with oliguria. The average duration of the oliguric phase is about 10 days but is extremely variable.

b. The **diuretic phase** heralds the start of recovery of renal tubular function. A noticeable increase in daily urine output is accompanied by a stabilization or slow fall in plasma creatinine. Although urine output improves, renal concentrating ability and resorption are far from normal, and large losses of sodium, potassium, or both can occur, but this is rare.

c. The **recovery phase** may last from 3 to 12 months, during which GFR and tubular function gradually improve to nearly baseline levels.

3. Postrenal azotemia refers to obstruction in the collecting ducts, renal pelvis, ureter, or bladder outlet. A variety of causes must be considered, depending on the age and sex of the patient (Table 25.3). With acute obstruction, hydrostatic pressure in the collecting system rises and leads to a fall in GFR. Initially, tubular function tends to be preserved. After a period of about 4 weeks, the pressure in the collecting system gradually returns to normal as the GFR falls and lymphatic channels of egress from the renal pelvis become established.

Table 25.3.   Major causes of postrenal azotemia

Children
   Posterior urethral valves
   Bilateral ureteropelvic junction obstruction
   Renal agenesis
   Meatal stenosis
   Neurogenic bladder (myelodysplasia)

Adults
   Pregnancy
   Retroperitoneal neoplasms
   Bilateral calculi
   Neurogenic bladder dysfunction
   Impaired detrusor contractility
   Benign prostatic hypertrophy
   Prostate cancer
   Gynecologic malignancies

Despite the fall in intrapelvic pressure, dilatation of the collecting systems tends to persist, presumably because of loss of smooth muscle tone from chronic overdistension. With established obstructive uropathy, tubular function becomes impaired, leading to renal salt wasting, decreased concentrating ability, and polyuria. Thus, partial obstruction may be associated with normal urine output accompanied by azotemia. Complete anuria occurs only in the presence of complete obstruction. In general, complete recovery of function occurs after obstruction lasting <2 weeks, and little or no recovery occurs after 12 weeks. In intermediate cases, the prognosis depends on the level of preexisting renal function and the presence of additional insults such as infection.

E.   Differential diagnosis of acute oliguria. Acute or chronic urinary retention should be ruled out by physical examination or urethral catheterization. If urethral access to the bladder is not possible in a patient with bladder distention, ultrasonography (US) of the bladder can be performed. If no evidence of bladder distention is found, the diagnosis of prerenal azotemia and ATN should be considered, which together account for 75% of all cases of acute renal failure. Examination of the urine under the microscope and urine chemistry studies will allow differentiation of these two conditions in many instances (Table 25.4). These indexes are most useful in patients with oliguria and less definitive in patients with nonoliguric renal failure. A therapeutic trial of fluid replacement is probably the most important test in this situation. If no diuresis is observed, renal causes (most likely ATN) or bilateral ureteral obstruction should be considered. A plain film of the abdomen may reveal the presence of urinary calculi. Renal US is extremely useful in identifying the presence of obstruction. Retrograde pyelography is sometimes indicated, even in the presence of normal renal US results, if ureteral obstruction is suspected clinically. This is because the fornix may rupture in an acutely obstructed kidney and reduce the degree of hydronephrosis.

F.   Treatment of acute renal failure. In many patients, it is not possible to establish whether acute renal failure is caused by hypovolemia or ATN before treatment is started. The treatment of acute renal failure should be focused on reversing the underlying cause, preventing further renal injury, correcting

Table 25.4.   Differential diagnosis of acute renal failure

	Urine Sodium (mEq/L)	Urine Osmolality (mOsm)	Urine/Plasma Creatinine (mg/dL)
Prerenal	<20	>500	>20
Renal	>40	<350	<20
Postrenal			
Acute	<20	>500	>20
Chronic	>40	<350	<20

Table 25.5.   Mortality rate of acute tubular necrosis

Type	Mortality (%)
Oliguric	
Postoperative	60
Medical disease	40
Nonoliguric	30

fluid and electrolyte imbalances, and providing supportive measures until renal recovery has occurred. Whether renal failure is caused by hypovolemia or ATN, the initial therapy in acutely oliguric patients should be aggressive fluid repletion. In patients with normal serum sodium levels and no evidence of congestive heart failure, it is generally safe to give half-normal saline solution at a rate of 500 mL/h. If oliguria persists after administration of 500 to 1,000 mL of fluids, a loop diuretic such as furosemide (200 mg IV) or an osmotic diuretic such as mannitol (25 g IV) should be given. A presumptive diagnosis of prerenal azotemia can be made if these maneuvers produce a persistent diuresis. It should be remembered, however, that a loop diuretic may also produce diuresis in some cases of ATN. The difference is that in prerenal azotemia, renal function should return to nearly normal levels within 48 to 72 hours after correction of hypovolemia. In ATN, no significant improvement in renal function will occur despite adequate fluid repletion or increased urine output. Treatment of established renal failure caused by ATN is largely supportive. Nephrotoxic drugs should be discontinued or avoided. Hyperkalemia can be treated with hydration, oral or rectal binding resins, or the intravenous administration of glucose and insulin. Metabolic renal acidosis may be corrected with sodium bicarbonate. A low-protein diet with additional calories is generally recommended in renal failure and should be ordered in consultation with the dietitian. Anemia is a common finding and is often secondary to decreased production of erythropoietin, decreased red blood cell survival, and phlebotomy. Bleeding disorders secondary to uremia can be reversed with blood products, estrogens, or vasopressin analogues. Patients with severe and prolonged acute renal failure are best treated by peritoneal dialysis or hemodialysis. The overall mortality rate of ATN is approximately 80% (Table 25.5). Continuous therapies with venovenous access and more permeable membranes may facilitate fluid removal in critically ill patients with acute renal failure.

III.   CRF

A.   Definition. CRF is defined as an established, slowly progressive decrease in GFR and tubular function. Generally, the term "end-stage renal disease" (ESRD) is applied in cases of irreversible renal failure severe enough to require renal replacement therapy such as dialysis or transplantation. ESRD is more common in elderly, male, and African American individuals. The most common causes are diabetic nephropathy, hypertension, and glomerulonephritis (Table 25.6; Fig. 25.2). Native Americans

Table 25.6.   Causes of chronic renal failure

Diabetic nephropathy
Hypertension (nephrosclerosis)
Glomerulonephritis
Hereditary renal disease
  Polycystic kidney disease
  Alport's syndrome
Obstructive uropathy
Interstitial nephritis
Chronic pyelonephritis

have a higher prevalence of diabetes, whereas hypertension disproportionately high among African Americans.

B.   Clinical findings in CRF are caused by uremia itself an by compensatory mechanisms that attempt to restore wate and electrolyte balance.

1.   Constitutional symptoms are usually the first appear in CRF. Patients often complain of fatigue, lack energy, and insomnia.

2.   Gastrointestinal symptoms are common in CRF an include anorexia, nausea, and vomiting. These sympton tend to improve with dialysis.

3.   Cardiovascular changes include pericarditis, conge tive heart failure, and hypertension. Pericarditis is an ind cation for immediate, aggressive dialysis. Dialysis usuall reverses pericarditis within 1 to 2 weeks. Cardiovascular cor plications are a common cause of death in dialysis patient for example, cerebrovascular accidents account for 30% deaths in dialysis patients under the age of 50.

4.   Hematologic changes are common in CRF and inclu anemia and coagulopathy. Both of these may complicate su gical therapy in uremic patients. Anemia is caused by a re ative lack of erythropoietin, decreased red cell survival, an phlebotomy. A platelet dysfunction, usually correctable k dialysis, accounts for the bleeding tendency observed in 60 of patients with CRF.

5.   Neurologic changes include both encephalopathy an peripheral neuropathy. Early encephalopathy in uremia ma manifest as impaired mental concentration, insomnia, an emotional lability. Later, disorientation and confusion ma develop, progressing to coma. Uremic encephalopathy ofte is accompanied by tremor and asterixis. The mental change disappear rapidly with dialysis. Uremic polyneuropathy usu ally presents as sensory changes, particularly paresthesia and later progresses to motor weakness. The sensory change are usually reversible by dialysis, but the motor neuropath is less reversible. The appearance or worsening of motor neu ropathy is usually considered an indication to begin or in crease the frequency of dialysis. Autonomic neuropathy common in CRF, accounting for postural hypotension an erectile dysfunction. Dialysis does not restore potency, how

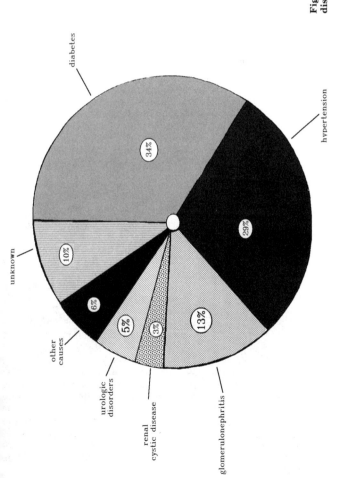

Fig. 25.2. Etiologies of end-stage renal disease.

ever, which suggests that other factors, such as vascular disease and decreased libido, are involved.

6.   Endocrine changes. Depression of plasma testosterone, oligospermia, and elevation of luteinizing hormone and follicle-stimulating hormone levels are common in male dialysis patients and consistent with primary testicular failure. Amenorrhea is very common in female patients. Successful renal transplantation often reverses these changes.

7.   Renal osteodystrophy is a consequence of either (a) secondary hyperparathyroidism induced by hyperphosphatemia, hypocalcemia, deficient production of calcitriol, and skeletal resistance to parathyroid hormone or (b) low-turnover bone disease generally associated with aluminum retention from aluminum-containing binders. Renal osteodystrophy manifests radiologically as subperiosteal bone resorption, best seen in the bones of the fingers. Clinical findings include bone pain and pathologic fractures. Metastatic calcification may occur in dialysis patients and lead to calcium deposits in peripheral vessels, around joints, and in the myocardium.

8.   Acquired cystic kidney disease is a disorder recently recognized to occur in up to 40% of patients with CRF, especially, but not exclusively, in those undergoing hemodialysis for longer than 3 years. Small, multiple cysts develop in both kidneys and may cause hematuria or retroperitoneal hemorrhage. More importantly, the incidence of renal adenocarcinoma is increased in patients with acquired cystic kidney disease to between 4% and 10%. Although most of these tumors are of low malignant potential and rarely metastasize, patients with acquired cystic kidney disease should be followed with yearly renal US to detect any new growths.

9.   Erectile dysfunction may be secondary to hormonal or vascular changes and to anemia.

C.   Treatment of CRF is the responsibility of nephrologists; only selected aspects of treatment that are relevant to urologic practice are discussed.

1.   Anemia. A normochromic, normocytic anemia is very common in CRF. In most dialysis patients, the hematocrit is between 15% and 30%; however, only about 25% of patients are symptomatic and require regular transfusions. Patients with angina pectoris or other signs of ischemia should be treated with transfusions of packed red cells until adequate oxygen-carrying capacity is restored. Treatment with recombinant human erythropoietin often increases the hematocrit within a few weeks.

2.   Coagulopathy. The bleeding time is prolonged in approximately 50% of patients with CRF. Although there is no simple relationship between the degree of azotemia and the degree of coagulopathy, circulating antibodies that interfere with platelet function are probably present. Another factor is the anemia commonly present in CRF. Simply raising the hematocrit to 30% will improve the bleeding time in many patients, presumably by increasing platelet–endothelial cell interaction. Several treatment options are available for patients being prepared for surgery or other invasive procedures.

a. Dialysis is effective in more than two-thirds of patients. Either hemodialysis or peritoneal dialysis may be used. In patients already undergoing dialysis, increased frequency of treatment may be indicated. The efficacy of dialysis is one of the arguments supporting the presence of a circulating platelet toxin.

b. Administration of 1-deamino-8-D-arginine-vaso-pressin (desmopressin) improves bleeding time within 1 hour of infusion, and the effect lasts up to 8 hours. The dose is 0.3 µg/kg dissolved in 50 mL of normal saline solution given intravenously over 30 minutes. The mechanism appears to involve release of factor VIII from endothelial cells.

c. Cryoprecipitate appears to act by improving platelet adhesion to endothelial cells. The onset of action is at 12 to 24 hours, and the effect lasts up to 24 hours. The usefulness of this mode of therapy is limited by the risk for transmitting hepatitis and acquired immunodeficiency syndrome (AIDS).

d. Transfusions may correct the coagulopathy if the hematocrit remains above 30%. This form of therapy carries risks for transmission of infectious disease and requires at least several hours to accomplish in most cases.

e. Estrogens. Conjugated estrogens given intravenously in a dosage of 0.6 mg/kg/day for 5 days may be used if a delay in onset of action is acceptable. The onset occurs within 6 hours, but the effect does not reach a peak until the fifth day. The duration may be as long as 2 weeks. The mechanism of action is unknown.

3. Protein restriction (0.6 to 0.7 g/kg/day) will reduce the accumulation of nitrogenous waste products. Adequate caloric intake (30 to 50 kcal/kg/day) is strongly recommended to avoid catabolism of endogenous protein. Consultation with a dietitian is beneficial in the management of these patients.

4. Potassium should be restricted to 40 mEq/day when the GFR falls below 20 mL/min.

5. Sodium restriction should be individualized, but in general a diet with "no added salt" is adequate.

6. Fluid intake in stable patients should equal the daily urine output plus 500 mL for insensible losses.

7. Acidosis may be treated, when indicated, with oral sodium bicarbonate (300 to 600 mg three times daily).

8. Renal osteodystrophy is a complex problem and may require correction of hyperphosphatemia and hypocalcemia, management of aluminum toxicity, and (occasionally) parathyroidectomy.

IV. Dialysis

A. Definition. Dialysis is any process that changes the concentration of solutes in the plasma by exposure to a second solution (the dialysis solution) across a semipermeable membrane. In-center hemodialysis accounts for about 60% of all treated ESRD patients.

B. Indications for dialysis are summarized in Table 25.7. In many instances, clinical judgment must be used in deciding whether it is appropriate to initiate dialysis. In contrast-induced ATN, for example, dialysis is usually not necessary, even in

Table 25.7.   Indications and contraindications for dialysis

Indications	Contraindications
Pericarditis	Irreversible dementia or coma
Altered mental status	Hepatorenal syndrome
Prolonged bleeding time	Advanced malignancy
Neuropathy	
Hyperkalemia	
Acidosis	
Fluid overload	
Drug overdose	
Urea nitrogen >100 mg/dL *or*	
Creatinine clearance <0.10 mL/ min/kg body wt	

symptomatic patients, because renal function typically begins t recover within 5 days. In postischemic ATN, however, many fe that dialysis should be started even in asymptomatic patien when the BUN reaches 100 mg/dL because many weeks ma pass before recovery occurs.

C.   Peritoneal dialysis versus hemodialysis. Both form of dialysis are effective when properly used. Hemodialys: achieves more rapid clearance of the plasma and is especiall useful in treating hyperkalemia, fluid overload, and drug ove doses. About 10% of ESRD patients are treated with chron peritoneal dialysis. Peritoneal dialysis is preferred in patien who cannot tolerate hypotensive episodes or the heparinizatio required to perform hemodialysis. In many cases, the choice : a matter of patient preference based on the significant adva tages of peritoneal dialysis over hemodialysis (Table 25.8). Co traindications for peritoneal dialysis are listed in Table 25.9.

D.   Peritoneal dialysis is performed by introducing 1 to 8 of a dextrose-containing dialysis solution into the peritone:

Table 25.8.   Advantages and disadvantages of peritoneal dialysis

Advantages
  Portability, safety
  Fewer symptoms
  Fewer medications
  Higher hematocrit
  No routine anticoagulation
  Better control of parathyroid hormone levels

Disadvantages
  Increased risk of infection, malnutrition, hypertriglyceridemia
  Less efficacious
  Catheter-related problems
  Potential pulmonary complications

Table 25.9. Contraindications for peritoneal dialysis

Absolute
  Peritoneal fibrosis
  Pleuroperitoneal fistula

Relative
  Presence of colostomy or nephrostomy
  Cardiac prosthesis (e.g., valve)
  Fungal or tuberculous peritonitis
  Inguinal or abdominal hernias
  Obesity
  Peripheral vascular disease
  Hyperlipidemia
  Diverticulosis
  Polycystic kidney disease
  Mental or physical incapacity

cavity. The peritoneum acts as a semipermeable membrane, and the dextrose creates an osmotic gradient with respect to plasma. The length of time the dialysate remains in the peritoneal cavity is called the **dwell time.** Access to the peritoneal cavity is most commonly achieved via a surgically implanted catheter. As in hemodialysis, small molecules such as urea diffuse rapidly, whereas larger protein molecules diffuse slowly, if at all. Hemodialysis membranes are more efficient at excluding proteins, and in general more protein is lost in peritoneal dialysis than in hemodialysis.

1. Peritoneal dialysis solutions closely approximate normal plasma in respect to electrolyte concentrations. Although many commercial solutions are available, most contain sodium chloride, sodium lactate, calcium chloride, and magnesium chloride. Dextrose is added to provide an osmotic gradient, and lactate or acetate is added as a source of bicarbonate (Table 25.10).

2. Dialysis schedules. Peritoneal dialysis is commonly administered according to one of four schedules:

Table 25.10. Composition of hemodialysate and peritoneal dialysate solutions

	Hemodialysate	Peritoneal Dialysate
Glucose (g/dL)	0–0.20	1.4–3.9
Sodium (mmol/L)	140	132
Potassium (mmol/L)	2.0	0
Calcium (mEq/L)	2.5	1.5–3.5
Magnesium (mEq/L)	0.5	0.5–1.5
Chloride (mEq/L)	105	95–102
Lactate (mEq/L)	—	35–40
Bicarbonate (mEq/L)	25–40	—

   a. Acute dialysis is achieved by instilling and draining
dialysate every 1/2 to 2 hours over a 2- to 3-day period.
   b. Chronic intermittent peritoneal dialysis involve
a short dwell time (30 minutes) repeated over 8 to 10 hour
per session. The dialysate is infused and drained with
cycle machine. Three to four sessions per week are usual
required. The abdomen contains no dialysate betwee
sessions.
   c. Continuous ambulatory peritoneal dialysis
carried out by the patient by means of gravity infusion ar
drainage. Dialysate is always present in the abdomen ar
is exchanged three to five times daily.
   d. Continuous cycle assisted peritoneal dialysis
similar to chronic intermittent dialysis except that dial
sis takes place overnight while the patient sleeps. Fres
dialysate is left in the abdomen during the day.
3. **Complications**
   a. The most important complication of peritoneal dialys
is **peritonitis,** which should be suspected in any patien
undergoing peritoneal dialysis in whom abdominal pai
nausea, vomiting, or diarrhea develops. The peritoneal flu
becomes cloudy, and gram stain will reveal the presence
bacteria. Approximately 70% of instances are caused b
gram-positive organisms (*Staphylococcus aureus, Staph
lococcus epidermidis,* and *Streptococcus* sp), and coli form
account for most of the remainder. Five percent of the in
fections are fungal and are caused by *Candida albican
Nocardia asteroides, Aspergillus* sp, and *Mycobacteriun
The treatment of these infections is based on immediate a
dominal lavage with rapid flushes of dialysate fluid, empir
administration of intraperitoneal antibiotics (Table 25.11
and empiric administration of broad-spectrum systemic ant
biotics depending on the results of peritoneal gram stai
until definitive cultures and sensitivities are obtained. Gen
erally, the peritoneal catheter can remain in place in case
of bacterial peritonitis, whereas fungal peritonitis almo
always requires removal of the peritoneal catheter. Othe
indications for catheter removal are infection by *Pseud
monas* sp, persistence of symptoms, and failure of dialysa
cell count to decline.
   b. Obesity may result from absorption of glucose in th
dialysis solution across the peritoneal membrane.

Table 25.11. Empiric regimens for peritonitis

Gram positive	Vancomycin alone
Gram negative	Aminoglycoside alone or third-generation cephalosporin
Mixed organisms	Vancomycin + aminoglycoside + metronidazole
Gram stain negative	Vancomycin + aminoglycoside
Fungal infections	Fluconazole IP or amphotericin IP/IV

c. **Protein loss** averaging 9 g/day can occur in peritoneal dialysis. Both protein loss and hyperglycemia can be addressed by attention to dietary intake. Other metabolic complications include hyperosmolar nonketotic coma, hyperkalemia or hypokalemia, hyperlipidemia, metabolic alkalosis, and sodium imbalances.

d. **Mechanical problems** include pain with inflow or outflow, fluid leakage, poor outflow drainage, and scrotal edema.

e. Atelectasis, hydrothorax, and aspiration pneumonia are the most common pulmonary problems seen in patients undergoing peritoneal dialysis.

f. The most common cardiovascular complication is fluid overload, followed by hypertension and dysrhythmias.

E. Hemodialysis requires access to the bloodstream and use of a hemodialysis machine.

1. The **hemodialysis machine** pumps blood from the patient through a dialysis cartridge (Fig. 25.3). In the dialyzer, the patient's blood is exposed to the dialysis solution across a semipermeable membrane. The blood is then pumped back to the patient through a return circuit. Treatment schedules are typically 3 to 5 hours three times a week. Despite the many

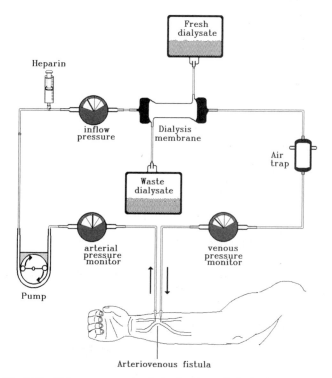

Fig. 25.3. Major components of a typical hemodialysis circuit.

technical advances in hemodialysis technology, patients undergoing this treatment continue to have a mortality rate of 5% to 10% while on maintenance dialysis.

2. Dialysis solutions typically contain sodium, potassium, calcium, magnesium, chloride, and bicarbonate or acetate (Table 25.10). The potassium concentration is somewhat lower than in plasma, phosphorus is absent, and bicarbonate is higher than in plasma, resulting in removal of potassium and phosphorus from the bloodstream with the addition of bicarbonate. In instances of acute hyperkalemia, solutions containing little or no potassium can be used to hasten removal of potassium from the bloodstream.

F.   Hemofiltration, first described in 1977, relies on ultrafiltration of solutes across a highly porous, semipermeable membrane. It is useful as a method for treatment of overly hydrated patients who are resistant to diuretics. Large volumes of ultrafiltrate can be taken from the patient and replaced by a fluid not containing urea or other nitrogenous wastes. Thus, uremia can be slowly reduced but at a much slow rate than using hemodialysis. If additional clearance is desired, a dialysis circuit can be added to the hemofilter.

G.   Vascular access. Temporary access for patients requiring acute dialysis or hemofiltration may be obtained through a percutaneous venous cannula placed into the subclavian, jugular, or femoral vein. This form of access should be replaced by a more permanent form as soon as possible. The two most common forms of permanent vascular access are the arteriovenous fistula and the prosthetic shunt (Fig. 25.4).

1. Arteriovenous (Cimino–Brescia) fistula involves anastomosis of the cephalic vein and radial artery. Such a fistula usually requires 3 to 6 weeks to mature before it can be used for dialysis. The long-term patency rate is high (75% at 2 years), although revisions and declotting of the fistula may be required periodically in many patients. In many cases, permanent vascular access becomes difficult or impossible once all the veins in the forearm have been used.

2. A prosthetic fistula or shunt made with a Gore-Tex graft can be used to connect an artery and vein in the upper arm. Such artificial grafts can be used for dialysis immediately if necessary, but a period of maturation and healing should be allowed whenever possible. Such a shunt has a patency rate of 30% at 2 years; the most common cause of shunt failure is intimal hyperplasia, resulting in stenosis of the venous anastomosis.

3. Complications of vascular access

a.   Occlusion and thrombosis of vascular access are suspected by loss of pulsation in an arteriovenous fistula or high pressure in the venous line during dialysis. Fistulography may be performed to identify the site of occlusion. A percutaneous transluminal angioplasty may be successful in correcting the problem. A thrombosed access site may be cleared with urokinase injection. If these maneuvers are unsuccessful, surgical reconstruction of the site is necessary.

b.   Infection of vascular access site is usually manifested by fever with little or no sign of local inflammation.

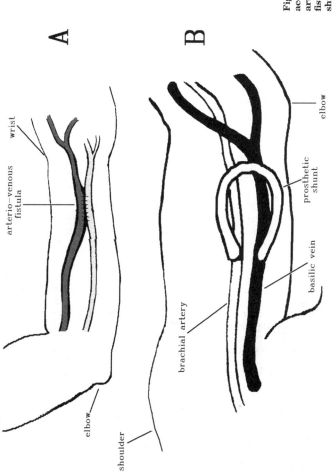

Fig. 25.4. Two common forms of vascular access for dialysis. A: Direct side-to-side arteriovenous fistula. B: Arteriovenous fistula using prosthetic, usually Gore-Tex, shunt.

Broad-spectrum antibiotics should be administered until the results of blood culture are available. If a rapid response is not obtained, the vascular access should be removed or ligated.

4. **Complications of dialysis**

a. The **disequilibrium syndrome** consists of headache, nausea, confusion, or seizures during or soon after hemodialysis. It is thought to be caused by removal of urea more rapidly from the extracellular fluid than from the brain, leading to cerebral edema. The problem can be managed by infusion of mannitol or reduction of the rate of dialysis.

b. Hypotension occurs during up to 50% of dialysis treatments and is usually caused by volume depletion; it can be corrected by administration of intravenous fluids.

c. Muscle cramps are common during high-volume hemodialysis. Common therapeutic approaches include fluid restriction, stretching exercises, and administration of quinine sulfate.

d. Arrhythmias are generally seen in predisposed patients and are often secondary to a combination of factors such as hypoxemia, removal of antiarrhythmic drugs during dialysis, and rapid changes of bicarbonate, sodium, potassium, calcium, and magnesium concentrations.

e. Acquired renal cystic disease develops in approximately 80% of patients with ESRD who undergo dialysis for >3 years.

f.   Other complications are bleeding, anemia, transfusion-related diseases, metabolic bone disease, and pericarditis.

H. Surgery and anesthesia in the patient with CRF are complicated by the need for regular dialysis, electrolyte and acid–base imbalance, and increased cardiac risk. Based on the current American College of Cardiology/American Heart Association guidelines on perioperative cardiovascular evaluation of noncardiac surgery, patients with a creatinine level of ≥ 2 mg/dL are considered to have at least intermediate probability of increased perioperative cardiovascular risk. In addition, azotemia is associated with platelet dysfunction (see above), acidosis, and inability to handle fluid overload. Dosage adjustments or drug avoidance is very important in patients with CRF. Meperidine (Demerol) should be avoided in patients with CRF because the active metabolite (normeperidine) can accumulate and cause seizures. Various drugs may cause hyperkalemia in patients with CRF (Table 25.12).

1. **Effect of anesthetic agents in patients with CRF.** Fluorinated compounds such as methoxyflurane and enflurane are nephrotoxic and should be avoided in patients with CRF. Succinylcholine, a depolarizing blocker, causes hyperkalemia. The effect of neuromuscular blocking agents may be prolonged.

2. **Effect of surgery in persons with CRF.** Tissue trauma, surgery, hemolysis, or rhabdomyolysis may lead to hyperkalemia. Ringer's lactate solution contains potassium and should be avoided in patients with CRF. Most patients with CRF have chronic acidosis that may be worsened by surgery and/or anesthesia.

Table 25.12. Drugs associated with hyperkalemia in patients with chronic renal failure

Inhibitors of renin synthesis
  β blockers (e.g., metoprolol, atenolol)
  Clonidine
  Methyldopa
  Nonsteroidal antiinflammatory drugs
  Cyclooxygenase-2 inhibitors (e.g., celecoxib, rofecoxib)
Angiotensin-converting enzyme inhibitors
  Enalapril
  Fosinopril
Angiotensin II receptor blockers
  Losartan
  Candesartan
Heparin
Low-molecular-weight heparin
  Enoxaparin
  Nadroparin
Immunosuppressive drugs
  Cyclosporin
  Tacrolimus
Potassium-sparing diuretics
  Spirolactone
  Triamterene
  Amiloride
Antibiotics
  Trimethoprim/sulfamethoxazole
  Pentamidine
Succinylcholine
Haloperidol
Digoxin (overdose)

V. Renal transplantation

Renal transplantation remains the only treatment of ESRD that reverses the underlying pathophysiology. Approximately 200,000 patients are receiving dialysis in the United States while awaiting renal transplantation. Nearly 20,000 kidney transplants are performed annually, of which about two-thirds are from living related donors and one-third are cadaveric in origin.

A. Immunology of transplantation. The major histocompatibility (MHC) antigens are responsible for allowing the host to recognize the graft as foreign. These antigens are located on the short arm of chromosome 6 and encode polymorphic cell surface molecules called human leukocyte antigens (HLAs). The HLA type is inherited in a Mendelian fashion. The HLA types are divided into class I and class II according to cellular location and their structure. The MHC antigens are involved in forming complexes of foreign proteins that can be recognized by T cells and B cells.

B. Rejection. Acute graft rejection is a T cell-dependent process that occurs through either a direct or an indirect pathway. In the direct pathway, cytotoxic T cells, referred to as CD8+ T cells, are involved and lead to early graft rejection by direct cell contact, during which cytoplasmic granules containing cytotoxic substances are released. In the indirect pathway, cells known as CD4+ T cells recognize the donor MHC allopeptides presented by the antigen-presenting cells. Once activated, these cells initiate rejection and destroy the graft by recruiting B cells, which bind to the cell surface of the allograft and destroy the cells by complement-mediated lysis. In addition, cells known as natural killer cells participate in tissue destruction by producing cytokines and phospholipases.

C. Evaluation and selection of the recipient. With current advances in critical care and significant reduction in acute and chronic rejection consequent to newer immunosuppressive therapies, the number of potential renal transplant recipients has increased. The accepted age range of recipients is approximately 1 to 70 years.

   1. The **pretransplantation work-up** of recipients begins with a detailed history and physical examination. Laboratory studies should include a complete blood cell count with differential, measurement of serum electrolytes, liver function tests, determination of prothrombin and partial thromboplastin time and levels of calcium, magnesium, and phosphorus, ABO blood typing, and viral serologies, including titers for toxoplasmosis, rubella, cytomegalovirus infection, and herpes (TORCH). In addition, the patient should be screened for hepatitis and infection with human immunodeficiency virus (HIV). If the patient is not anuric, a urine specimen should be obtained for analysis and culture. Tissue typing, chest roentgenography, and electrocardiography complete the routine initial evaluation. In certain cases, an echocardiogram, exercise or thallium cardiac stress test, pulmonary function test, and coronary angiogram may be appropriate. A dental evaluation and psychosocial assessment may be indicated. Evaluation of the lower urinary tract is crucial, as the success of the transplant depends on appropriate bladder function and the absence of obstruction (e.g., obstructing prostate, urethral strictures, congenital urethral valves). A voiding cystourethrogram (VCUG) and urodynamic studies are performed to rule out obstruction and determine bladder capacity and compliance. Cystoscopy may be useful as well in selected patients if bladder tumors are suspected. A VCUG is generally avoided in the presence of polycystic kidney disease, for fear of introducing infection.

   2. **Immunologic evaluation.** Because the histocompatibility system is based on the ABO blood group and HLA systems, the donor and recipient should be ABO compatible. ABO incompatibility may result in hyperacute rejection. However, studies have shown that successful transplantation of kidneys from both living and cadaveric sources without ABO compatibility has been performed. This requires removal of anti-A and anti-B antibodies by immunoadsorption, plasmapheresis, or splenectomy. HLA matching is routinely performed to assess

the degree of compatibility between donor and recipient. Through the years, it has been observed that transplants between HLA-identical siblings have the longest survival in comparison with mismatched transplants. The survival of one-haplotype-matched grafts is second best. Studies have demonstrated the relevance of HLA matching in cadaveric kidney transplants. The rate of loss of allograft is constant after the first year of transplantation. At 8 years, approximately one-half of cadaveric renal transplants are still viable. Perfectly HLA-matched transplants represent only about 7% of cases, but half are still viable at 19 years. However, it has also been observed that the rate of graft survival varies among the different centers, from 60% to 90%. With the development of newer immunosuppressive agents, graft survival will continue to improve.

D. Preparation for renal transplant recipient

1. Exclusion criteria. Active malignancy, sepsis, active tuberculosis, severe vasculitis, significant vascular disease, AIDS, active hepatitis, recent myocardial infarction, active lupus, extremes of age (<1 year and generally >70 years), and impaired mental function generally preclude transplantation.

2. Nephrectomy. Indications for pretransplant nephrectomy include uncontrolled hypertension, renal infection, renal calculi, obstruction of the upper tract, severe ureteral reflux, and renal malignancy. Polycystic kidney disease may require nephrectomy if persistent infection is present or if the sheer size of the native kidneys precludes implantation of the allograft.

3. Urologic procedures. Vesicoureteral reflux remains the most common abnormality of the lower urinary tract. This condition may predispose the patient to infection in the native kidneys, especially after transplantation. Reflux can be treated by injecting Teflon or collagen at the ureteral orifice or by ureteral reimplantation. In cases of prior cystectomy, the ureter of the transplanted kidney may be anastomosed to the existing urinary diversion. Obstructing conditions such as benign prostatic hyperplasia or congenital urethral valves should be corrected surgically.

E. Living related kidney donor. Living renal transplants offer significant advantages over cadaveric grafts. Living related kidney allografts have been shown to have better survival during the first year. The average "half-life" of a fully matched living related transplant is 25 years. With the advent of newer immunosuppressive agents, however, the gap between cadaveric and living related graft survival continues to narrow. Unfortunately, there is a considerable shortage of cadaveric allografts. On average, it takes 3 to 4 years for a patient on dialysis to receive a kidney allograft. The graft survival of spousal living unrelated transplants is comparable with that of one-haplotype-matched living related grafts. In the United States, living related transplants represent 35% of all renal transplants.

1. Evaluation. A potential living donor is extensively evaluated. The evaluation closely parallels that of the recipient, with the addition of a test called a mixed lymphocyte culture,

Table 25.13. Exclusion criteria for living-related donors

Age	<18 or >65 y
Hypertension	>140/90 mm Hg
Diabetes	Abnormal glucose tolerance test
Urine protein	>250 mg/24 h
Renal stones	Positive history
Creatinine clearance	<80 mL/min
Hematuria	Present
Obesity	>30% above ideal weight
Medical illness	Malignancy, pulmonary or cardiac disease, HIV, hepatitis

HIV, human immunodeficiency virus.

in which lymphocytes from the proposed donor are incubated in serum from the recipient to anticipate a possible rejection episode. Further, imaging of the aorta and renal vessels with angiography allows the surgeon to select the more technically appropriate kidney. Magnetic resonance angiography may soon replace conventional angiography. The left kidney is often chosen because of the extra length of the renal vein.

2. Inclusion criteria. Qualified living donors must have two normally functioning kidneys and are usually between 18 and 65 years of age. One of the most important aspects is the donor's willingness to donate an organ. Every patient should understand the inherent risks of undergoing a nephrectomy under general anesthesia. With 20 years of follow-up, the life expectancy of a donor and that of a person with two native kidneys have not been found to differ.

3. Exclusion criteria. Potential donors are excluded if there is any history of hypertension, renal disease, diabetes mellitus, hepatitis, HIV infection, or malignancy (Table 25.13).

4. Living related donor nephrectomy. Laparoscopic hand-assisted donor nephrectomy is now the standard approach in most transplant centers. As discussed in Chapter 12, the procedure has been demonstrated to greatly decrease postoperative discomfort and shorten hospital stay. During the operation, great care is taken to preserve even the smallest accessory renal arteries (e.g., branches of the lower pole). Length of the renal vein is maximized to facilitate reimplantation. Careful preservation of the periureteral adventitia helps maintain the ureteral blood supply. Often, diuresis is induced with mannitol and furosemide just before division of the main renal vessels to help avoid ATN.

F. Cadaveric renal donors. Cadaveric renal transplants now account for approximately one-third of all transplants performed.

1. Criteria for brain death. Although the laws defining brain death vary from state to state, it is usually defined as the complete and irreversible loss of all cerebral and brainstem functions (Table 25.14). This determination is usually based on a thorough physical examination followed by results of confirmatory diagnostic tests such as the absence of any re-

Table 25.14.   Criteria for brain death

Cerebral unresponsiveness
  No response to painful stimuli
Apnea
  No spontaneous respiration
Absent brainstem reflexes
  Pupillary, corneal, oculocephalic, oculovestibular, oropharyngeal
Confirmatory tests
  Electroencephalography, radionuclide brain scan, cerebral angiography

sponse to noxious stimuli. An observation period of 24 hours is often required before the declaration is made. An apnea test is performed by ventilating the patient with 100% oxygen for 10 minutes and then disconnecting the ventilator for 3 to 5 minutes, with oxygen supplied passively through a tracheal cannula. This normally results in hypercarbia, which in turn stimulates spontaneous breathing. After 5 minutes, arterial blood gases are measured, and the patient is reconnected to the ventilator. The test result is considered positive if the arterial carbon dioxide tension is >60 mm Hg and no spontaneous respiration is observed during the test. On occasion, an electroencephalogram or measurement of cerebral blood flow (nuclear scan or cerebral angiogram) may be performed. Donor acceptance criteria vary between transplant centers but are usually based on parameters as such as age, weight, ABO compatibility, serology, results of liver function tests, and general health status of the potential donor.

2.   Preparation of cadaveric donor. The donor should be carefully maintained in a hemodynamically stable state to facilitate adequate perfusion of the organs. The serum osmolarity is measured at frequent intervals to assess fluid status. An arterial line for continuous monitoring of blood pressure and a central or pulmonary artery catheter can be used to monitor the patient further. The ventilator parameters are monitored by arterial blood gas measurements, and the oxygen saturation is maintained at 100%. As hypothalamic control is lost, wide variations in body temperature may be seen. The core temperature should be maintained above 34°C. Any coagulopathy should be corrected by the use of fresh frozen plasma.

3.   Surgical technique. A long midline incision from sternal notch to pubis is routinely used. The kidneys are often harvested at the same time that other teams harvest the eyes, heart, pancreas, and liver. The peritoneal contents are examined to rule out any intraabdominal sepsis or neoplasm. The abdominal aorta and inferior vena cava are then exposed by mobilization of the right side of the colon. The pancreas along with the duodenum is retracted upward and the celiac axis exposed. The proximal aorta is freed from surrounding structures for cross-clamping at this segment. The aorta and vena cava are cannulated at a point proximal to their bifurcation

(Fig. 25.5), and 300 U of heparin/kg of body weight is given intravenously. The aorta and vena cava are cross-clamped. The cold preservation solution is infused through the cannulas. The kidneys are removed en bloc with Gerota's fascia intact. The ureter is bluntly dissected along its course and divided at the bladder. The vena cava and aorta are divided in the midline, and the kidneys are separated. Currently, the kidneys are preserved by simple static cold storage.

G.   Technique of transplantation. After induction of general anesthesia, the bladder is distended with 100 to 150 mL of a solution containing bacitracin (50,000 U) and 1 g of kanamycin/L to improve intraoperative identification. A Gibson incision is made either in the right or in the left lower quadrant. The subcutaneous tissue and the external oblique, internal oblique, and transverse muscles are divided with electrocautery. The inferior epigastric vessels are divided and ligated. In women, the round ligament can be divided and ligated. The spermatic cord is identified and preserved. The retroperitoneum is entered, and the lymphatics over the iliac vessels are ligated and divided to prevent a lymphocele. The transplant kidney is inspected and the vessels prepared for anastomosis. Generally, the renal vein is anastomosed to the external iliac vein, then the renal artery to the internal iliac artery (Fig. 25.6). At completion of the vascular anastomosis, 40 mg of furosemide and 12.5 mg of mannitol are given to initiate diuresis. On release of the cross-clamp, the kidney is expected to be perfused homogeneously and become firm. The ureter is then passed posteriorly to the spermatic cord and anastomosed to the bladder by an extravesical or intravesical (less commonly performed) method. A submucosal tunnel is created by using the overlying detrusor muscle and perivesical pad of fat to prevent reflux. Postoperatively, hemodynamic monitoring is essential to optimize graft function and fluid management. Monitoring of blood pressure is critical, as the initial arterial blood flow to the graft depends on the mean systemic arterial pressure. A pulmonary artery catheter may be required in some patients for the initial 48 hours. Managing blood pressure in these patients is somewhat complicated, as most have long-standing systemic hypertension. High systolic blood pressure in the immediate postoperative period increases the risk for cerebrovascular accidents. On the other hand, reduced arterial blood pressure may increase the risk for ATN in the graft and vascular thrombosis. If the systolic blood pressure is consistently elevated, pharmacologic intervention is required.

1.   Postoperative orders. Typical postoperative orders are as follows:

a.   Bed rest for 48 hours (patient supine or lying on same side as transplant).

b.   Measure vital signs and input and output every hour for the first 24 hours, then every 4 hours from the second postoperative day.

c.   Nothing by mouth.

d.   Obtain body weight every morning.

e.   Replace fluids intravenously. If urine output is <200 mL/h, replace hourly output and insensible water loss (5% dextrose in half-normal saline solution at 30 mL/h). I

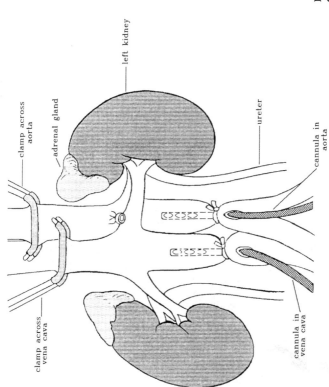

Fig. 25.5. Technique of en bloc kidney harvest in cadaveric donor.

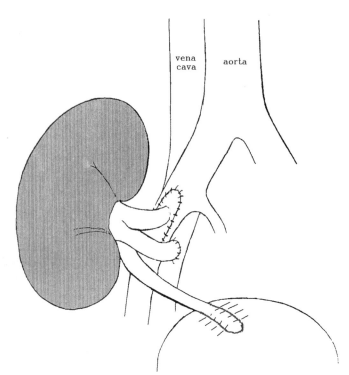

Fig. 25.6.   Technique of vascular and ureteral anastomosis in renal transplantation.

output is >200 mL/h, replace 200 mL plus two-thirds of amount of output in excess of 200 mL.
f.   Irrigate Foley catheter with normal saline solution as needed if blood clots are noted in urine or if acute drop in urine output occurs.
g.   Check dialysis fistula every 4 hours.
h.   No blood pressure measurement or intravenous line in extremity with fistula.
i.   Obtain complete blood cell count and measure electrolytes (chem 7) every 6 hours, then every morning.
j.   Determine cyclosporin level every other day.
k.   Perform urine culture twice a week.
l.   Obtain nuclear renal scan on postoperative day 1.
m.   Obtain renal US on postoperative day 5.
n.   Obtain cystogram on postoperative day 5.
o.   Immunosuppression as ordered.
2.   Postoperative care. The insensible fluid loss is replaced with dextrose solution, and urine replacement should be with half-normal saline solution. A bolus of saline solution can be given to those patients who are assessed to be hypovolemic or euvolemic to increase the urine output. If the urine output de-

clines or stops abruptly, the Foley catheter should be flushed to clear any blood clots. If the patient remains oliguric or anuric, the fluid status should be assessed carefully. If the patient fails to respond to furosemide or volume challenge, further studies are required, including a Doppler scan and US of the graft to assess blood flow and rule out extravasation of urine. The nuclear scan is performed routinely on postoperative day 1 and may be repeated to assess renal function. In patients who become hypotensive, after assessment of fluid status, early postoperative bleeding should be considered. Most hematomas resolve spontaneously and do not require surgical intervention. If generalized bleeding develops secondary to uremia-induced platelet dysfunction, desmopressin acetate can be used. In oliguric patients, postoperative dialysis may be required until the kidney functions. Persistently hyperkalemic patients may also require dialysis. A nuclear scan with 99mTc-mercaptoacetyltriglycine is obtained on day 1 to assess the perfusion and function of the graft. A cystogram and US are obtained on day 5. If the cystogram is unremarkable, the Foley catheter is removed. Most patients are discharged to home by postoperative day 6. About 30% to 50% of the cadaveric kidneys function immediately. When graft function is delayed, some studies report that 1-year graft survival is reduced by 20%. Various factors such as donor age above 55 years, ATN, prolonged duration of graft ischemia, intraoperative hypotension, previous transplants, early use of the monoclonal antibody muromanab-CD3 (OKT3), and high doses of cyclosporin play a role in delayed graft function. Rejection episodes are managed as described in the section on immunosuppression.

H. Immunosuppression. At the present time, triple immunosuppression with cyclosporin or tacrolimus, prednisone or other glucocorticoid, and mycophenolate mofetil (CellCept) or azathioprine continues to be commonly used. Antilymphocyte antibody preparations are sometimes used as immunosuppression primers. The following is a brief overview of the most commonly used immunosuppressive agents.

1. Cyclosporin is available in two forms: Sandimmune and the microemulsion form called Neoral. Cyclosporin impairs expression of critical T-cell activation genes, including those coding for interleukin-2 and its receptor and for the proto-oncogenes H-*ras* and c-*myc*. The expression of transforming growth factor-β is enhanced by cyclosporin, which again inhibits interleukin-2 and the production of cytotoxic T lymphocytes. Cyclosporin leaves the phagocytic activity of neutrophils intact and does not affect antigen recognition. Cyclosporin is available in both liquid and capsule form. Absorption of cyclosporin is incomplete and varies from patient to patient. Bioavailability is about 35% to 45%. A steady blood level is reached in about 4 to 8 weeks. **Neoral** is formulated in a microemulsion form and is found to have improved bioavailability. The half-life of cyclosporin is 8 hours, and it is metabolized by the cytochrome P-450 microsomal enzyme system in the liver and gastrointestinal system. It is primarily excreted in bile and does not require dose alteration in the case of renal dysfunction resulting from ATN or rejection.

2. Drug interactions. Drugs that may reduce cyclosporin levels include rifampin, isoniazid, barbiturates, phenytoin, carbamazepine, nafcillin, trimethoprim, sulfadimidine (intravenous), cephalosporins, and imipenem. Drugs that may increase cyclosporin levels include calcium channel blockers (verapamil, diltiazem, nicardipine). Use of these drugs for hypertension control in the posttransplant period may help to reduce the dosage up to 40%. The antifungal drugs ketoconazole, fluconazole, and itraconazole increase cyclosporin levels significantly. Some centers use this combination routinely to reduce the cost of cyclosporin. Erythromycin, histamine blockers, and hormones (corticosteroids, testosterone, oral contraceptives, norethindrone) all may increase cyclosporin levels. Amphotericin, aminoglycosides, NSAIDs, enalapril, metoclopramide, colchicine, cholestyramine, and lovastatin should be used with caution, as they may increase the nephrotoxicity of cyclosporin.

3. Toxicity. Nephrotoxicity induced by cyclosporin may be manifested by a wide variety of syndromes (Table 25.15), including acute and chronic decreases in glomerular filtration, acute microvascular disease, worsening of early graft dysfunction, hypertension, hypomagnesemia, hyperchloremic acidosis, hyperuricemia, and gout. It may be difficult to differentiate cyclosporin toxicity from acute rejection (Table 25.16). Other complications may include hepatotoxicity, cholelithiasis, hypertrichosis, hyperlipidemia, impairment of glucose tolerance, tremor, bone pain, headache, and deep venous thrombosis.

4. Mycophenolate (CellCept). Approved in 1995, this drug reversibly inhibits the enzyme inosine monophosphate dehydrogenase and exerts a selective antiproliferative effect on lymphocytes. Mycophenolate is found to be effective in

Table 25.15. Toxicity of cyclosporin A

Nephrotoxicity

Hypertension

Biochemical effects
  Hyperbilirubinemia
  Hyperkalemia
  Hyperuricemia
  Increased alkaline phosphatase

Neurologic effects
  Seizure
  Tremor
  Paresthesias

Miscellaneous
  Hirsutism
  Anorexia
  Nausea
  Gingival hypertrophy
  Breast fibroadenoma

Table 25.16.   Differentiating acute rejection
from cyclosporin A nephrotoxicity

	Acute Rejection	Cyclosporin A
Serum creatinine	>50% rapid increase	<25% slow increase
Intrarenal pressure	Elevated	Normal
Fever	May be present	Usually absent
Cyclosporin A level	<100 ng/mL	>250 ng/mL

treating ongoing rejection and is able to prevent rejection
episodes effectively when used in conjunction with cyclosporin
and steroids. Diarrhea occurs in about one-third of patients
receiving mycophenolate. Esophagitis, gastritis, and gastrointestinal bleeding are observed in 4% to 5% of treated patients. Leukopenia, anemia, and rarely lymphomas occur in
<1% of patients.

5.   Polyclonal antibodies. Antithymocyte globulin is the
only polyclonal antibody currently available in the United
States. The monoclonal antibody muromanab-CD3 (OKT3)
has been used for many years. Antithymocyte globulin is derived from immunizing either horses or rabbits with human
lymphoid tissue and then harvesting the γ-globulin fractions.
Once routinely administered for induction in the immediate
posttransplant period, antithymocyte globulin is now used
mostly for treating rejection. When it is given intravenously, a
drop in the total lymphocyte count is noted as T cells are lysed
and driven into the reticuloendothelial system. The usual dose
of 10 to 20 mg/kg/day is given for 7 to 14 days through a central vein. The patient will require premedication with 30 mg
of prednisone, 50 mg of diphenhydramine (Benadryl) IV, and
650 mg of oral acetaminophen (Tylenol) 30 minutes before administration of antithymocyte globulin. Adverse effects may
include fever, chills, and arthralgias.

6.   Monoclonal antibodies are produced by the hybridization of murine antibody-secreting B lymphocytes with
nonsecreting myeloma cell lines. Currently, OKT3 is the only
available agent approved for human therapeutic use. This
drug attacks the CD3 antigen complex of mature T cells and
is used most commonly for steroid-resistant rejection. It is
also used less frequently for induction, primary rejection
treatment, and rejection prophylaxis. The standard dose is
5 mg given intravenously through a Millipore filter. The
usual course is for 10 days. Before the first dose of OKT3, patients should undergo chest roentgenography to rule out congestive heart failure. Patients in congestive heart failure
may require dialysis. Patients may require premedication
with 5 to 8 mg of methylprednisolone/kg, 50 mg of diphenhydramine IV, and 650 mg of acetaminophen PO.

I.   Management of acute rejection

1.   Pulse steroids. The first episode of acute rejection can
be managed successfully about 75% of the time with high

doses of steroids. Often, 500 to 1,000 mg of methylpred nisolone (Solu-Medrol) IV is given once a day for 3 days. Some centers use low-dose pulsing with 120 to 250 mg of prednisone PO for 3 to 5 days. The patients are then placed back on their usual immunosuppression regimen following pulsing.

2.   If patients fail to respond to pulsing with steroids alone, **intravenous OKT3** is used for 10 to 14 days. About 90% of acute rejections can be treated successfully with OKT3. For patients with refractory rejection, a second course of OKT3 may be used. However, long-term graft function is achieved in only about 40% to 50% of patients. High levels of OKT3 antibodies may develop, which limits the further use of this agent.

J.   Complications have been declining in frequency following renal transplantation during the last two decades. Improve ments in surgical technique, better diagnostic methods to eval uate postoperative problems, and better immunosuppressive agents are likely responsible.

1.   Vascular complications. The overall reported incidence ranges between 6% and 30%. Arterial complications are more frequent than venous complications.

The incidence of renal artery thrombosis, which manifests by abrupt anuria in a previously well-functioning allograft is about 1%. Other causes such as an occluded Foley catheter or prerenal azotemia should be excluded before a renal scan is obtained. Delay in diagnosis results in a 50% to 60% mor tality rate secondary to occult sepsis.

a.   Renal artery thrombosis is attributed to technical problems such as dissection or an intimal flap, occlusion re sulting from technique or atherosclerotic vessels, or kinking or torsion of the vessels. Renal artery stenosis may be caused by occlusive atherosclerotic disease or intimal hyperplasia of the recipient or donor artery. The reported incidence varies from 2% to 10%. Renal artery stenosis manifests by refrac tory hypertension, decline in renal function of the allograft, and an audible bruit over the allograft. Several imaging modalities are available to evaluate and diagnose the steno sis. These include a duplex scan, captopril scan, and digital subtraction angiography. The sensitivity of these studies varies from 50% to 80%. Arteriography remains the gold standard for confirming the diagnosis. Treatment options include percutaneous transluminal angioplasty and surgi cal revision.

b.   Renal vein thrombosis is a rare complication follow ing renal transplantation, with a reported incidence of 0.3% to 4%. Thrombosis of the renal vein results in irreversible graft damage. The signs and symptoms include graft swell ing and pain or tenderness over the graft, hematuria, and oliguria. Diagnosis can be made by duplex sonography or renal scintigraphy. However, it is difficult to differentiate renal vein thrombosis from acute rejection based on these studies, as the findings are similar for both conditions. Most often, renal vein thrombosis is diagnosed at exploration. Successful recovery of graft function with infusion of strepto kinase has been reported.

c. Vascular anastomotic disruption is a rare complication following transplantation that may result from mycotic aneurysm or infection of the anastomosis. Technical factors such as overt tension on the anastomotic site, missed arterial or venous laceration, or disrupted ligature after the transplant may be responsible. This condition manifests with symptoms of hemorrhage and back pain. Operative exploration for possible salvage of the graft is required. However, repair is associated with a high rate of rebleeding, and most often nephrectomy is required. A mortality rate of 35% to 50% has been reported.

2. Ureteral complications. Ureteral complications can be classified according to whether they are caused by leakage or obstruction. The donor ureter depends solely on the hilar vasculature of the graft for its blood supply. The donor ureter should be handled with care to prevent devascularization, from the time of donation to the time of implantation.

a. Ureteral leakage from the hilum or anastomotic site occurs in from 3% to 10% of cases. This is usually secondary to tension at the anastomosis, which causes ischemia of the distal segment. Less likely are changes in the ureter resulting from rejection. These patients usually have a wide variety of symptoms such as pain and swelling of the graft, fever, oliguria, elevated serum creatinine, cutaneous drainage, or sepsis. US may identify peritransplant fluid collections in about 67% of patients. Percutaneous antegrade pyelography has a sensitivity of 85%. Management depends on the site and amount of the fluid collection. Percutaneous drainage with ureteral stenting may be adequate. Surgical exploration and correction of the problem ensure good drainage and reduce the risk for development of sepsis. Depending on the findings, either revision of the anastomosis with an indwelling stent or a diverting nephrostomy or creation of a flap by using the recipient's bladder to replace the necrotic ureter may be necessary. The stents are removed 2 weeks after a cystogram demonstrates no extravasation.

b. Obstruction of the transplanted ureter without leakage may also be seen. During the early postoperative period, this may be caused by edema of the ureter, hematoma in the wall of the distal ureter, or malrotation or kinking. Obstruction that develops over time is related to fibrosis resulting from chronic ischemia or to extrinsic compression by a lymphocele or a mass. Patients present with oliguria, sepsis, rising creatinine, and graft tenderness. US is useful in making the diagnosis. Antegrade pyelography will delineate the actual site and degree of obstruction. The Whitaker test can be useful in making the diagnosis. Surgical exploration with revision of the ureteroneocystostomy is preferable to percutaneous balloon dilatation.

3. Bladder complications usually appear soon after transplantation.

a. Extravasation from the bladder suture line may manifest as a rise in serum creatinine, a palpable suprapubic mass, a tender graft, and/or dysuria. Pelvic US or cystogram can confirm the diagnosis. Complications are usually managed by surgical repair.

b. Lymphoceles may occur in the pelvis following transplantation. The incidence ranges from 0.6% to 18%. Lymphoceles may develop as a result of inadequate ligation of the lymphatics during dissection or as a result of decapsulation of the kidney transplant. Most lymphoceles are small and resolve spontaneously. Larger lymphoceles may exert pressure on adjacent structures such as the bladder, ureter, iliac vein, or lymphatics. The presence of lymphoceles can be confirmed by US. If resolution does not occur after a period of observation, intervention may be required. US-guided laparoscopic or open drainage is effective in managing lymphoceles.

4. Pelvic hematoma may result from uremic coagulopathies, unrecognized minor trauma to the donor hilar vessels, or the use of heparin intraoperatively and during preoperative dialysis. Symptoms may include pain over the graft site, a palpable mass, and a drop in hematocrit. US is useful in making the diagnosis. Large, expanding hematomas require surgical intervention. Smaller hematomas may resolve spontaneously.

5. Infectious and other complications. Renal transplant patients are at a high risk for infection because of their immunocompromised status. The antiinflammatory properties of steroids delay wound healing. Other risk factors that predispose to infection include diabetes mellitus, hepatitis and C, leukopenia, splenectomy, and the use of cadaveric organs. The incidence of posttransplant infectious complications has decreased during the last several years. It is known that recipients are at a higher risk for common infections as well as opportunistic infections. Opportunistic infections occur from 1 to 6 months postoperatively. Unusual infections with bacteria and slow-growing fungi become clinically apparent between 6 months and 1 year after transplantation. Identification and prophylaxis of infection begin at the time of the transplant evaluation. Patients are screened for active infection and for exposure before transplant to any organisms that could become active following immunosuppression. As described in the section on preoperative evaluation, routine screening is performed for toxoplasmosis, hepatitis, herpes simplex, and infection with Epstein–Barr virus, cytomegalovirus, varicella-zoster virus, and HIV. All donors, both living and cadaveric, are screened in the same way. During the operative procedure, patients benefit from administration of intravenous antibiotics. Most commonly, a cephalosporin or penicillin antibiotic is administered to cover *S. aureus*. Preoperative bladder washing or instillation has no proven value.

K. Malignancy in transplant patients is an important issue. Some form of cancer will develop in about two-thirds of patients with transplants for >20 years.

1. The incidence of **lymphoma** in renal transplant patients is about 1% to 2%; the most common type is non-Hodgkin B-cell lymphoma. Epstein–Barr virus infection has been found to be a great risk factor, especially in seronegative patients who receive a seropositive organ. Epstein–Barr virus binds to epithelial oropharyngeal cells and replicates, inducing a latent infection. This results in transformation of B cells and production of lymphoblastoid cells. The mortality rate in transplanted patients is almost 50 times that of the general population. Polyclonal B-cell lesions respond to discontinuation of immunosuppression and antiviral therapy. Monoclonal lesions are malignant and may represent later stages of the disease; they sometimes respond to cessation of immunosuppression and chemotherapy. Patients with polyclonal B-cell lesions are most likely to respond to therapy with acyclovir. Unfortunately, discontinuation of immunosuppression usually leads to rapid loss of the graft.

2. Skin cancers are about 20 times more common in transplant patients than in the general population. Male sex, mismatched transplants at the HLA-B locus, and recipient homozygosity for HLA-DR have been found to be associated with higher risk for development of squamous cell cancer. The incidence of squamous cell carcinoma is more common than that of basal cell carcinoma. Malignant melanomas account for about 5% of skin cancers in these patients. Kaposi's sarcoma is rare and tends to respond to withdrawal of immunosuppression coupled with chemotherapy and radiotherapy. Avoidance of excessive exposure to sun, use of topical sunscreens and low-dose retinoids, surgical excision of suspected lesions, and aggressive dermatologic surveillance are the keys to management and prevention of skin cancers in this patient population.

3. Other malignancies. The incidence of cancers of the lung, prostate, colon, rectum, and breast in transplant patients is not increased in comparison with the incidence in the general population. Women with kidney transplants should undergo a pelvic examination and Papanicolaou smear every year. Those with a history of genital warts require more frequent examinations.

SUGGESTED READING

Barry JM. Unstented extravesical ureteroneocystostomy in kidney transplantation. *J Urol* 1983;129:918–919.

Basile JJ, McCullough DL, Harrison LH, et al. End-stage renal disease associated with acquired cystic disease and neoplasia. *J Urol* 1988;140:938–943.

Berman SJ. Infections in patients with end-stage renal disease: an overview. *Infect Dis Clin North Am* 2001;15:709–720.

Brady HR, Singer GG. Acute renal failure. *Lancet* 1995;346:1533–1540.

Brayman KL, Matas AJ, Schmidt W, et al. Analysis of infectious complications occurring after solid organ transplantation. *Arch Surg* 1992;127:38–48.

Brennan J, Babayan RK, Siroky MB. Acquired cystic kidney disease: urologic implications. *Br J Urol* 1991;67:342–348.

Cooper K, Bennett WM. Nephrotoxicity of common drugs used in clinical practice. *Arch Intern Med* 1987;147:1213–1218.

Dunn JF, Nylander WA, Richiere RE, et al. Living related kidney donors: a 14-year experience. *Ann Surg* 1986;203:637–643.

Forni LG, Hilton PJ. Continuous hemofiltration in the treatment of acute renal failure. *N Engl J Med* 1997;336:1303–1309.

Hyman A, Mendelssohn DC. Current Canadian approaches to dialysis for acute renal failure in the ICU. *Am J Nephrol* 2002;22:29–3.

Ifudu O. Care of patients undergoing hemodialysis. *N Engl J Me* 1998;339:1054–1062.

Kellum JA, Angus DC, Johnson JP, et al. Continuous versus intermittent renal replacement therapy: a meta-analysis. *Intensi Care Med* 2002;28:29–37.

Khauli RB, Stoff JS, Lovewell T. Post-transplant lymphoceles: a critical look into the risk factors, pathophysiology and managemen *J Urol* 1993;150:22–26.

Mehta RL, Letteri JM. Current status of renal replacement therap for acute renal failure: a survey of US nephrologists. *Am J Nephr* 1999;19:377–382.

Mehta R, McDonald B, Gabbai F, et al. A randomized clinic trial continuous versus intermittent dialysis for acute renal failur *Kidney Int* 2001;60:1154–1163.

Nolph KD, Kindblad AS, Novak JW. Current concepts: continuous an bulatory peritoneal dialysis. *N Engl J Med* 1988;318:1595–1600.

Palder SB, Kirkman RL, Whittemore AD, et al. Vascular access f hemodialysis. *Ann Surg* 1985;202:235–239.

Palevsky PM. Acute renal failure. *J Am Soc Nephrol* 2003;2:41–76.

Pastan S, Bailey J. Dialysis therapy. *N Engl J Med* 1998;33 1428–1437.

Rabbat CG. Comparison of mortality risk for dialysis patients and c daveric first renal transplant recipients in Ontario, Canada. *J A Soc Nephrol* 2000;11:917–922.

Swartz RD, Messana JM, Orzol S, et al. Comparing continuous hem filtration with hemodialysis in patients with severe acute ren failure. *Am J Kidney Dis* 1999;34:424–432.

Thadhani R, Pascual M, Bonventre JV. Acute renal failure. *N Engl Med* 1996;334:1448–1460.

U.S. Renal Data System. *USRDS 2000 annual data report: atl of end-stage renal disease in the United States*. Bethesda, M National Institute of Diabetes and Digestive and Kidney Disease NIH, 2000.

Van de Noortgate N, Verbeke F, Dhondt A, et al. The dialytic ma agement of acute renal failure in the elderly. *Semin Dialys* 2002;15:127–132.

Wyner LM, Novick AC, Streem SB. Improved success of living u related renal transplantation with cyclosporin immunosuppressio *J Urol* 1993;149:706–708.

Perioperative Care
of the Patient

Rie Aihara

I. Preoperative risk assessment is necessary to identify and minimize the risk of major cardiopulmonary complications and death in patients undergoing elective surgery. General determinants of surgical risk are patient age and physical health as well as the type of surgery (major, minor, elective, emergent). The classification of the American Society of Anesthesiologists is commonly used as a nonspecific indicator of risk based on patient status (Table 26.1). The varying risk associated with various surgical procedures is presented in Table 26.2. The confluence of these two types of risk—that due to the patient and that due to the procedure—determines the actual risk to the patient.

A. Cardiac complications following surgery include myocardial infarction, congestive heart failure (pulmonary edema), and cardiac arrhythmias. The risks of postoperative pulmonary edema and cardiac arrhythmias are each 7% in patients with cardiac disease undergoing noncardiac surgery. In patients with evidence of cardiac disease, the risk of myocardial infarction following noncardiac surgery is about 1% in contrast to a risk of about 0.2% for patients without cardiac disease. However, the risk of myocardial infarction can be as high as 35% in patients with poor cardiac function undergoing major surgery. Other factors include the patient's functional status (Table 26.3). Perioperative cardiac risk is significantly increased in patients who cannot exercise to a level of 4 metabolic equivalents during normal activities of daily living (Table 26.3).

B. Preoperative cardiac evaluation may result in various clinical decisions to reduce the risk to the patient, including (a) optimizing preoperative medical management, (b) reevaluating the decision to perform surgery, (c) pursuing further cardiac evaluation (including cardiac catheterization), and (d) monitoring the patient postoperatively in the intensive care unit (ICU) or coronary care unit. Specific techniques of cardiac evaluation will not be considered here.

1. History seeks to identify risk factors for coronary heart disease, such as prior angina, recent or past myocardial infarction, heart failure, symptomatic arrhythmias, and use of cardiac pacemaker. Documenting the presence of other conditions such as peripheral vascular disease, cerebrovascular disease, diabetes mellitus, renal impairment, and chronic pulmonary disease is important. Note any recent worsening of angina. Document all current medications and their doses as well as the use of alcohol, tobacco, and nonprescription drugs. Determine the patient's functional capacity by asking about the example activities in Table 26.3.

2. Physical examination should be tailored to identify conditions that increase operative risk, such as heart failure,

Table 26.1.   ASA classification of physical status

ASA class I	A normal healthy patient
ASA class II	A patient with mild systemic disease
ASA class III	A patient with severe systemic disease that limits activity but is not incapacitating
ASA class IV	A patient with incapacitating systemic disease that is a constant threat to life
ASA class V	A moribund patient not expected to survive 24 h with or without surgery
E	Designates an emergency surgical procedure

ASA, American Society of Anesthesiologists.

Table 26.2.   Risk of cardiac complications in various procedures

High Risk (>5%)	Intermediate Risk (<5%)	Low Risk (<1%)
Major emergency operation	Carotid endarterectomy	Endoscopic procedures
Aortic/major vascular surgery	Head/neck surgery	Skin procedures
Peripheral vascular surgery	Abdominal/thoracic surgery	Cataract surgery
Procedures with large fluid	Orthopedic surgery	Breast surgery
Shifts/blood loss	Prostate surgery	

Table 26.3.   Functional status assessment

Excellent (>7 METs)	Moderate (4–7 METs)	Poor (<4 METs)
Squash	Cycling	Vacuuming
Jogging (10-min mile)	Climbing flight of stairs	Activities of daily living (e.g., eating, dressing, bathing)
Scrubbing floors	Golf (without cart)	Walking 2 mph
Singles tennis	Walking 4 mph	
Yard work	Writing	

METs, metabolic equivalents (70-kg, 40-year-old man resting).

valvular disease, and peripheral vascular disease. Measure the vital signs, including blood pressure in both arms. Palpate the carotid pulse and listen for bruits. Document any distended jugular veins. Auscultation of the lungs should be performed to detect any wheezing or hyperinflation. Precordial auscultation should be done to detect any murmurs or gallop. Palpate the abdomen, looking for organomegaly or abdominal aneurysm. Examine the lower extremities for edema and palpate the peripheral pulses.

3. Electrocardiogram (ECG) is recommended in asymptomatic patients based on patient age and gender. Preoperative ECGs should be obtained in all male patients older than 40 years and female patients older than 50 undergoing any procedure that requires general or spinal anesthesia. Younger patients should have preoperative ECG if there is a history of hypertension, hypercholesterolemia, smoking, diabetes, obesity, cardiac disease in family members, pulmonary disease, radiation therapy, and alcohol or drug abuse. An ECG >2 months old is not adequate for preoperative risk assessment.

4. Cardiac risk indexes. The original Goldman risk index identified nine preoperative factors that were found to be associated with cardiac complications and perioperative cardiac death: myocardial infarction within 6 months, S3 gallop or jugular venous distension, age over 70, rhythm other than sinus on preoperative ECG, >5 preventricular contractions/ min, important aortic stenosis, poor general medical status, emergency surgery, and intraperitoneal, intrathoracic, or aortic surgery. Although validated in many studies, the data, derived from the 1970s, do not reflect current advances. The Goldman index was later modified by Detsky et al. (1986). In 1999, Lee et al. described the revised cardiac risk index. This index uses six independent risk factors: ischemic heart disease, congestive heart failure, cerebral vascular disease, high-risk surgery, preoperative insulin treatment for diabetes mellitus, and preoperative creatinine level >2 mg/dL (Table 26.4). Patients without any risk factors are assigned to the

Table 26.4.   Revised cardiac risk index

Risk factors
  High-risk surgery
  Ischemic heart disease
  History of congestive heart failure
  History of cerebrovascular disease
  Insulin therapy for diabetes
  Preoperative serum creatinine >2.0 mg/dL

Risk Class	No. of Risk Factors	Cardiac Complication Rate (%)
I	0	0.5
II	1	1.3
III	2	3.6
IV	3–6	9.1

lowest risk class (I) and have cardiac complication rates
0.5%. In contrast, patients with three or more risk factors a
assigned to the highest risk class (IV) and have cardiac com
plication rates of about 10%. This type of index can be used t
decide whether patients carry inordinate risk and should hav
diagnostic or therapeutic intervention prior to surgery.

C.   Pulmonary complications include pneumonia, respira
tory failure, bronchospasm, atelectasis, and exacerbation of ur
derlying chronic lung disease. **Smoking** increases the risk
pulmonary complications even in the absence of chronic lun
disease, and all patients undergoing elective surgery shou
be counseled to stop smoking for at least 2 months prior t
surgery. **Chronic obstructive pulmonary disease** increase
the risk of pulmonary complications by a factor of 2.5 to 5. Fc
asthma, current guidelines from the National Heart, Lun
and Blood Institute state that a patient without wheezing an
at >80% of predicted peak flow can proceed to surgery withou
increased risk.

II.   Prophylaxis against endocarditis is indicated in surg
cal patients with prosthetic heart valve, prior history of infectiv
endocarditis, cyanotic congenital heart defect, hypertrophic ca
diomyopathy, or mitral valve prolapse with regurgitation or valv
thickening or both. Endocarditis prophylaxis is not recommende
for atrial septal defect, surgically repaired ventricular septal de
fect, patent ductus arteriosus, mitral valve prolapse without re
gurgitation, mild tricuspid regurgitation, or cardiac pacemake
defibrillator.

The following antimicrobial regimen is suggested for prophy
laxis of genitourinary or gastrointestinal surgery: ampicillin 2
IV and gentamicin 1.5 mg/kg 30 min prior to procedure, followe
by amoxicillin 1 g PO/IV/IM 8 hours later; if allergic to penicillir
alternatives include vancomycin 1 g IV and gentamicin 1.5 mg/k
1 to 2 hours prior to the procedure.

III.   Postoperative care of a patient begins the moment th
surgical procedure is completed. Recovery from surgery can be d
vided into the following stages: (a) emergence from anesthesia [re
covery room or postanesthesia care unit (PACU)], (b) short-ter
recovery during hospital admission, and (c) long-term recover
which takes place at home or in a rehabilitation setting. Th
length of recovery and the level of postoperative care depend o
the type of anesthesia administered (local, regional, general), th
type of procedure performed, the associated comorbidities, and th
occurrence of intraoperative/postoperative complications. Plar
ning for the postoperative period should begin well in advance c
the operation, for example, arranging for an ICU bed when th
need for one is anticipated.

A.   Care in the recovery room or PACU aims at monito
ing the patient for anesthesia-related complications that ma
arise as the patient emerges from anesthesia, for example, acut
pulmonary and hemodynamic events. The staff-to-patient rati
is much higher and monitoring devices are available in thi
acute setting to ensure close observation of the patients. Pai
control is another important aim. Therefore, management i
usually dictated by the anesthesiologist.

1.   Postoperative orders should be written by a membe
of the surgical team at some point between the patient's leav

ing the operating room and arrival in the recovery room. The following is an example of postoperative orders:

Admit: Location (ward, ICU, telemetry, transitional care), service, and the admitting surgeon/team.

Diagnosis: Status/postsurgical procedure performed.

Condition: State the condition of the patient as good (stable) or poor (unstable).

Allergies: Medication, especially to pain medicines and antibiotics; contact allergies such as latex and contrast medium should be mentioned here.

Vital signs: The frequency of the vital signs to be taken should be specified as well as any other exams such as neurologic and vascular checks. Typical is vital signs q5min until stable, then q15min for the first hour, then q30min.

Activity: State whether the patient is to be at bedrest, out of bed to chair, or ambulatory. Any special requirements such as assistance by physical therapy or elevation of head of bed should also be mentioned here.

Nursing: Fluid balances, daily weights, instructions on drains and tubes, venodynes, and dressing orders should be specified under this section.

Diet: NPO (nothing by mouth), clear liquids, regular diet or whether there are any restrictions such as a renal or diabetic diet, tube feedings (specify clearly which tube is to be used).

Intravenous fluids: Type and rate of maintenance intravenous fluid, total parenteral nutrition orders, if applicable.

Medications: Orders for both around-the-clock and as-needed (prn) medications.

Laboratory: Orders for blood tests should be written here. Do not order daily lab orders here—these should be determined on daily rounds.

2. Discharge from PACU. Discharge criteria vary but should include the return of preoperative consciousness level and protective reflexes, maintenance of a clear airway, satisfactory oxygenation (oxygen saturation >93% on room air), and stable pulse and blood pressure. Once discharged from the recovery room by the anesthesiologist, the patient will generally be transferred to the ward under the care of the operating surgical team. Patients who require cardiopulmonary supportive care (such as ventilators and vasopressors), close monitoring, and intensive nursing care will be sent to the ICU until ready for the floor.

B. The **ICU** is necessary for those patients who require close monitoring and/or support of the cardiovascular and pulmonary systems, neurovascular monitoring, frequent assessment of wounds, and a high level of nursing care. Care is provided using a multidisciplinary approach including the intensivists, consulting specialists, nursing staff, respiratory therapists, nutritionists, and pharmacists.

1. Ventilatory support. Postoperative patients may require assistance with ventilation for a variety of reasons including prolonged anesthesia time, underlying pulmonary disease, hemodynamic instability, and airway edema due to

Table 26.5. Criteria for ventilatory support

Blood Gases	Pulmonary Function Tests
$P_{O_2} < 55$ mm Hg	Vital capacity < 10 mL/kg
$P_{CO_2} > 50$ mm Hg	Maximum inspiratory force > -25 cm H_2O
pH < 7.32	$FEV_1 < 10$ mL/kg

FEV_1, forced expiratory volume in 1 s.

traumatic or difficult intubation. Clinical criteria indicating the need for ventilatory support include apnea, respiratory distress with altered mentation, clinically apparent increased work of breathing, and need for airway protection. Other criteria are given in Table 26.5. However, clinical decision making should always overrule laboratory criteria. Patients will require some level of sedation to tolerate the ventilator. A fine balance must be maintained to allow for extubation when that becomes possible. Current ventilators are capable of operating using volume-cycled as well as pressure-cycled volume delivery modes.

   a. Pressure-controlled ventilators are regulated by the peak inspiratory pressure. The delivered volume varies according to the airway resistance and the thoracic compliance. A major advantage of pressure-cycled modes is a decelerating inspiratory flow pattern, in which inspiratory flow tapers off as the lung inflates. This usually results in a more homogeneous gas distribution throughout the lungs. A major disadvantage is that the volume delivered may be quite variable.

   b. Volume-controlled ventilators. The most commonly used modes of ventilation are based on volume control. In these modes, the tidal volume and ventilatory rate are predetermined to give constant minute ventilation (rate × tidal volume). The patients are allowed to take spontaneous breaths in between these predetermined or mandatory machine breaths, in which case the minute ventilation will be the sum of the patient-initiated breaths and the machine-initiated breaths. A major disadvantage of volume-controlled respiration is that high pressures may be generated, resulting in barotrauma to the lungs, especially when high peak inflation pressures (>40 cm H_2O) are delivered. Barotrauma produces alveolar cellular dysfunction, surfactant depletion, and atelectasis as well as an increased risk of pneumothorax.

2. Criteria for extubation. As the patient awakens, the patient can be weaned off the ventilator such that the work of breathing comes increasingly from the patient. This can be accomplished either by gradually decreasing the machine-initiated breaths until every breath taken is initiated by the patient (machine rate of 0) or by gradually decreasing the pressure support given by the ventilator. Once the patient has demonstrated an ability to generate spontaneous breaths

Table 26.6.   Criteria to consider extubation

Blood Gases	Pulmonary Function Tests
$Po_2 > 65$ *on* $F_io_2 < 40\%$ $Pco_2 < 50$ mm Hg	Respiratory rate < 30/min Vital capacity > 10 mL/kg Tidal volume > 5 mL/kg Maximum inspiratory force < –25 cm H_2O

without excessive stress, extubation may be considered. Some criteria to consider for extubation are given in Table 26.6.

3.   Invasive hemodynamic monitoring is indicated in patients who have underlying cardiac or pulmonary disease, renal failure, or any other condition, such as shock, that requires quantitative monitoring of cardiac function and intravascular volume.

a.   Central venous pressure. A central venous catheter can be placed in either the internal jugular vein or the subclavian vein to permit monitoring of the central venous pressure or the right atrial pressure of the patient (Fig. 26.1). Measuring the end-diastolic pressure of the right heart will provide information on the patient's intravascular volume, thus helping to direct fluid management. It must be kept in mind, however, that certain conditions such as liver disease, right heart failure, tricuspid regurgitation, and pericardial tamponade can lead to an elevated central venous pressure (Table 26.7).

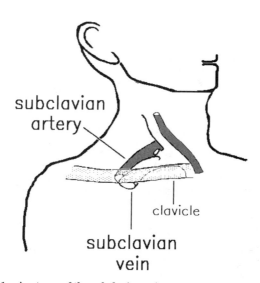

Fig. 26.1.   Anatomy of the subclavian vein.

Table 26.7.   **Interpretation of central venous pressure**

Central Venous Pressure Reading	Other Features	Diagnosis
Low	Rapid pulse Blood pressure normal or low Low urine output Poor capillary refill	Hypovolemia
High	Unilateral breath sounds Asymmetric chest movement Tracheal deviation Rapid pulse	Tension pneumothorax
High	Breathlessness Third heart sound Pink frothy sputum Edema	Heart failure
Very high	Rapid pulse Muffled heart sounds	Pericardial tamponade

   b.   Left heart function. Central venous pressure monitoring cannot provide any information on the patient's left heart function. To overcome this drawback, a pulmonary artery catheter can be used to provide indirect information about left heart function. The ballooned catheter tip is guided by the blood flow into the pulmonary artery via the internal jugular, subclavian, or sometimes the femoral veins. Once the catheter tip with the inflated balloon reaches the part of the pulmonary artery where it becomes wedged, an occlusion pressure can be obtained. Since there are no valves in the pulmonary vasculature, this maneuver can, in theory, provide information on left heart pressure. Thus, the pressure measured by the catheter tip beyond the region of the inflated balloon is a good estimate of the pressure in the left heart. In addition to pressure measurements, the pulmonary artery catheter can calculate other parameters such as cardiac output and index and systemic vascular resistance. Again, as with central venous pressure monitoring, underlying conditions such as pulmonary hypertension, mitral regurgitation, and addition of high levels of peak end-expiratory pressure on the ventilator may alter the measurements, leading to a falsely elevated number. Thus, these measurements must be interpreted carefully and integrated with the clinical exam.
   C.   Postoperative ward care. This phase of care is aimed at resolving the acute postoperative medical needs of the patient. The goal is to reach a functional and stable state so that the patient may be safely discharged to home or a rehabilitation facility

ity. This implies the presence of a stable cardiopulmonary status, adequate pain control, full nutritional support, stable surgical wounds and drains, and treated or controlled infection status. The postoperative course varies in length and acuity depending on the procedure performed and the comorbidities and the complications that can occur during the hospital stay. However, the following are some of the basic issues that are universal to all postoperative patients.

1. Hemodynamics. Surgical patients often enter the operating room in a mild state of dehydration due to NPO status preoperatively and bowel preparation. Postoperatively, a significant amount of fluid shift takes place, rendering the patient further volume depleted despite administration of full maintenance fluids.

a. Hypovolemia is by far the most common cause of immediate postoperative hypotension with low urine output. After examining the patient for other possible causes, a 500-mL bolus of normal saline or lactated Ringer's solution should be given intravenously. If this improves the blood pressure, the rate of maintenance fluids may be increased. For patients with low hematocrit (≤30%), blood transfusion should be considered in addition to fluids. If a patient has a central venous pressure catheter, this can be a useful corroboration of hypovolemia. If the hypotension continues or is only transiently responsive to fluid administration, internal bleeding should be suspected. This is especially the case in the postnephrectomy patient.

b. Hemorrhage must also be considered as a possible cause of hypovolemia; this should be ruled out with a stat hematocrit. The surgical dressing/site should be examined for staining and hematomas, and volume of drain output should be checked to assess for acute bleeding.

c. Acute cardiopulmonary events include such events as a myocardial infarction. Cardiac arrhythmias and pulmonary embolus should also be considered. Thus, it is important to obtain a history from the patient regarding symptoms such as chest pain and dyspnea and to examine the patient at the bedside. Appropriate tests must be ordered to investigate these possible diagnoses.

d. Medications are also important causes of postoperative hypotension. Antihypertensive medications and opioids are prime candidates in this regard. If a patient has an epidural catheter, the anesthesiologist should be consulted for possible adjustment in the dosing.

2. Pain management is an extremely important aspect of postoperative patient care. If pain is untreated or inadequately treated, it can lead to complications such as pneumonia, atelectasis, deep vein thrombosis (DVT), pulmonary emboli, and poor control of hypertension. Pain is, of course, an extremely subjective perception that varies between individuals and across different cultures.

a. Aspirin and nonsteroidal antiinflammatory drugs (NSAIDs) (Table 26.8) are first-line therapy for mild to moderate pain in patients who can take oral medication. Unlike

Table 26.8.   Examples of NSAIDs and opioids

Drug	Dosage Forms	Daily Dose Range (mg)	Half-Life (h)
Ibuprofen	Tablet, syrup	600–1,200	1–2
Indomethacin	Capsule, suspension, suppository	50–200	4
Naproxen	Tablet, suspension, suppository	500–1,000	14

Drug Name	Route of Delivery	Dose (mg)	Length of Action (h)
Meperidine	IM	100–150	1–2
Morphine	IM/SC	10–15	2–4
Methadone	IM	7.5–10	4–6
Buprenorphine	SL	0.2–0.4	6–8

opioids, aspirin and NSAIDs act peripherally to decrease levels of many inflammatory mediators generated at the site of tissue injury, including prostaglandins. Because aspirin and NSAIDs (but not acetaminophen) inhibit platelet aggregation, this raises concern about potential bleeding complications when they are used perioperatively. NSAIDs have several advantages over opioids. They do not cause hypotension, do not cause respiratory depression, and do not inhibit gastric or small bowel motility. For some of them however, the cost is significantly greater than that of morphine. NSAIDs may cause significant renal impairment particularly in patients with renal disease or decreased circulating blood volume. Finally, aspirin and NSAIDs tend to have a narrow therapeutic range; that is, after a certain dose level is reached, there is little increase in analgesia with increased dose, but there is a considerable increase in toxicity

(1)   **Aspirin** is an effective analgesic that is active orally within a short period of time. It is rapidly metabolized into salicylic acid, which has analgesic and antiinflammatory activity. Salicylic acid has a half-life of about 4 hours. The length of action may be reduced if aspirin is given with antacids. Doses range from a minimum of 300 mg PO q4h to a maximum of 8 g PO qd.

(2)   **Acetaminophen** has analgesic and antipyretic properties but little antiinflammatory effect. It is well absorbed orally and is metabolized almost entirely in the liver. It has few side effects in normal dosage. With high doses, it may cause hepatotoxicity by overloading the normal metabolic pathways with the formation of a toxic metabolite. Doses range from a minimum of 500 mg PO q4h to a maximum of 4 g PO qd. Acetaminophen is often contained in combinations containing opioids such as codeine or oxycodone.

(3) NSAIDs have both analgesic and antiinflammatory actions. They may be combined with opioids because of their different modes of action. The choice of an NSAID should be made on the basis of availability, cost, and length of action. All NSAIDs have antiplatelet activity, leading to increased bleeding time. These drugs also inhibit prostaglandin synthesis in the gastric mucosa and may thus produce gastric bleeding as a side effect. Extreme care should be exercised when using these drugs in patients with asthma or moderate to severely impaired renal function. Other relative contraindications include a history of peptic ulceration, gastrointestinal bleeding or bleeding diathesis, operations associated with high blood loss, dehydration, and any history of hypersensitivity to NSAIDs or aspirin. Ibuprofen is the drug of choice if the oral route is available. It is clinically effective and low cost and has a lower side effects profile than other NSAIDs. Where the oral route is not available, the drug may be given as a rectal suppository or via nasogastric tube. Aspirin and most of the NSAIDs are available as suppositories and are well absorbed from the rectum.

(4) Cyclooxygenase-2 inhibitors. Long-term use of NSAIDs can cause upper gastrointestinal bleeding. In response to this, the drug industry has produced a new class of NSAIDs: the cyclooxygenase-2 inhibitor. Presently, three of these medications are on the market: celecoxib (Celebrex), rofecoxib (Vioxx), and valdecoxib (Bextra). Because these medications have been on the market for a short time, few studies are available documenting their use in the postoperative setting. These medications have not been shown to be more efficacious than ibuprofen, acetaminophen, or naproxen.

b. Opioids are commonly used postoperatively and may be given by a variety of routes. Opioids are often significantly underdosed because of a widespread fear of overdosage and dependency. Furthermore, many opioid orders are written on a prn pain basis that requires the patient to ask for pain medication. It is better to order that these drugs be offered on a q4h basis if adequate analgesia is to be obtained. With the administration of opioids, a bowel regimen to avoid constipation is indicated.

(1) Oral administration causes less discomfort than intramuscular injections but is associated with a delayed onset of action. Codeine phosphate, oxycodone, and meperidine may be given orally and are effective for mild to moderate pain. Tramadol (Ultram) is a weak opioid with an analgesic potency roughly similar to meperidine, but without cardiovascular or respiratory depression and with very low dependency potential. It can also be given by parenteral injection.

(2) Intramuscular administration of opioids, particularly morphine sulfate and meperidine hydrochloride, has been the mainstay of postoperative analgesia for many years. It is often difficult to find an intramuscular dose that will provide pain relief for >4 hours.

(3) Subcutaneous administration may be very effective as the onset of pain relief occurs at about the same time as with intramuscular injection, the injection is less painful, and the effect lasts longer.

(4) Intravenous administration is most commonly given in the form of **patient-controlled analgesia** (PCA). Continuous intravenous administration provides pain control as long as effective, steady-state blood concentrations of drug are maintained. This usually occurs after about 24 hours of administration. Both meperidine and morphine are suitable drugs for continuous intravenous infusions. The PCA device limits the number of activations per unit time and the minimum time that needs to elapse between activations to avoid patient overdose. PCA has been shown to provide superior analgesia with less total drug use, less sedation, more rapid return to physical activity, and superior patient satisfaction because patients feel that they have control over their therapy. A major drawback is that PCA is less useful in confused or debilitated patients.

c. Continuous epidural analgesia may be required in some cases in which other techniques are ineffective. The epidural catheter can be used to give continuous infusion of local anesthetic such bupivacaine or in some cases opioids.

3. Fever. Fever occurs in nearly half of postoperative patients. In most instances, low-grade fevers resolve spontaneously without a specific underlying source identified. However, serious infections can manifest as fever, and therefore it is extremely important to evaluate patients who develop fever during their postoperative course. Low-grade fevers occurring in the first 2 days after surgery are most likely due to atelectasis of the lungs. Use of the incentive spirometer and ambulation will often allow the fever to resolve without further intervention. The wound should also be examined to rule out any necrotizing infections caused by gas-forming organisms such as *Clostridium,* which can occur in the immediate postoperative period. A full work-up including blood cultures is generally not indicated during the first 48 hours, unless the patient has been hospitalized preoperatively for a long period of time. Beyond 48 hours, however, infectious causes of fever must be sought out. A thorough physical exam, urinalysis as well as urine culture, blood culture, sputum culture, complete blood count, chest x-ray, and assessment of all catheters must be performed. In addition to the most common causes of fever such as pneumonia, urinary tract infections, and catheter-related infections, other diagnoses such as sinusitis and *C. difficile* colitis must be kept in mind. If supported by positive culture data, the appropriate antibiotic or antifungal therapy should be initiated. At about 7 days after surgery, intra-abdominal abscess and anastomotic leak must be ruled out. Other sources of fever include DVT, pulmonary embolism, and medications ("drug fever"). In all postoperative patients, it is important to remove catheters and drains as soon as possible to avoid serious infectious complications.

4. Nutrition. Nutritional support is an extremely important component of postoperative recovery, yet it is often placed lower on the priority list of postoperative issues. A state of malnutrition may exist secondary to the disease process and may be exacerbated by the catabolic state imposed by the surgery.

   a. Oral feeding. Although parenteral options for providing nutrition exist, the use of the gastrointestinal tract is the preferred route of nutritional intake. If patients can eat, it is best to feed them by mouth. If the gastrointestinal tract is functioning but other factors are interfering with feeding, such as ventilator dependency, need for sedation, altered mental status, or disruption in the swallowing mechanism, a feeding tube can be placed either in the stomach or in the jejunum. Temporary access may be accomplished via a nasogastric or nasojejunal tube. If permanent access is needed, consider placing a gastrostomy tube or a surgically placed jejunostomy tube. Patients who are known to aspirate should have a jejunostomy tube placed.

   b. Parenteral feeding. For patients who cannot be fed through the gastrointestinal tract because of a prolonged ileus, bowel surgery, or other postoperative complications such as severe pancreatitis, parenteral nutrition must be provided. Total parenteral nutrition is based on giving a highly concentrated solution of lipids, amino acids, and carbohydrates along with electrolytes, minerals, and vitamins that must be delivered through a central vein. Peripheral parenteral nutrition utilizes a less concentrated solution that can be administered through a peripheral vein. Enteral nutrition may be associated with many complications including catheter-related infections, venous thromboses, hepatic cholestasis, and atrophy of the gut mucosa.

5. Care of the gastrointestinal tract

   a. Ileus. Bowel motility ceases after anesthesia and handling of the bowel, resulting in postoperative ileus that may last for 48 to 72 hours. In addition, bowel resection and anastomosis disrupt normal bowel peristalsis. Although small bowel function returns within 24 hours, the stomach can take longer. Without decompression of the stomach, the patient will experience nausea and vomiting from the accumulation of gastric secretions. Thus, the postoperative patient will most likely require a nasogastric tube (NGT) to decompress the stomach during this period. Once NGT output decreases and bowel sounds return, the NGT may be taken off wall suction to make sure that the patient will be able to tolerate ceasing active decompression of the stomach. If residuals are low and there are no complaints of nausea or vomiting, the tube may be removed. Once the tube is removed, the patient's diet must be advanced. The patient initially begins with a tray of clear liquid, which usually consists of water, juices (such as cranberry and apple), gelatin dessert, and broth. Once the patient tolerates the clear liquid tray, the diet can be advanced as tolerated to a regular diet.

   b. Constipation. Patients in the hospital are subject to constipation for a number of reasons. As mentioned above, anesthesia and the operative procedure will in itself slow the activity of the gastrointestinal tract. Second, pain medications prescribed postoperatively, especially opioids, slow peristalsis. Third, although patients are encouraged to ambulate as much as possible, the lack of activity in the hospital puts them at risk for constipation. General measures to reduce constipation include ambulation, stool softeners (docusate sodium 100 mg PO qd), and avoiding opioid analgesics. Mild constipation may be handled with a glycerin or Dulcolax suppository. More severe constipation may require a Fleet enema, mineral oil enema, or manual disimpaction.

6. Prophylaxis for DVT. Objective tests have shown that 8% to 15% of untreated patients develop venous thrombosis after major abdominal surgery. Thrombosis of deep leg veins is the cause of fatal pulmonary embolism in about 2 in 1,000 postoperative patients each year. Most patients who die from pulmonary embolism do so within 30 minutes of the acute event, making treatment after the event very difficult. Thus, the only effective way to prevent pulmonary embolism is to prevent DVT. General risk factors for the development of DVT are described in Table 26.9. Risk for DVT and fatal pulmonary embolism is further stratified in Table 26.10.

a.   Low-risk patients. Nonpharmacologic prophylaxis is recommended for low-risk patients throughout the preoperative and postoperative period until they are ambulatory (Table 26.11). Elastic stockings and early ambulation have few, if any, complications and are effective for patients who have low risk of thromboembolism. Intermittent pneumatic compression is indicated during surgery, especially when patients have their legs supported by stirrups. Intermittent pneumatic compression is not indicated outside the operating room.

b.   Medium-risk patients. In medium-risk patients, mechanical methods such as stockings should be combined with drug treatment (Table 26.11). Either low-dose heparin or low-molecular-weight heparin (LMWH) regimens may be used. Antiplatelet agents such as aspirin are considered less effective in preventing DVT.

c.   High- and highest-risk patients. In high-risk patients, the most effective drugs are LMWHs (Table 26.11).

**Table 26.9. Some important risk
factors for deep vein thrombosis**

Age >40 y
Trauma or surgery (especially pelvis, hip, and lower limb)
Severe obesity
Malignancy (especially pelvic or abdominal)
Immobility (bed rest >4 d) or paralysis
Heart failure
Pregnancy
Recent myocardial infarction
Puerperium
High-dose estrogens
Severe infection
Previous deep vein thrombosis or pulmonary embolism

Table 26.10. Stratification of risk (%) for deep venous thrombosis and pulmonary embolism

Event	Risk (%)			
	Low	Medium	High	Very High
Calf vein thrombus	2	10–20	20–40	40–80
Proximal vein thrombosis	0.4	2–4	4–8	10–20
Clinical pulmonary embolism	0.2	1–2	2–4	4–10
Fatal pulmonary embolism	0.002	0.1–0.4	0.4–1.0	0.2–5

Low risk

Uncomplicated minor surgery; age <40 y; no clinical risk factors

Medium risk

Any surgery in patients aged 40–60 y with no additional risk factors; major surgery in patients <40 y with no additional risk factors; minor surgery in patients with risk factors

High risk

Major surgery in patients >60 y without additional risk factors or patients aged 40–60 y with additional risk factors; patients with myocardial infarction; medical patients with risk factors

Very high risk

Major surgery in patients >40 y with prior venous thromboembolism, malignant disease, or hypercoagulable state; patients undergoing elective major lower-extremity orthopedic surgery, hip fracture, stroke, multiple trauma, or spinal cord injury

These can and should be combined with mechanical methods such as elastic stockings and intraoperative pneumatic compression. Heparin and LMWH are equivalent in preventing DVT, although LMWH has a longer duration of anticoagulant effect in fixed doses and little requirement for laboratory monitoring. Use of LMWH is associated with a lower frequency of bleeding complications (1% versus 3.5%) and a lower incidence of DVT (10% versus 15%) than with postoperative unfractionated heparin.

D. Discharge from the hospital. Once the patient's immediate postoperative medical issues have been resolved or stabilized and the patient has a functioning gastrointestinal tract and good pain control, he or she is ready for discharge from the acute hospital setting. This does not mean, however, that recovery is complete. Further recuperation and physical therapy may be necessary either at home or at a rehabilitation facility. The determination of whether or not the patient may be safely discharged home depends on such things as the availability of family support and the assessments by the physician, physical therapist, and social services. At the time of discharge, it is

Table 26.11. Drug regimens for thromboembolism prophylaxis

Regimen	Dose
Low-dose heparin	Heparin 5,000 U administered SC q8h (high risk) to SC q12h (moderate risk), starting 1–2 h preoperatively
Adjusted-dose heparin	Heparin 3,500 U administered SC q8h, postoperatively adjust ±500 U to maintain 1.5–2 times normal activated partial thromboplastin time
Low-molecular-weight heparin	**Medium risk:** 2,000 U (20 mg) SC 1–2 h preoperatively, then SC qd postoperatively **High/highest risk:** 4,000 U (40 mg) SC 1–2 h preoperatively, then SC qd postoperatively, *or* 3,000 U (30 mg) SC q12h starting 8–12 h postoperatively Major trauma: 3,000 U (30 mg) SC q12h starting 12–36 h after injury
Warfarin	**High/highest risk:** Adjust dose to maintain international normalized ratio at 2.0–3.0

important to provide information to patients on their medications, dressing/drain care, restrictions on activity or diet, and follow-up plans. It is also helpful to provide instructions to patients should any emergencies arise.

SUGGESTED READING

Agnelli G, Sonaglia F. Prevention of venous thromboembolism. *Thromb Res* 2000;97:V49–V62.

Attia J, Ray JG, Cook DJ, et al. Prophylaxis of venous thromboembolism in the critically ill. *Arch Intern Med* 2001;161:1268–1279.

Bick RL, Haas SK. International consensus recommendations. Summary statement and additional suggested guidelines. European Consensus Conference, November 1991. American College of Chest Physicians consensus statement of 1995. International Consensus Statement, 1997. *Med Clin North Am* 1998;82:613–633.

Braunschweig CL, Levy P, Sheean PM, et al. Enteral compared with parenteral nutrition: a meta-analysis. *Am J Clin Nutr* 2001;74: 534–542.

Davies AR, Froomes PR, French CJ, et al. Randomized comparison of nasojejunal and nasogastric feeding in critically ill patients. *Crit Care Med* 2002;30:586–590.

Detsky AS, Abrams HB, McLaughlin JR, et al. Predicting cardiac complications in patients undergoing non-cardiac surgery. *J Gen Intern Med* 1986;1:211–219.

Eagle KA, Brundage BH, Chaitman BR, et al. Guidelines for perioperative cardiovascular evaluation for noncardiac surgery. Report of the American College of Cardiology/American Heart Association Task Force on Practice Guidelines (Committee on Perioperative

Cardiovascular Evaluation for Noncardiac Surgery). *J Am Coll Cardiol* 1996;27:910–948.

Eggimann P, Pittet D. Infection control in the ICU. *Chest* 2001;120: 2059–2093.

Fletcher GF, Balady G, Froelicher VF, et al. Exercise standards: a statement for healthcare professionals from the American Heart Association. *Circulation* 1995;91:580–615.

Gammon RB, Strickland JH Jr, Kennedy JI Jr. Mechanical ventilation: a review for the internist. *Am J Med* 1995;99:553–562.

Geerts W, Cook D, Selby R, et al. Venous thromboembolism and its prevention in critical care. *J Crit Care* 2002;17:95–104.

Holte K, Kehlet H. Postoperative ileus: a preventable event. *Br J Surg* 2000;87:1480–1493.

Lee TH, Marcantonio ED, Mangione CM, et al. Derivation and prospective validation of a simple index for prediction of cardiac risk of major noncardiac surgery. *Circulation* 1999;100:1043–1049.

Li JM. Pain management in the hospitalized patient. *Med Clin North Am* 2002;86:771–795.

MacFie J. Enteral versus parenteral nutrition. *Br J Surg* 2000;87: 1121–1122.

Palda VA, Detsky AS. Perioperative assessment and management of risk from coronary artery disease. *Ann Intern Med* 1997;127: 313–328.

Shoemaker WC, Ayres SM, Grenvik A, et al. *Textbook of critical care.* Philadelphia: Saunders, 2000.

Tobin MJ. Mechanical ventilation. *N Engl J Med* 1994;330:1056–1061.

Appendix I. American Urological Association Symptom Score Index

Last Name	First Name						Date		Your score
		Not at all	< 1/5 the time	< 1/2 the time	~ 1/2 the time	> 1/2 the time	Almost always		
1. **Incomplete emptying:** Over the past month, how often have you had a sensation of not emptying your bladder completely after you finished urinating?		0	1	2	3	4	5		
2. **Frequency:** Over the past month, how often have you had to urinate again less than 2 hours after you finished urination?		0	1	2	3	4	5		
3. **Intermittency:** Over the past month, how often have you found that you stopped and started again several times when you urinated?		0	1	2	3	4	5		
4. **Urgency:** Over the past month, how often have you found it difficult to postpone urination?		0	1	2	3	4	5		

	0	1	2	3	4	5	
5. **Weak stream:** Over the past month, how often have you had a weak stream?	0	1	2	3	4	5	
6. **Straining:** Over the past month, how often have you had to push or strain to begin urination?	0	1	2	3	4	5	
	None	1 time	2 times	3 times	4 times	> 5 times	
7. **Nocturia:** Over the past month or so, how many times did you get up to urinate from the time you went to bed until the time you got up in the morning?	0	1	2	3	4	5	
						Total score =	

Quality of life due to urinary symptoms: If your were to spend the rest of your life with your urinary condition just the way it is now, how would you feel about that?

Appendix II. Modified Partin Table for Predicting Pathological Stage in Prostate Cancer

Gleason sum	$0 \le PSA \le 2.5$				$2.6 \le PSA \le 4.0$				$4.1 \le PSA \le 6.0$				$6.1 \le PSA \le 10.0$				$PSA \ge 10.1$				Pathology
	T1c	T2a	T2b	T2c	T1c	T2a	T2b	T2c	T1c	T2a	T2b	T2c	T1c	T2a	T2b	T2c	T1c	T2a	T2b	T2c	
2–4	95	91	88	86	92	85	80	78	90	81	75	73	87	76	69	67	80	65	57	54	OC
	5	9	12	14	8	15	20	22	10	19	25	27	13	24	31	33	20	35	43	46	CP
	0	0	0	0	0	0	0	0	0	0	0	0	0	0	0	0	0	0	0	0	SV+
	0	0	0	0	0	0	0	0	0	0	0	0	0	0	0	0	0	0	0	0	LN+
5,6	90	81	75	73	84	71	63	61	80	66	57	55	75	58	49	45	62	42	33	30	OC
	9	17	22	24	15	27	34	36	19	32	39	40	23	37	44	46	33	47	52	51	CP
	0	1	2	1	1	2	2	2	1	1	2	2	2	4	5	5	4	6	8	6	SV+
	0	0	1	1	0	0	1	1	0	1	2	3	0	1	2	3	2	4	8	13	LN+
3+4=7	79	64	54	51	68	50	41	38	63	44	35	31	54	35	26	24	37	20	14	11	OC
	17	29	35	36	27	41	47	48	32	46	51	50	36	49	52	52	43	49	47	42	CP
	2	5	6	5	4	7	9	8	3	6	7	6	8	13	16	13	12	16	17	13	SV+
	1	2	4	6	1	2	3	5	2	4	7	12	2	3	6	10	8	14	22	33	LN+
4+3=7	71	53	43	39	58	39	30	27	52	33	25	21	43	25	19	16	27	14	9	7	OC
	25	40	45	45	37	52	57	57	42	56	60	57	47	58	60	58	51	55	50	43	CP
	2	4	5	5	4	6	7	6	3	5	5	4	8	11	13	11	11	13	13	10	SV+
	1	3	6	9	1	2	4	7	3	6	10	16	2	5	8	13	10	18	27	38	LN+
8–10	66	47	37	34	52	33	25	23	46	28	21	19	37	21	15	13	22	11	7	6	OC
	28	42	46	47	40	53	57	57	45	58	59	57	48	57	57	56	60	52	46	41	CP
	4	7	9	8	6	10	12	10	5	8	9	7	13	17	19	16	17	19	19	15	SV+
	1	3	6	10	1	3	5	8	3	6	10	18	3	5	8	13	11	17	27	38	LN+

CP, ...

Subject Index

Page numbers in *italics* denote figures; page numbers followed by a *t* denote tables.

A

Abdominal compression, 23
Abrams–Griffiths nomogram, *96, 97*
Abscess
  periurethral, 175–176
  of the prostate, 100, 224
  renal/perirenal, 217–218
Absent testis syndrome, 376
Absorbent aids
  for treatment of urinary incontinence, 132
  underpants, 132
Acetaminophen, for postoperative pain management, 500
Acidosis
  pediatric, 367
  in treatment of chronic renal failure, 467
Acquired immunodeficiency disease syndrome (AIDS), 423–424
Acquired renal cystic disease, 474
Acute bacterial cystitis, 220, 222
  multiple recurrent infections, 222
  relapse or bacterial persistence, 222
Acute epididymitis, 226–227
Acute glomerulonephritis, 39
Acute interstitial nephritis, 39, *41*
Acute poststreptococcal glomerulonephritis, 9
Acute pyelonephritis, 213–214
Acute renal failure, 459–463
  causes, 460t, 461
  classification, 459–462, 460t
  definition, 459
  differential diagnosis, 462t
  drugs associated with, 461t
  oliguria, 459
  symptomatic uremia, 459
  treatment, 462–463, 463t
Acute tumular necrosis, *38*

Adenocarcinoma
  bladder, 258
  kidney, 249–255
    diagnosis, 250, 252
    etiology and risk factors, 249–250
    hereditary syndromes, 251t
    incidence, 249
    staging, 252, *253,* 254t
    treatment, 252–255
    tumor classification and histology, 250
  prostate, 100, 270
  ureter, 256
Adrenal adenoma, 431–432
  diagnosis, 431
  treatment, 432
Adrenal carcinoma, 433–436
  diagnosis, 434–435
  endocrine manifestations, 434t
  prognosis, 436
  staging, 433t
Adrenal cysts, 432
Adrenal gland, 426–440
  benign lesions, 431–433
  masses
    differential diagnosis, 427t
    incidentally discovered, 429–431, *430,* 431t
    metastatic lesions, 440
    common primary sites, 427t
    primary malignant lesions, 433–440
  radiology, 426–429
    computed tomography, 427–428
    fine-needle aspiration biopsy, 429
    magnetic resonance imaging, 29, 428
    plain radiography, 426–427
    radioisotope scanning/positron emission tomography, 428–429
    ultrasound, 427
    vascular studies, 429

Adrenal gland (*contd.*)
surgical anatomy and embryology, 426, *428*
AIDS. *See* Acquired immunodeficiency disease
syndrome
AJCC. *See* American Joint Committee on Cancer
Albarran (deflecting) bridge, 69,
70
Alkylating agents
mechanism of action, 305
for medical management of
genitourinary malig-
nancy, 304–306, *305*
toxicities, 305–306
α-adrenergic agents
as cause of erectile dysfunction, 151*t*
effect on bladder, 102
for treatment of LUTS, 109,
109*t*
for treatment of stress urinary incontinence, 132
α-Methyldopa, as cause of erectile dysfunction, 151*t*
Alport's syndrome (progressive
familial nephropathy), 10
Alprostadil, for treatment of
sexual dysfunction, 159,
160
Alum, for hemorrhagic cystitis,
12
Amenorrhea, after alkylating
agents, 306
American Heart Association
recommendations for prophylaxis for prostate surgery,
227
web site, 227
American Joint Committee on
Cancer (AJCC)
staging system for bladder
carcinoma, *262,* 263*t*
staging system for penile cancer, 294*t*
staging system for prostate
cancer, *276,* 277*t*
staging system for renal carcinoma, *253,* 254*t*
staging system for testicular
cancer, *286,* 287*t*
staging system for
ureteral–pelvic tumors
and 5-year survival, 257*t*

American Society of Anesthesiologists (ASA), classification of physical status,
491, 492*t*
American Urological Association (AUA)
standardized symptom scores,
103, 104*t*
symptom score index, 508–510
AML. *See* Angiomyolipoma
Ampicillin
antibiotic prophylaxis for
valvular cardiac and
prosthetic devices, 228*t*
for treatment of acute
pyelonephritis, 213
for treatment of genitourinary
infections, 215*t*–216*t*
Anaphylaxis, following antimicrobial agents, 309
Anderson–Hynes dismembered
pyeloplasty, 361
Androgen, replacement for
treatment of sexual dys-
function, 157
Anemia, 466
Anesthesia. *See also* Surgery
chronic renal failure and, 474,
475*t*
Angiography
for diagnosis of adrenal
masses, 429
for diagnosis of renal masses,
57
Angiomyolipoma (AML), 51–53
clinical features and diagnosis, 51–52
radiologic diagnosis, 52
treatment, 52–53
Antiandrogenic agents, 321*t*
as cause of erectile dysfunction, 151*t*
Antibiotics. *See also* individual
drug name
preoperative administration
for endoscopy, 191
prophylaxis in urologic
surgery, 228*t*
for treatment of bacteremia,
212
for treatment of Fournier's
gangrene, 185
for treatment of genitourinary
tract infections, 215*t*–216*t*

for treatment of scrotal injuries, 183
Anticholinergic agents. *See also* individual drug name
as cause of erectile dysfunction, 151t
for treatment of LUTS, 117
Anticoagulants
as cause of priapism, 407
hematuria and, 13–14
Antihistamines
as cause of erectile dysfunction, 151t
effect on bladder, 102
Antihypertensive drugs, as cause of priapism, 407
Antimetabolites
mechanism of action, 307
for medical management of genitourinary malignancy, 307
toxicity, 307
Antimicrobial agents
mechanism of action, 309
for medical management of genitourinary malignancy, 309
toxicities, 309
Antimuscarinic agents
for treatment of LUTS, 117
for treatment of urinary incontinence, 133–134
for treatment of voiding dysfunction, 349–350
Antipsychotic drugs, as cause of priapism, 407–408
Antispasmodic agents, for treatment of LUTS, 117
Argyle catheter, 72
Arrhythmias, 474
ART. *See* Assisted reproductive technologies
Arterial disease, as cause of erectile dysfunction, 147–148
Arterial priapism, 410
definition, 407
diagnosis, 410
etiology, 410t
treatment, 412
Artificial urinary sphincter, for treatment of urethral incompetence, 353
ASA. *See* American Society of Anesthesiologists

Aspirin, for postoperative pain management, 499–501
Assisted reproductive technologies (ART), 380, 405–406
AUA. *See* American Urological Association
Augmentation cystoplasty
for treatment of urge urinary incontinence, 138
for treatment of voiding dysfunction, 350
Autologous fat, for treatment of stress urinary incontinence, 134
Autonomic dysreflexia, 347–348, 348
male infertility and, 400
management, 353
Azithromycin
for treatment of chancroid, 422
for treatment of lymphogranuloma venereum, 423
for treatment of nongonococcal urethritis, 416
Azoospermia
after alkylating agents, 306
male infertility and, 392–394
Azotemia, 206
pediatric, 367
postrenal, 461–462, 461t
prerenal, 459
renal, 459–461, 461t

B
Bacille Calmette Guérin (BCG)
for medical management of genitourinary malignancy, 310, 316
for treatment of bladder cancer, 264–265
Bacilluria, 210
Bacteremia, 211–212
diagnosis, 211–212
etiology, 211
septic shock, 212
treatment, 212
Bacteria, in urine, 5
Bacterial endocarditis, antimicrobial prophylaxis for surgery, 227–228
Bacteriuria, 3, 206
treatment, 211
unresolved, 206

Bacteroides fragilis, 185
Bacteroides spp., 54
β-Adrenergic blockers, as cause
    of erectile dysfunction,
    151*t*
Balanitis xerotica obliterans,
    292
Balloon dilators, 81
Basal cell carcinoma, penile, 293
BCG. *See* Bacille Calmette
    Guérin
Behavioral modification, for
    treatment of urinary
    incontinence, 129
Benign essential hematuria
    (Berger's disease), 9–10
Benign familial hematuria, 10
Benign prostatic hyperplasia
    (BPH), 100
    endoscopy and, 193–194
    indications for, 194*t*
Berger's disease (benign essen-
    tial hematuria), 9–10
Bethanechol
    supersensitivity testing, 89
    for treatment of LUTS, 119
Bicalutamide, for medical man-
    agement of genitourinary
    malignancy, 310
Biofeedback therapy
    for treatment of LUTS, 119
    for treatment of urinary in-
        continence, 130
    for treatment of voiding dys-
        function, 350
Biologic agents, in medical man-
    agement of malignancies,
    310, 316
Biopsy
    for diagnosis of adrenal
        masses, 429
    for diagnosis of renal masses,
        57–58
    with endoscopy, 76
    mucosal, 76
    prostate, 77, *271,* 271–273
Bipolar electrode prostatic re-
    section, 196
Birt–Hogg–Dube syndrome, 53
Bladder
    calculi, 103
        clinical presentation, 238,
            239
        diagnosis, 239
        treatment, 239–240

cancer, radiation therapy for,
    332–333
cellule formation, 103
complications in renal trans-
    plantation, 487–488
decompensation, 102
differential diagnosis in
    LUTS, 100–103
diverticulum formation, 103
effects of radiation therapy,
    339
imaging, 21–22
instability, 102
neck obstruction, 100, 197
neoplasms, 258–269
    cancer screening, 259*t*
    diagnosis, 259–260, 259*t*
    etiology, 258–259
    incidence, 258
    prognostic factors, 266*t*
    tumor classification, 258
neural control, 124
neuromuscular dysfunction,
    100
pediatric exstrophy, 372–373
perforation, 77–78
peripheral neuropathy, 102
physiology of urinary inconti-
    nence, 123
response to outflow obstruc-
    tion, 102
trabeculation, 102–103
trauma, 172–174, *174*
    complications of injury, 173
    diagnosis, 173
    treatment, 173
tumors, 198
urinary calculi, 238–240, *239*
Bladder tumor antigen (BTA),
    260
Bleeding. *See* Hemorrhage
Bleomycin
    hypersensitivity, 309
    for medical management of
        genitourinary malig-
        nancy, 309
    for medical management of
        testicular cancer, 324
    toxicity, 309
Blood, in urine, 3
Blood urea nitrogen (BUN), 458
Body temperature. *See* Fever
Bone marrow transplantation,
    for medical management
    of testicular cancer, 326

Bone scan
  for detection of metastatic disease, 274–275
  for evaluation of bladder neoplasms, 261
Bosniak classification, 60t
Botulinum toxin
  for treatment of external sphincter dyssynergia, 352
  for treatment of voiding dysfunction, 350–351
Bougies, 65–67, 66, 67
Bowen's disease, 293
BPH. See Benign prostatic hyperplasia
Brachytherapy, 331
  for treatment of prostate cancer, 279–280
Brain death, 478–479, 479t
Bretylium, as cause of erectile dysfunction, 151t
Bronchospasm, 26
Brown–Wickham technique, 90, 92, 94
  normal uroflow values, 92t
BTA. See Bladder tumor antigen
BUN. See Blood urea nitrogen
Burch colposuspension, for treatment of stress urinary incontinence, 135

C

C. perfringens, 185
Calcium disorders, 453–455
Calcium gluconate, for treatment of hypermagnesemia, 456
Calculi. See Urinary calculi
Calyceal diverticula, 61
Cancer
  bladder, 258–269
    radiation therapy, 332–333
  clinical criteria for treatment, 304t
  complications in renal transplantation, 488–489
  genitourinary tract, 249–299
  kidney, 249–255
    metastatic lesions, 59
  medical management of malignancies, 300–327
  penile, 291–297
    medical management, 326

radiation therapy, 335–338, 337
prostate, 195t, 197, 269–284
  magnetic resonance imaging, 28
  medical management, 319–323, 321t
  radiation therapy, 333–335, 334
  proteins and, 8–9
renal adenocarcinoma, 54–58
  medical management, 316–317
skin, 489
testes, radiation therapy, 335
testicle, 284–291
  medical management, 323–326
ureter, 255–258
urothelial, medical management, 317–319, 318t
Candida albicans, 210, 222–223
Candidiasis, 424
Cannon's law, 89
Captopril, renal study, 34, 37
Carcinoma
  adrenal, 433–436
  in situ, 258
Cardiac evaluation
  cardiac risk indexes, 493–494, 493t
  preoperative, 491–494
  risk of cardiac complications in various procedures, 492t
Cardiovascular support, with treatment of bacteremia, 212
Castration, for treatment of prostate cancer, 283–284
Catheterization
  in female patients, 74
  indwelling, 117
  instrumentation, 72–74
  intermittent self-, 117
  in male patients, 72, 74
  specimen collection, 208
  for treatment of LUTS, 119
    technique, 120
  for treatment of voiding dysfunction, 351–352
  ureteral, 76
  with urethral trauma, 175
Catheters, 63–65, 64, 130–131
  cone-tip, 79, 80

Catheters (*contd.*)
indwelling, for treatment of urinary incontinence, 130
microwave, *113*
open-ended, 79, *80*
spiral-tip, 79, *80*
in treatment of LUTS, 117
whistle-tip, 79, *80*
Cavernosography, for evaluation of sexual dysfunction, 154
Cavernosometry, for evaluation of sexual dysfunction, 154
CBAVD. *See* Congenital bilateral absence of the vas deferens
Cefazolin, antibiotic prophylaxis for endoscopic surgery, 228*t*
Cefixime, for treatment of gonorrhea, 418–419
Cefoxitin, antibiotic prophylaxis for colon and small bowel surgery, 228*t*
Ceftriaxone
for treatment of acute pyelonephritis, 213
for treatment of chancroid, 422
for treatment of genitourinary infections, 215*t*–216*t*
for treatment of gonorrhea, 418
for treatment of syphilis, 422
Celecoxib (Celebrex), for postoperative pain management, 501
Cells
cycle, 300, *301*
examination in urine, 4
germ, 381, *382*
Leydig, 381
Sertoli, 383
Cephalosporins, for treatment of bacteremia, 212
Chancroid, 422
diagnosis, 422
treatment, 422
Chemolysis, for treatment of struvite stones, 244–245
Chemotherapy
agents in medical management of malignancies, 304–309, *305,* 308*t*
combination therapy, 304

guidelines, 303–304, 303*t*
in locally advanced disease, 318
in metastatic disease, 318–319
for treatment of bladder cancer, 262–263, 267
for treatment of Wilms' tumor, 357
Children. *See* Pediatric urology
Chlamydia trachomatis, 210, 415–416
Chromophilic carcinoma, 250
Chronic interstitial nephritis, 214
Chronic obstructive pulmonary disease, 494
Chronic pyelonephritis, 214, 217
Chronic renal failure (CRF), 463–467
causes, 464*t*
definition, 463–464
drugs associated with, 475*t*
etiology, *465*
treatment, 466–467
Cimetidine, as cause of erectile dysfunction, 151*t*
Ciprofloxacin
for treatment of chancroid, 422
for treatment of genitourinary infections, 215*t*–216*t*
for treatment of granuloma inguinale, 422
Cisplatin
for medical management of testicular cancer, 324
for medical management of urothelial cancer, 319
Clear cell tumors, 250
Clindamycin
for treatment of bacteremia, 212
for treatment of Fournier's gangrene, 185
Clitoral priapism, 412
Clomiphene citrate, for treatment of oligoasthenoteratospermia, 404
Clonidine, as cause of erectile dysfunction, 151*t*
Coagulopathy, in treatment of chronic renal failure, 466
Coaxial dilators, 66
Cobalt–chromium stent, 110, *111,* 112

Cocaine, as cause of priapism, 408
Cockroft–Gault equation, 457–458
Collecting duct tumors, 250
Colon, antimicrobial prophylaxis for surgery, 227
Colon conduit, 449
Colostomy, for treatment of Fournier's gangrene, 185
Complete gonadal dysgenesis, 376
Computed tomography (CT)
  for diagnosis of adrenal masses, 427–428
  for diagnosis of renal masses, 57
  for evaluation of bladder neoplasms, 260–261
  for evaluation of genitourinary trauma, 165
  for evaluation of hematuria, 8
  for evaluation of metastatic disease, 275
  for evaluation of the genitourinary tract, 19–22
  intravenous contrast agent and, 20
  protocols, 20–22
  technique, 19–20
Condom catheter, for treatment of urinary incontinence, 130
Congenital adrenal hyperplasia, 376–377
Congenital bilateral absence of the vas deferens (CBAVD), 390
Conn's syndrome, 432
Conray 60, 24*t*
Constipation, postoperative, 503–504
Contact laser, for treatment of LUTS, 116
Continent urinary diversion, 450
Continuous incontinence, 125
Contrast agents
  characteristics, 24*t*
  in computed tomography, 20
  delayed reactions, 25–26
  drug interactions, 27
  for evaluation of bladder neoplasms, 260–261
  for evaluation of genitourinary trauma, 165

guidelines for administration, 23*t*
  high-osmolality, 23–24
  iodinated, 23–27, 24*t*
  local effects, 25
  low-osmolarity, 23–24
  mortality, 27
  nephrotoxicity, 25
  prophylaxis, 26
  systemic reactions, 24–25
  treatment of reactions, 26–27
Cortical agents, radionuclide imaging and, 33–34, *35*
Corticosteroids
  for medical management of prostate cancer, 323
  for treatment of bacteremia, 212
  for treatment of Fournier's gangrene, 185
Coude catheter, 63, *64, 65*
Councill catheters, *64,* 65
Counseling, with treatment of sexual dysfunction, 161
CPPS, 226
Crede maneuver, for treatment of voiding dysfunction, 352
CRF. *See* Chronic renal failure
Cryoablation, for treatment of renal neoplasms, 255
Cryoprecipitate, in treatment of chronic renal failure, 467
Cryotherapy, for treatment of prostate cancer, 280–281
Cryptorchidism, 367–369
Crystals, microscopic examination in urine, 5
CT. *See* Computed tomography
Cunningham clamp, for treatment of urinary incontinence, 130, *131*
Cushing's syndrome, 432
Cyclooxygenase-2 inhibitors, for postoperative pain management, 501
Cyclophosphamide (Cytoxan)
  hemorrhagic cystitis and, 12
  for medical management of genitourinary malignancy, 304–306, *305*
Cyclosporin
  immunosuppression in renal transplantation, 483
  toxicity, 484*t,* 485*t*

Cyproterone acetate, as cause of erectile dysfunction, 151*t*
Cystectomy, indications, 266*t*
Cystinuria, 246
Cystitis, antibiotic therapy, 216*t*
Cystocath, 72
Cystocele, 100
  urinary incontinence and, 127, *127*
Cystography, for evaluation of genitourinary trauma, 165
Cystolithotomy, for treatment of bladder calculi, 240
Cystometrogram, 87–90, *88*
  characteristics, 88–90
  for evaluation of urinary incontinence, 128
Cystometry
  ambulatory, 107
  for evaluation of LUTS, 107
Cystoprostatectomy
  as cause of erectile dysfunction, 150
  for treatment of bladder cancer, 266–267
Cystoscopy
  flexible, 76
  for hemorrhagic cystitis, 12
Cystostomy, for treatment of Fournier's gangrene, 185
Cystourethroscopy, 67, *68*, 74–76, 188
  for evaluation of hematuria, 8
  for evaluation of LUTS, 106
Cysts
  adrenal, 432
  Bosniak classification, 60*t*
  multilocular cystic nephroma, 60–61
  renal, 59–60
Cytology, for evaluation of hematuria, 8
Cytoxan (cyclophosphamide), hemorrhagic cystitis and, 12

D

Deep vein thrombosis (DVT), postoperative, 504–505, 504*t*, 505*t*
Desmopressin, in treatment of chronic renal failure, 467
Detrusor, pharmacologic therapy for overactivity, 117–119, 118*t*

Detumescence, 146
Diabetes mellitus
  acute pyelonephritis and, 213
  as cause of erectile dysfunction, 148
  vesicourethral dysfunction, 349
Dialysis
  acute, 470
  complications, 470–471, 470*t*, 474
  composition of solutions, 469*t*
  continuous, 470
  definition, 467
  indications/contraindications, 467–468, 468*t*, 469*t*
  peritoneal, 468–469
    advantages/disadvantages, 468*t*
    versus hemodialysis, 468, 468*t*, 469*t*
    peritoneal solutions, 469, 469*t*
  solutions, 472
  in treatment of chronic renal failure, 467
Diapers, for treatment of urinary incontinence, 132
Dicyclomine (Bentyl)
  for treatment of LUTS, 117, 118*t*
^{99m}Tc-DTPA (^{99m}Tc-diethylkenetriaminepentaacetic acid), 30, *32, 33*
Diet
  postoperative, 502–503
  prostate cancer and, 269
  renal carcinoma and, 249
  for treatment of recurrent stone disease, 240
Digital rectal examination (DRE), 270–271
Digoxin, as cause of erectile dysfunction, 151*t*
Dihydrotestosterone, for medical management of genitourinary malignancy, 310
Dilation, for treatment of LUTS, 107
Dilators, 65–67, *66*
^{99m}Tc-DMSA (^{99m}Tc-dimercaptosuccinic acid), 33, 34, *35*
Disequilibrium syndrome, 474
Disopyramide, as cause of erectile dysfunction, 151*t*

Disseminated intravascular co-agulation, 14

Distilled water, for sickle cell–associated hematuria, 11

Diuretics, for sickle cell–associated hematuria, 11

Docetaxel, for medical management of prostate cancer, 323

Donovanosis (granuloma inguinale), 422

Dorsal rhizotomy, for treatment of voiding dysfunction, 351

Doxazosin (Cardura), for treatment of LUTS, 109t

Doxorubicin, for treatment of bladder cancer, 263

Doxycycline
  for treatment of granuloma inguinale, 422
  for treatment of lymphogranuloma venereum, 423
  for treatment of nongonococcal urethritis, 416
  for treatment of syphilis, 422

DRE. See Digital rectal examination

Drugs. See also individual drug name
  associated with hyperkalemia, 475t
  associated with vesicourethral dysfunction, 345t
  as cause of erectile dysfunction, 150, 151t
  in medical management of malignancies, 300–303, 302
  postoperative, 499
  regimens for thromboembolism prophylaxis, 506t
  resistance, 301–303
  for treatment of urethral incompetence, 352
  for treatment of voiding dysfunction, 347, 349–350

Duplication, 361–364

DVT. See Deep vein thrombosis

Dwell time, 469

Dysgenetic male pseudohermaphroditism, 375

Dysuria, 219–220, 219t

E

EACA. See ε-Aminocaproic acid

ε-Aminocaproic acid (EACA)
  as cause of erectile dysfunction, 151t
  for hemorrhagic cystitis, 12
  for sickle cell–associated hematuria, 11–12

ECG. See Electrocardiogram

ED. See Erectile dysfunction

Ejaculation, 143
  antegrade propulsion, 384
  bladder neck closure, 384
  duct obstruction, 395
  emission, 384
  following TURP, 196
  neurophysiology, 384

Electrical stimulation
  for treatment of LUTS, 119
  for treatment of voiding dysfunction, 350

Electrocardiogram (ECG), preoperative, 493

Electrohydraulic lithotripsy, 83

Electrolyte disorders, 441–456

Electromyography, 90, 93, 94
  for evaluation of urinary incontinence, 129

Electrosurgery. See also Surgery
  general principles, 188–191, 189, 190

Emergencies, renal vascular, 170–171

Endocarditis, prophylaxis against, 494

Endocrine disorders, as cause of erectile dysfunction, 149–150

Endoscopy. See also Surgery
  antibiotic prophylaxis, 228t
  complications, 77–78
  contraindications, 74
  cystourethroscopy, 74–76
  general principles of transurethral surgery, 191–193
  indications, 74
  instrumentation, 74–76
  of the lower urinary tract, 188–205
  precautions, 74–75
  preoperative preparation, 191
  sterilization of instruments, 75

Endoscopy (*contd.*)
  technique, 75–76
  transurethral procedures,
    191–198, *192, 194*
Endourologic techniques,
    246–247
End-stage renal disease
    (ESRD), 463–464
  etiology, *465*
Enema, preoperative admnis-
    tration for endoscopy, 191
Enterobacter sp., 210
Enterococcus, 185
Ephedrine, 102
Epididymitis, *49,* 416
  acquired immunodeficiency
    disease syndrome and,
    423
  acute, 226–227
  chronic, 227
Epididymoorchitis, 196
Epirubicin, for treatment of
    bladder cancer, 263
Epitaxy, 232
Erectile dysfunction (ED)
  causes, 147–151, 148*t*, 151*t*
  effects of radiation therapy,
    339
  impotence, following TURP,
    196
  neurophysiology, 146–147
  vascular physiology, 146
  venoocclusive, 148
Erection, physiology, 143–147,
    144, 145, 147*t*
Erythromycin
  for treatment of chancroid, 422
  for treatment of granuloma
    inguinale, 422
  for treatment of lymphogran-
    uloma venereum, 423
  for treatment of syphilis, 422
  for treatment of *Trichomonas
    vaginalis,* 416
Erythroplasia of Queyrat, 293
Escherichia coli, 2, 54, 185, 210
Estramustine, for medical man-
    agement of prostate can-
    cer, 323
Estrogens, *313*
  as cause of erectile dysfunc-
    tion, 151*t*
  for medical management of
    genitourinary malig-
    nancy, 310

renal carcinoma and, 249
  in treatment of chronic renal
    failure, 467
  for treatment of stress urinary
    incontinence, 132–133
ESWL. *See* Extracorporeal
    shock wave lithotripsy
Ethanol, as cause of erectile
    dysfunction, 151*t*
Etoposide, for medical manage-
    ment of testicular cancer,
    324
Excretory urogram. *See* Intra-
    venous urogram
Exercise, hematuria and, 10
External sphincterotomy, for
    treatment of external
    sphincter dyssynergia,
    352
Extracorporeal shock wave
    lithotripsy (ESWL),
    247–248, 247*t*
  characteristics of third-
    generation shock wave
    lithotriptors, 247*t*
  for treatment of struvite
    stones, 244
  for treatment of urinary cal-
    culi, 247–248
Extragonadal germ cell cancer,
    medical management,
    323–326
Extravasation necrosis, follow-
    ing antimicrobial agents,
    309
Extubation, 496–497, 497*t*

F

Famciclovir, for treatment of
    herpes simplex virus, 418
Female pseudohermaphro-
    ditism, 376
Fever
  endoscopy and, 190–191
  postoperative, 502
Filiforms, 65–66, *67*
Finasteride, for treatment of
    LUTS, 109
Fine-needle aspiration biopsy,
    for diagnosis of adrenal
    masses, 429
Fistula, urinary incontinence
    and, 122–123
Flare reaction, 310

Flavoxate (Urispas), for treatment of LUTS, 117, 118*t*

Fluid and electrolyte disorders, 441–456
  calcium, 453–455
  causes of volume excess, 443*t*
  magnesium, 455–456
  metabolic acid-base disorders, 447–451
  potassium, 451–452
  sodium and volume disorders, 441–447

5-Fluorouracil, for treatment of human papilloma virus, 415

Flutamide, *315*
  for medical management of genitourinary malignancy, 310

Foley catheter, 63, *64*

Folinic acid, for treatment of oligoasthenoteratospermia, 404

Followers, 65–66, *67*

Formalin, for hemorrhagic cystitis, 12–13

Forskolin, for treatment of sexual dysfunction, 159

Four-corner bladder neck suspension, for treatment of stress urinary incontinence, 135–136

Fournier's gangrene, 183–185
  comorbidity, 184*t*
  etiology, 184*t*
  prognosis, 185
  treatment, 185

Fracture, penile, 181–182

Free-beam laser, for treatment of LUTS, 114, 116

Furosemide, radionuclide imaging and, *43*

G

Gallium 67, 34

Ganglioneuromas, adrenal, 433

Gastrocystoplasty, 450–451

Gastrointestinal tract
  effects of radiation therapy, 339–340
  postoperative care, 503–504

Gatifloxacin, antibiotic prophylaxis for endoscopy, 228*t*

Gemcitabine, for medical management of urothelial cancer, 319

Genetics
  assessment of the infertile male, 390, *390, 391*
  influence on prostate cancer, 269

Genital molluscum contagiosum, 419

Genitourinary tract
  acquired immunodeficiency disease syndrome and, 423–424
  bacterial infection, 226–227
  imaging, 16–29
  infections, 206–231
    antibiotic therapy, 215*t*–216*t*
    antimicrobial prophylaxis in urologic surgery, 227–228, 228*t*
    bacteremia, 211–212
    classification, 206–207
    general principles, 206
    indications for evaluation, 211
    laboratory diagnosis, 207–211, 207*t*, *209*, 209*t*
    of the lower urinary tract, 219–223, 219*t*, *221*
    prostatic, 223–226, 223*t*
    scrotal contents, 226–227
    septic shock, 211–212
    of the upper urinary tract, 213–218
  medical management of malignancies, 300–327
    biologic and immunologic agents, 310, 316
    carcinoma of the penis, 326
    chemotherapeutic agents, 304–309, *305,* 308*t*
    chemotherapy
      in locally advanced disease, 318
      in metastatic disease, 318–319
    chemotherapy guidelines, 303–304, 303*t*
    combination therapy, 304
    hormonally active agents, 310, *311–315*
    mechanisms of drug activity, 300–303, *302*
    prostate cancer, 319–323, 321*t*
    renal cell carcinoma, 316–317

Genitourinary tract, medical
    management of malig-
    nancies (*contd.*)
  selective toxicities, 300,
    301, 303
  testicular and extragonadal
    germ cell cancer,
    323–326
  urothelial cancer, 317–319,
    318*t*
neoplasms, 249–299
  bladder, 258–269
  kidney, 249–255
  penile, 291–297
  prostate, 269–284
  renal pelvis and ureter,
    255–258
  testicular, 284–291
radiation therapy for treat-
    ment of malignancy,
    328–340
  clinical radiotherapy,
    331–338, *334, 336, 337*
  complications, 338–340
  physics of radiation,
    328–329
  radiobiology, *329*, 329–331
trauma and emergencies,
    164–187
Gentamicin
  for treatment of acute
    pyelonephritis, 213
  for treatment of Fournier's
    gangrene, 185
GFR. *See* Glomerular filtration
    rate
Gittes needle suspension, for
    treatment of stress uri-
    nary incontinence, 135
Gleason system, 270
Glide wires, 80
Glomerular filtration rate
    (GFR), 457–458, *458*
Glucocorticoids, for treatment of
    hypercalcemia, 454
Glucose, 3
  for treatment of hyperkalemia,
    452
^{99m}Tc-Glucoheptonate, 30, 33
Glutaraldehyde cross-linked
    highly purified bovine
    collagen, for treatment of
    stress urinary inconti-
    nence, 134

Gonads
  effects of radiation therapy,
    339
  mixed gonadal dysgenesis, 375
  pure gonadal dysgenesis, 376
  Turner's syndrome, 374–375
Gonorrhea, 418–419, 420*t*–421*t*
  diagnosis, 418
  treatment, 418–419
Goodpasture's syndrome, 10
Granulocytopenia, after cis-
    platin, 306
Granuloma inguinale (dono-
    vanosis), 422
Guanethidine, as cause of erec-
    tile dysfunction, 151*t*
Guide wires, 79–80

H
Haloperidol, as cause of erectile
    dysfunction, 151*t*
Hamartomas, adrenal, 433
Hammock hypothesis, 124
Hematologic disorders, as cause
    of priapism, 409
Hematuria, 5–15. *See also*
    Sickle cell anemia
  anticoagulation and, 13–14
  causes, 5, 6*t*
  diagnosis, 8–9
  endoscopy and, 77
  factitious, 5
  false, 5
  malignancy risk, 7
  of obscure origin, 9–10
  renal causes, 9–10
Hemiacidrin, 455
Hemodialysis, *471,* 471–472
  for treatment of hyper-
    kalemia, 452
  for treatment of hypermagne-
    semia, 456
Hemofiltration, 472–474, *473*
Hemophilia, 14
Hemorrhage
  adrenal, 433
  following TURP, 196
  postoperative, 499
Hemorrhagic cystitis, 12–13
  after cyclophosphamide ther-
    apy, 305–306
  treatment, 12–13
Herpes simplex virus (HSV),
    416, 418

clinical features, 416
diagnosis, 418
treatment, 418
High-osmolality contrast material (HOCM), 23–24
HIV. *See* Human immunodeficiency virus
HOCM. *See* High-osmolality contrast material
HOLEP. *See* Holmium laser enucleation of prostate
Holmium laser enucleation of the prostate (HOLEP), 116, 197
Hormones
    evaluation in adrenal gland masses, 429, 431
    evaluation in male infertility, 389–390
    influence on prostate cancer, 269
    for treatment of cryptorchidism, 368
Hospitalization, discharge, 505–506
HPV. *See* Human papilloma virus
HSV. *See* Herpes simplex virus
Human papilloma virus (HPV), 414–415
    diagnosis, 414
    epidemiology, 414
    prevention, 415
    treatment, 414–415
    virology, 414
Hurwitz trocar, 72
Hydronephrosis, 39, 41, *43*
Hydroureteronephrosis, 103
Hyoscyamine (Levsin), for treatment of LUTS, 117
L-Hyoscyamine (Levsin)
    for treatment of LUTS, 118*t*
    for treatment of urinary incontinence, 134
Hyperbaric oxygen therapy, for treatment of Fournier's gangrene, 185
Hypercalcemia, 453
Hypercalciuria, 240–242
    absorptive, 241–242
    classification, 241*t*
    renal, 242
    resorptive, 240–241
    treatment, 241
Hypergonadotropic hypogonadism

as cause of erectile dysfunction, 149
male infertility and, 394
Hyperkalemia, 451–452. *See also* Potassium disorders
    drugs associated in patients with chronic renal failure, 475*t*
    drugs associated with, 475*t*
    manifestations, 452
    treatment, 452
Hypermagnesemia, 455–456
    treatment, 456
Hyperoxaluria, 243
    enteric, 243
    exogenous, 243
    primary, 243
Hyperprolactinemia, as cause of erectile dysfunction, 149–150
Hyperprolactinemic agents, as cause of erectile dysfunction, 151*t*
Hyperuricosuria, 242–243
    etiology, 242
    treatment, 242–243
Hypocalcemia, 454–455
Hypocitraturia, 243
Hypogonadotropic hypogonadism
    as cause of erectile dysfunction, 149
    male infertility and, 394–395
Hypokalemia, 451. *See also* Potassium disorders
    manifestations, 451
    treatment, 451
Hypomagnesemia, 455
Hypospadias, *373,* 373–374
Hypotension, 474
Hypothalamic–pituitary–gonadal axis
    effect of exogenous estrogenic compounds, *313*
    effect of luteinizing hormone-releasing hormone agonists, *314*
    effect of nonsteroidal antiandrogens, *315*
    effect of orchiectomy, *312*
    normal, *311,* 380–383, *381, 382*
Hypovolemia, postoperative, 499

I

Ifosfamide
  hemorrhagic cystitis and, 12
  for medical management of
      genitourinary malig-
      nancy, 304–306, *305*
IgA nephropathy, 9–10
IGF-1. *See* Insulin-like growth
      factor-1
IL-2, for medical management
      of renal cell carcinoma,
      316–317
Ileal conduit, 448–449
Ileus, postoperative care, 503
ILs, for medical management of
      genitourinary malig-
      nancy, 316
Imaging. *See also* individual
      imaging modality
  for evaluation of urinary in-
      continence, 129
  of the genitourinary tract,
      16–29
  radionuclide, 30–50
  testicular, 44, *46, 47, 48, 49,*
      50
  utility of various modalities,
      17*t*
Imipramine (Tofranil)
  as cause of erectile dysfunc-
      tion, 151*t*
  for treatment of LUTS, 117,
      118*t*, 119
  for treatment of urinary in-
      continence, 134
Immunotherapy
  future, 317
  in medical management of
      malignancies, 310, 316
  metastatic disease and, 255
Impotence. *See also* Erectile
      dysfunction
  following TURP, 196
Indinavir, 234
Indium-111, 34
Indwelling catheters, for treat-
      ment of urinary inconti-
      nence, 130
Infections
  complications in renal trans-
      plantation, 488
  following penile prosthetic
      surgery, 162–163
  genitourinary tract, 206–231
  instrumentation and, 78

probability based on single-
      specimen colony counts,
      207*t*
  radionuclide imaging, 34
  recurrent, 206–207
  reinfection, 207
Infertility, 369
  clinical evaluation of the in-
      fertile couple, 385–392
  definitions, 380
  in men, 380–406
  reproductive male dysfunc-
      tion, 380–406
Inhibitors, 232–233
Instrumentation, 63–78. *See*
      also Lithotripsy
  balloon dilators, 81
  bougies, 65–67, *66*
  for catheterization, 72–74
  catheters, 63–65, *64*, 79, *80*
  diagnostic and operating in-
      struments, 67–71, *68, 69,*
      70, 71
  dilators, 65–67, *66*
  for endoscopic diagnosis,
      74–76
  for evaluation of urethral
      trauma, 178
  flexible, 69, 71
  glide wires, 80
  guide wires, 79–80
  infections and, 78
  laparoscopic, *201*
  for percutaneous cystostomy,
      76–77
  percutaneous cystostomy tro-
      cars, 71–72, *73*
  for perineal urethrostomy, 77
  resectoscope, *190*
  sterilization, 75
  upper tract, 79–86
  ureteral access sheaths,
      80–81, *81*
  ureteral stent, 83–84
  ureteroscopes, 81–83, *82*
  video monitoring, 71, *71*
Insulin, for treatment of hyper-
      kalemia, 452
Insulin-like growth factor-1
      (IGF-1), prostate cancer
      and, 269
Interferons
  for medical management of
      genitourinary malig-
      nancy, 316

for medical management of renal cell carcinoma, 317

Interleukin-2, contrast agents and, 27

Interstitial laser, for treatment of LUTS, 116

Interstitial nephritis, 39, *41*

Intrauterine insemination, 405

Intravenous pyelogram (IVP). *See also* Intravenous urogram
for evaluation of hematuria, 8

Intravenous urogram (IVU), 22–27. *See also* Intravenous pyelogram
for evaluation of bladder neoplasms, 260
for evaluation of genitourinary trauma, 165, 166
indications, 23
technique, 22–23, *23t*

Intrinsic sphincteric deficiency (ISD), physiology of urinary incontinence and, 124

In vitro fertilization, 405

Iohexol 180 (Omnipaque 180), *24t*

Iohexol 300 (Omnipaque 30), *24t*

Ion-exchange resins, for treatment of hyperkalemia, 452

Iopamidol 128 (Isovue 128), *24t*

Iopromide 240 (Ultravist 240), *24t*

Iridium-192, for treatment of penile cancer, 295

Irradiation, as cause of erectile dysfunction, 150

Irrigation
endoscopy and, 190
for sickle cell–associated hematuria, 12

Ischemic priapism
definition, 407
diagnosis, 410
etiology, *408t*
management, 410–412, *412*
pathophysiology, 409–410

ISD. *See* Intrinsic sphincteric deficiency

IVP. *See* Intravenous pyelogram

IVU. *See* Intravenous urogram

J

Jackson staging system, 294, *294t*

Jejunal conduit, 448, *449*

Juxtaglomerular tumor, 54

K

Kallikrein, for treatment of oligoasthenoteratospermia, 404

Kallmann syndrome, male infertility and, 394

Kaposi's sarcoma, 423–424

Karnofsky Performance Scale, *303t*

Kegel exercises, 129–130

Ketoconazole, as cause of erectile dysfunction, *151t*

Kidneys
acquired immunodeficiency disease syndrome and, 423
blunt trauma, 166
treatment, 168–169
classification of renal injury, 167, *168*
CT angiography, 21
duplication, 361–364
effects of radiation therapy, 338–339
living related donor, 477–478, *478t*
metastatic lesions, 59
neoplasms, 249–255
penetrating trauma, 166–167, *167t*
treatment, 169
sarcoma, 59
trauma, 166–171, *167t, 168, 169t, 170t*

Klebsiella, 54, 185, 210

Klinefelter's syndrome, 374
as cause of erectile dysfunction, 149
male infertility and, 394

L

Laboratory tests
for evaluation of genitourinary tract infections, 207–211, *207t, 209, 209t*
for evaluation of genitourinary trauma, 165

Laboratory tests (*contd.*)
  for evaluation of LUTS, 105
  for evaluation of sexual dys-
    function, 153
  for evaluation of the infertile
    male, 386–390, 387*t*
Lactic acidosis, contrast agents
    and, 27
Laparoscopic nephrectomy
    (LRN), 199, 202–203
  approach, 202–203
  complications, 203
  contraindications, 202
  donor, 204, *204*
  indications, 202
  postoperative care, 203
Laparoscopic pelvic lymph node
    dissection (LPLND),
    203–204
  approach, 203–204
  complications, 204
  contraindications, 203
  indications, 203
  postoperative care, 204
Laparoscopy, 198–204. *See also*
    Surgery
  approaches, 201–202
  contraindications, 199
  instruments, *201*
  patient preparation and posi-
    tioning, 199
  preoperative preparation,
    198–199
  techniques, 199–201, *200*
Laser prostatectomy, for treat-
    ment of LUTS, 114, 116
Laser vaporization of the
    prostate, 197
Laurence–Moon–Biedl syn-
    drome, as cause of erec-
    tile dysfunction, 149
Leukemia, 59
Leukocytes, 3
Leukopenia, toxicity, 305
Leukoplakia, 292
LGV. *See* Lymphogranuloma
    venereum
LH-releasing hormone (LHRH),
    for medical management
    of genitourinary malig-
    nancy, 310
LHRH. *See* LH-releasing
    hormone
Libido, 143

Lithotripsy, 83. *See also*
    Extracorporeal shock
    wave lithotripsy;
    Instrumentation
  electrohydraulic, 198
    for treatment of bladder cal-
      culi, 239–240
    for treatment of urinary
      calculi, 247
  laser, 198
    for treatment of bladder cal-
      culi, 239
    for treatment of urinary
      calculi, 247
  mechanical, 197
  percutaneous, for treatment
    of struvite stones, 244
  pneumatic
    for treatment of bladder cal-
      culi, 240
    for treatment of urinary
      calculi, 247
  pneumohydraulic, 198
  ultrasound, 83, 197–198
    for treatment of bladder cal-
      culi, 240
    for treatment of urinary
      calculi, 246–247
Lithotrites, for treatment of
    bladder calculi, 239
LOCM. *See* Low-osmolarity
    contrast material
Lower urinary tract
  endoscopic surgery, 188–205
  infections, 219–223, 219*t, 221*
  obstruction, pediatric,
    365–367
Lower urinary tract symptoms
    (LUTS), 98–121
  causes, 99*t*
  definitions, 98
  diagnostic approach, 103–107
  differential diagnosis, 99–103,
    99*t*
  pathogenesis, 98
  treatment, 107–120
Low-osmolarity contrast mater-
    ial (LOCM), 23–24. *See
    also* Contrast agents
LPLND. *See* Laparoscopic pelvic
    lymph node dissection
LRN. *See* Laparoscopic
    nephrectomy
LUTS. *See* Lower urinary tract
    symptoms

Lymphadecectomy, for evaluation of metastatic disease, 275
Lymphogranuloma venereum (LGV), 422–423
  diagnosis, 423
  treatment, 423
Lymphoma. *See* Renal lymphoma in renal transplantation, 488–489

M

Magnesium disorders, 455–456
Magnetic resonance angiography (MRA), of renal vasculature, 28
Magnetic resonance imaging (MRI)
  contraindications, 28
  for diagnosis of adrenal masses, 428
  for diagnosis of renal masses, 57
  for evaluation of bladder neoplasms, 261
  for evaluation of the genitourinary tract, 27–29
  for evaluation of urinary incontinence, 129
  indications, 28
  of prostate cancer, 28
  spinal cord compression from metastatic prostate cancer, *336*
Magnetic resonance urography, 29
Malecot catheter, *64, 65*
Marijuana
  as cause of erectile dysfunction, 151*t*
  as cause of priapism, 408
Marshall–Marchetti–Krantz procedure, for treatment of stress urinary incontinence, 135
Matrix, 233
McGuire urinal, 130, 131
Meatal stenosis, 99
Megaureter, 364–365
  diagnosis, 365
  pathophysiology, 364–365
  treatment, 365
Megestrol acetate, for medical management of genitourinary malignancy, 310

Meglumine diatrizoate (Cystografin), 24*t*
Meglumine diatrizoate 60 (Hypaque 60), 24*t*
Meglumine iothalamate (Cysto-Conray), 24*t*
Melanoma, penile, 293
Men. *See also* Penis
  catheterization, 72, 74
  collection of urine specimen, 1
  dysuria, 219–220
  erectile dysfunction in, 147–151, 148*t*, 151*t*
  examination of genitalia, for evaluation of LUTS, 104
  life expectancies, 272*t*
  reproductive dysfunction, 380–406
    abnormalities, 392–395
    therapy, 395–406
  sexual dysfunction, 143–163
  specimen collection, 208
  urinary retention following instrumentation, 78
MEN-1. *See* Multiple endocrine neoplasia type 1
99mTc-MAG3 (99mTc-mercaptoacetyltriglycine), 30, *31, 32*
MESA, 396
Mesenchymal tumors, 54
MESNA (2-mercaptoethanesulfonic acid), hemorrhagic cystitis and, 12
Metabolic acidosis, 447, 450–451
Metabolic disorders, 447–451
  as cause of priapism, 409
Metastatic disease
  adrenal, 427*t*, 440
  medical management, 318–319
  from prostate cancer, 334–335
  renal cell carcinoma and, 254
  spinal cord compression from metastatic prostate cancer, *336*
  ureter, 258
Metformin, contrast agents and, 27
Methylprednisolone, in management of rejection in renal transplantation, 485
Metoclopramide, as cause of erectile dysfunction, 151*t*

Metronidazole
    for treatment of bacteremia,
        212
    for treatment of Fournier's
        gangrene, 185
    for treatment of *Trichomonas
        vaginalis*, 416
    for treatment of vaginitis,
        219–220
Microsurgery, reconstruction,
    396
Microwave therapy, for treatment of LUTS, 112–114,
    113, 115
Mithramycin, contraindication,
    454
Mitomycin C, for treatment of
    bladder cancer, 263
Mitoxantrone, for medical management of prostate cancer, 323
Mixed gonadal dysgenesis, 375
Mixed urinary incontinence, 125
Mohs surgery, for treatment of
    penile cancer, 296
Monoclonal antibodies, immunosuppression in
    renal transplantation,
    485
MRA. *See* Magnetic resonance
    angiography
MRI. *See* Magnetic resonance
    imaging
Multilocular cystic nephroma,
    60–61
Multiple endocrine neoplasia
    type 1 (MEN-1), 429
Multiple sclerosis, vesicourethral
    dysfunction and, 349
Mumps orchitis, 226
Muscle cramps, 474
M-VAC, for medical management of urothelial cancer,
    319
Mycobacterium tuberculosis, 210
Mycophenolate (CellCept),
    484–485
Myelolipomas, 432–433
Myelosuppression, following antimicrobial agents, 309

N
Na-EDTA. *See* Sodium ethylenediaminetetraacetic
    acid

Nafcillin
    for treatment of genitourinary
        infections, 215*t*–216*t*
    for treatment of renal/
        perirenal abscess, 218
Naproxen, as cause of erectile
    dysfunction, 151*t*
National Institutes of Health
    (NIH), chronic prostatitis
    symptom index, 230–231
NCNGU. *See* Nonchlamydial,
    nongonococcal urethritis
Neodymium-YAG laser, for
    treatment of penile cancer, 296
Neoplasms, genitourinary tract,
    249–299
Nephrectomy
    renal transplantation and,
        477
    for treatment of renal neoplasms, 252–255
    for treatment of ureteropelvic
        junction obstruction, 361
Nephritis, 9–10
    chronic interstitial, 214
Nephropathy, 9–10
Nephrotoxicity
    contrast agents and, 25
    immunosuppression in renal
        transplantation, 484
Nephroureterectomy, for treatment of neoplasms of the
    ureter, 256–257
Neuroblastoma, 439–440
    diagnosis, 439
    pediatric, 357
    prognosis, 440
    treatment, 439–440
Neurologic disorders, as cause
    of priapism, 409
Neurologic examination
    for evaluation of LUTS, 105
    for evaluation of sexual dysfunction, 153
    for evaluation of urinary incontinence, 128
Neurologic lesions, as cause of
    erectile dysfunction, 149
Neuromodulation, for treatment
    of voiding dysfunction,
    351
Neurotoxicity, following antimicrobial agents, 309
Neurourology, 341–354

classification, 344–349, 346t, 347t, 348

diagnosis, 343–344, 345t

treatment of voiding dysfunction, 349–353

vesicourethral unit, 341–343, 342, 343, 344

NGU. *See* Nongonococcal urethritis

NIH. *See* National Institutes of Health

Nilutamide, for medical management of genitourinary malignancy, 310

Nitric oxide, 146

Nitrofurantoin, contraindications, 213

NMPs. *See* Nuclear matrix proteins

Nocturia, 98

Nocturnal enuresis, 98, 125

Nocturnal penile tumescence (NPT), for evaluation of sexual dysfunction, 153

Nonchlamydial, nongonococcal urethritis (NCNGU), 415

Nongonococcal urethritis (NGU), 415–416

clinical features, 415

diagnosis, 415–416

treatment, 416

Nonsteroidal antiandrogens, 315

for medical management of genitourinary malignancy, 310

Nonsteroidal antiinflammatory drugs (NSAIDS)

acute renal failure and, 460, 460t

for postoperative pain management, 499–501, 500t

Norfloxacin, for treatment of genitourinary infections, 215t–216t

NPT. *See* Nocturnal penile tumescence

NSAIDS. *See* Nonsteroidal antiinflammatory drugs

Nuclear matrix proteins (NMPs), 260

Nutrition

oral, 503

parenteral, 503

postoperative, 502–503

O

Obesity, as complication of dialysis, 470

Obturators, 67

OKT3, in management of rejection in renal transplantation, 485

Oligoasthenospermia, male infertility and, 395

Oligoasthenoteratospermia, 404–406

Oliguria, 459

differential diagnosis, 462, 462t

Oncocytomas, 250

Opiates, as cause of erectile dysfunction, 151t

Opioids

as cause of erectile dysfunction, 151t

for postoperative pain management, 500t, 501–502

Orchiectomy, 312

cancer treatment following, 289–291, 290

for treatment of prostate cancer, 283

Orchitis, 226

Orgasm, 143

Ototoxicity, 306

Overflow incontinence, 125

Oxybutynin (Ditropan)

for treatment of LUTS, 117, 118t

for treatment of urinary incontinence, 133

for treatment of voiding dysfunction, 350

P

Paclitaxel, for medical management of urothelial cancer, 319

Pain

postoperative management, 499–502

with treatment of sexual dysfunction, 160

PAP. *See* Prostatic acid phosphatase

Papaverine hydrochloride, for treatment of sexual dysfunction, 158, 158t

Papillary cystadenocarcinoma, 61

Papillary necrosis, 206
from bacterial infection of the kidney, 217

Papillary transitional cell carcinoma, 258

Paraphimosis, 182

Parathyroid hormone (PTH), 453

Parenchymal abnormalities, radionuclide imaging, 34–39, *38, 40, 41, 42*

Paresthesias, 454

Partial nephrectomy, for treatment of renal neoplasms, 255

PCNL. *See* Percutaneous nephrostolithotomy

Pediatric urology, 355–379
bladder, exstrophy, 372–373
catheterization, 74
causes of postrenal azotemia, 461t
collection of urine specimen, 1
disorders of sexual differentiation, 374–378
hypospadias, *373,* 373–374
neuroblastoma, 357
obstruction
of the lower urinary tract, 365–367
of the upper urinary tract, 359–365, 361t, 362t, 363t
specimen collection, 208
testes
maldescent, 367–369
torsion, 369–372, *370, 371,* 371t
vesicoureteral reflux, 357–359, 357t, 359t
Wilms' tumor (nephroblastoma), 355–357, 356t

Pediculosis pubis, 424

Pelvic examination
for evaluation of LUTS, 104
for evaluation of urinary incontinence, 126

Pelvic floor therapy, for treatment of urinary incontinence, 129–130

Pelvic lymphadenectomy, for evaluation of metastatic disease, 275

Pelvic organ prolapse, 125–126
classification, 127

Pelvic Organ Prolapse Quantification System, 127

Penectomy, for treatment of penile cancer, 294–295

Penicillin, for treatment of syphilis, 422

Penile vibratory stimulation (PVS), 398–400, *400*

Penis. *See also* Men
anatomy, *144*
blood supply to, 145, *145*
cancer, radiation therapy, 335–338, *337*
carcinoma, 326
erection, 143–147, *144, 145,* 147t
fracture, 181–182
medical management of malignancies, 326
neoplasms, 291–297
classification, 292–293
diagnosis, 293
etiology, 292
incidence, 291–292
prognosis, 297
route of spread, 293
staging, 294
treatment, 294–297
trauma, 181–183
venous drainage, 145–146

Pentoxifylline, for treatment of oligoasthenoteratospermia, 404

Percutaneous cystostomy, instrumentation, 76–77

Percutaneous cystostomy trocars, 71–72, *73*

Percutaneous nephrostolithotomy (PCNL), 238

Pereyra needle syspension, for treatment of stress urinary incontinence, 135

Pereyra–Raz needle syspension, for treatment of stress urinary incontinence, 135

Perineal urethrostomy, instrumentation, 77

Perioperative care, 491–507
care in the recovery room, 494–495
postoperative care, 494–506
preoperative risk assessment, 491–494, 492t

prophylaxis against endo-
carditis, 494
Peritoneal dialysis solutions,
469, 469*t*
Peritonitis, 470, 470*t*
Pessary, for treatment of urinary incontinence, 130
PET. *See* Positron emission tomography
Pezzar catheter, *64, 65*
Pharmacologic agents. *See also*
individual drug names
as cause of urinary incontinence, 125
effect on bladder, 102
Phenothiazines
as cause of erectile dysfunction, 151*t*
effect on bladder, 102
Phentolamine mesylate, for
treatment of sexual dys-
function, 158–159
Phenylpropanolamine, 102
Pheochromocytoma, 429,
436–439
biochemical abnormalities,
437, 437*t*
diagnosis, 436–437
management, 438
prognosis, 438–439
radiologic diagnosis, 437–438
Phimosis, 182
Physical examination
for evaluation of Fournier's
gangrene, 184–185
for evaluation of genitourinary trauma, 164–165
for evaluation of LUTS, 104
for evaluation of sexual dysfunction, 152
for evaluation of urethral
trauma, 178
for evaluation of vesi-
courethral dysfunction,
343–344
of the infertile male, 385–386,
386*t*
preoperative cardiac evaluation, 491, 493
Phytotherapy, for treatment of
LUTS, 109–110
PIN. *See* Prostatic intraepithelial neoplasia
Piperacillin, for treatment of
Fournier's gangrene, 185

Plain radiography
for diagnosis of adrenal
masses, 426–427
for evaluation of bladder neoplasms, 261
for evaluation of genitourinary trauma, 165
for evaluation of the genitourinary tract, 16
indications, 16
technique, 16
Platinum agents
mechanism of action, 306
for medical management of
genitourinary malig-
nancy, 306
toxicities, 306
Podofilox, for treatment of
human papilloma virus,
415
Podophyllin, for treatment of
human papilloma virus,
414–415
Polyclonal antibodies, immunosuppression in renal
transplantation, 485
Polyuria, 98
Positioning, during laparoscopy,
199
Positron emission tomography
(PET), for diagnosis of
adrenal masses, 428–429
Postobstructive diuresis,
443–444
Postrenal abnormalities, radionuclide imaging,
39–50, *43, 44, 45, 46, 47,
48, 49*
Postrenal azotemia, 461–462,
461*t*
Posttransurethral resection syndrome, 445–446, 445*t*
Potassium, restriction in treatment of chronic renal failure, 467
Potassium disorders, 451–452
hyperkalemia, 451–452
hypokalemia, 451
Prader–Willi syndrome
as cause of erectile dysfunction, 149
male infertility and, 394
Prazosin (Minipress), for treatment of LUTS, 109*t*

Prednisone, for treatment of hypercalcemia, 454
Pregnancy
  spinal cord injury and, 399t
  treatment of asymptomatic bacteriuria during, 211
Prerenal azotemia, 459
Pressure–flow studies, 95–97
  for evaluation of LUTS, 107
Priapism, 143, 160, 182, 407–413
  arterial, 407, 410, 410t, 412
  classification, 407
  definition, 407
  diagnosis, 410
  etiology, 407–409
    hematologic disorders, 409
    idiopathic, 409
    metabolic disorders, 409
    neurologic disorders, 409
    pharmacologic agents, 407–409, 408t
  management, 410–412
  pathophysiology, 409–410
  prognosis, 412
  with transurethral resection of the prostate, 193
Primary fibrinolysis, 14
Progressive familial nephropathy (Alport's syndrome), 10
Prostate, 384
  abscess, 100
  acquired immunodeficiency disease syndrome and, 423
  acute prostatitis, 100
  adenocarcinoma, 100
  benign enlargement, 107, 108
  cancer, 197
  differential diagnosis in LUTS, 100, 100, 101
  effects of heat on, 112–114, 113, 115
  effects of radiation therapy, 339
  examination for evaluation of LUTS, 104–105
  infections, 223–226, 223t
  magnetic resonance imaging of cancer of, 28
  medical management of malignancies, 319–323, 321t
  needle biopsy, 77
    antimicrobial prophylaxis, 227

neoplasms, 269–284
  secretions, 208, 209, 209t
  transabdominal ultrasound, 18–19
  transurethral resection, 113–114
Prostate cancer, 269–284
  chemoprevention, 320
  cytotoxic chemotherapy, 322–323
  diagnosis and staging, 270–275
  etiology, 269
  hormonal therapy, 320–322, 321t
  incidence, 269
  indications for laparoscopic pelvic lymph node dissection, 195t
  radiation therapy, 333–335, 334
  screening, 281
  spinal cord compression from metastatic prostate cancer, 336
  survival, 279t
  treatment, 275–284
    modalities, 278t
  tumor histology and grading, 269–270
Prostatectomy
  as cause of erectile dysfunction, 150
  open, for treatment of LUTS, 116–117
  quality of life after, 278t
  retropubic, 116–117
  simple perineal, 117
  suprapubic, 116
Prostate-specific antigen (PSA), 270–271
  parameters suggesting need for biopsy, 272t
Prostatic abscess, 224
Prostatic acid phosphatase (PAP), 274
Prostatic intraepithelial neoplasia (PIN), 269–270
Prostatic stents, for treatment of LUTS, 110, 110–112, 111
Prostatitis
  acute, 100, 224
  antibiotic therapy, 216t
  chronic, 225
    nonbacterial, 225

classification, 223, 223*t*
granulomatous, 225
NIH chronic prostatis symptom index, 230–231
treatment, 224
Prostheses
antibiotic prophylaxis for surgery, 228*t*
antimicrobial prophylaxis for surgery, 227
penile
for treatment of sexual dysfunction, 161–163
types, 161*t, 162*
Proteins
cancer-related, 8–9
loss, as complication of dialysis, 471
restriction in treatment of chronic renal failure, 467
in urine, 3
Proteus mirabilis, 54
Proteus sp., 2, 210, 233
Prune-belly syndrome, 358
PSA. *See* Prostate-specific antigen
Pseudoephedrine, 102
for treatment of stress urinary incontinence, 132
Pseudohermaphroditism
female, 376–377
male, 375, 377–378
Pseudohyperparathyroidism, 453
Pseudomonas sp., 54, 185, 210
Psychological examination, for evaluation of sexual dysfunction, 152
PTH. *See* Parathyroid hormone
Pubovaginal sling, for treatment of stress urinary incontinence, 136
Pudendal nerves, 147
Pulmonary support
preoperative evaluation, 494
with treatment of bacteremia, 212
Pulmonary thrombosis, after alkylating agents, 306
PVS. *See* Penile vibratory stimulation
Pyelonephritis, 39, *41, 42*
acute, 213–214
antibiotic therapy, 215*t*–216*t*
chronic, 214, 217

diagnosis, 54
treatment, 54
xanthogranulomatous, 53–54, 214, 217
Pyeloplasty, for treatment of ureteropelvic junction obstruction, 361
Pygeum africanum, for treatment of LUTS, 110
Pyrolytic carbon-coated zircondium oxide beads, for treatment of stress urinary incontinence, 134
Pyuria, 209–210

Q
Quality of life
after prostatectomy, 278*t*
urinary incontinence and, *142*
Quinolone, for treatment of acute pyelonephritis, 213

R
Radiation cystitis, 12
Radiation therapy, 328–340
clinical radiotherapy, 331–338, *334, 336, 337*
complications, 338–340
physics, 328–329
radiobiology, *329,* 329–331
for treatment of penile cancer, 295
types, 328–329
Radical nephrectomy, for treatment of renal neoplasms, 252–255
Radical prostatectomy, for treatment of prostate cancer, 275–276
Radiobiology, *329,* 329–331
Radiofrequency ablation, for treatment of renal neoplasms, 255
Radioisotope scanning, for diagnosis of adrenal masses, 428–429
Radiologic examination
for evaluation of Fournier's gangrene, 184
for evaluation of genitourinary trauma, 165–166
for evaluation of urethral trauma, 178, *179*
of the infertile male, 392

Radionuclide cystography (RNC), 41, 44, *45*
Radionuclide imaging, 30–50
    with cortical agents, 33–34, *35*
    for evaluation of genitourinary trauma, 166
    flow and function evaluation, 30–33, *31, 32, 33*
    of parenchymal abnormalities, 34–39, *38, 40, 41, 42*
    of postrenal abnormalities, 39–50, *43, 44, 45, 46, 47, 48, 49*
    of renal infection, 34
    of vascular abnormalities, 34, *36, 37*
Radiopharmaceuticals, 30
Radiotherapy, 331–338, *334, 336, 337*
    for treatment of bladder cancer, 266
    for treatment of Wilms' tumor, 357
RCC. *See* Renal adenocarcinoma; Renal cell carcinoma
Rectal probe electroejaculation, 400–401
Red blood cells, microscopic examination in urine, 4
Reifenstein's syndrome, 378
Renal adenocarcinoma (RCC), 54–58
    clinical diagnosis, *56,* 56–57
    etiology, 55–56
    radiologic diagnosis, 57–58
    treatment, 58
Renal arterial embolus, radionuclide imaging, 34, *36*
Renal arterial stenosis, radionuclide imaging, 34, *37*
Renal arteriography, for evaluation of genitourinary trauma, 166
Renal artery thrombosis, 486
Renal azotemia, 459–461, 461*t*
Renal cell carcinoma (RCC)
    chemotherapy, 316
    hormonal therapy, 316
    immulologic therapy, 316–317
    medical management, 316–317
    paraneoplastic syndromes, 252*t*
    radiation therapy, 332

Renal cysts, 59–60
    radiologic diagnosis, 59
    treatment, 60
Renal failure, 454, 457–490
    acute, 459–463
    as cause of erectile dysfunction, 148–149
    chronic, 463–467
    dialysis, 467–474
    renal function tests, 457–458
    renal transplantation, 475–489
Renal infection
    radionuclide imaging, 34
    ultrasound and, 21
Renal injuries
    classification, 167, *168*
    complications, 169–170
    diagnosis, 167–168
    emergencies, 170–171
    treatment, 168–169
Renal lymphoma, 59
Renal masses, 52*t*
    benign lesions, 51–54, 59–61
    cystic, 59–61
    diagnostic decision tree for evaluation, *55*
    evaluation, 51–62
    magnetic resonance imaging, 28
    malignant, 54–59, 61
    ultrasound and, 21
Renal oncocytoma, 53
    clinical diagnosis, 53
    radiologic diagnosis, 53
    treatment, 53
Renal osteodystrophy, 467
Renal pelvis, duplication, 361–364
Renal transplant, 475–489
    as cause of erectile dysfunction, 150
    complications, 486–488
    donor
        cadaveric, 478–480, 479*t,* *481*
        living related, 477–478, 478*t*
    immunology of transplantation, 475
    immunosuppression, 483–485, 485*t*
    malignancy in transplant patients, 488–489

recipient
  evaluation and selection,
      476–477
  preparation, 477
  rejection, *40,* 476
    management, 485–486
    technique, 480–483, *482*
  ultrasound and, 18
Renal tubular acidosis, 245–246
Renal tubular dysfunction, 234
Renal vein thrombosis
  diagnosis, 171
  radionuclide imaging, 34
  renal transplantation and, 486
  treatment, 171
Renogram, normal, *32*
Reno-M-60, 24*t*
Reproduction, dysfunction in
    men, 380–406
Resectoscopes, *190,* 191
Reserpine, as cause of erectile
    dysfunction, 151*t*
Retention
  acute, 98
  chronic, 98
  with trauma
    diagnosis, 174
    treatment, 174, *174*
Retrograde ejaculation,
    402–404, 402*t*
Retrograde urethrogram (RUG)
  for evaluation of genitouri-
      nary trauma, 165
  for evaluation of LUTS,
      105–106
Retroperitoneal lymph node dis-
    section, 401–402
Retropubic syspension proce-
    dures, for treatment of
    stress urinary inconti-
    nence, 134–135
RNC. *See* Radionuclide
    cystography
Robinson catheter, 63, *64*
Rofecoxib (Vioxx), for postopera-
    tive pain management,
    501
RUG. *See* Retrograde urethro-
    gram
Rusch trocar, 72

S

Sacral neuromodulation, for
    treatment of urge urinary
    incontinence, 138

Saline diuresis, for treatment of
    hypercalcemia, 453–454
Sarcomas
  of the kidney, 59
  penile, 293
  of the prostate, 270
Saw palmetto, for treatment of
    LUTS, 110
Scabies, 424
Scrotal patch, for treatment of
    sexual dysfunction,
    157–158
Scrotum
  epididymitis, *49*
  evaluation of male infertility
      and, 392
  infections, 226–227
  trauma, 183–185, 184*t*
  ultrasound and, 18
Secondary neoplasia, 306
Semen, analysis in male infer-
    tility, 386–388, 387*t*
Septic shock, 211–212
  pediatric, 367
Sessile transitional cell carci-
    noma, 258
Sex therapy, 155
Sexual differentiation, disor-
    ders, 374–378
  absent testis syndrome, 376
  complete gonadal dysgenesis,
      376
  dysgenetic male pseudoher-
      maphroditism, 375
  female pseudohermaphro-
      ditism, 376
  Klinefelter's syndrome, 374
  male pseudohermaphro-
      ditism, 377–378
  mixed gonadal dysgenesis,
      375
  pure gonadal dysgenesis, 376
  true hermaphroditism,
      375–376
  Turner's syndrome (gonadal
      dysgenesis), 374–375
  XX male syndrome, 374
Sexual dysfunction, male,
    143–163
  causes of erectile dysfunction,
      147–151, 148*t,* 151*t*
  definitions, 143
  evaluation, 152–155
  neurologic pathways of sexual
      response, 147*t*

Sexual dysfunction, male (*contd.*)
physiology of erection, 143–147, *144, 145,* 147*t*
treatment, *155,* 155–163, 158*t, 159,* 161*t, 162*
Sexually transmitted diseases (STDs), 414–425
acquired immunodeficiency disease syndrome, 423–424
antibiotic therapy, 420*t*–421*t*
candidiasis, 424
chancroid, 422
Chlamydia trachomatis, 415–416
clinical features, 417*t*
diagnosis, 219
epididymitis and, 226, 416
genital molluscum contagiosum, 419
gonorrhea, 418–419, 420*t*–421*t*
granuloma inguinale (donovanosis), 422
herpes simplex virus, 416, 418
human immunodeficiency virus, 414–415
lymphogranuloma venereum, 422–423
new cases annually, 415*t*
pediculosis pubis, 424
scabies, 424
syphilis, 419, 422
Trichomonas vaginalis, 416, 417*t*
Sickle cell anemia, 10–12. *See also* Hematuria
diagnosis, 11
treatment, 11–12
Sildenafil citrate
adverse effects, 156–157
contraindications, 156
dosing, 156
for treatment of sexual dysfunction, 156–157
Silicone (polydimethylsiloxane elastomer suspension), for treatment of stress urinary incontinence, 134
Silver nitrate, for hemorrhagic cystitis, 12
Sipple's syndrome, 436
Skin cancer, in renal transplantation, 489

Sling procedures, for treatment of urethral incompetence, 352–353
Small bowel, antimicrobial prophylaxis for surgery, 227
Smoking
as cause of carcinoma of the bladder, 259
renal carcinoma and, 250
Sodium bicarbonate, for treatment of hyperkalemia, 452
Sodium diatrizoate 50 (Hypaque 50), 24*t*
Sodium disorders, 441–447
causes of hypovolemic states, 442*t*
causes of volume depletion, 442*t*
Sodium ethylenediaminetetraacetic acid (Na-EDTA), 454
South African star grass, for treatment of LUTS, 110
Spectinomycin, for treatment of gonorrhea, 419
Sperm, analysis in male infertility, 388–389
Spermatocytogenesis, 385
Spermatogenesis, 384–385
cycle, *382*
Spermatotoxins, 386*t*
elimination, 404
Spermiogenesis, 385
Sphincter, intrinsic sphincteric deficiency, 124
Sphincterotomy, endoscopy and, 193
Spinal cord injury
classification, 346–347
male infertility and, 398–400
pathophysiology, 344, 346
pregnancy rates and, 399*t*
vesicourethral dysfunction and, 344–348
Spironolactone, as cause of erectile dysfunction, 151*t*
Squamous cell carcinoma
bladder, 258
penile, 293, *337*
ureter, 256
Stamey needle suspension, for treatment of stress urinary incontinence, 135
Stamey trocar, 72, *73*

Staphylococcus aureus, 185

Staphylococcus sp., 210

STDs. *See* Sexually transmitted
    diseases

Stents
    for treatment of external
        sphincter dyssynergia,
        352
    ureteral, 83–84

Steroidal antiandrogens, for
    medical management of
    genitourinary malig-
    nancy, 310

Steroids
    male infertility and, 395
    in management of rejection in
        renal transplantation,
        485
    replacement for adrenalec-
        tomy, 436*t*

Stress urinary incontinence, 124
    treatment, 132

Struvite stones, 243–245. *See
    also* Urinary calculi
    diagnosis, 244
    prevention, 245
    treatment, 244–245

Stuttering priapism, 409

Stylets, 65

Sulfisoxazole, for treatment of
    lymphogranuloma
    venereum, 423

Supravesical urinary diversion,
    for treatment of voiding
    dysfunction, 350

Surgery. *See also* Electro-
    surgery; Endoscopy;
    Laparoscopy
    antimicrobial prophylaxis in
        urologic surgery,
        227–228, 228*t*
    chronic renal failure and, 474,
        475*t*
    discharge from the hospital,
        505–506
    perioperative care, 491–507
    postoperative care, 494–506
    postoperative ward care,
        498–505
    preoperative risk assessment,
        491–494, 492*t*
    prophylaxis against endo-
        carditis, 494
    reconstructive microsurgery,
        396

for renal masses, 58

for renal oncocytoma, 53

risk of cardiac complications in
    various procedures, 492*t*

for treatment of adrenal carci-
    nomas, 435–436, 436*t*

in treatment of chronic renal
    failure, 474, 475*t*

for treatment of crypt-
    orchidism, 368–369

for treatment of neuroblas-
    toma, 439–440

for treatment of oligoas-
    thenoteratospermia,
    404–405

for treatment of pheochromo-
    cytoma, 438

for treatment of priapism, 411,
    412

for treatment of prostatitis,
    224

for treatment of scrotal in-
    juries, 183

for treatment of sexual dys-
    function, 160–163

for treatment of stress uri-
    nary incontinence,
    134–138

for treatment of struvite
    stones, 244

for treatment of ureteropelvic
    junction obstruction, 361

for treatment of urge urinary
    incontinence, 138

for treatment of vesicoureteral
    reflux, 358–359

for treatment of Wilms'
    tumor, 356–357

for urinary calculi, 238

video monitoring, 71, *71*

for xanthogranulomatous
    pyelonephritis, 54

Sympatholytic agents, as cause
    of erectile dysfunction,
    151*t*

Syndromes of vasal aplasia, 390

Syphilis, 419, 422
    diagnosis, 419, 422
    pathology, 419
    treatment, 422

T

Tadalafil, for treatment of sex-
    ual dysfunction, 157

Tamoxifen citrate, for treatment of oligoasthenoteratospermia, 404

Tamsulosin (Flomax), for treatment of LUTS, 109*t*

Tazobactam, for treatment of Fournier's gangrene, 185

Teflon (polytetrafluoroethylene), for treatment of stress urinary incontinence, 134

Telescopes, 67, *69*

Telomerase, 260

Temperature, endoscopy and, 190–191

Tension-free transvaginal tape (TVT), for treatment of stress urinary incontinence, 136

Terazosin (Hytrin), for treatment of LUTS, 109*t*

Testes
  absent testis syndrome, 376
  acquired immunodeficiency disease syndrome and, 423
  cancer, 284–291
    diagnosis, 284–285
    frequency of elevated tumor markers, 288*t*
    incidence, 284
    pathology and classification, 284*t*
    radiation therapy, 335
    route of spread, 285
    staging, 285–288
    treatment
      after orchiectomy, 289–291, *290*
      primary, 288
  pediatric
    maldescent, 367–369
    torsion, 369–372, *370, 371,* 371*t*
  trauma, 185–186

Testicles
  medical management of malignancies, 323–326
  chemotherapy
    in advanced disease, 324–326
    in early disease, 323–324
  complications of treatment, 325
  follow-up after treatment, 325

neoplasms, 284–291
  pediatric, 369
  normal anatomy, 383–384, *384*
  radionuclide imaging, 44, *46, 47, 48, 49,* 50
    acute testicular torsion, *47*
    clinical application, 44, *46, 47, 48, 49,* 50
    delayed torsion, *48*
    normal scan, *46*
    technique, 44

Testosterone
  for medical management of genitourinary malignancy, 310
  for treatment of sexual dysfunction, 157

Tetracycline, for treatment of syphilis, 422

Thiazides, as cause of erectile dysfunction, 151*t*

Thiotepa, for treatment of bladder cancer, 262–263

Thrombocytopenia, 13–14
  after cisplatin, 306
  toxicity, 305

Thromboembolism, drug regimens for prophylaxis, 506*t*

Titanium–nickel stent, 112

TMP/SMX, for treatment of acute bacterial cystitis, 222

Tolterodine (Detrol)
  for treatment of LUTS, 117, 118*t*
  for treatment of urinary incontinence, 133–134

Tomograms, 23

Topoisomerase-interactive agents
  mechanism of action, 307
  for medical management of genitourinary malignancy, 307, 309
  toxicity, 307, 309

Torsion of the testis, 369–372
  diagnosis, 372
  extravaginal, 369–370
  intravaginal, *370,* 370–372, *371,* 371*t*
  treatment, 372

Toxic agents
  as cause of carcinoma of the bladder, 258–259

as cause of priapism, 409
male infertility and, 394
in medical management of
malignancies, 300, *301*,
303
renal carcinoma and, 250
spermatotoxins, 386*t*
Transabdominal ultrasound
(TRUS), 18–19
indications, 18–19
technique, 19
Transfusions, in treatment of
chronic renal failure, 467
Transitional cell carcinoma,
255–256
Transplants. *See* Renal transplant
Transrectal prostate needle
biopsy, antimicrobial prophylaxis, 227
Transrectal ultrasound (TRUS),
for evaluation of male infertility, 392
Transurethral alprostadil, for
treatment of sexual dys-
function, 160
Transurethral balloon dilation
catheter, for treatment of
LUTS, 107
Transurethral incision of the
prostate (TUIP), 196
Transurethral microwave thermotherapy (TUMT), for
treatment of LUTS,
112–114, *113, 115*
Transurethral needle ablation
(TUNA), for treatment of
LUTS, 114, *115*
Transurethral resection of the
prostate (TURP)
incidence, 445*t*
post-TURP syndrome,
445–446, 445*t*
preoparative preparation, 191
for treatment of LUTS,
113–114
Transurethral sphincterotomy,
as cause of erectile dys-
function, 150
Transurethral vaporization of
the prostate, 196
Transvaginal bladder neck
syspensions, for treat-
ment of stress urinary incontinence, 135–136

Trauma
bladder, 172–174, *174*
as cause of erectile dysfunction, 150
genitourinary, 164–187
kidney, 166–171, 167*t, 168,*
169*t,* 170*t*
penile, 181–183
principles of management,
164–166
scrotum, 183–185, 184*t*
testes, 185–186
ureter, 171–172
urethra, 175–181, *177, 179,*
180*t*
Traumatic lymphangitis, 182
Trazodone, as cause of priapism,
407
Triamterene, 234
Trichomonas vaginalis, 416,
417*t*
diagnosis, 416
treatment, 416
Tricyclic antidepressants
as cause of erectile dysfunction, 151*t*
for treatment of voiding dysfunction, 350
Trimethoprim/sulfamethoxazole,
for treatment of granu-
loma inguinale, 422
TRUS. *See* Transabdominal ultrasound; Transrectal ul-
trasound
TS. *See* Tuberous sclerosis
Tuberous sclerosis (TS), 51
Tubular function tests, 458
TUIP. *See* Transurethral incision of the prostate
Tumor markers, urinary, 259
Tumors. *See also* Cancer
benign, 51–54, 59–61
adrenal gland, 431–433
mesenchymal, 54
bladder, 198
urethral, 198
TUMT. *See* Transurethral microwave thermotherapy
TUNA. *See* Transurethral needle ablation
Turner's syndrome (gonadal
dysgenesis), 374–375
TURP. *See* Transurethral resection of the prostate
TVT. *See* Tension-free transvaginal tape

U

Ultrasonic lithotripsy, 83

Ultrasonography
  for evaluation of genitourinary trauma, 166
  for evaluation of sexual dysfunction, 154

Ultrasound (US)
  for diagnosis of adrenal masses, 427
  for diagnosis of renal masses, 57
  for evaluation of bladder neoplasms, 260
  for evaluation of the genitourinary tract, 16–19
  indications, 18
  renal transplant and, 18
  scrotal, 18
  technique, 18
  TRUS, 18–19

Upper urinary tract
  calculi, 234–238
    clinical presentation, 234
    diagnosis, 234–235
    management, 236–238, 237
    treatment, 235
  duplication, 361–364
  infections, 213–218
  obstruction
    pediatric, 359–365, 361t, 362t, 363t
  specimen collection, 208
  urinary calculi, 234–238, 237

Ureaplasma, 210

Ureter
  complications in renal transplantation, 487
  duplication, 361–364
  effects of radiation therapy, 339
  external penetrating injury, 172
  iatrogenic injury, 172
  imaging, 21–22
  neoplasms, 255–258
    diagnosis, 256
    follow-up care, 258
    incidence, 255
    metastatic disease, 258
    staging and prognosis, 256
    treatment, 256–258
    tumor classification, 255–256

trauma, 171–172
  complications, 172
  treatment, 172

Ureteral access sheaths, 80–81, *81*

Ureteral catheterization, 76

Ureteral ectopia, urinary incontinence and, 123

Ureteral reflux studies, 41, 44, *45*

Ureteral stent, 83–84

Ureterocele, duplication and, 362–363, 363t

Ureterography, retrograde, 79, *80*

Ureteropelvic junction obstruction, pediatric, 359–361, 363–364

Ureteroscopes, 81–83, *82*

Ureteroscopy, 84–85
  for evaluation of hematuria, 8

Ureterosigmoidostomy, 449–450

Ureterostomy, for treatment of megaureter, 365

Urethra
  differential diagnosis in LUTS, 99
  incompetence
    treatment, 352–353
  perforation, 77–78
  physiology of urinary incontinence, 124
  pressure measurement, 90–95
  trauma, 175–181, *177, 179,* 180t
    catheterization, 175
    complication rate, 180t
    diagnosis, 176–178
    periurethral abscess, 175–176
    treatment, 180–181
  trauma in the female patient, 181
  tumors, 198

Urethral bulking agents
  for treatment of stress urinary incontinence, 134
  for treatment of urethral incompetence, 353

Urethral inserts, for treatment of urinary incontinence, 130

Urethral pressure profile, for evaluation of urinary incontinence, 129

Urethral stenosis, 99
Urethral strictures, 78, 99
   endoscopy and, 193
Urethral syndrome, 219
Urethroplasty, for treatment of
      LUTS, 107
Urge urinary incontinence, 124
Urinalysis
   abnormal, 1–15
   specimen collection, 1
Urinary alkalinization, for
      sickle cell–associated
      hematuria, 11
Urinary calculi, 232–248. *See
      also* Struvite stones
   acquired immunodeficiency
      disease syndrome and,
      424
   in the bladder, 238–240, *239*
   composition, frequency, and
      characteristics, 233*t*
   endourologic techniques,
      246–247
   epidemiology, 232
   etiology, 232–234, 233*t*, 234*t*
   extracorporeal shock wave
      lithotripsy, 247–248, 247*t*
   extraction, 238
   pathogenesis, 232–234, 233*t*,
      234*t*
   percutaneous nephrostolithot-
      omy, 238
   recurrent stone disease,
      240–246
   surgery, 238
   types, 234*t*
   in the upper urinary tract,
      234–238, *237*
Urinary diversion, 447–448,
      448*t*
   for hemorrhagic cystitis, 13
   for treatment of stress uri-
      nary incontinence, 138
   urinary incontinence and, 123
Urinary incontinence, 122–142
   assessment, 125–129
   classification, 124–125
   definition, 122
   differential diagnosis,
      122–123
   following TURP, 195
   impact questionnaire, *141*
   physiology of continence,
      123–124

   quality-of-life visual analog
      scale, *142*
   risk factors, 122
   sample voiding diary, *140*
   treatment, 129–138
      nonsurgical, 129–132
      with pharmacologic agents,
         132–134
      surgical, 134–138
   urogenital distress inventory,
      142
Urinary leakage, 41, *44*
Urinary sphincter, artificial, for
      treatment of stress uri-
      nary incontinence, 136,
      137, 138
Urinary stones. *See* Urinary
      calculi
Urine. *See also* Hematuria
   chemical characteristics, 2–3,
      3*t*
      acid, 2
      alkaline, 2
      pH level, 2
   microscopic examination,
      3–5, *4*
      differentiating causes of re-
         colored urine, 3*t*
      red blood cells, 4
   physical characteristics, 1, 2*t*
      color, 1, 2*t*
      gravity/osmolality, 1
      turbidity/nontransparency, 1
   retention following instru-
      mentation, 78
Urine culture
   false–negative results,
      210–211
   false–positive results, 211
   interpretation, 210–211
Urodynamic studies, 87–97
   cystometrogram, 87–90
   electromyography, 90
   for evaluation of urinary in-
      continence, 128
   pressure–flow studies, 95–97
   urethral pressure measure-
      ment, 90–95
   uroflowmetry, 90
   video urodynamics, 95–97
Uroflowmetry, 90, *91, 92*
   for evaluation of LUTS, 106,
      106
   for evaluation of urinary in-
      continence, 128
   normal values, 92*t*

Urolithiasis, factors associated with, 233t
Urothelial cancer
    chemotherapy, 318–319
    intravesical therapy, 317–318
    medical management, 317–319
US. *See* Ultrasound

V

Vacuum erection device (VED), *155,* 155–156
    complications, 156
Vagina
    effects of radiation therapy, 339
    examination for evaluation of urinary incontinence, 127, *127*
    reflux of urine, 123
Vaginitis, 219–220
Valdecoxib (Bextra), for postoperative pain management, 501
Valrubicin, for treatment of bladder cancer, 263
Valsalva maneuver, for treatment of voiding dysfunction, 352
Van Buren sounds, 65, *66*
Vardenafil, for treatment of sexual dysfunction, 157
Varicocelectomy, for treatment of oligoasthenoteratospermia, 404–405
Vasal aplasia, 395–396
Vascular abnormalities, radionuclide imaging, 34, *36, 37*
Vascular injuries, penile, 182
Vascular studies, for diagnosis of adrenal masses, 429
Vascular surgery, as cause of erectile dysfunction, 150
Vascular testing, for evaluation of sexual dysfunction, 154
Vas deferens, 383, 390
Vasectomy, reversal, *397,* 397–398
Vasoepididymostomy, 397
Vasography, for evaluation of male infertility, 392
Vasovagal reaction, 26–27
Vasovasostomy, 397
Ventilatory support, 495–496, *496t*

Vesicosphincter dyssynergia, 90, *94*
    treatment, 349–353
    vesicourethral dysfunction and, 347
Vesicostomy, for treatment of megaureter, 365
Vesicoureteral reflux
    duplication and, 362
    pediatric, 357–359, 357t, 359t
        diagnosis, 358
        etiology, 357–358
        incidence, 357
        treatment, 358–359
Video monitoring, 71, *71*
Video urodynamics, 95–97
    for evaluation of urinary incontinence, 129
    interpretation, 97
    technique, 95, *96*
Visual urethrotomy, for treatment of LUTS, 107
Vitamin D, 453
Voiding
    classification systems, 346t
    dysfunction, acquired immunodeficiency disease syndrome and, 424
    frequency, 98
    neurourology and, 349–353
    psychogenic dysfunction, 102
    sample diary, *140*
Voiding cystourethrogram (VCUG), 41, 44
    for evaluation of LUTS, 106
    for evaluation of urinary incontinence, 129
Voiding pressure study, for evaluation of urinary incontinence, 128–129
Von Hippel–Lindau disease, 55, 429
    renal carcinoma and, 250
von Willebrand's disease, 14

W

Warfarin (Coumadin), preoperative administration for endoscopy, 191
Whistle-tip catheter, *64,* 65
Whitaker test, 360
White blood cells
    microscopic examination in urine, 4
    radionuclide imaging, 34

Wilms' tumor (nephroblastoma)
    pediatric, 355–357, 356t
        diagnosis, 355
        histology, 355
        incidence, 355, 356t
        staging, 355, 356t
        treatment, 356–357
    radiation therapy, 332
Women. *See also* Pregnancy
    catheterization, 74
    collection of urine specimen, 1
    dysuria, 219–220, 219t
    female sounds, *66*, 67
    pelvic examination, for evalu-
        ation of LUTS, 104
    specimen collection, 208
    urethral injury, 181
    vaginitis, 219–220
Wounds, care following debride-
    ment, 185
Wunderlich's syndrome, 52

X
Xanthogranulomatous
        pyelonephritis (XGP),
        53–54, 214, 217
Xenograft sling, for treatment of
        stress urinary inconti-
        nence, 136
XGP. *See* Xanthogranulomatous
        pyelonephritis
XX male syndrome, 374
    male infertility and, 394

Y
Y-chromosome microdeletions,
        male infertility and, 394
Yohimbine hydrochloride, for
        treatment of sexual dys-
        function, 157